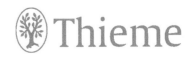

Pharmacology

An Essential Textbook

Second Edition

Mark A. Simmons, PhD
Professor of Pharmacology
Department of Pharmaceutical Sciences
School of Pharmacy
University of Maryland Eastern Shore
Princess Anne, Maryland
and
Professor of Pharmacology (Retired)
Department of Integrative Medical Sciences
Northeast Ohio Medical University
Rootstown, Ohio

206 illustrations

Thieme
New York • Stuttgart • Delhi • Rio de Janeiro

Library of Congress Cataloging-in-Publication Data

Names: Simmons, Mark A., author.

Title: Pharmacology : an essential textbook / Mark A. Simmons.

Description: Second edition. | New York : Thieme, [2020] | Includes index. | Summary: "Pharmacology: An Essential Textbook covers the facts of pharmacology–the study of the effects of drugs on the body–and integrates the concepts to master for success in the classroom, in the laboratory and for board examinations. It provides a focused text for pharmacology courses. It can also be used as a source of key knowledge for daily clinical practice"– Provided by publisher.

Identifiers: LCCN 2020045503 (print) | LCCN 2020045504 (ebook) | ISBN 9781626237384 (paperback) | ISBN 9781626237414 (ebook)

Subjects: MESH: Pharmacological Phenomena | Examination Questions | Outline

Classification: LCC RM301.13 (print) | LCC RM301.13 (ebook) | NLM QV 18.2 | DDC 615.1076–dc23

LC record available at https://lccn.loc.gov/2020045503

LC ebook record available at https://lccn.loc.gov/2020045504

Thieme Medical Publishers, Inc.
333 Seventh Avenue, 18th Floor
New York, NY 10001, USA
+1 800 782 3488, customerservice@thieme.com

Thieme Publishers Stuttgart
Rüdigerstrasse 14, 70469 Stuttgart, Germany
+49 [0]711 8931 421, customerservice@thieme.de

Thieme Publishers Delhi
A-12, Second Floor, Sector-2, Noida-201301
Uttar Pradesh, India
+91 120 45 566 00, customerservice@thieme.in

Thieme Revinter Publicações Ltda,
Rua do Matoso, 170 – Tijuca
Rio de Janeiro RJ 20270-135 - Brasil
+55 21 2563-9702, www.thiemerevinter.com.br

Cover design: Thieme Publishing Group
Typesetting by DiTech Process Solutions, India

Printed in the United States of America by King Printing Co., Inc.   5 4 3 2 1

ISBN 978-1-62623-738-4

Also available as an e-book:
eISBN 978-1-62623-741-4

Important note: Medicine is an ever-changing science undergoing continual development. Research and clinical experience are continually expanding our knowledge, in particular our knowledge of proper treatment and drug therapy. Insofar as this book mentions any dosage or application, readers may rest assured that the authors, editors, and publishers have made every effort to ensure that such references are in accordance with **the state of knowledge at the time of production of the book.**

Nevertheless, this does not involve, imply, or express any guarantee or responsibility on the part of the publishers in respect to any dosage instructions and forms of applications stated in the book. **Every user is requested to examine carefully** the manufacturers' leaflets accompanying each drug and to check, if necessary in consultation with a physician or specialist, whether the dosage schedules mentioned therein or the contraindications stated by the manufacturers differ from the statements made in the present book. Such examination is particularly important with drugs that are either rarely used or have been newly released on the market. Every dosage schedule or every form of application used is entirely at the user's own risk and responsibility. The authors and publishers request every user to report to the publishers any discrepancies or inaccuracies noticed. If errors in this work are found after publication, errata will be posted at www.thieme.com on the product description page.

Some of the product names, patents, and registered designs referred to in this book are in fact registered trademarks or proprietary names even though specific reference to this fact is not always made in the text. Therefore, the appearance of a name without designation as proprietary is not to be construed as a representation by the publisher that it is in the public domain.

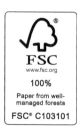

To the teachers who cultivated my interest in pharmacology,
To the colleagues who have collaborated with me in teaching and research,
To the students who have made the teaching of pharmacology so rewarding,
and To Robin, my eternal inspiration.

Contents

Preface

Pharmacology, the study of the effects of drugs on the body, is one of the most important disciplines that must be mastered by health care practitioners and biomedical scientists. The prevention or treatment of almost every disease involves the use of drugs. Furthermore, many patients seek medical help as a result of drug side effects or toxicities, effects that can be avoided if prescribers have a good knowledge of pharmacology.

Pharmacology: An Essential Textbook covers the facts of pharmacology and integrates the concepts that you must master for success in the classroom, in the laboratory, and for board examinations. It provides a focused text for pharmacology courses. It can also be used as a source of key knowledge for daily clinical practice.

One of the perennial issues that instructors face in teaching pharmacology is how to manage and evaluate the wealth of scientific information on drugs, which can seem overwhelming to students. To this end, the authors have made a concerted effort to focus on fundamental concepts and the most important aspects of pharmacology.

Students in pharmacology are challenged by the necessity to learn many drug names and to remember their effects. To help meet this challenge, the authors have put the drugs in context, focused on concepts, and grouped similar drugs together into classes and subclasses.

Summary tables are provided throughout the text. Hundreds of full-color figures are used to illustrate pharmacological processes and modes of action.

Many drug properties are presented in a streamlined bullet-point format. For each pharmaceutical agent or group of agents, mechanisms of action, pharmacokinetics, uses, contraindications, and side effects are discussed. Callout boxes connect pharmacological concepts in the text with foundational (green), clinical correlations (blue), and notes (yellow).

For self-testing, the text includes both factual and board-type questions. All of the questions are accompanied by detailed answer explanations. Over 400 questions and answers in the text can also be accessed online at MedOne.thieme.com via the scratch-off code in the book. The questions provide intensive practice, offer immediate feedback, and allow you to quickly identify areas for further study. I tell the students in my pharmacology courses that if they can answer the questions in this book and online correctly, they will have no problem with the pharmacology portions of the licensing exams.

As you use this book, please send comments or suggestions you have for improvement to simmons@neomed.edu.

Mark A. Simmons

Acknowledgments

I am most grateful to the contributors who have provided their expertise, time, and effort to this project. I would like to thank the editorial staff at Thieme, who have made significant contributions to this work. In particular, I wish to thank Mary Wilson, the developmental editor, who has organized and improved the text and illustrations; Torsten Scheihagen, Managing Editor at Thieme, who has worked tirelessly on the production of this volume; and Delia DeTurris, Acquisitions Editor at Thieme, for her unwavering support.

Mark A. Simmons

Contributors

Katharina Brandl, PhD
Associate Teaching Professor
Skaggs School of Pharmacy and Pharmaceutical Sciences
University of California San Diego
La Jolla, California

Edwin C. Johnson, PhD
CNS Biotech Consultant
Bella Vita LLC
Green Cove Springs, Florida

Dennis M. Peffley, PhD, JD
Professor of Physiology and Pharmacology
Department of Biomedical Sciences
Philadelphia College of Osteopathic Medicine Georgia
Suwanee, Georgia

Mark A. Simmons, PhD
Professor of Pharmacology
Department of Pharmaceutical Sciences
School of Pharmacy
University of Maryland Eastern Shore
Princess Anne, Maryland
and
Professor of Pharmacology (Retired)
Department of Integrative Medical Sciences
Northeast Ohio Medical University
Rootstown, Ohio

T. Sean Vasaitis, PhD
Associate Professor
Department of Pharmaceutical Sciences
School of Pharmacy
University of Maryland Eastern Shore
Princess Anne, Maryland

June Yun, PhD
Associate Professor
Department of Integrative Medical Sciences
Northeast Ohio Medical University
Rootstown, Ohio

Unit I

General Principles of Pharmacology

I

1 Introduction and Pharmacokinetics

Summary

Pharmacology is the study of drugs and their effects. A drug is a compound that has an effect on an organism or blocks the effects of other drugs on that organism. A receptor is a macromolecule on or within a cell to which a drug binds to produce an effect. Signal transduction is the process by which the binding of a ligand to a receptor leads to changes in cellular function. Pharmacokinetics is concerned with the movement of drugs into and out of the body and includes the processes of absorption, distribution, metabolism, and elimination. Routes of drug administration include enteral, parenteral, topical, transdermal, by inhalation, and by subcutaneous implant. To reach their site of action, drugs must cross biological membranes by either passive (down a concentration gradient) or active (energy-requiring) mechanisms. Bioavailability is the fraction of the administered dose of a drug that reaches the systemic circulation in an unchanged form. Drug metabolism usually inactivates therapeutic agents, transforming them into products that are more readily excreted. Metabolism consists of a phase 1 reaction (oxidation, reduction, or hydrolysis) to a less active form, followed by a phase 2 conjugation reaction. Conjugated compounds are generally inactive, especially glucuronide, sulfate, and glutathione conjugates, which are highly water soluble and are readily excreted in urine. Elimination mainly occurs via urine and feces, although other minor routes of elimination exist, including saliva, sweat, tears, breast milk, and expired air. Drug interactions may occur at any stage between absorption and elimination. Competition for binding to plasma albumin and induction/inhibition of the CYP-450 enzymes are the most common interactions. The rate of drug dosing depends primarily on the rate of drug elimination. Most drugs are removed from plasma by processes that are concentration-dependent (i.e., metabolism, secretion, and filtration) and result in "first-order" kinetics of elimination. With zero-order kinetics, a constant amount of drug is eliminated per unit of time regardless of its concentration. This usually occurs because the route of elimination has become saturated.

Keywords: receptor, administration, distribution, metabolism, elimination, dosing

1.1 What Is Pharmacology?

Pharmacology is the study of drugs and their effects. A drug is a compound that has an effect on an organism or blocks the effects of other drugs on that organism.

Why is it important for you to know the fundamentals of drug action? Knowing how a drug acts will allow you to understand its effects on the body, predict its side effects, and understand its interactions with other drugs. An understanding of today's drugs will provide a foundation for lifelong learning by allowing you to more easily comprehend future developments in the field. In summary, knowledge of pharmacology will allow you to understand the clinical effects of drugs.

Pharmacokinetics is concerned with the movement of drugs into and out of the body and includes the processes of absorption, distribution, metabolism, and elimination (ADME). Knowledge of a drug's pharmacokinetic profile allows the clinician to select the correct agent, mode of administration, and dosing regimen to achieve a timely drug effect.

1.2 Historical Perspective

Drugs have been used since prehistoric times, sometimes for therapeutic reasons and sometimes for superstitious or ritualistic reasons. Until the 1800s, most therapeutic drug use was the result of trial and error with natural products. Almost all of the drugs used prior to this time were from plants. A Greek physician, Pedanius Dioscorides, cataloged the uses of plants in the first century AD in a treatise called *De Materia Medica*. This manuscript continued to be used for 1500 years. It had many editions and translations and eventually was printed following the invention of the printing press. Some drugs in use today that were originally isolated from plants include morphine from poppies, aspirin from willow bark, digitalis from foxglove, and quinine from cinchona.

The discipline of pharmacology became established as a science in the late 1800s and early 1900s and was closely connected to advances in both chemistry and biology at the time.

The first pharmacology department was established in the mid-1800s by Rudolf Buchheim at the University of Dorpat in what was Germany at the time, now the University of Tartu in present-day Estonia. In 1867 he moved to the University of Giessen, which claims to be the "First Department of Pharmacology in Germany and birthplace of Experimental Pharmacology."

Oswald Schmiedeberg, known as the father of pharmacology, was one of Buchheim's students. In 1872, Schmiedeberg became a professor of pharmacology at the University of Strasburg (then part of Germany, now Strasbourg in France), where he remained for the next 46 years.

In his 46 years at Strasburg, Schmiedeberg trained most of the men who became professors at other German universities and in several foreign countries. He was largely responsible for the preeminence of the German pharmaceutical industry up to World War II. Many of Schmiedeberg's trainees went on to establish pharmacology departments throughout the world. These trainees included John Jacob Abel, who went on to establish the first pharmacology department in the United States at the University of Michigan in 1891, as chair of Materia Medica and Therapeutics. Abel moved to Johns Hopkins University in 1893, which was just establishing its medical school and was basing medicine on science and linking basic science to treatments and clinicians to scientists. He remained there as chair until 1932 and as professor until he died. He cofounded the *Journal of Biological Chemistry* with Christian Archibald Herter in 1905, the American Society for Pharmacology and Experimental Therapeutics in 1908 and the *Journal of Pharmacology and Experimental Therapeutics* in 1909.

The receptor is the target molecule to which a drug binds. The historical development of the receptor concept occurred in the late 1800s and early 1900s in two separate groups headed by John Langley at Cambridge University in England and Paul Ehrlich in Germany.

1.3 Definitions

- **Receptor:** A macromolecule on or within a cell that recognizes and binds to a specific ligand to produce an effect or transduce a signal. It can be a membrane receptor, enzyme, transporter, carrier protein, ion channel, or even nonprotein. Receptors can be endogenous or exogenous (e.g., viral or bacterial). Most, but not all, drugs work through receptors. Examples of drugs that do not act via receptors are osmotic diuretics, bulk-forming laxatives, and antacids.
- **Ligand:** A molecule that is able to bind and form a complex with another molecule.
- **Signal transduction:** The processes by which the binding of a ligand to a receptor leads to changes in cellular function.
- **Effector:** In cellular terms, these are the molecules involved in signal transduction. In body terms, an organ that is activated by stimulation, usually of nerves.

1.3.1 Measurement of Drug–Receptor Interactions

Direct (saturation) or indirect (competition) binding studies are used to determine whether a given drug binds to a specific receptor. Physiological responses of organs to drugs can be measured. For example, the contraction of a muscle, a change in the force or rate of the heartbeat, dilation or contraction of the pupil, or an increase or decrease in blood pressure. Biochemical studies can measure drug-induced changes in cellular messengers, including intracellular ions, cyclic adenosine monophosphate (cAMP), cyclic guanosine monophosphate (cGMP), inositol trisphosphate (IP3), and almost any other chemical. Reporter systems couple receptor activation to lacZ, green fluorescent protein (GFP), or luciferase reporter enzymes.

These studies can reveal if the receptor is in the cells or tissues of interest, determine if a drug is acting on the desired receptor, and determine the interactions of the drug with endogenous compounds.

1.4 Characteristics of Drugs

Drugs can be divided into small molecules and large molecules; the latter are sometimes called biologics (drugs created by biological rather than purely chemical processes). Traditionally, most drugs were small molecules (< 500 Da). Such molecules were amenable to becoming drugs because of their stability, ability to be isolated, ability to be synthesized, and ability to be taken orally.

There were a few large molecules, such as insulin, growth hormone, and blood clotting factors for hemophilia, all of which were isolated from human or animal products, which sometimes led to problems. For example, patients occasionally experienced allergic reactions to insulin isolated from porcine or bovine pancreas. Several hundred patients contracted Creutzfeldt–Jacob disease from growth hormone that was isolated from human pituitary at autopsy. From the late 1970s to the mid 1980s, about half of all people with hemophilia became infected with human immunodeficiency virus (HIV) through blood products. HIV transmission by any factor VIII or IX product in the United States has not occurred since 1986 due to viral inactivation (viral killing) methods that are used to treat blood products. These include heat treatment, solvent-detergent cleansing, and monoclonal purification. Insulin and growth hormone are now synthesized using recombinant DNA technologies. With advances in biotechnology, there are now many large molecules available that are used as therapeutics, and many more are under investigation.

These advances have occurred in several areas. Discoveries made through basic research on the biochemistry of DNA and RNA has led to an ability to control and manipulate DNA and RNA. Advances in the ability to control and manipulate bacteria, mainly *Escherichia coli*, and viruses has led to the development of methods to transfect DNAs and RNAs into bacteria, thus programming them to make more DNAs, RNAs, or proteins. Methods have also been developed to synthesize large peptides and proteins, and drug delivery systems have been improved.

As a result of these scientific discoveries, our therapeutic armamentarium has increased dramatically both in size and in effectiveness.

1.5 Routes of Drug Administration

1.5.1 Enteral

Enteral administration is the term used to describe drugs given via the gastrointestinal (GI) tract. Oral administration (PO) is by far the most common enteral route. The predominant site of absorption for drugs given orally is the duodenum, due to its large surface area. Drugs may also be absorbed in the stomach.

1.5.2 Parenteral

In **parenteral administration**, a drug is delivered by injection; therefore, the drug bypasses the GI tract. This method is used for medications that are poorly absorbed in the GI tract or when rapid onset of action or tight control of pharmacokinetic parameters (e.g., plasma concentration) is required.

1.5.3 Other Methods of Drug Administration

Other methods of drug administration are **topical**, **transdermal**, by **inhalation**, and by subcutaneous **implant**. See ▶ Table 1.1 for a comparison of the different routes of drug administration and ▶ Fig. 1.1 for the time course of plasma concentration with each route.

1.6 Absorption of Drugs

1.6.1 Factors that Affect Drug Absorption

Following are several factors that influence the absorption of drugs given orally:
- Stomach acid can destroy many drugs unless they are coated with an acid-resistant enteric coating.
- Slowed gastric transit of the drug due to the presence of food in the stomach or decreased gastric motility may delay or decrease absorption of the drug.

Table 1.1 Routes of drug administration

Route	Advantages	Disadvantages
Enteral		
Oral	Convenient Cost-effective Relatively safe Desired therapeutic concentration is achieved gradually	Often low bioavailability following first-pass metabolism by liver More difficult to adjust plasma concentration Requires a functional GI tract Requires compliance by patients
Rectal	Useful when patient is vomiting Can be used in the unconscious patient Limited first-pass metabolism Relatively painless Tolerated well in children	Not well accepted Irregular absorption can compromise safety Irritation to rectal mucosa
Sublingual (buccal)	Rapid absorption Avoids first-pass metabolism	Only useful for small amount of drug Requires prolonged contact with mucosa Unpleasant taste
Parenteral		
Intravenous	Allows for rapid administration of a precise amount of drug Avoids first-pass metabolism Dosage is easily adjusted Suitable for large volumes Very useful in the unconscious patient No issues with compliance by patients	Drug cannot be recalled once administered More complications from administration (e.g., infection and hematoma) Adverse reactions more likely, so monitoring by clinician is vital IV access often difficult to establish
Intramuscular	Relatively easy to administer Fairly rapid absorption under normal circumstances May be used to deliver depot injections, where the active compound of a drug is released consistently over time	Painful Can cause nerve damage Can cause bleeding, so contraindicated in bleeding disorders Can only be used for relatively small injection volumes
Subcutaneous	Easy to administer Slow and constant absorption Minimal pain involved May be used to deliver depot injections, where the active compound of a drug is released consistently over time	Can only be used for very small volumes of drug Potential tissue irritation
Other methods		
Topical	Applied to various surfaces, commonly the skin, eyes, nose, and vagina to produce a local effect	May cause irritation
Transdermal	Controlled release preparations may be used via this mode of application Can achieve systemic effects	Rate of absorption variable May cause irritation
Inhalation	Rapid absorption Ideal for drugs that can be administered as an aerosol Ideal for treating lung disease, as drug is essentially exerting a local effect	Variable systemic distribution (not considered a disadvantage for the current drugs administered by this route) May cause irritation of the respiratory tract
Implant	Sustained absorption of long duration (months to years) No peaks/troughs in blood levels Obviates problems with patient adherence to contraceptive and antiaddiction regimens May be applied locally to tumors	Local inflammation or injury after insertion or removal Serious adverse reactions require removal of device

Abbreviations: GI, gastrointestinal; IV, intravenous.

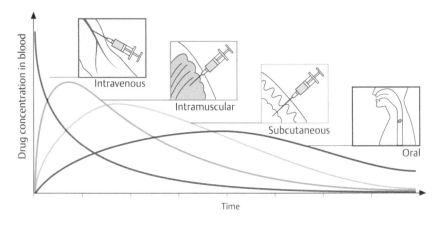

Fig. 1.1 Mode of drug administration and time course of plasma drug concentration.
Drugs given intravenously (*red*) reach their peak plasma drug concentration almost immediately, but this declines rapidly as the drug is distributed and eliminated. Drugs given intramuscularly (*green*) take longer time to reach their peak plasma concentration, followed by drugs given subcutaneously (*blue*). Drugs taken orally (*purple*) are the slowest to reach their peak plasma concentration, the value of which is determined by bioavailability following first-pass metabolism.

Clinical Correlation

Drug Absorption and Food in the Stomach

Certain drugs can cause irritation to the stomach unless they are taken with food. Food delays the absorption until the drug (e.g., aspirin) reaches the duodenum, where it is more easily tolerated. Other drugs (e.g., ampicillin) must be taken on an empty stomach, as food may decrease their absorption.

- Digestive enzymes (e.g., pepsins, lipases, proteases) may break down drugs.
- All orally administered drugs will enter the hepatic portal system and be subject to metabolism in the liver.

Foundations

Portal Circulation

A portal system is one in which veins from one capillary bed drain into another capillary bed, instead of emptying into the heart. The hepatic portal system is one such example of this. In this system, the hepatic portal vein, formed from the superior mesenteric and splenic veins, drains blood from the stomach, intestines, pancreas, and spleen. This nutrient-rich blood drains into the hepatic sinusoids, and the substrates it contains are then metabolized by hepatocytes. Blood leaves the liver via the hepatic vein, which empties into the inferior vena cava, then into the right atrium of the heart. This system ensures that ingested substances are metabolized before entering the systemic circulation.

Foundations

First-pass Metabolism

When a drug is given orally, it must traverse the intestinal epithelium and travel in the portal system to the liver before it gets to the systemic circulation. If a drug is metabolized to an inactive form at any point in this journey prior to entering the systemic circulation, it is said to have undergone "first-pass metabolism." This process has also been termed "presystemic elimination." The liver is the main site of first-pass metabolism. This mainly involves drugs that are taken orally, but can also affect the drugs that are administered rectally to a lesser extent. Parenteral administration of drugs avoids first-pass metabolism.

Drugs given intravenously (IV) gain direct access to the bloodstream, so their absorption is complete. Drugs given by other methods have to cross biological membranes to reach the bloodstream, leading to partial absorption. The amount and rate of absorption are critical factors in therapeutics.

Absorption of a drug from the site of administration to the bloodstream and from the bloodstream to target organs depends on both the properties of the drug and physiological variables. The factors that govern whether a drug crosses a biological membrane include size, charge, and hydrophobicity. In general, low molecular weight, nonionized, water-soluble molecules are more readily absorbed.

The mechanisms by which molecules can cross biological membranes include passive (down a concentration gradient) and active (energy-requiring) mechanisms.

- **Passive diffusion**: It is the most common method of absorption and occurs when a concentration gradient exists across a membrane such that the drug will move from the side with a high concentration to that with the lower concentration. Water-soluble drugs and those with low molecular weights are able to diffuse directly through pores in cell membranes.
- **Facilitated diffusion**: It is a passive process by which transmembrane proteins facilitate the movement of a molecule down its concentration gradient across a membrane. The carrier proteins have high specificity for their target molecule substrate. Few drugs utilize this pathway.
- **Active transport**: It is an energy-requiring process that occurs when a drug is moved against its concentration gradient or when the properties of the drug do not allow it to penetrate the cell by diffusion. Transmembrane carrier proteins with high structural specificity are responsible for active transport by utilizing energy from adenosine triphosphate (ATP) hydrolysis. The rate of carrier-mediated transport may show saturation at high solute concentrations because the number of carrier proteins is finite and the cycling of carrier proteins is limited.
- **Endocytosis**: This process occurs when a drug is engulfed by the cell membrane and internalized. This mechanism may occur when a drug binds to a membrane receptor and the drug–receptor complex is then internalized.

Effect of Ionization on Drug Absorption

Most drugs exist as weak acids or weak bases; however, unionized forms will be absorbed more readily. The fraction of drug in the unionized form depends on the pK_a of the drug and the pH of the environment. This can be determined using the Henderson–Hasselbalch equation. For a weak acid, A, the equation is as follows:

$$pH = pK_a + \log[A^-]/[HA]$$

Where
$pH = -\log_{10}[H^+]$ (pH units).
$pK_a = -\log_{10}$ equilibrium constant.
$[A^-]$ = concentration of the unprotonated, or ionized, form of the acid.
$[HA]$ = concentration of the protonated, or unionized, form of the acid.
For a weak base, B, the equation is as follows:

$$pH = pK_a + \log[B]/[BH^+]$$

Where
$pH = -\log_{10}[H^+]$ (pH units).
$pK_a = -\log_{10}$ equilibrium constant.
$[B]$ = concentration of the unprotonated, or unionized, form of the acid.
$[BH^+]$ = concentration of the protonated, or ionized, form of the acid.
When the pH equals the pK_a, the drug is 50% ionized and 50% unionized. When the pH is less than the pK_a the protonated forms HA and BH^+ predominate; conversely, when the pH is greater than the pK_a, the unprotonated forms A^- and B predominate. At gastric pH, acidic drugs tend to unionize and are

absorbed well through the stomach, whereas basic drugs tend to ionize in the stomach and are absorbed only when they reach the duodenum, where they will exist in their more unionized form.

Ion trapping occurs when the ionized form of a drug accumulates due to the difference between the pK_a of the drug and the pH of the environment. This property can be exploited to enhance drug elimination. For example, methylenedioxymethamphetamine (MDMA or ecstasy) has a $pK_a = 10$. In alkaline urine its half-life of elimination ($t_{1/2}$) is 16 to 31 hours. Acidification of the urine will increase the proportion of the drug in the ionized form, trapping it in the urine and enhancing its elimination ($t_{1/2} = 7$ to 10 hours).

1.6.2 Bioavailability

Bioavailability (F) is the fraction of the administered dose of a drug that reaches the systemic circulation in an unchanged form. It is calculated by comparing the plasma concentration of a drug over time after an IV dose (where all of the drug reaches the plasma, $F = 1$) with the plasma concentration of the drug over time following administration of the same dose of the drug given by another route (e.g., orally). Absorption and first-pass metabolism are the main factors that influence bioavailability.

1.7 Drug Distribution

1.7.1 Factors that Affect Distribution

Following its absorption, a drug is distributed in the bloodstream before it leaves this compartment and enters the extracellular fluid and/or the cells of tissues (▶ Fig. 1.2). This process is primarily affected by the blood flow to a particular tissue, the permeability of capillaries to the drug, and the degree of drug binding to proteins in plasma and tissues. A drug will tend to move from the bloodstream to tissues along a concentration gradient until equilibrium is established. When blood levels of a drug fall, the process reverses, and the drug is eliminated from the tissues.

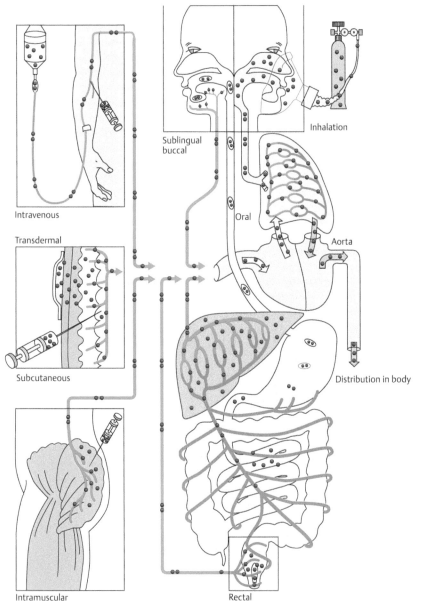

Fig. 1.2 Distribution following different modes of administration.
Drugs given intravenously, transdermally, subcutaneously, intramuscularly, sublingually, and buccally enter the venous circulation following administration and reach the general circulation after passing through the heart and lungs. Oral drugs are absorbed from the stomach or duodenum into the portal circulation, where they undergo first-pass metabolism in the liver before reaching the venous and then the general circulation. Drugs given rectally are mainly transported directly to the venous circulation, but some of the drug enters the portal circulation to the liver. Drugs given by inhalation have a local effect on the lungs and may also reach the general circulation (e.g., general anesthetics).

Intravenous

Transdermal

Subcutaneous

Intramuscular

Sublingual buccal

Oral

Inhalation

Aorta

Distribution in body

Rectal

Blood Flow

Initial distribution will tend toward those tissues with a higher blood flow (brain or central nervous system [CNS], liver, and kidneys). The drug will then gradually be redistributed to less vascularized tissues (e.g., skin, bone, and adipose tissue).

Permeability of Capillaries

Capillary endothelial cells that line blood vessels are, in general, separated by junctions that allow drugs to pass between them quite readily (▶ Fig. 1.3). In the liver, these junctions are larger than usual allowing drugs to pass even more readily. This is useful as the liver is the major site of drug metabolism. Conversely, the capillary endothelial cells of the brain have very tight junctions between them, which, along with glial cells,

form the blood–brain barrier. For drugs to enter the brain, they must diffuse through the endothelial cells (i.e., must be lipophilic) or be transported across the endothelial cell membrane via a carrier molecule.

Plasma Protein Binding

Drugs that are bound to plasma proteins (usually albumin but also α_1-acid glycoprotein [AAG]) cannot be distributed into tissues or eliminated, thus are pharmacologically inactive. However, the bound drugs act as a reservoir such that when the concentration of free drug in plasma falls (due to redistribution, metabolism, or elimination), the bound drug proportionally dissociates from albumin to maintain a constant bound-to-free drug ratio.

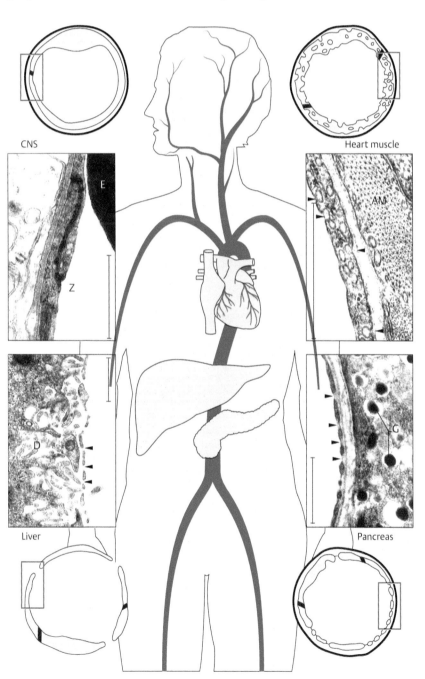

CNS

Heart muscle

Liver

Pancreas

Fig. 1.3 Blood–tissue barriers.
The penetrability of the capillary wall depends on the tissue. In cardiac muscle (*top right*), there is endocytotic and transcytotic activity (*arrowheads* in micrographs) that transports fluid and macromolecules into and out of the interstitium. Drugs that are in the fluid will also be transported, regardless of their physiochemical properties. In the endocrine glands (e.g., the pancreas, *lower right*) and the gut, the endothelial cells have fenestrations (*arrowheads*) that are closed by diaphragms. These diaphragms, along with the basement membrane, can readily be penetrated by low-molecular-weight substances (i.e., most drugs), but macromolecule penetration will depend on molecular weight and ionization. The liver (*lower left*) has large fenestrations that are not closed by diaphragms or basement membranes, so drugs are able to move freely into the interstitium. Finally, the central nervous system (*top left*) has no pores, fenestrations, or transcytotic activity, so drugs must either diffuse or be transported through the endothelial cells to gain access. AM, actomyosin; D, Disse space; E, erythrocyte; G, insulin storage granule; Z, tight junction. *Solid black line* in schematic drawings are basement membranes.

Different drugs have different affinities for albumin. Competition for binding occurs when two drugs with a high affinity for albumin are given at the same time. This will increase plasma free drug concentration that may lead to increased side effects or toxicity. Displacement of plasma protein binding of one drug by another is a common cause of drug interactions.

Foundations

Albumin

Serum albumin is the most abundant plasma protein in the body. It is synthesized by the liver and is an important transport molecule for endogenous substances such as steroid hormones, bilirubin, bile salts, free fatty acids, and calcium. It also acts as a transporter of many drugs. Albumin plays a critical role in regulating blood volume by maintaining the oncotic pressure of blood, which allows fluid to be retained in the vascular compartment. The concentration of albumin falls in liver disease, kidney disease (e.g., nephrotic syndrome, where kidney damage causes proteins to leak into urine), in inflammatory states, and in cases of malnutrition.

Foundations

α₁-Acid Glycoprotein

AAG is an acute-phase protein whose levels increase in acute inflammatory states and tissue injury. Like albumin, AAG is synthesized in the liver and acts as a transport protein for endogenous substances, such as steroid hormones, and many drugs.

Clinical Correlation

Hypoalbuminemia

Lower than normal levels of albumin in the blood is known as hypoalbuminemia. This leads to decreased plasma protein binding and it may occur in the following conditions: liver disease (e.g., hepatitis, cirrhosis, or hepatocellular necrosis), ascites, nephrotic syndrome, malabsorption syndromes (e.g., Crohn disease), extensive burns, and pregnancy.

► Table 1.2 lists the drug types that bind to albumin and AAG and gives specific examples of such drugs.

Volume of Distribution

Volume of distribution (V_d) is a pharmacological term that is defined as the volume in which a drug would need to be uni-

Table 1.2 Plasma protein binding

Plasma protein	Drug type	Examples
Albumin	Acidic drugs Neutral drugs	Warfarin, naproxen, phenytoin, sulfamethoxazole
α₁-acid glycoprotein	Basic drugs	Alprenolol, amitriptyline, imipramine, lidocaine

Note: Plasma protein binding is reversible.

formly distributed to produce the same concentration throughout the body as found in plasma. It is an arbitrary value that is useful as a guide when comparing the relative concentration of the drug in plasma with the rest of the body and should not be thought of as an actual physical volume of fluid. A low V_d (e.g., 4 L) indicates that the drug is mainly distributed in plasma, whereas a larger V_d (> 10 L) means that the drug has been distributed to additional compartments (e.g., interstitial or intracellular fluid). In reality, a drug will not be exclusively contained within one fluid compartment but distributed unevenly throughout one or more of them. ► Fig. 1.4 illustrates the compartments for drug distribution. ► Table 1.3 lists the physiochemical features of drugs that cause them to predominate in a certain compartment and provides examples.

The apparent V_d of a drug relates to the amount of drug administered to the plasma concentration according to the equation:

$$V_d = \text{Dose (mg)}/\text{plasma concentration (mg/L)}$$

Calculating the Amount of Drug to Administer from V_d

The V_d is used to calculate the amount of drug needed to achieve a desired plasma concentration by rearrangement of the above equation:

$$\text{Dose (mg)} = \text{plasma concentration (mg/L)} \times V_d(L)$$

This assumes, for simplicity, that the bioavailability of the drug is complete, distribution is instantaneous, and the drug is not being eliminated.

Effect of V_d on the Half-life of a Drug

For a drug to be eliminated, it must be present in its free form in plasma so that it may pass through the liver or kidney for excretion in bile or urine. The higher the V_d, the less a drug is contained in the plasma compartment, so its half-life will be prolonged.

1.8 Metabolism of Drugs

Drug metabolism usually inactivates therapeutic agents, transforming them into products that are more readily excreted. However, metabolism can also produce active agents from inactive prodrugs or can produce toxic metabolites.

The liver and intestinal wall are the main sites of metabolism, but drug metabolism can also occur in the kidneys, lungs, and gonads.

1.8.1 Phase 1 Metabolism

Metabolism generally consists of a phase 1 reaction that converts a drug to a less active form, followed by a phase 2 conjugation reaction (► Fig. 1.5). Phase 1 metabolism involves the oxidation, reduction, or hydrolysis of a drug, making it more polar by adding or exposing a functional group (e.g., −OH, −NH₂, −SH, −COO⁻). These functional groups can then act as the site of conjugation in phase 2 metabolism.

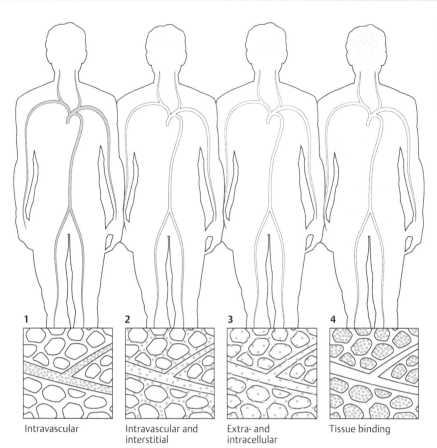

Fig. 1.4 Fluid compartments for drug distribution.
Drugs may be distributed to different body compartments depending on their physiochemical properties. See ▶ Table 1.3 for the V_ds and examples of drugs that distribute to each compartment.

1	2	3	4
Intravascular	Intravascular and interstitial	Extra- and intracellular	Tissue binding

Table 1.3 Features of drugs that cause them to predominate in each fluid compartment

Fluid compartment	Drug features	Examples
Intravascular (plasma) (4 L) (▶ Fig. 1.4–1)	High molecular weight Bound to plasma albumin	Heparin Warfarin Benzodiazepines Penicillin Sulfonamides Tetracyclines
Interstitial fluid (14 L) (▶ Fig. 1.4–2)	Low molecular weight Hydrophilic	Epinephrine Amikacin
Intracellular fluid (42 L) (▶ Fig. 1.4–3)	Low molecular weight Hydrophobic	Ethanol
Tissue binding (49 L) (▶ Fig. 1.4–4)	Binds to high affinity site in those tissues High lipid solubility	Digoxin (myocardial and skeletal muscle) Thiopental (adipose tissue) Tetracyclines Lead (bone and teeth)

Oxidation Reactions

In the liver, the most important site of metabolism is the microsomal enzyme system. This includes the mixed function oxidases located in the smooth endoplasmic reticulum. Pharmacologically, the most important of these is the cytochrome P-450 family of enzymes (▶ Fig. 1.6).

Each cytochrome P-450 enzyme is denoted by the abbreviation CYP followed by a number related to the family, then an upper-case letter related to its subfamily, followed by a number to specify the particular enzyme. Each enzyme has the capacity to catalyze the metabolism of many drugs with some overlap between them for substrates. More than 50% of drugs are catalyzed by the CYP3A family, about 30% by CYP2D6 and 15% by CYP2C. This system can be induced or inhibited by drugs which creates a huge potential for drug interactions (▶ Fig. 1.7).

Clinical Correlation

Drug–Grapefruit Interactions

Grapefruit juice is a powerful inhibitor of CYP3A4-mediated drug metabolism. This can lead to elevated plasma concentrations of many drugs, including benzodiazepines, codeine, and amiodarone (a potent antiarrhythmic drug), and the possible toxicity of these drugs.

The cytochrome P-450-dependent oxidation reactions include
- Aromatic and aliphatic hydroxylation.
- Alkyl oxidations and desulfuration.
- Oxidative deamination.
- N-dealkylation from nitrogen, oxygen, and sulfur.
- Sulfoxidation.
- Epoxidation.

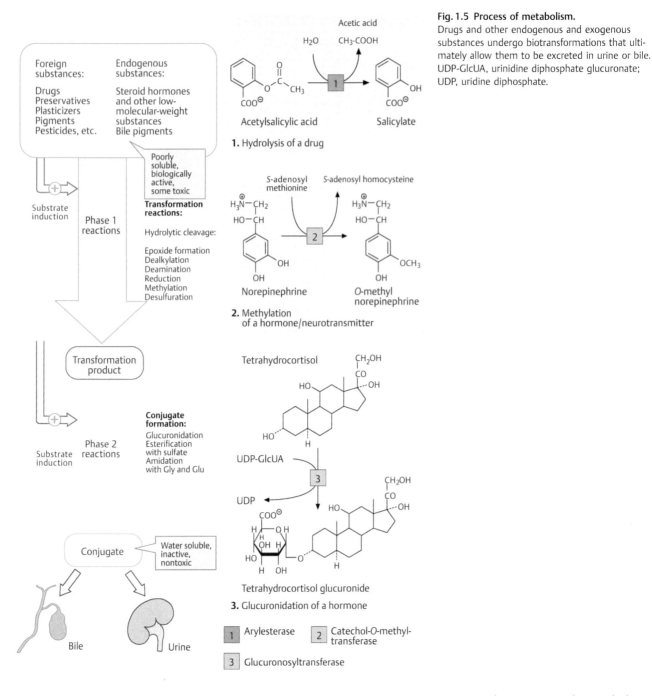

Foreign substances:

Drugs
Preservatives
Plasticizers
Pigments
Pesticides, etc.

Endogenous substances:

Steroid hormones and other low-molecular-weight substances
Bile pigments

Poorly soluble, biologically active, some toxic

Substrate induction

Phase 1 reactions

Transformation reactions:

Hydrolytic cleavage:

Epoxide formation
Dealkylation
Deamination
Reduction
Methylation
Desulfuration

Transformation product

Substrate induction

Phase 2 reactions

Conjugate formation:

Glucuronidation
Esterification with sulfate
Amidation with Gly and Glu

Conjugate

Water soluble, inactive, nontoxic

Bile

Urine

Acetic acid

H_2O $CH_3\text{-}COOH$

Acetylsalicylic acid

Salicylate

1. Hydrolysis of a drug

S-adenosyl methionine

S-adenosyl homocysteine

Norepinephrine

O-methyl norepinephrine

2. Methylation of a hormone/neurotransmitter

Tetrahydrocortisol

UDP-GlcUA

UDP

Tetrahydrocortisol glucuronide

3. Glucuronidation of a hormone

1 | Arylesterase
2 | Catechol-O-methyl-transferase
3 | Glucuronosyltransferase

Fig. 1.5 Process of metabolism.
Drugs and other endogenous and exogenous substances undergo biotransformations that ultimately allow them to be excreted in urine or bile. UDP-GlcUA, urinidine diphosphate glucuronate; UDP, uridine diphosphate.

Substrates

Inducer

Protein synthesis

CYP

Inhibitors

mRNA

Transcription factors

CYP gene

Fig. 1.6 Cytochrome P-450 synthesis in the liver.
Inducer substances activate transcription factors in the *CYP* gene, producing more cytochrome P-450. Cytochrome P-450 enzymes are then able to metabolize substrates unless they are acted upon by an inhibitor. Inhibitors bind to cytochrome P-450 enzymes with high affinity and cause the substrates of cytochrome P-450 enzymes to be metabolized more slowly. mRNA, messenger RNA.

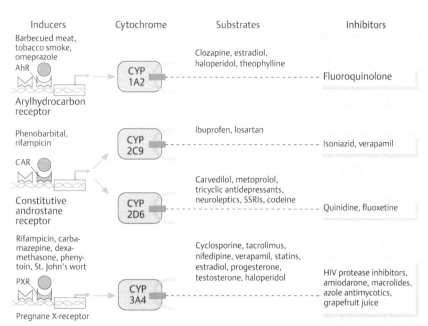

Fig. 1.7 Substrates, inducers, and inhibitors of cytochrome P-450 enzymes.
Inducer substances can be environmental compounds, endogenous substances, or they may be drugs themselves. The cytochrome enzyme that they induce is then able to metabolize specific substrates (drugs) more rapidly, so the substrate drugs may not reach their effective therapeutic concentration. Inhibitors interfere with substrate metabolism and may cause toxic accumulation of a drug in the body. HIV, human immunodeficiency virus; SSRIs, selective serotonin reuptake inhibitors.

When a drug is oxidized, oxygen is reduced to water as a byproduct. This type of reaction requires energy in the form of NADPH to drive the conversion. The enzyme cytochrome P-450 reductase transfers electrons from NADPH to CYP.

Some drugs are metabolized by noninducible, nonmicrosomal enzymes. Examples include monoamine oxidase (in mitochondria) in the metabolism of sympathomimetic amines, such as epinephrine, norepinephrine, dopamine; alcohol dehydrogenase (in cytosol) in the metabolism of ethanol; and xanthine oxidase (in cytosol) in the catabolism of purines and xanthines.

Reduction Reactions

Reduction reactions generally require anaerobic conditions and may be catalyzed by bacteria in the gut or urinary tract. Microsomal enzymes can also reduce drugs under appropriate conditions. Examples of reduction reactions include the formation of nitrites from organic nitrates and amine formation from the reduction of nitro ($-NO_2$) containing compounds.

Hydrolysis Reactions

Drug hydrolysis predominantly occurs in plasma and cellular cytosol as a result of chemical or enzymatic reactions. Examples of enzymes that catalyze these reactions include esterases which metabolize acetylcholine, atropine, and procaine; amidases which metabolize procainamide and lidocaine; and peptidases which metabolize insulin and vasopressin. Metabolites produced by these reactions are usually more water soluble than the parent compound and may be excreted in this form or processed further by conjugation.

1.8.2 Phase 2 Metabolism

Drug conjugations are referred to as phase 2 reactions because they often occur after initial drug oxidation, reduction, or hydrolysis; however, drugs can bypass phase 1 metabolism and go straight to phase 2. Conjugated compounds are generally inactive,

Table 1.4 Phase 2 conjugation reactions

Type of conjugation	Method of conjugation	Examples
Glucuronidation*	Glucose is used to form UDPGA which transfers a glucuronide to the functional group of the drug in the presence of glucuronyl transferase	Majority of drugs Steroid hormones Bilirubin
Sulfation	Catalyzed by sulfotransferases	Estradiol, acetaminophen
Amino acids	Conjugated by glycine and glutamine	Simple aromatic acids (e.g., salicylates)
Glutathione	Catalyzed by glutathione S-transferase	Acetaminophen
Acetylation	Catalyzed by acetyltransferases	Limited to drugs with primary amino groups (e.g., sulfonamides)
Methylation	Catalyzed by N-methyl-transferases, catechol-O-methyl-transferase (methylates, dopamine, methyldopa, and L-dopa), and a thiopurine methyltransferase	Azathioprine 6-mercaptopurine Thioguanine

Abbreviation: UDPGA, uridine diphosphate glucuronic acid.
*This is the only phase 2 reaction that can be induced by other pharmacological agents and has a potential for drug interactions.
Note: All conjugations, except glucuronidation, are catalyzed by transferases, located mainly in the cytosol.

especially glucuronide, sulfate, and glutathione conjugates, which are highly water soluble and readily excreted in urine.

▶ Table 1.4 lists the types of phase 2 conjugation reactions and gives examples of drugs that undergo each type of conjugation.

11

Creatinine

Creatinine is formed in a nonenzymatic reaction from creatine phosphate in skeletal muscle. It is excreted with minimal reabsorption in the kidneys, and its clearance rate is an excellent indication of glomerular filtration and, therefore, renal function.

1.9 Elimination of Drugs

Elimination of drugs and their metabolites mainly occurs via urine and feces, although many other minor routes of elimination also exist such as saliva, sweat, tears, breast milk, and expired air (from the lungs).

1.9.1 Renal Elimination

To undergo renal elimination, a drug must be filtered or actively transported into the urine and must resist reabsorption back into plasma and subsequent reentry into the systemic circulation.

Glomerular Filtration

Drugs are filtered into the urine from plasma depending on their molecular weight, ionization, and degree of protein binding.
- Low-molecular-weight and/or ionized drugs are more readily filtered.
- Drugs that are highly bound to plasma proteins are too large to be filtered.
- Drugs that are filtered in the glomerulus and not reabsorbed are eliminated at a rate that equals creatinine clearance (125 mL/minute).

Active Transport in the Proximal Tubule

Drugs that are acids or bases in plasma can be actively secreted into the tubular lumen against a concentration gradient by anionic and cationic transport systems. This process requires energy.

Reabsorption in the Distal Tubule

Unionized drugs are able to passively diffuse back into plasma, especially if they are lipid soluble and there is a favorable concentration gradient. The ionization of a drug is affected by changes in urinary pH. For example, if the urine is made more alkaline by administration of bicarbonate, weak acids will become more ionized, thereby slowing their reabsorption and increasing their elimination (see Henderson–Hasselbalch equation page 3).

1.9.2 Hepatic Elimination

Conjugated drugs (mainly glucuronic acid derivatives) are actively secreted into bile. Unconjugated drugs are liberated in the small intestine by bacterial enzyme hydrolysis and reabsorbed into the portal circulation. This is the enterohepatic cycle. Some of the drug escapes reabsorption and appears in feces. Antibiotic-induced decreases in intestinal bacterial flora will decrease the hydrolysis of conjugated drugs thus interfering with enterohepatic cycling and decreasing the drug concentration below its therapeutic range (e.g., steroids used for contraception).

1.10 Drug Interactions

Drug interactions may occur at any stage between absorption and elimination, but competition for plasma albumin binding and induction/inhibition of the CYP-450 enzymes (▶ Fig. 1.8) are by far the most common interactions. ▶ Table 1.5 lists some common mechanisms of interactions and gives examples of drugs that can cause them.

1.11 Determinants of Plasma Concentration and Dosing

The rate of drug dosing depends primarily on the rate of drug elimination. Most drugs are removed from plasma by processes that are concentration-dependent (i.e., metabolism, secretion, and filtration) and result in "first-order" kinetics of elimination.

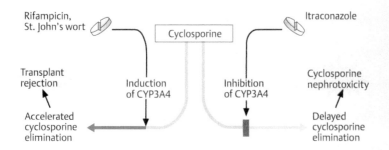

Fig. 1.8 Drug interactions involving cytochrome P-450 enzymes.
In patients taking cyclosporine (an immunosuppressant drug used to prevent organ rejection), concomitant use of rifampicin (an antibiotic) or St. John's wort (an herbal drug used to treat depression) will induce CYP3A4, increasing cyclosporine metabolism and elimination. In this case, plasma levels of cyclosporine are not maintained at the therapeutic level leading to transplant rejection. Conversely, if itraconazole (an antifungal agent) is taken with cyclosporine, CYP3A4 is inhibited, and cyclosporine metabolism and elimination are slowed, leading to toxic accumulation in the kidneys.

Table 1.5 Pharmacokinetic stage and mechanisms of drug interactions

Stage	Mechanism of interaction	Drug example(s)
Absorption	Change in GI pH	H$_2$ blockers, antacids
	Changes in GI motility	Laxatives, anticholinergics
	Changes in GI perfusion	Vasodilators
	Chelation	Tetracycline, calcium
	Inactivation of drug by adsorption	Activated charcoal
Distribution	Competition for plasma albumin binding	Warfarin, NSAIDs, nifedipine
	Changes in perfusion	Vasodilators, ACE inhibitors
	Changes in V_d	Diuretics
Metabolism	Increased by inducers of CYP-450	Carbamazepine, rifampin, phenytoin
	Decreased by inhibitors of CYP-450	Erythromycin, ketoconazole, fluoxetine
	Increased by inducers of glucuronidation	Rifampin
Elimination	Changes in urinary pH	Bicarbonate
	Competition for binding to active transporters in the proximal tubule	Salicylate, furosemide, penicillin G

Abbreviations: ACE, angiotensin-converting enzyme; GI, gastrointestinal; NSAIDs, nonsteroidal anti-inflammatory drugs.

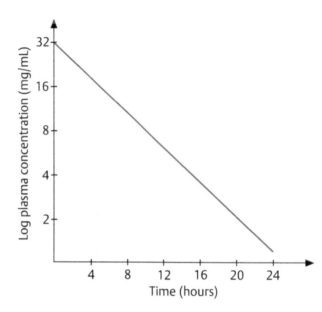

Fig. 1.9 First-order elimination.
With first-order kinetics, a constant percentage of the drug is eliminated per unit of time. Note that plasma concentration is plotted on a logarithmic scale and that the $t_{1/2}$ of this drug is 4 h.

Foundations

Blood, Plasma, and Hematocrit

Blood consists of cells suspended in plasma. The plasma is an aqueous solution containing proteins, electrolytes, vitamins, metabolites, gases, and hormones. The cells are primarily red blood cells (erythrocytes) along with some white blood cells (leukocytes) and platelets (thrombocytes). The hematocrit is a measure of the percentage of blood volume that is cellular, and it is normally about 45%.

1.11.1 First-Order Elimination

With first-order kinetics,
- A constant percentage of the drug is eliminated per unit of time. This is known as the elimination rate constant (K_e).
- The elimination half-life ($t_{1/2}$) is the time it takes for the plasma concentration to be reduced by 50%. It is constant and is independent of the dose.
- Half-life is related to K_e by the following:

$$t_{1/2} = 0.693/K_e$$

- Clearance (CL) is the volume of fluid from which the drug is eliminated per unit of time.

$$CL = V_d \times K_e$$

Substituting $0.693/t_{1/2}$ for K_e gives

$$CL = (0.693 \times V_d/t_{1/2})$$

- A plot of log plasma concentration against time is a straight line (▶ Fig. 1.9). The y-intercept is an extrapolated value and would be the plasma concentration of drug at time 0 assuming instantaneous distribution.
- Most drugs exhibit first-order kinetics unless they are given in very high doses.

1.11.2 Zero-Order Elimination

With zero-order kinetics,
- A constant amount of drug is eliminated per unit of time regardless of its concentration. This usually occurs because the route of elimination has become saturated.
- The half-life is not constant but depends on the concentration (i.e., the higher the concentration, the longer the half-life).
- Drugs in this category will demonstrate first-order kinetics whenever the drug concentration falls substantially below the saturation level of the elimination process.
- Examples of drugs that exhibit zero-order kinetics include ethanol and heparin, plus other drugs at high doses (e.g., salicylates such as aspirin).

1.12 Pharmacokinetics of Drug Administration in Practice

It is important that clinicians understand the factors that affect the total amount of drug in the body, how much drug is in plasma, and how this changes over time so that an appropriate therapeutic regimen can be devised. To illustrate these concepts, we will discuss the two different types of drug administration: continuous IV infusion and repeated dosing.

1.12.1 Kinetics of Continuous IV Infusion

If a drug is given by continuous IV infusion, a constant amount of the drug enters the plasma and a constant percentage is eliminated (cleared from the blood) per unit of time (if elimination is first-order); that is, plasma concentration and elimination are proportional such that any increase in plasma concentration of a drug will lead to an increase in its elimination. At the start of an IV infusion, plasma drug concentration will rise until it reaches the point where elimination exactly matches administration. At this point, the plasma concentration will remain constant and is referred to as the steady-state concentration (C_{ss}) (▸ Fig. 1.10). For drugs that are given by continuous IV infusion, the equation for calculating C_{ss} is

$$C_{ss} = R_0/CL$$

where
  R_o = the infusion rate (mg/minute).
  CL = clearance (mL/minute).

- Note that the time to reach C_{ss} is solely determined by the half-life of the drug. It takes roughly four half-lives for a drug to be eliminated from the body, and because C_{ss} and elimination are proportional, it takes about four half-lives to reach C_{ss}.
- Increasing the rate of infusion will increase the C_{ss}, but not the rate at which the new C_{ss} is achieved.
- Increasing the rate of infusion will increase the rate at which a given concentration of drug lower than C_{ss} is achieved.

1.12.2 Kinetics of Repeated Dosing

Fixed-Dose/Fixed-Time-Interval Regimens

The most common drug dosing regimen is to take a drug orally one or more times per day. However, compared to continuous infusion, a repeated dosing regimen introduces issues related to fluctuations in plasma drug concentration that occur between doses. With any fixed-dose/fixed-time-interval regimen, a C_{ss} is ultimately reached, but it is not achieved in a smooth, exponential

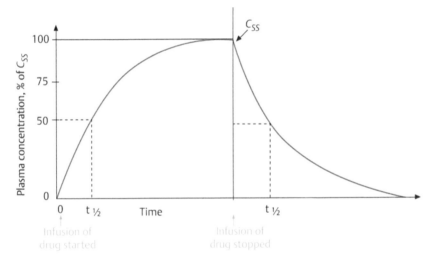

Fig. 1.10 Time for drug that obeys first-order kinetics to reach plasma steady-state concentration and be eliminated.
When a drug that is eliminated according to first-order kinetics is given by IV infusion, 50% of plasma steady-state concentration (C_{ss}) is achieved after one half-life and 75% after two half-lives; C_{ss} is complete after approximately four half-lives. If the infusion is stopped, the drug is eliminated in these same proportions (i.e., 50% is eliminated after one half-life and so on until it is almost completely eliminated after four half-lives). On this graph plasma concentration is plotted on a linear scale, resulting in an exponential curve. Compare this to the log plot of first-order elimination in ▸ Fig. 1.9, which gives a straight line.

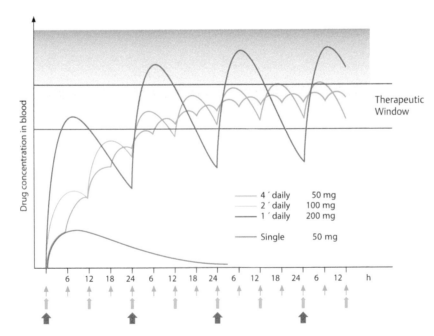

Fig. 1.11 Accumulation: dose, dose interval, and fluctuation of plasma level.
When a large dose of a drug is given once per day, the plasma concentration fluctuates greatly. Toxic levels are obtained (*pink area*) at peak plasma concentrations and subtherapeutic levels (below the *green area*) are obtained at the trough. If the drug is given in smaller, more frequent doses (2 times daily and 4 times daily), the peaks and troughs become smaller. The C_{ss} will be the same and will be obtained in four half-lives, independent of the frequency of dosing. The range of blood or plasma concentrations that are sufficient to provide a therapeutic response without producing toxic effects is termed the *therapeutic window* for the drug.

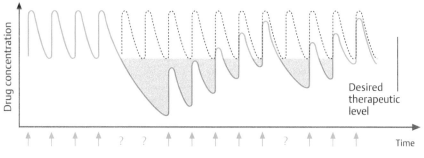

Fig. 1.12 Plasma concentration of drugs with irregular dosing.
Irregular dosing, such as occurs with the increased nocturnal dosing interval during fixed-dose/fixed-time-interval regimens or due to missed doses (poor patient adherence), results in the plasma drug concentration falling below the desired therapeutic level (*pink areas*). It then takes several doses to reach the desired therapeutic level once again. Note that the arrows (↑) signify when each dose of drug is taken and the question mark (?) represents a missed dose.

way as with continuous infusion, but rather by way of fluctuating around a mean (▶ Fig. 1.11). This is because most intermittent doses of drugs are given in fewer than four half-lives (i.e., before the preceding dose has been completely eliminated), so the drug will accumulate until the C_{ss} is achieved. The magnitude of the peaks and troughs around the mean will depend on the dosing interval (see ▶ Table 1.6). Smaller doses at shorter intervals will minimize these fluctuations, but will not alter the C_{ss} or the rate at which it is attained.

For drugs that are taken orally on a fixed-dose/fixed-time-interval regimen, the equation for calculating the C_{ss} is

$$C_{ss} = \left[F \times \left(\frac{D}{T}\right)\right]/CL$$

where
C_{ss} = steady-state concentration (mg/mL).
F = bioavailability.
D = dose (mg).
T = dosing interval (minute).
CL = clearance (mL/minute).
Note:
- To change the C_{ss}, it is generally better to increase the frequency of dosing rather than the amount of drug given to avoid toxic effects related to larger excursions around the mean concentration (i.e., larger peak and trough values).
- For orally administered drugs, bioavailability must be taken into account in the calculation of C_{ss}.
- No simple prediction of C_{ss} can be made for drugs eliminated by zero-order kinetics. In this case, toxic concentrations can accumulate more quickly and be eliminated more slowly than for drugs that follow first-order kinetics.

Use of a Loading Dose

It is often desirable to achieve the C_{ss} more quickly than four half-lives, especially if the half-life of the drug is long. In these cases, a loading dose (*LD*) can be used. Loading doses can be given as a single bolus injection, but the high initial plasma concentrations achieved can sometimes lead to adverse effects. These adverse effects may be avoided by staggering the loading dose over a short period, which allows time for some redistribution of the drug to occur. Loading dose (mg) is calculated as follows:

$$LD = (V_d) \times (\text{desired } C_{ss})$$

For an orally administered loading dose, bioavailability must be considered.

Table 1.6 Effect of dosing interval on time to reach steady-state concentration, the degree of fluctuation of plasma drug concentration, and the most useful mode of administration to combat these variables

Half-life (h)/ dosing interval	Time to reach C_{ss}	Plasma concentration fluctuation	Mode of administration
< 4	Short	Large	IV infusion sustained-release preparation
6–24	Medium	Medium	Usually oral fixed dose at interval equal to $t_{1/2}$
> 24	Long	Small	Sustained-release preparation ± loading dose

Abbreviations: C_{ss}, steady-state concentration; IV, intravenous.

1.12.3 Irregular Dosing Regimens

Irregular dosing occurs to some extent during fixed-dose/fixed-time-interval regimens because patients do not take a drug dose during the night. It also commonly occurs when patients do not adhere strictly to the prescribed dosing interval. As a consequence of irregular dosing, plasma drug concentrations often fall below the therapeutic level (▶ Fig. 1.12).

▶ Table 1.7 summarizes the factors that should be considered when choosing a dosing regimen.

1.13 Drug Dosage in Renal Disease

Renal disease must be taken into consideration when drugs are excreted primarily (> 50%) unchanged by the kidney.
- The initial dose is the same as for any patient, but because clearance is decreased, the maintenance dose is decreased or the dosing interval is increased in proportion to the decrease in renal clearance of creatinine. In doing this, the percentage of drug eliminated by the kidney remains unchanged.

1.14 Drug Dosage in Hepatic Disease

Hepatic disease has the potential to affect the pharmacokinetics of many drugs; however, because hepatic reserves are large, the disease has to be severe for changes in drug metabolism to

Table 1.7 Summary of factors to consider when choosing a dosing regimen

Factor	Comments
Steady-state plasma concentration (C_{ss})	This will be the desired therapeutic plasma concentration and will lie within the therapeutic index
Clearance (CL)	This is the same as creatinine clearance in a healthy adult patient (125 mL/min)
Half-life ($t_{1/2}$)	This dictates the time taken to reach the steady-state concentration and therefore the dosing interval
Therapeutic index (TI)	The therapeutic index is a means of comparing the amount of a drug required to attain the therapeutic level in 50% of patients to the amount that is lethal to 50% of patients. A large TI allows for a variety of dosing regimens. A small TI often necessitates that a drug is given by IV infusion or as a sustained-release preparation
Bioavailability (F)	This must be factored in when considering all methods of administration of drugs except for IV (100% bioavailability). It is especially important in determining oral dosing regimens
Volume of distribution (V_d)	This will affect the concentration of free drug in plasma which, in turn, determines how much is available for elimination. V_d is usually constant and can be largely ignored when calculating a dosing regimen, but it gains significance in disease states
Route of administration	This is determined by patient factors and the biochemical properties of the drug
Drug interactions	Clinicians should always consider drug interactions, especially the most serious and clinically relevant ones

Abbreviation: IV, intravenous.

occur. The mechanisms by which the pharmacokinetics may be altered include the following:

- Reduced hepatic blood flow reduces first-pass metabolism of drugs taken orally.
- Reduced plasma protein binding affects both distribution and elimination.
- Plasma clearance of a drug is reduced if it is eliminated following metabolism and/or following excretion into bile.

A dose reduction will be necessary in hepatic disease, but it should be calculated for each individual patient.

Clinical Correlation

Nephrotoxic Drugs

An example of a nephrotoxic drug is gentamicin, an aminoglycoside antibiotic used to treat severe bacterial infections. It is excreted in unchanged form, mostly by glomerular filtration, in the kidney. In renal impairment, gentamicin will accumulate in the kidney causing destruction of kidney cells (nephrotoxicity). When gentamicin is prescribed, the dosage and treatment period should be minimized and plasma concentration should be closely monitored.

2 Mechanisms of Drug Action and Pharmacodynamics

Summary

Pharmacodynamics are the pharmacological principles that describe drug effects on the body. Most drug effects are produced by interaction of the drug with specific receptors to produce a response. There are 5 major types of receptors: ligand-gated ion channels, G protein-coupled receptors (GPCRs), voltage-dependent ion channels, enzyme-linked membrane receptors and intracellular receptors. Agonists bind to a receptor and produce an effect. *Full agonists* are drugs of high intrinsic efficacy. *Partial agonists* are drugs with efficacy lower than full agonists. Antagonists bind to a receptor, do not produce a response (they lack efficacy), and block the effects of agonists. *Competitive antagonists* compete with the agonist for binding to the receptor. *Noncompetitive antagonists* either prevent the agonist from binding to the receptor or prevent the agonist from activating the receptor. *Chemical antagonists* are drugs that inhibit the effects of other compounds by a direct chemical interaction. *Physiological antagonism* occurs when two drugs act by different mechanisms to produce opposite physiological effects. Inverse agonists are drugs that cause an effect opposite that of conventional agonists. Both allosteric inhibitors and allosteric potentiators are known to exist. Receptor activation can also lead to *desensitization, resensitization, down-regulation,* and *up-regulation.* Potency refers to the amount of drug required to produce an effect of a given intensity. The therapeutic index is the ratio $LD_{50}:ED_{50}$. A high therapeutic index indicates a safe drug. The certain safety factor is $LD_1:ED_{99}$. It indicates the degree of overlap of the lethal and therapeutic effect curves.

Keywords: receptor, signal transduction, agonist, antagonist, dose-response curve

2.1 Pharmacodynamics

Pharmacodynamics are the pharmacological principles that describe drug effects on the body, explaining both mechanism of action and dose–response relationship.

2.2 Effects of Drugs on Receptors

Most drug effects are produced by interaction of the drug with specific plasma membrane or intracellular receptors, leading to molecular changes that produce a given response (▶ Fig. 2.1). Drug receptors are mainly proteins or nucleic acids. A drug binds to a specific binding site on its receptor. The binding is usually reversible and occurs by low-energy forces (e.g., hydrogen bonds, hydrophobic bonds, and van der Waals bonds) or ionic bonds. Some drugs (e.g., aspirin and penicillin) form irreversible covalent bonds with their receptors. Binding requires structural specificity of the drug for the receptor and often exhibits stereospecificity (specificity for one stereoisomer of the drug).

Drugs may also exert their effects by physical or chemical interactions that do not involve receptors. Examples include antacids that work by neutralizing gastric pH; chelators that bind to heavy metals, inactivating them; and osmotic diuretics that act by absorbing water into the lumen of the kidney to maintain osmotic balance.

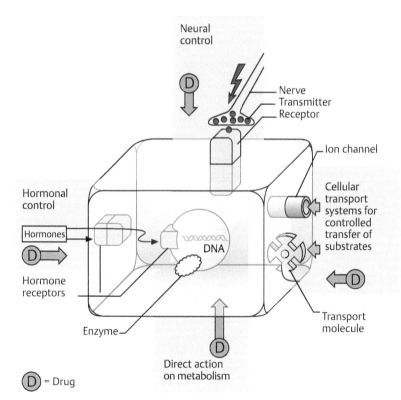

Fig. 2.1 Sites at which drugs act to modify cell function. Drugs may act at the same receptors as endogenous neurotransmitters or on ion channels to cause direct effects (e.g., opening of an ion channel), or receptor binding may activate a signal transduction system, leading to the cellular response. Drugs may also act by altering the activity of a cellular transport system or by activating or inhibiting enzymes that control intracellular metabolism. They may also act on DNA to damage it or to alter the transcription of proteins.

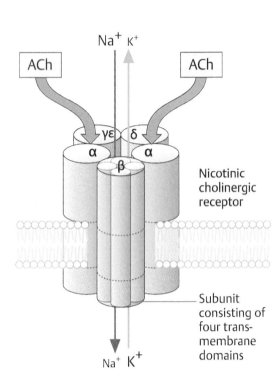

Fig. 2.2 Ligand-gated ion channel.
An example of a ligand-gated ion channel is the nicotinic cholinergic receptor on the motor end plate. When two acetylcholine (Ach) molecules bind to this receptor simultaneously (at the α-subunits) and the inner pore opens, Na⁺ enters the cell and K⁺ leaves the cell. This causes membrane depolarization and action potential generation, resulting in muscle contraction.

2.2.1 Receptors and Their Signal Transduction

Types of Receptors

- **Ligand-gated ion channels.** These are specialized membrane pores made up of multisubunit proteins. Binding of ligands, for example, endogenous compounds or drugs, to these receptors opens or closes the pores, thus changing the permeability of Na⁺, K⁺, Cl⁻, or other ions (▸ Fig. 2.2).
- **Voltage-dependent ion channels.** These normally open or close in response to changes in the membrane potential, but they can also function as receptors for drugs. For example, the local anesthetic agents bind to and block voltage-dependent Na⁺ channels in neuronal cell membranes (▸ Fig. 2.3).
- **Enzyme-linked membrane receptors.** One subgroup of these receptors consists of an extracellular hormone-binding domain, a hydrophobic segment of the polypeptide that crosses the lipid bilayer of the plasma membrane, and a cytoplasmic enzyme domain, which may be a protein tyrosine kinase, a serine kinase, or a guanylyl cyclase. When a drug binds to this type of receptor, it causes the enzyme to become

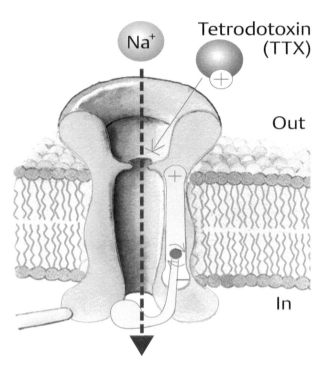

Fig. 2.3 Voltage-gated ion channel.
An example of a voltage-gated ion channel is the tetrodotoxin (TTX)-sensitive Na channel in nerve axons. Membrane depolarization leads to channel opening, allowing Na⁺ to enter the cell. Voltage-dependent Na channels are involved in conducting neuronal impulses. These channels are blocked by TTX (the paralytic toxin from pufferfish) and by local anesthetics (see **Fig. 8.3**).

"switched on" intracellularly. This enzyme then catalyzes the formation of other signal proteins that ultimately lead to the cellular response (▸ Fig. 2.4).
In a related subgroup, the enzyme activity is not intrinsic to the receptor molecule. The activated receptor binds to a separate intracellular protein tyrosine kinase leading to the cellular response (▸ Fig. 2.5).

- **Intracellular receptors.** Lipid-soluble drugs diffuse through cell membranes and bind either in the cellular cytosol or in the nucleus. Gene expression is altered and protein synthesis is either increased or decreased, which causes the cellular response (▸ Fig. 2.6). This mechanism is the slowest and effects can usually be measured in terms of hours rather than minutes or seconds.
- **G protein-coupled receptors (GPCRs).** The GPCRs are a large family of integral membrane proteins that are receptors for many endogenous signaling molecules and drugs. These receptors couple to guanine nucleotide-binding proteins (G proteins) which transduce the signal from ligand-bound GPCRs to the formation of several intracellular second messengers that culminate in a cellular response. The mechanisms of G protein signal transduction are discussed further below.

2.2.2 G Protein Signal Transduction

It has been estimated that 40 to 50% of currently marketed drugs target GPCRs. As the name implies, when these receptors are activated, they couple to heterotrimeric G proteins (▶ Fig. 2.7). The activated α-subunit and βγ dimers then interact with other proteins in the membrane to produce second messengers. These second messengers include cyclic adenosine monophosphate (cAMP), diacylglycerol (DAG), and inositol 1, 4, 5-trisphosphate (IP$_3$) (▶ Fig. 2.8).

- G$_s$ proteins activate cAMP.
- G$_i$ proteins inhibit cAMP.
- G$_q$ proteins activate phospholipase C, which increases DAG and IP$_3$.

Adenylate Cyclase System

Ligands that bind to a GPCR that activates G$_s$ stimulate adenylate cyclase to convert adenosine triphosphate (ATP) to cAMP (▶ Fig. 2.9a). cAMP then activates protein kinase A, which phosphorylates proteins, resulting in the physiologic response. cAMP is degraded to 5'AMP by phosphodiesterases. Ligands that bind to a GPCR that activates G$_i$ inhibit adenylate cyclase (↓ cAMP), therefore protein kinase A is not activated and downstream proteins are not phosphorylated.

Diacylglycerol and Inositol 1, 4, 5-trisphosphate System

GPCRs may also couple to G$_q$. G$_q$ activates the enzyme phospholipase C, which produces the second messengers IP$_3$ and DAG from phosphatidylinositol 4, 5-bisphosphate (PIP$_2$) (▶ Fig. 2.9b).

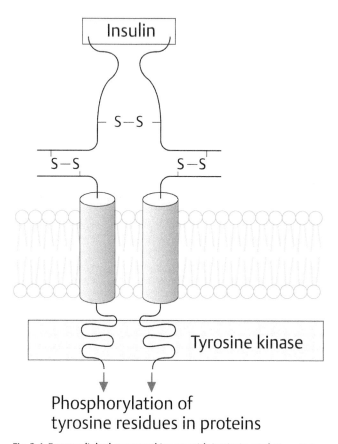

Fig. 2.4 Enzyme-linked receptor kinases with intrinsic catalytic activity. Insulin binding to the extracellular side of the receptor tyrosine kinase (RTK) leads to receptor dimerization and activation of the enzyme which phosphorylates tyrosine residues on specific intracellular proteins. This leads to a protein activation cascade, eventually resulting in glucose uptake into the cell.

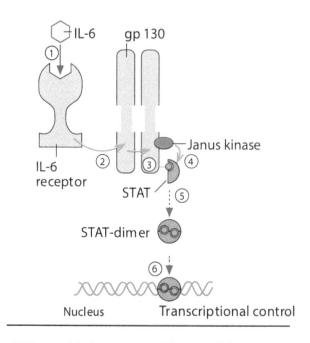

Fig. 2.5 Enzyme-linked receptors coupled to intracellular kinases. Activation of cytokine receptors (**1**), by interleukin 6 (IL-6), promotes dimerization of the signal transduction protein gp130 (**2**) which binds to Janus kinase (**3**). The Janus kinase phosphorylates (**4**) the receptor, gp130, and STAT molecules, leading to the formation of STAT-dimers (**5**) which translocate to the nucleus and alter transcription (**6**).

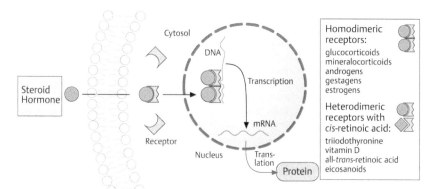

Fig. 2.6 Intracellular receptor. Lipophilic substances, such as steroid hormones and thyroid hormones, can diffuse through the cell membrane and interact with receptors in the cytoplasm or nucleus. The hormone–receptor complex then alters gene transcription, causing the synthesis of effector proteins. The hormone–receptor complex interacts with DNA in pairs; these may be identical (homodimeric) or nonidentical (heterodimeric) pairs.

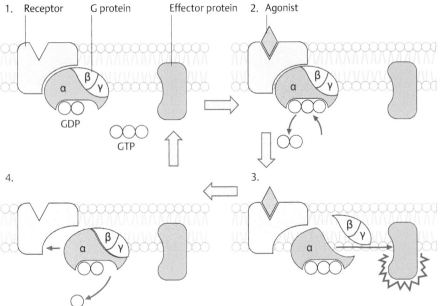

1. Receptor   G protein   Effector protein   2. Agonist

GDP

GTP

4.

3.

Fig. 2.7 G protein-mediated effect of an agonist.
(**1**) This shows the G protein-coupled receptor in the resting state. (**2**) When an agonist binds to the G protein-coupled receptor, it causes the receptor and G protein to change conformation. The α-subunit exchanges GTP for GDP and dissociates from the βγ subunits. (**3**) The α-subunit interacts with an effector protein (adenylate cyclase or phospholipase C) that stimulates or inhibits second messenger molecules to produce a physiological effect. (**4**) The α-subunit then hydrolyses the bound GTP to GDP and reassociates with the other subunits. GDP, guanosine diphosphate; GTP, guanosine triphosphate.

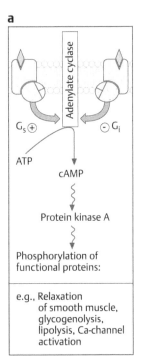

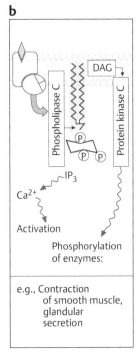

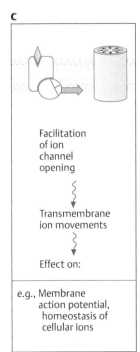

a

Adenylate cyclase

$G_s \oplus$ $\ominus G_i$

ATP

cAMP

Protein kinase A

Phosphorylation of functional proteins:

e.g., Relaxation of smooth muscle, glycogenolysis, lipolysis, Ca-channel activation

b

Phospholipase C

DAG

Protein kinase C

IP_3

Ca^{2+}

Activation

Phosphorylation of enzymes:

e.g., Contraction of smooth muscle, glandular secretion

c

Facilitation of ion channel opening

Transmembrane ion movements

Effect on:

e.g., Membrane action potential, homeostasis of cellular ions

Fig. 2.8 G proteins, second messengers, and effects.
(**a**) G proteins can stimulate or inhibit adenylate cyclase. G_s stimulates adenylate cyclase to produce the second messenger cAMP which activates protein kinase A (PKA) which catalyzes phosphorylation of proteins, leading to the physiological effects. Inhibition of adenylate cyclase by G_i decreases PKA activity and produces opposite effects. (**b**) G_q proteins activate phospholipase C which converts the membrane phospholipid phosphatidylinositol 4, 5-bisphosphate to DAG and IP_3. DAG activates protein kinase C while IP_3 causes the intracellular release of Ca^{2+} to cause physiological effects. (**c**) G proteins can also cause ion channels to open. The movement of ions may then initiate an action potential, or it may normalize intracellular ion content. ATP, adenosine triphosphate; cAMP, cyclic adenosine monophosphate; DAG, diacylglycerol; IP_3, inositol trisphosphate.

Hydrophilic IP_3 diffuses from the membrane to the endoplasmic reticulum and releases Ca^{2+}. The Ca^{2+} released can then produce physiologic effects in the following ways:
- Activation of protein kinase C (with DAG) leading to the phosphorylation of proteins.
- Binding to calmodulin with the resultant complex mediating further effects, for example, production of nitric oxide (NO).

Lipophilic DAG has two functions:
- Activation of protein kinase C. This process is Ca^{2+}-dependent.
- Formation of arachidonic acid (an eicosanoid precursor) following its degradation by DAG lipase.

Other Effects of G Proteins

G protein α-subunit and βγ dimers subunits may also interact directly with ion channels to alter ionic conductance and cellular excitability (► Fig. 2.9c).

► Table 2.1 gives examples of each of the types of receptors discussed above and substances that bind to these receptors.

2.3 Dose–Response Relationships

Quantitative mathematical descriptions of a drug's binding to its receptor, its effects on cellular signal transduction, and the responses of animals, including humans, to the drug are

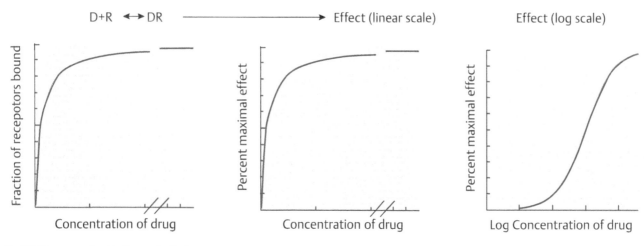

Fig. 2.9 Drug–receptor binding and effect.
Increasing the concentration of drug D increases the fraction of receptors to which the drug will bind DR (*left panel*) and the effect of the drug (*center panel*). In both of these panels, concentration of drug is plotted on a linear scale, leading to hyperbolic curves. On these graphs, it is difficult to see the rapid changes occurring at low concentrations of drug while there is little change in the curve at high concentrations. If the concentration of drug is plotted on a logarithmic scale, the concentration–effect curve becomes sigmoidal (S-shaped). With this curve, it is easier to ascertain threshold and maximal concentrations of the drug.

Table 2.1 Types of receptors

Type of receptor	Examples
Ligand-gated ion channels	Nicotinic receptors (bind ACh); glutamate receptor; GABA$_A$ receptor
G protein-coupled receptor	Muscarinic receptors (bind ACh)
Voltage-dependent ion channels	Ca^{2+} channels on cardiac or smooth muscle
Enzyme-linked membrane receptor	Tyrosine kinase receptor (binds insulin)
Intracellular receptors	Steroid hormones; thyroid hormone (thyroxine)

Abbreviations: GABA$_A$, gamma-aminobutyric acid, type A; ACh, acetylcholine.

important for understanding the mechanism of action of a drug and its clinical effectiveness at various doses.

2.3.1 Drug Binding to Receptor

Drug–receptor binding and effect resemble enzyme–substrate interactions and can be modeled similarly.

$$D + R \leftrightharpoons DR \rightarrow Effect(D = drug; R = receptor)$$

The drug is analogous to the substrate, with the exception that it is not changed by the receptor. The reactions follow the law of mass action such that increasing [D] leads to an increase in [DR] and a greater effect (▶ Fig. 2.9). The ability of a drug to bind to its receptor is indicated by its equilibrium dissociation constant, or K_d, the concentration of drug at which 50% of receptors are occupied. The lower the concentration required to bind to half of the receptors, the higher the drug's affinity for that receptor. Thus, affinity is inversely proportional to the K_d (affinity $\propto 1/K_d$). High affinity compounds typically have K_d's in the low nM or pM range.

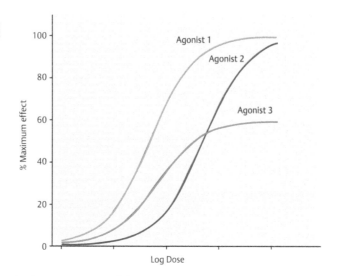

Fig. 2.10 Comparison of dose–response curves for agonists with different potencies and efficacies.
Agonists 1 and 2 have the same efficacy (100%) while agonist 3 has lower efficacy (60%). In terms of potency, agonist 1 is more potent than agonist 2 because it takes less drug to reach the same percentage effect, although at higher concentrations agonist 2 can reach the same level of effect. For low percentage effects, for example, 20% of maximum, agonist 3 is more potent than agonist 2 while at about 55% of maximum agonist 2 and agonist 3 are equipotent (where the lines cross). At high percentage effects, the potencies of agonists 2 and 3 cannot be compared because agonist 3 does not reach those effect levels even at high doses.

Responses to drugs may be graded (response magnitude is on a continuous scale) or quantal (response is all or none). Graded concentration–response curves are most commonly used in preclinical studies to assess the cellular and molecular actions of a drug (▶ Fig. 2.10). Quantal dose–response curves are most commonly used to measure the effects of drugs on a population of individuals (▶ Fig. 2.11).

2.4 Drug Classification Based on Receptor Interactions

2.4.1 Agonists

Agonists bind to a receptor and produce an effect. Agonist binding causes a change in receptor conformation that leads to a cellular response. The magnitude of the response for any given concentration of drug is determined by its **efficacy**, which is the maximum effect a given drug can produce, and by its **affinity**, which is the propensity of a drug to bind to a receptor, measured as the K_d (see above) (▶ Fig. 2.10).

- **Full agonists** are drugs of high intrinsic efficacy (100% efficacy).

- **Partial agonists** are drugs with efficacy lower than full agonists (< 100% efficacy).
- Tissue factors (receptor number and/or receptor coupling to transduction mechanisms) may cause markedly different relative responses for the same partial agonist when applied to different tissues. Increased receptor numbers in a tissue or more effective receptor coupling will lead to larger responses.
- Partial agonists may antagonize the effects of full agonists at sufficient concentrations and may have greater affinity than full agonists for the same receptor.

2.4.2 Antagonists

Antagonists bind to a receptor, usually with high affinity, but they do not produce a cellular response (they lack efficacy). Antagonists occupy the receptor and block the effects of agonists. When given simultaneously with agonists, **competitive antagonists** will compete with the agonist for binding to the receptor (▶ Fig. 2.12). The respective affinities and concentrations of the two drugs will determine the degree of antagonism produced.

Noncompetitive antagonists either prevent the agonist from binding to the receptor or prevent the agonist from activating the receptor. This antagonism cannot be overcome by increasing the agonist concentration.

▶ Fig. 2.13 compares the effects of competitive and noncompetitive antagonists on dose–response curves.

Other modes of antagonism are:
- **Chemical antagonists** are drugs that inhibit the effects of other compounds by a direct chemical interaction. For example, protamine is a highly basic peptide heparin antagonist. It binds to heparin, forming an inactive salt and thus inhibits the anticoagulant activity.
- **Physiological antagonism** occurs when two drugs act by different mechanisms to produce opposite physiological effects. This is most commonly observed in the opposing actions on smooth and cardiac muscle of the sympathetic and parasympathetic divisions of the autonomic nervous system (see Section II).

2.4.3 Inverse Agonists

These are drugs that cause an effect opposite to that of conventional agonists (▶ Fig. 2.14). The receptor must have a basal

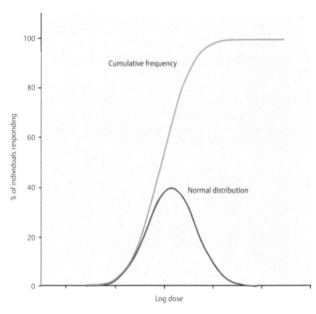

Fig. 2.11 Quantal dose–response relationships.
Quantal dose–response curves are constructed by measuring a defined response in a population of subjects. The response could be a therapeutic response, a toxic effect, or a side effect (see ▶ Fig. 2.16). Each subject is given a single dose and whether or not the subject responds at that dose is recorded. Typically, a plot of the number of individuals responding versus log dose gives a bell-shaped curve (normal distribution). If the cumulative frequency, i.e., the number of individuals responding at or below a given dose, is plotted, a sigmoidal curve is obtained.

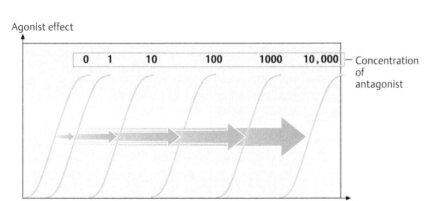

Fig. 2.12 Competitive antagonism.
Agonists and competitive antagonists compete for binding to the same receptor. Their affinities for the receptor and their concentrations will determine which one predominates; therefore, an increase in agonist concentration can overcome the blockage of the competitive antagonist and allow it to reach its maximal effect.

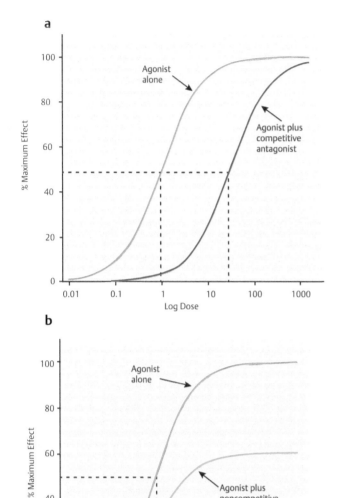

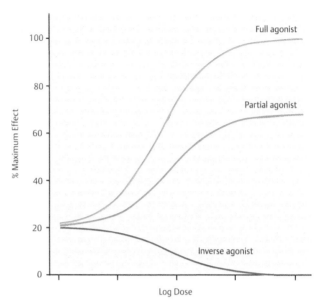

Fig. 2.14 Dose–response curves for a full agonist, partial agonist, and inverse agonist.
Full agonists have high intrinsic efficacy (can produce a 100% effect). Partial agonists are drugs with efficacy lower than full agonists (<100% effect). Inverse agonists are drugs that cause an effect opposite that of conventional agonists. The receptor must have a basal level of spontaneous activity in order for the effect of an inverse agonist to be observed.

Fig. 2.13 Comparison of competitive and noncompetitive antagonism.
To obtain the data for these curves, a dose–response curve for an agonist was constructed. The experiment was then repeated in the presence of a fixed concentration of an antagonist.
(**a**) The competitive antagonist shifts the dose–response curve for the agonist to the right and this can be overcome by increasing the concentration of agonist (i.e., it is surmountable). (**b**) A noncompetitive antagonist does not shift the dose–response curve but decreases the effectiveness of the agonist. This usually occurs because the binding of the antagonist is irreversible or at least takes a long time to reverse (pseudoirreversible), and is therefore insurmountable.

level of spontaneous activity in order for the effect of an inverse agonist to be observed.

2.4.4 Allosteric Effects

The classifications discussed above relate to the actions of agonists and antagonists binding to the same receptor site. Drugs

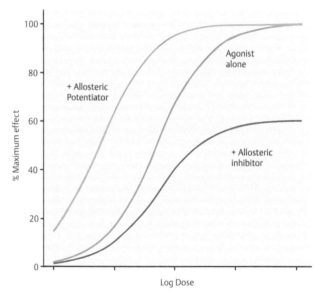

Fig. 2.15 Dose–response curves for an agonist alone and in the presence of an allosteric potentiator and an allosteric inhibitor.
Allosteric modulators are drugs that bind at a different site on the receptor molecule than the normal activator of the receptor. An allosteric potentiator will shift the dose–response curve to the right, while an allosteric inhibitor will produce a downward shift in the dose–response curve, as seen with noncompetitive antagonists.

may also alter receptor signaling by binding at alternative sites on the receptor protein to produce allosteric effects. Both allosteric inhibitors and allosteric potentiators are known to exist (▶ Fig. 2.15).

23

2.4.5 Receptor Regulation

In addition to eliciting a cellular response, receptor activation can also lead to changes in the number and/or sensitivity of receptors. Such changes are more commonly observed after repeated or prolonged applications of drugs and include **desensitization, resensitization, downregulation,** and **upregulation**. Desensitization occurs when the response to a drug decreases due to continuous or repeated exposure to that drug. Resensitization occurs when the responsiveness returns. Desensitization can follow receptor phosphorylation or agonist-induced conformational changes leading to a receptor that is either uncoupled from cellular signaling or unable to be activated. Reversal of these processes leads to resensitization. Desensitization and resensitization can occur within seconds to minutes of drug exposure. Longer-term exposures may lead to receptor downregulation that consists of endocytosis, internalization and lysosomal breakdown of receptors, and decreasing the number of receptors on the cell membrane. Desensitization and downregulation typically occur in response to agonists.

Prolonged exposure of a receptor to an antagonist drug can lead to increased cellular expression of that receptor, a process known as upregulation.

There are several clinical correlates of receptor regulation processes. Tachyphylaxis is a rapid, usually acutely observed, decrease in the response to a drug that may correlate to rapid receptor desensitization. Tolerance is a decreased responsiveness to drug that occurs over a longer time course and may include both desensitization and downregulation components. Upregulation is more commonly associated with drug side effects. For example, receptor upregulation in response to D2-antagonist antipsychotics can lead to abnormal movement disorders.

2.4.6 Signal Amplification

Amplification can occur between ligand binding to a receptor and the ultimate cellular response. For example, one agonist-activated GPCR can activate many G proteins, which in turn can activate many adenylate cyclase molecules that will produce multiple cAMP molecules that, further, will activate protein kinase A. Signaling cascades like this can lead to large responses with activation of a relatively small proportion of receptors.

2.4.7 Potency

Potency refers to the amount of drug required to produce an effect of a given intensity. It is convenient to set this intensity value at median effective dose (ED_{50}) that corresponds to 50% of the maximal response. The higher the potency of a drug, the lower the concentration needed to reach ED_{50}. A drug that is more potent in producing a therapeutic effect is usually also more potent in producing adverse effects and toxicities. Therefore, a more potent drug is not necessarily a better drug.

2.4.8 Therapeutic Index

The therapeutic index is a means of comparing the amount of a drug required to attain the therapeutic level in 50% of patients to the amount that is lethal to 50% of patients (▶ Fig. 2.16). It is expressed as the ratio LD_{50}/ED_{50}. A high therapeutic index is preferable, as the margin of safety between the dose that would be sufficient to achieve therapeutic levels and the dose that would produce toxic effects is high.

2.4.9 Certain Safety Factor

The certain safety factor is defined as the ratio $LD_1:ED_{99}$ (i.e., the amount that would be lethal to just 1% of patients compared with the amount that would elicit a therapeutic effect in 99% of patients). It is another estimate of risk that indicates the degree of overlap of the lethal and therapeutic effect curves.

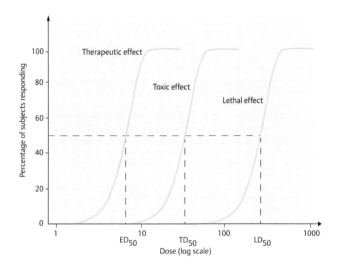

Fig. 2.16 Safety of a drug as determined by quantal dose–response curves.
This graph illustrates the ED_{50}, which is the dose that provides a therapeutic effect (e.g., vasodilation) in 50% of patients; the TD_{50}, which is the dose producing a toxic effect in 50% of patients (e.g., arrhythmia); and the LD_{50}, which is the lethal dose in 50% of patients.

3 Pharmacogenetics, Drug Development, and Special Populations

Summary

The pharmacokinetics and pharmacodynamics of a drug may be affected by genetic conditions, age-related conditions, and pregnancy, altering drug effects and influencing drug choice and dosing regimens. *Pharmacogenetics* is concerned with hereditary differences that contribute to variations in responses to drugs. *Pharmacogenomics* is a related but broader term concerned with how all of the genes in the genome influence responses to drugs. Application of the knowledge of a patient's genome to tailor a therapy is termed *personalized medicine*. There are four phases of clinical trials required for the marketing of new drugs, phase I–phase IV. To appropriately treat the pediatric patient, the clinician must appreciate that children differ physiologically and psychologically from adults. In addition to the physiological changes that occur as a person ages, chronic diseases are more common. The use of multiple drugs, or *polypharmacy*, is also more common in this population. Polypharmacy can increase the chance of adverse reactions and drug interactions, leading to morbidity and mortality. It has also been shown to decrease compliance. During pregnancy, any drug given to the mother that crosses the blood-brain barrier will also cross the placenta and exert an effect on the unborn child. Some of these effects can be predicted from our understanding of the pharmacokinetics of the drug given, but others cannot. The clinician should assess the risks to the unborn child of a drug for use during pregnancy. The physiology of a neonate (child younger than 30 days old) is markedly different from older children and adults. Low-molecular-weight, non-ionized, non-protein-bound drugs passively diffuse into breast cells and may be ingested by the neonate via breast milk.

Keywords: pharmacogenomics, target, pediatric, elderly, pregnancy, breastfeeding

3.1 Pharmacokinetics and Pharmacodynamics

The pharmacokinetics and pharmacodynamics of a drug may be affected by genetic conditions, age-related conditions, and pregnancy. Such conditions alter the drug effects and influence drug choice and dosing regimens.

3.2 Pharmacogenetics

Pharmacogenetics is concerned with hereditary differences that contribute to variations in responses to drugs. **Pharmacogenomics** is a related but broader term concerned with how all of the genes in the genome influence responses to drugs. Application of the knowledge of a patient's genome to tailor a therapy is termed **personalized medicine**. Although pharmacogenetic disorders are inherited, they may not be recognized until the individual is challenged with a drug and exhibits an abnormal response (▸ Fig. 3.1). Some common examples of pharmacogenetic disorders are listed in ▸ Table 3.1.

3.3 Drug Development Process

Modern drug discovery efforts usually arise from basic biomedical research findings related to diseases and their mechanisms.

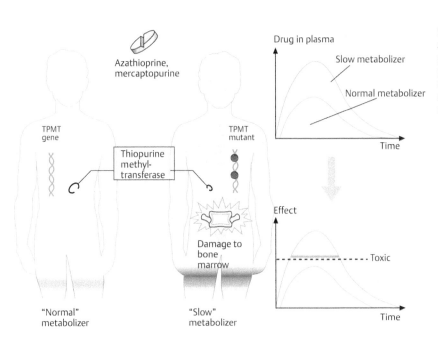

Fig. 3.1 Genetic variants in pharmacokinetics. Azathioprine and mercaptopurine (immunosuppressant drugs) are metabolized more slowly in people with a genetic disorder affecting the enzyme thiopurine methyltransferase (TPMT). This causes toxic plasma drug levels to accumulate, resulting in damage to bone marrow.

Table 3.1 Pharmacogenetic disorders

Disorder	Cause
Abnormally low amounts of enzymes or defective proteins	
Succinylcholine apnea	Caused by an atypical plasma cholinesterase, resulting in prolonged muscle relaxation and apnea after administration of succinylcholine
Acetylation polymorphism	Rapid and slow acetylators differ by a single autosomal gene. Slow acetylation is a recessive trait. The phenotype determines the rate of N-acetylation of drugs such as isoniazid and sulfonamides Drug-induced lupus erythematosus is more common in slow acetylators following exposure to hydralazine and procainamide due to their slow metabolism
Hemolytic anemia	Glucose-6-phosphate dehydrogenase deficiency, an X-linked defect, may result in hemolytic anemia after exposure to primaquine and certain other oxidizing drugs
Abnormalities in cytochrome P-450	Debrisoquine-4-hydroxylase deficiency was one of the first adverse effects attributed to low levels of a form of cytochrome P-450 (CYP 2D6), which metabolizes many drugs
Increased resistance to drugs	
Heritable insensitivity to warfarin anticoagulants	This condition is probably related to abnormal proteins which synthesize vitamin K-dependent clotting factors. Affinity is decreased for warfarin, but not for vitamin K
Responses indirectly related to drug metabolism	
Induction of drug-metabolizing enzymes	This increases heme biosynthesis through increased activity of aminolevulinic acid synthetase. This may result in various types of porphyria in people who are slow to metabolize heme precursors

Such research reveals specific steps in disease processes to which potential therapeutics can be targeted (▶ Fig. 3.2). This leads to the initial step in the drug discovery process, which is termed as **target identification and validation**. The target is whatever the drug is designed to bind to (i.e., the receptor that is targeted by the drug). The next step is to identify compounds that will interact with the target through screening. Screening involves the synthesis of a large number of compounds that are tested to see which of them bind to the target. Off-target binding of a drug frequently leads to side or toxic effects. This is called lack of selectivity. **Selectivity** is the ability of a drug to bind to the desired target molecule but not to other molecules. A drug is said to be **specific** if it has high selectivity (specificity is the ultimate of selectivity). A compound that is found through screening to bind to a target is called a **hit**. Hits are then typically tested further in binding assays to assess their affinity for the target and in cellular or subcellular screening assays for biological activity. These studies are accompanied by computer modeling of hit and target structures and predicted binding properties known as in silico studies. Screening may be repeated in an iterative manner to further refine structures of interest or **leads**. The next step is **lead optimization** through which the chemical structure of the drug is further improved. The pharmacological properties and toxicology of the leads are studied in a battery of preclinical studies. The two most important features required for a lead to proceed to clinical development are safety (lack of toxicity) and effectiveness in nonhuman disease models. Only a few compounds will make it through this final stage of discovery and will be slated for clinical development which involves giving the drugs to humans.

There are four phases of clinical trials required for the marketing of new drugs. Phase I studies are "first in man" studies in 10 to 100 patients to test the safety and tolerability of the drug. Pharmacokinetics will also be measured to determine dosing for further studies. Phase I trials are usually done with healthy volunteers, although in cases of rare or serious disease these may also be done in patients.

Phase II is usually the "first in patient" trial designed to test the effectiveness of the drug in 50 to 500 diseased patients and, thus, provide "proof of concept" that the chosen therapeutic approach is valid. These studies are designed to show what the potential product does and study dose ranges.

Drugs that show promise in phase II will proceed to phase III which will test the drug in hundreds to thousands of patients in randomized, well-controlled trials that compare a drug with either a placebo or another treatment. Phase IV studies are the postmarketing studies during which the safety of the drug is monitored.

Foundations

Glucose-6-phosphate Dehydrogenase

Glucose-6-phosphate dehydrogenase catalyzes the conversion of glucose to ribose 5-phosphate in the pentose phosphate pathway. Nicotinamide adenine dinucleotide phosphate (NADPH) and H^+ are also produced. Ribose 5-phosphate is a precursor of nucleotide biosynthesis, and NADPH is involved in the biosynthesis of fatty acids and in protecting cells from oxidative damage.

3.4 The Pediatric Patient

Children are not just small adults. To appropriately treat the pediatric patient, the clinician must appreciate that children differ physiologically and psychologically from adults. When prescribing drugs for children, the following factors should be kept in mind:
- A "child" usually refers to someone 12 years of age or under.
- Dosages of drugs for children are usually expressed per kilogram of body weight to account for age and weight differences.
- If possible, painful intramuscular injections should be avoided.

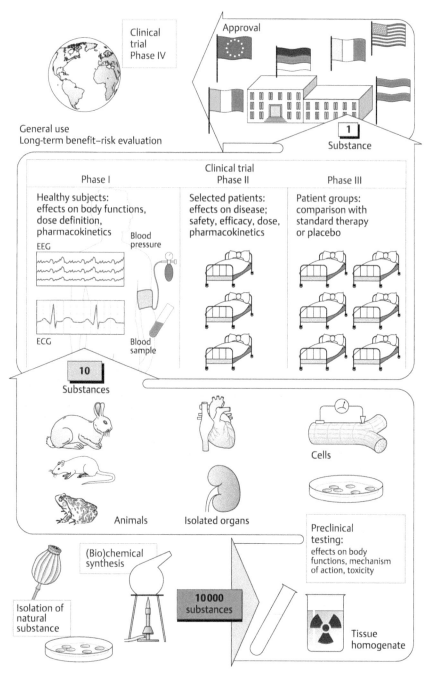

Fig. 3.2 Steps in drug discovery and development.

Clinical trial Phase IV

Approval

General use
Long-term benefit–risk evaluation

1
Substance

Clinical trial

Phase I | Phase II | Phase III

Healthy subjects: effects on body functions, dose definition, pharmacokinetics

EEG

ECG

Blood pressure

Blood sample

Selected patients: effects on disease; safety, efficacy, dose, pharmacokinetics

Patient groups: comparison with standard therapy or placebo

10
Substances

Cells

Animals

Isolated organs

Preclinical testing:
effects on body functions, mechanism of action, toxicity

(Bio)chemical synthesis

Isolation of natural substance

10 000
substances

Tissue homogenate

Clinical Correlation

Porphyria

Porphyrias are a rare group of diseases in which there are errors in the pathway of heme biosynthesis. This causes the precursors of heme, porphyrins, to build up in the body. Porphyrias primarily affect the nervous system (acute porphyria) and skin (cutaneous porphyria). Symptoms of acute porphyria include colicky abdominal pain with vomiting or constipation, peripheral neuritis (especially motor), seizures, and mental disturbances, such as psychosis, depression, and anxiety. Skin manifestations include itching, blistering, erythema (redness of the skin), and skin edema. Treatment for both types of porphyria involves avoiding/treating precipitating factors. Acute porphyria may also require the administration of pain medication, intravenous (IV) fluids to correct electrolyte imbalances and treat dehydration, and the IV injection of hemin or hematin (heme arginate), which are forms of heme. Cutaneous porphyria may require repeated blood draws to reduce the iron content of the body which reduces porphyrins, activated charcoal to absorb excess porphyrins and facilitate faster excretion, and beta carotene (a vitamin A precursor) to promote healthy skin.

Drug-induced Lupus Erythematosus

Drug-induced lupus erythematosus (DIL) is an autoimmune disease caused by the chronic use of certain drugs, most commonly hydralazine (an antihypertensive drug), procainamide (an anticonvulsant drug), and isoniazid (an antibiotic). DIL is thought to be caused by slow acetylation of the drug by a portion of the population. Symptoms are similar to those caused by systemic lupus erythematosus (SLE), the more common and more serious form of lupus. These include joint pain (arthralgia), swelling, and stiffness; muscle pain (myalgia), fatigue, pericarditis (inflammation of the pericardium surrounding the heart), and pleuritis (inflammation of the pleura surrounding the lungs). Treatment involves discontinuing the causal drug, nonsteroidal anti-inflammatory drugs (NSAIDs) to treat pain and inflammation, and corticosteroids to treat inflammation.

3.5 The Elderly Patient

In addition to the physiological changes that occur as a person ages, chronic diseases are more common. The use of multiple drugs, or **polypharmacy**, is also more common in this population. Polypharmacy can increase the chance of adverse reactions and drug interactions that may lead to morbidity and mortality. It has also been shown to decrease compliance.

When prescribing drugs for the elderly, factors mentioned in subsequent text should be kept in mind.

1. **Minimize polypharmacy.**
   - Avoid excessive or inappropriate consumption of drugs but do prescribe adequately when necessary.
   - Review and simplify drug regimens periodically.
2. **Consider the form of the drug.**
   - Some elderly patients may have difficulty swallowing tablets, so prescribe liquid preparations when possible.
3. **Consider sensitivity.**
   - As we age, our target organs, especially the central nervous system, become more susceptible to drugs, so all drugs should be used with caution.
4. **Reduce the dose.**
   - It is prudent to assume at least mild renal impairment when prescribing for any elderly patient. Generally, the doses given should be lower than those for healthy adults.
   - Dose reduction should be proportional to creatinine clearance in more severe cases.
   - Drugs with long half-lives should be avoided.

Acute illness may lead to a rapid decline in renal function, especially if coupled with dehydration. This is particularly relevant when prescribing drugs with a narrow therapeutic index (e.g., digoxin, a cardiac glycoside used to treat heart failure).

3.6 The Pregnant Patient

During pregnancy, any drug given to the mother that crosses the blood–brain barrier will also cross the placenta and exert an effect on the unborn child. Some of these effects can be predicted from our understanding of the pharmacokinetics of the drug, but not all. The clinician should assess the risks of a drug to the unborn child during pregnancy.

When prescribing a drug for a pregnant patient, consider the following factors:

1. **Stage of development of the unborn child.**
   - A severe consequence of a drug given in the first trimester would be malformation of the unborn child, as this is the stage when organ development is occurring (▶ Fig. 3.3). After the first trimester, drugs may cause functional disturbances, as the child has formed but is growing and maturing. Drugs given at term or during labor may affect the neonate.
2. **Ability of the drug to pass through the placenta.**
   - The placental syncytiotrophoblast forms a diffusion barrier between the maternal circulation and the capillaries of the fetal umbilical cord (▶ Fig. 3.3). However, it is permeable to most drugs (especially low-molecular-weight, nonionized, nonprotein-bound drugs), so any systemically acting drug given to the mother during pregnancy can reach the fetus.
3. **Teratogenicity of the drug.**
   - Drugs that are known teratogenic agents are listed in any pharmacopeia and the clinician should become familiar with these. This will allow for an educated analysis of the risk of teratogenesis to be made. Unfortunately, the teratogenic potential of new drugs often cannot be established.
4. **The effect on the fetus of discontinuing the drug.**
   - The clinician must also consider the effect of discontinuing a drug on the unborn child (this may happen if the mother continues receiving the drug, but the child is born, thus severing its supply of the drug). The child may suffer from withdrawal effects and should be treated accordingly.

Physiological Changes in Pregnancy

Maternal physiology changes during pregnancy. In the cardiovascular system, blood volume increases (> 50% of prepregnancy levels), heart rate increases (10–15%), stroke volume increases (30%), cardiac output increases (up to 60%), and blood pressure (especially diastolic) drops in the first and second trimesters but rises to nonpregnant levels at term. In the respiratory system, ventilation increases (40%) and oxygen consumption increases (20%). In the kidneys, glomerular filtration increases (60%), renal plasma flow increases (50–70%), and there is glycosuria (as glucose reabsorption mechanisms become saturated). In the gastrointestinal tract, there is decreased esophageal tone, decreased gastric acid production, increased mucus production, and decreased gut motility. These physiological parameters return to normal after parturition.

I

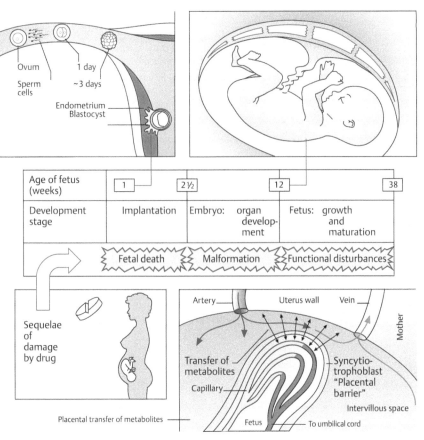

Fig. 3.3 Pregnancy: fetal damage due to drugs. The sequelae of a drug taken during pregnancy depends on the stage of fetal development and the ability of the drug to cross the placenta.

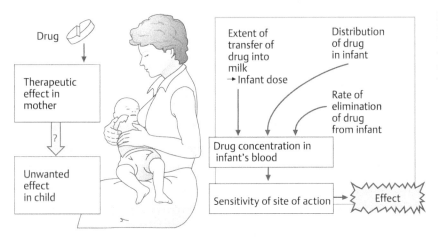

Fig. 3.4 Lactation: maternal intake of drugs. Drugs taken by a nursing mother can be secreted in breast milk and ingested by the baby. The effect that this has on the baby will depend on the extent of drug transfer into the milk (which determines the dose to the baby), and how the baby metabolizes and eliminates the drug.

Clinical Correlation

Physiology of Neonates

The physiology of neonates differs from that of older children and adults. Notably, neonates have immature active transport systems for organic anions and cations, an immature liver microsomal system for drug metabolism, a lower glomerular filtration rate, a reduced ability to glucuronidate phase 1 metabolism products causing delayed elimination of drugs, and a differing target organ sensitivity to drugs.

3.7 The Breastfeeding Child

The physiology of a neonate (child younger than 30 days old) is markedly different from older children and adults. Low-molecular-weight, nonionized, nonprotein-bound drugs passively diffuse into breast cells and may be ingested by the neonate via breast milk (▶ Fig. 3.4). A drug that is considered relatively safe during pregnancy due to its relative inability to cross the placenta may be more readily secreted into breast milk and is therefore not safe for the breastfeeding infant (e.g., chloramphenicol can accumulate to toxic levels in breastfeeding infants causing bone marrow suppression).

Unit I Review Questions

1. What is the term used to describe the fraction of a drug dose that reaches the systemic circulation?
   A. Plasma half-life.
   B. Bioavailability.
   C. Enterohepatic cycling.
   D. Biotransformation.
   E. Biliary excretion.

2. A new antiarrhythmic agent is given intravenously to a patient with premature ventricular contractions in a dose of 500 mg. The electrocardiogram (ECG) is monitored and blood samples are taken for analysis of plasma concentrations. The concentrations reported from the laboratory are given in the table below. The ECG tracing showed changes in myocardial conduction for 30 minutes after administration that were indicative of the toxic effect of the drug. The patient's premature ventricular contractions were not apparent on the ECG until 5 hours after the drug was given intravenously. The information from the drug company contains no data on the metabolism or renal clearance of the drug. The patient has no preexisting liver or kidney disease. What is the apparent volume of distribution (V_d) of the drug?
   A. 40 L.
   B. 100 L.
   C. 200 L.
   D. 400 L.

Time after administration (hours)	Concentration of free drug (µg/mL)
0.5	4.5
1	4.0
2	3.4
3	2.8
4	2.4
5	2.0
6	1.7
7	1.4
8	1.3

3. The patient in question 2 is sent home with an oral preparation of the drug. You have decided to maintain the average plasma concentration halfway between the toxic and minimal therapeutic plasma concentrations and give the drug every 8 hours. What would be the dose within 50 mg that the patient would take?
   A. 100 mg.
   B. 200 mg.
   C. 350 mg.
   D. 800 mg.
   E. 1 g.

4. A patient who has been taking secobarbital (a barbiturate that induces the liver microsomal enzyme system) for several weeks is stabilized on warfarin (an oral anticoagulant that is inactivated by side-chain hydroxylation). The patient then discontinues the secobarbital but continues to take the warfarin. How should the patient's warfarin dose be changed?
   A. The dose should be increased.
   B. The dose should be decreased.
   C. The dose should not be changed.

5. For a drug that is eliminated by a first-order process, which parameter is dependent upon the dose?
   A. Clearance.
   B. Elimination rate constant.
   C. Steady-state plasma concentration.
   D. Elimination half-life.
   E. Time required to reach steady-state plasma concentration.

6. A patient with seizures is started on phenytoin, 300 mg daily. Frequent plasma level monitoring is done as part of a clinical study. After 5 days, phenytoin concentration in plasma is stabilized below the desired range, and the patient still has seizures. The dose is increased to 450 mg daily. It now takes 9 days for plasma levels to stabilize, and although seizures are controlled, the drug concentration in plasma is higher than predicted and the patient shows signs of phenytoin toxicity. Which one of the following is the most likely explanation for the higher-than-predicted drug concentration?
   A. The enzymes that hydroxylate phenytoin are saturated, so its biotransformation is no longer a first-order process.
   B. There is accumulation of an active metabolite.
   C. Phenytoin is not very water soluble, so its distribution becomes limited at higher plasma concentrations.
   D. Phenytoin has induced the cytochrome P-450 enzymes, increasing its own biotransformation.
   E. The patient has a genetic inability to parahydroxylated phenytoin.

7. The total body clearance of theophylline in an adult weighing 70 kg is 48 mL/min. If theophylline is administered by continuous intravenous (IV) infusion at a rate of 60 mg/hour, what will be the approximate steady-state plasma concentration (C_{ss})?
   A. 1 mg/dL.
   B. 2 mg/dL.
   C. 5 mg/dL.
   D. 10 mg/dL.
   E. 20 mg/dL.

8. A 53-year-old man has swollen ankles, shortness of breath, and fatigue upon mild exercise. He is observed to have severe pitting edema of the lower extremities, distended neck veins with prominent pulsation, a sinus tachycardia of 105 beats/min at rest, and a normal blood pressure. He is diagnosed as being in congestive heart failure. It is noted, however, that his renal function is relatively normal (creatinine clearance = 115 mL/minute). If treatment is begun with oral digoxin ($t_{1/2}$ = 36 hours) with a usual daily maintenance dose of 0.125 mg, how long should you wait before increasing the dose in case his initial response appears inadequate?
   A. Approximately 2 hours.
   B. Approximately 1 day.

C. Approximately 2 days.
D. Approximately 1 week.

9. A patient with impaired renal function (creatinine clearance = 40 mL/minute) is being treated for a urinary tract infection with a cephalosporin antibiotic. The drug is normally excreted unchanged by the kidneys with a clearance rate approximately equal to creatinine clearance (120 mL/min). The typical oral dose of the drug is 240 mg every 6 hours. Which of the following dosing regimens would be appropriate for this patient to achieve the same drug level as a patient with normal renal function?
A. 80 mg every 18 hours.
B. 120 mg every 6 hours.
C. 240 mg every 12 hours.
D. 80 mg every 6 hours.
E. 240 mg once a day.

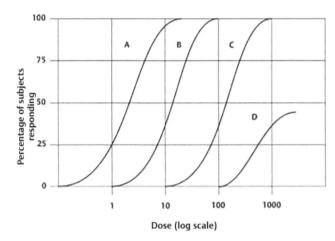

Dose (log scale)

10. Which one of the following statements is true concerning the dose–response curves in the graph?
A. Curves A, B, and C represent responses to weak agonists, with C being the most potent.
B. Curve A represents the responses to a full agonist, and curves B and C represent the responses to the agonist in the presence of two concentrations of a competitive antagonist.
C. Curves A, B, and C show that the three drugs are acting at different receptors because their potencies are different.
D. Curve D shows the response to agonist A in the presence of a competitive inhibitor.
E. Curve D represents an agonist with a high intrinsic efficacy, as the dose needed for a given effect is larger than that of agonists A, B, or C.

11. Which of the following provides information about the sensitivity of a population to a drug?
A. Graded dose–response curve.
B. Quantal dose–response curve.
C. Therapeutic index.
D. Efficacy.

12. An experiment was performed to determine the median effective dose of a drug required to produce hypnosis in 50% of the population (ED$_{50}$) and the median lethal dose for 50%

of the population (LD$_{50}$) of a drug. The ED$_{50}$ was found to be 1 mg. The LD$_{50}$ was found to be 300 mg. What is the therapeutic index for this drug?
A. < 1.
B. 1.
C. 3.
D. 30.
E. 300.

The following table shows the drug dosages that produce a therapeutic effect (bronchodilation), a toxic effect (cardiac arrhythmia), and death in 1, 50, or 99% of patients. Use it to answer questions 13-16.

Percentage of patients showing effect	Dose causing bronchodilation (mg)	Dose causing cardiac arrhythmia (mg)	Dose causing death (mg)
1	1	200	2,000
50	15	750	6,000
99	200	900	9,000

13. What is the median effective dose for 50% of the population (ED$_{50}$)?
A. 1 mg.
B. 15 mg.
C. 200 mg.
D. 750 mg.
E. 6,000 mg.

14. What is the median lethal dose for 50% of the population (LD$_{50}$)?
A. 1 mg.
B. 15 mg.
C. 200 mg.
D. 750 mg.
E. 6,000 mg.

15. At a dose of 200 mg, what percentage of patients experienced an adverse effect?
A. 1%.
B. 10%.
C. 50%.
D. 75%.
E. 99%.

16. If a patient overdoses on 9 g of the drug, what is the probability that the patient will die?
A. 1%.
B. 10%.
C. 50%.
D. 75%.
E. 99%.

17. A patient with Lyme disease is to be treated with tetracycline (500 mg, taken orally twice daily). Tetracycline is normally well absorbed after oral administration. Absorption is decreased by calcium or other cations. The drug has a t$_{1/2}$ of 10 hours. A steady-state plasma concentration will be reached in about how many hours?
A. 10 hours.
B. 20 hours.

C. 40 hours.
D. 80 hours.

18. A patient with Lyme disease is to be treated with tetracycline (500 mg, taken orally twice daily). Tetracycline is normally well absorbed after oral administration. Absorption is decreased by calcium or other cations. The drug has a $t_{1/2}$ of 10 hours. If the patient takes the drug with a glass of milk, what will be the effect on the steady-state plasma concentration?
A. It will be increased.
B. It will be decreased.
C. It will be unchanged.
D. It will be reached more rapidly.
E. It will be reached more slowly.

19. A new antiarrhythmic agent is given intravenously to a patient with premature ventricular contractions in a dose of 500 mg. The electrocardiogram (ECG) is monitored, and blood samples are taken for analysis of plasma concentrations. The following concentrations were reported from the laboratory (see table below). The ECG tracing showed changes in myocardial conduction for 30 minutes after administration that were indicative of the toxic effect of the drug. The patient's premature ventricular contractions were not apparent on the ECG until 5 hours after the drug was given intravenously. The information from the drug company contains no data on the metabolism or renal clearance of the drug. The patient has no preexisting liver or kidney disease. The patient is sent home with an oral preparation of the drug. You have decided to maintain the average plasma concentration halfway between the toxic and minimal therapeutic plasma concentrations and to give the drug every 8 hours. What would be the dose within 50 mg that the patient would take?

Time after Administration (hours)	Concentration of Free Drug (µg/mL)
0.5	4.5
1	4.0
2	3.4
3	2.8
4	2.4
5	2.0
6	1.7
7	1.4
8	1.3

A. 100 mg.
B. 200 mg.
C. 350 mg.
D. 800 mg.
E. 1 g.

20. Your patient is receiving a new antiarrhythmic agent ($t_{1/2}$ = 12 hours) that needs to be dosed to achieve plasma concentrations of 2 to 6 mg/L. At the most recent office visit, the concentration is 1.2 mg/L. A dosage adjustment is made, and the patient is scheduled to have a follow-up concentration checked. How soon will steady state be achieved so that the new plasma concentration can be checked?

A. 2 days.
B. 7 days.
C. 2 weeks.
D. 6 weeks.
E. 6 months.

21. A young child has been brought to the emergency room with an apparent overdose of the weak acid acetylsalicylic acid (aspirin). What would be an effective method of enhancing the elimination of this toxin?
A. Acidify the urine.
B. Administer an anticholinergic agent to retard the movement of acetylsalicylic acid from the stomach.
C. Nothing can be done to enhance the drug's elimination.
D. Lower the blood pH to 6.0.
E. Alkalinize the urine.

22. What is the term used to describe the continuous passage of a drug between the gastrointestinal tract and the liver?
A. Plasma half-life.
B. Bioavailability.
C. Enterohepatic cycling.
D. Biotransformation.
E. Biliary excretion.

23. The major site at which drugs that are weak bases are absorbed following oral ingestion is the
A. Esophagus.
B. Stomach.
C. Small intestine.
D. Large intestine.
E. Rectum.

24. A drug has an elimination rate constant of 0.175 hour^{-1}. It is administered every 60 minutes. About how long will it take to achieve a steady-state concentration?
A. 0.87 hour.
B. 3 to 5 hours.
C. 16 to 20 hours.
D. 35 to 40 hours.

25. Zero-order kinetics of drug metabolism is
A. A fixed rate of metabolism.
B. Proportional to the amount of drug in plasma.
C. Nonsaturable.
D. Defined by the half-life of elimination.
E. A constant percent of metabolism per unit of time.

26. The affinity of a drug for its receptor indicates
A. Whether the drug is an agonist or antagonist.
B. The concentration of the drug necessary to produce a half-maximal response.
C. How tightly the drug is bound to the receptor.
D. Whether the drug will be useful clinically or not.
E. How likely the drug is to produce side effects.

27. The efficacy of a drug is
A. What percentage of patients will experience an effect with this drug.
B. How well the drug activates (stimulates) the receptor to which it is bound.
C. Whether or not the drug is effective in treating a particular disease.

D. Whether or not the drug is safe to use for a particular patient.

E. The dose of the drug necessary to treat the patient.

28. A partial agonist
   A. Has lower affinity than a full agonist.
   B. Has higher efficacy than a full agonist.
   C. Has a lower efficacy than a full agonist.
   D. Has higher affinity than a full agonist.

29. A competitive antagonist
   A. Binds to the same receptor site as does the agonist.
   B. Increases the metabolism of an agonist.
   C. Binds to a different receptor than the agonist.
   D. Is irreversible.

30. Binding of a drug to plasma proteins will tend to
   A. Decrease its half-life.
   B. Decrease its rate of glomerular filtration.
   C. Increase its rate of biotransformation.
   D. Increase its free concentration in the plasma.

31. Plasma is a major site for which biotransformation?
   A. Glucuronidation.
   B. Sulfation.
   C. Acetylation.
   D. Cytochrome P-450 oxidation.
   E. Ester hydrolysis.

32. A ligand that binds to constitutively active receptors and reduces the fraction of them in the active conformation is called a/an
   A. Antagonist.
   B. Full agonist.
   C. Inverse agonist.
   D. Partial agonist.
   E. Potentiator.

33. A macromolecule on or within a cell to which a drug binds to produce an effect is called a/an
   A. Effector.
   B. Hit.
   C. Ligand.
   D. Receptor.
   E. Transducer.

34. Referring to the attached figure, which drug has the lowest efficacy?

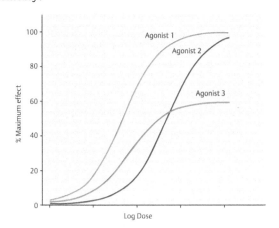

A. Agonist 1.
B. Agonist 2.
C. Agonist 3.

35. Using the data shown on the attached figure, indicate which of the following values corresponds to the ED_{50} for the agonist drug.

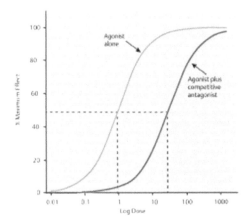

A. 0.1.
B. 1.
C. 10.
D. 100.
E. 1000.

36. The graph in the attached figure shows the effect of an agonist drug alone (curve labeled "0") and in the presence of increasing concentrations of another drug, (curves labeled "1," "10," "100," "1000," and "10,000"). Based on these data, one could conclude that the second drug is a/an

Agonist effect

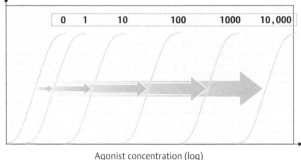

Agonist concentration (log)

A. Allosteric inhibitor.
B. Competitive antagonist.
C. Full agonist.
D. Inverse agonist.
E. Noncompetitive antagonist.

37. The attached graph shows the effect of Drug A alone and in the presence of another drug, A + B. Based on these data, one could conclude that Drug B is most likely a/an

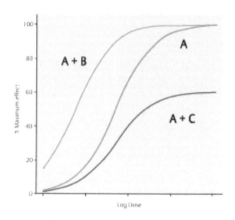

A. Allosteric inhibitor.
B. Allosteric potentiator.
C. Inverse agonist.
D. Noncompetitive antagonist.
E. Partial antagonist.

38. The attached graph shows concentration-response curves for three drugs, Agonist 1, Agonist 2, and Agonist 3, each given alone. Agonist 3 would best be characterized as which of the following?

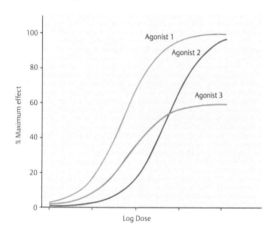

A. Allosteric inhibitor.
B. Noncompetitive inhibitor.
C. Antagonist.
D. Partial agonist.
E. Competitive inhibitor.

39. What percentage of receptors are occupied when the concentration of a drug is equal to the K_d?
   A. 1.
   B. 10.
   C. 50.
   D. 99.
   E. 100.

40. Etanercept binds to tumor necrosis factor-alpha and prevents it from interacting with its receptors, which are cytokine receptors. How do cytokine receptors differ from ligand-regulated transmembrane enzymes such as receptor tyrosine kinases?
   A. Cytokine receptors possess an extracellular binding domain.
   B. Cytokine receptors possess a hydrophobic segment of the polypeptide that crosses the lipid bilayer of the plasma membrane.
   C. Cytokine receptor enzyme activity is not intrinsic to the receptor molecule.
   D. Cytokine receptors dimerize after they bind the activating ligand.
   E. The signal transduction pathway activated by cytokine receptors involves phosphorylation steps.

41. To produce their therapeutic effects, lipid soluble agents such as dexamethasone and estradiol bind to
   A. Intracellular receptors.
   B. Ion channels.
   C. mRNA.
   D. Receptors in adipose tissue.
   E. The extracellular face of plasma membrane receptors.

42. Procaine inhibits a sodium channel that is normally activated by depolarization of the neuronal membrane. The receptor for procaine is a/an
   A. Ligand-gated ion channel.
   B. Voltage-gated ion channel.
   C. G protein-coupled receptor.
   D. Transmembrane enzyme.
   E. Intracellular receptor in the cell nucleus.

43. Diazepam binds to the benzodiazepine receptor, a specific binding site on the gamma subunit of the $GABA_A$ receptor, and potentiates the inhibitory effects of the endogenous neurotransmitter GABA (gamma amino butyric acid). The GABA binding site is on the alpha subunit of the $GABA_A$ receptor. Diazepam acts as a/an
   A. Allosteric potentiator.
   B. Competitive inhibitor.
   C. Direct channel opener.
   D. Insurmountable agonist.
   E. Noncompetitive inhibitor.

44. The ability of a ligand to bind to the desired target but not to other molecules is termed
   A. Selectivity.
   B. Efficacy.
   C. Throughput.
   D. Antagonism.
   E. Potency.

Unit I Answers and Explanations

1. B. Bioavailability is the fraction of the administered dose of a drug that reaches the systemic circulation in an unchanged form.

A. Plasma half-life is the time it takes for the drug level in the blood to decrease from its peak to one half of its peak.

C. Enterohepatic cycling occurs when conjugated drugs (mainly glucuronic acid derivatives) are actively secreted into bile, and unconjugated drugs are liberated in the small intestine by bacterial enzyme hydrolysis and reabsorbed into the portal circulation.

D. Biotransformation is the process by which drugs are metabolized to (usually) less active forms for excretion.

E. Biliary excretion occurs when drugs are delivered to the bile and then excreted.

2. B. V_d = dose (mg)/plasma concentration (mg/L) = 500 mg/4.5 mg/L ≈ 100 L.

3. C. Toxic effects were observed at 0.5 hour, when the plasma concentration was 4.5 µg/mL, and a therapeutic effect lasted until 4 hours, at which time the level was 2.4 µg/mL. Halfway between these two is ~3.5 µg/mL. The apparent volume of distribution of the drug was calculated from the initial dose given intravenously and its plasma concentration after 30 minutes as follows: V_d = dose (mg)/plasma concentration (mg/L) = 500 mg/4.5 mg/L ≈ 100 L. The amount of drug (taken orally) needed to achieve a desired plasma concentration by rearrangement of this equation is Dose = plasma concentration (mg/L) × V_d (L) = 3.5 mg/L × 100 L = 350 mg.

4. B. Induction of liver microsomal enzymes by secobarbital increases the metabolism of warfarin. Discontinuation of the secobarbital will lead to decreased microsomal enzyme activity, lower metabolism of warfarin, increased warfarin levels, and increased anticoagulant activity. Thus, the patient's dosage will have to be decreased to maintain the same degree of anticoagulant activity.

5. C. The only one of these that is dependent upon the dose is the steady-state plasma concentration, which equals $[F \times (D/T)]/CL$, where F is bioavailability, D is dose, T is dosing interval, and CL is clearance.

6. A. Zero-order kinetics of elimination usually occur because the route of elimination has become saturated. In this case, phenytoin originally exhibited first-order kinetics when the drug concentration was below the maximum rate of the elimination process. As elimination was saturated, the time to steady-state peak level, as well as the achievement of a higher than predicted drug level, was observed. Only answer **A** addresses these findings; none of the other answers can explain them.

7. B. For drugs that are given by continuous IV infusion, the equation for calculating C_{ss} is $C_{ss} = R_0/CL$, where R_0 is the infusion rate, and CL is clearance. C_{ss} = (60 mg/h)/(48 mL/min) = (1 mg/min)/(48 mL/min) = 0.02 mg/mL = 2 mg/dL.

8. D. The time to reach steady-state concentration (C_{ss}) is solely determined by the half-life ($t_{1/2}$). Because it takes roughly four half-lives for a drug to reach C_{ss}, for a drug with $t_{1/2}$ = 36 hours, 4 × 36 hours = 144 hours, or ~ 1 week, is required to reach C_{ss}. The C_{ss} coincides with the desired therapeutic concentration of a drug.

9. D. $C_{ss} = [F \times (D/T)]/CL$, where C_{ss} is the steady-state concentration, F is bioavailability, D is dose, T is dosing interval, and CL is clearance. Because clearance is decreased in this patient to approximately one-third of its normal value (= creatinine clearance), the maintenance dose must be decreased by one-third or the dose interval increased threefold to achieve the same steady-state drug concentration.

10. B. Because a competitive antagonist competes with the agonist for binding to the receptor, more of the agonist drug is required to elicit a given response in the presence of a competitive antagonist. This results in the dose–response curve being shifted to the right.

A. Curves A to C do not represent responses to a weak agonist because they all show 100% responses, which would not occur with a weak agonist. Also, C is the least potent, not the most potent.

C. Variations in potency do not indicate that different receptors are affected.

D. A competitive antagonist does not reduce the maximal response, instead increases the amount of agonist needed to obtain the same response.

E. Curve D, which does not reach a 100% response, represents a lower, not higher, efficacy for the agonist.

11. B. A quantal dose–response curve plots the proportion of a population that responds to different concentrations of a drug.

A. A graded dose–response curve plots the magnitude of a response as a function of the dose.

C. The therapeutic index is the ratio LD_{50}/ED_{50}, where LD_{50} is the drug dose that is lethal to 50% of the population and ED_{50} is the median effective dose for 50% of the population.

D. Efficacy is the maximum effect a given drug can produce.

12. E. The therapeutic index is the ratio LD_{50}/ED_{50}. In this example, the therapeutic index would be 300 (300/1), meaning that 300 times the median effective dose (ED_{50}) would need to be given to produce a lethal effect for 50% of the population.

13. B. The ED_{50} is the dose that causes bronchodilation, in this case, in 50% of patients. This is achieved with a dose of 15 mg.

14. E. The LD_{50} is 6,000 mg.

15. A. At a dose of 200 mg, only 1% of the patients experienced cardiac arrhythmia, the adverse effect.

16. E. At a dose of 9,000 mg (or 9 g), 99% of patients will die.

17. C. It takes approximately four half-lives to reach steady-state concentration (Css), or 4×10 hours = 40 hours.

18. B. Because absorption is decreased by calcium, the bioavailablity of the drug will be less if it is taken with milk. Steady-state concentration $(C_{ss}) = [F \times (D/T)] / CL$, where F is bioavailability, D is dose, T is dosing interval, and CL is clearance. Decreased bioavailability (F) will lead to decreased steady-state concentration (C_{ss}).

19. C. Toxic effects were observed at 0.5 hour, when the plasma concentration was 4.5 µg/mL, and a therapeutic effect lasted until 4 hours, at which time the level was 2.4 µg/mL. Halfway between these two is ~3.5 µg/mL. The apparent volume of distribution of the drug was calculated from the initial dose given intravenously and its plasma concentration after 30 minutes as follows: V_d = dose (mg)/plasma concentration (mg/L) = 500 mg/ 4.5 mg/L ≈ 100 L. The amount of drug (taken orally) needed to achieve a desired plasma concentration by rearrangement of this equation is: Dose = plasma concentration (mg/L) × V_d (L) = 3.5 mg/L × 100 L = 350 mg.

20. A. Because it takes roughly four half-lives for a drug to reach steady-state concentration (C_{ss}), for a drug with $t_{1/2}$ = 12 hours, 4×12 hours = 48 hours, or ~2 days to reach steady state.

21. E. To undergo renal elimination, aspirin must be filtered into the urine and must resist reabsorption back into plasma and reentry into the systemic circulation. Polar drugs are more readily filtered. Un-ionized drugs are able to diffuse passively back from urine into plasma, especially if they are lipid soluble and there is a favorable concentration gradient. Changes in urinary pH will affect reabsorption by altering the ionization of a drug. Making urine more alkaline by administering bicarbonate increases ionization of weak acids such as aspirin, slowing reabsorption and increasing elimination.

22. C. Drugs that are taken orally are absorbed in the gastrointestinal tract and enter the portal circulation to the liver. In the liver, drugs can be conjugated (usually by glucuronidation) and are actively secreted into bile. Bile is then secreted into the intestine where the drug may be reabsorbed into the portal circulation. Unconjugated drugs are liberated in the small intestine by bacterial enzyme hydrolysis and reabsorbed into the portal circulation. This is referred to as enterohepatic cycling.

A. Plasma half-life is the time it takes for the drug level in the blood to decrease from its peak to one-half of its peak.

B. Bioavailability is the fraction of the administered dose of a drug that reaches the systemic circulation in an unchanged form.

D. Biotransformation is the process by which drugs are metabolized to (usually) less active forms for excretion.

E. Biliary excretion occurs when drugs are delivered to the bile and then excreted.

23. C. Un-ionized drugs cross cell membranes more readily and are therefore absorbed more readily than ionized drugs. The fraction of drug in the un-ionized form depends on the pH of the environment. This can be determined using the Henderson-Hasselbach equation. Drugs that are weak bases do not exist primarily in their un-ionized form until they reach the duodenum, which is a basic environment.

A, D, and E. The esophagus, large intestine, and rectum have no role in drug absorption following oral administration.

B. At gastric pH, weak bases will tend to be ionized so little absorption occurs in the stomach. The stomach is the major site of absorption of weak acids since they will be un-ionized.

24. C. The time to reach steady-state concentration is solely determined by the half-life $(t_{1/2})$. Half-life $(t_{1/2})$ equals $0.693/K_e$, where K_e is the elimination rate constant. This, in turn, equals $0.693/(0.175 \text{ hour}^{-1}) \approx 4$ hours. It takes approximately four half-lives to reach steady-state concentration $(4 \times 4 \text{ hours} = 16 \text{ hours})$.

25. A. With zero-order kinetics, a constant amount of drug is eliminated per unit of time regardless of its concentration.

B-E. Metabolism that is proportional to the amount of drug in plasma is a first-order process. It is frequently the result of a saturable process and is not defined by the half-life of elimination. It is a fixed amount of drug metabolized per unit of time, not a constant percent of metabolism per unit of time.

26. C. Affinity is the propensity of a drug to bind to a receptor.

A. An agonist binds to a receptor with a given affinity causing a change in its conformation that ultimately leads to a cellular response. An antagonist binds to a receptor, often with high affinity, but does not produce a cellular response.

B. The concentration of a drug necessary to produce a half-maximal response (EC50) is a measure of relative potency.

27. B. Efficacy is the maximum effect a given drug can produce. This is a function of how well it stimulates the receptor to which it is bound.

A, C-E. It does not indicate what percentage of patients will experience an effect with this drug, whether or not the drug is effective in treating a particular disease, if the drug is safe to use for a particular patient, or the dose of the drug necessary to treat the patient.

28. C. A partial agonist is a drug whose efficacy is lower than that of a full agonist.

B. Answer B is the converse of C and so is wrong.

A and D. The affinity of a partial agonist may be lower, higher, or the same as a full agonist.

29. A. A competitive antagonist competes with the agonist for binding to the same receptor.

B. Competitive antagonists generally have no effect on the metabolism of an agonist.

C. Answer C is the converse of A, and so is wrong.

D. The binding of a competitive antagonist to a receptor is reversible and can be overcome by increasing the concentration of the agonist.

30. B. Proteins do not pass into the glomerular filtrate, and, thus, a drug bound to plasma proteins is not susceptible to glomerular filtration and so its clearance is decreased.

A. Decreased clearance will increase the drug's half-life.

C. Protein binding will also tend to make the drug less susceptible to biotransformation.

D. Binding of a drug to plasma proteins decreases the free concentration of the drug in plasma.

31. E. Drug hydrolysis by esterases predominantly occurs in plasma.

A–D. These biotransformations occur mainly in the liver.

32. C. Inverse agonists decrease the activity of constitutively active receptors.

A. Antagonists bind to the receptor but produce no effect.

B. Full agonists increase receptor activity with maximal efficacy.

D. Partial agonists increase receptor activity but cannot produce a maximal effect.

E. Potentiators increase the effects of agonists.

33. D. The cellular macromolecule to which a drug binds is its receptor.

A. An effector is a molecule that is activated or inhibited subsequent to receptor activation.

B. A hit is the term used in drug discovery for a ligand that binds to the target of interest.

C. A ligand is any molecule that binds to another molecule.

E. A transducer is a molecule that converts a signal from one form to another.

34. C. Agonist 3 has lower efficacy because its ability to produce an effect plateaus at 60% of maximum. Agonists 1 and 2 can both produce a maximum effect (100%).

35. B. The ED_{50} is the dose at which a drug produces 50% of its maximum effect. This is read directly from the graph by following the dashed line from the y-axis at 50% to the curve and then down to the x-axis to read the concentration.

36. B. Competitive antagonists compete with agonists for binding to the same receptor. In the presence of a competitive antagonist the concentration-response curve of an agonist drug is shifted to the right so that higher concentrations of the agonist are required to reach a given level of effect. Increasing the concentration of the agonist can overcome the blockage of the competitive antagonist and a maximal effect that can be reached at high concentrations of the agonist drug.

A. An allosteric inhibitor would be insurmountable and decrease the maximal effect of the agonist.

C. A full agonist would not decrease the response of another agonist.

D. An inverse agonist would not produce a large rightward shift of the curve or decrease the maximal effect.

E. An ideal noncompetitive antagonist would not shift the curve but would decrease the maximal effect of the agonist.

37. B. An allosteric potentiator increases the effectiveness of another drug, shifting the dose response curve to the left.

A. An allosteric inhibitor would be insurmountable and decrease the maximal effect of the agonist.

C. An inverse agonist would not produce a leftward shift of the curve.

D. An ideal noncompetitive antagonist would not shift the curve but would decrease the maximal effect of the agonist.

E. A partial agonist would produce a rightward shift of the curve.

38. D. Partial agonists are drugs with efficacy lower than full agonists (< 100% effect).

A, B, C, and E. All of the other choices are blockers (inhibitors or antagonists) that would have no effect on their own but block the effects of other drugs.

39. C. K_d is the equilibrium dissociation constant for a drug binding to its receptor as determined by a receptor binding study. By definition, when the drug concentration is equal to the K_d, 50% of the receptors are occupied.

40. C. The primary difference between receptor tyrosine kinases and cytokine receptors is that RTKs have enzymatic activity while cytokine receptors do not. Activated cytokine receptors couple to intracellular enzymes through intermediary JAK proteins.

A. Cytokine receptors and receptor tyrosine kinases both possess an extracellular binding domain.

B. Cytokine receptors and receptor tyrosine kinases both possess a hydrophobic segment of the polypeptide that crosses the lipid bilayer of the plasma membrane.

D. Cytokine receptors and receptor tyrosine kinases both dimerize after they bind the activating ligand.

E. The signal transduction pathway activated by both cytokine receptors and receptor tyrosine kinases involves phosphorylation steps.

41. A. Lipid-soluble drugs diffuse through cell membranes and bind either in the cellular cytosol or in the nucleus. Gene expression is altered and protein synthesis is either increased or decreased, which causes the cellular response.

B–D. Lipid-soluble drugs do not produce their therapeutic effect by binding to ion channels, mRNA, receptors in adipose tissue or to the extracellular face of plasma membrane receptors.

42. B. Sodium channels activated by depolarization are voltage-gated channels.

A. Ligand-gated channels are activated by ligand binding, not depolarization.

C-E. G protein-coupled receptors, transmembrane enzymes, and intracellular receptors in the cell nucleus are not sodium channels, nor are they activated by depolarization.

43. A. The key here is that diazepam is binding to a site distinct on the receptor from that to which GABA binds. This is defined as an allosteric interaction. Since diazepam increases GABA action, it is a potentiator.

B-E. None of these terms describe the effect of diazepam.

44. A. Selectivity is the ability of a drug to bind to the desired target molecule but not to other molecules. A drug is said to be specific for a target if it has high selectivity.

B. Efficacy is the ability of a drug to produce an effect.

C. Throughput is the number of assays that can be conducted in a given time.

D. Antagonism is the blocking of a drug's effect

E. Potency is the concentration or dose of a drug required to produce a specific effect.

Unit II

Drugs Acting on the Peripheral Nervous System

4 The Peripheral Nervous System

Summary

The peripheral nervous system (PNS) is composed of sensory (**afferent**) and motor (**efferent**) neurons that lie outside the brain and spinal cord. It also includes the autonomic nervous system (ANS) and the somatic nervous system (SNS). The **efferent** neurons of the ANS innervate the viscera and are responsible for involuntary homeostatic control of the organs. The ANS includes the sympathetic and parasympathetic divisions. Efferent neurons of the SNS originate in the spinal cord and synapse directly on skeletal muscle, mediating voluntary movements. The primary neurotransmitter/hormones of ANS and SNS include acetylcholine, norepinephrine, and epinephrine (EPI). Acetylcholine is the neurotransmitter released from preganglionic neurons that innervate all autonomic ganglia, postganglionic parasympathetic neurons, somatic motor neurons that innervate the neuromuscular junction, neurons that innervate the adrenal medulla, and postganglionic neurons that innervate sweat glands. Norepinephrine is the neurotransmitter released from postganglionic sympathetic neurons (except those to sweat glands which release acetylcholine). EPI is released into the bloodstream from the adrenal medulla. There are two broad categories of neurotransmitter receptors in the ANS: cholinergic and adrenergic. The cholinergic receptors can be further broken down into two types: nicotinic and muscarinic receptors. Nicotinic receptors are ligand-gated ion channels. Muscarinic receptors are G protein-coupled receptors (GPCRs). Adrenergic receptors are also GPCRs. There are two main subtypes of adrenergic receptors: α and β. Drugs that act on the ANS alter the physiological responses of the endogenous system. Most organs receive dual innervation from both the sympathetic and parasympathetic divisions, which generally have opposing effects.

Keywords: autonomic, somatic, sympathetic, parasympathetic, acetylcholine, norepinephrine

4.1 The Peripheral Nervous System

The PNS is composed of sensory (afferent) and motor (efferent) neurons that lie outside the brain and spinal cord. The PNS regulates and coordinates body physiology in conjunction with the endocrine system. The actions of the PNS are mediated by neurotransmitters acting on a diverse array of receptors at the effector organs such as smooth muscle of the viscera and blood vessels, cardiac muscle, glands, and skeletal muscle. Pharmacological agents act on the efferent nerves of the PNS by either mimicking or blocking the effects of these neurotransmitters.

4.1.1 Divisions of the Peripheral Nervous System

Autonomic Nervous System

The efferent neurons of the ANS innervate the viscera and are responsible for involuntary homeostatic control of the organs. The ANS includes the sympathetic and parasympathetic divisions that are summarized and compared in ▶ Table 4.1. The innervation of target organs by each subdivision are depicted in ▶ Fig. 4.1.

Table 4.1 Summary of the divisions of the autonomic nervous system

	Parasympathetic division	Sympathetic division
Region of spinal cord from which preganglionic neurons emerge	Cranial and sacral • Cell bodies of preganglionic neurons are in the midbrain, pons, and medulla giving rise to the autonomic components of cranial nerves III, VII, IX, and X • Cell bodies of preganglionic neurons are in S2–S4	Thoracolumbar • Cell bodies of preganglionic neurons are in T1–L3
Length of preganglionic neurons	Long	Short
Length of postganglionic neurons	Short	Long
Location of ganglia	Near target organs	Sympathetic chain ganglia (located parallel to the spinal cord on both sides) Abdominal prevertebral ganglia Adrenal medulla
Neurotransmitters and receptors	Preganglionic neurons release acetylcholine which acts at nicotinic receptors Postganglionic neurons release acetylcholine which acts at muscarinic receptors	Preganglionic neurons release acetylcholine which acts at nicotinic receptors Postganglionic neurons release norepinephrine which acts at adrenergic receptors
General functions	Principally concerned with maintenance, conservation, and protection of body resources (anabolic)	Principally involved with expenditure of body resources or energy (catabolic)
Comments	A functioning parasympathetic system is necessary to sustain life as it maintains essential bodily functions Parasympathetic nerves can act in isolation from the system as a whole, producing discrete effects at specific end organs	The sympathetic system is not strictly necessary to maintain life It is capable of a mass response, the emergency "fight or flight response." The neuronal basis of this widespread response lies in the wide divergence of preganglionic axons within the sympathetic chain ganglia

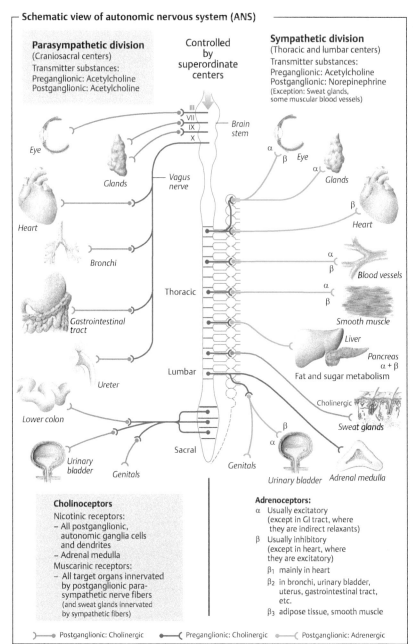

Schematic view of autonomic nervous system (ANS)

Parasympathetic division
(Craniosacral centers)
Transmitter substances:
Preganglionic: Acetylcholine
Postganglionic: Acetylcholine

Controlled by superordinate centers

Sympathetic division
(Thoracic and lumbar centers)
Transmitter substances:
Preganglionic: Acetylcholine
Postganglionic: Norepinephrine
(Exception: Sweat glands, some muscular blood vessels)

III
VII
IX
X

Brain stem

Eye

Glands

Vagus nerve

Heart

Bronchi

Thoracic

Gastrointestinal tract

Lumbar

Ureter

Lower colon

Urinary bladder   Genitals

Sacral

α
β   Eye
α
Glands

β   Heart

α
β   Blood vessels

α
β   Smooth muscle

Liver

Pancreas
α + β
Fat and sugar metabolism

Cholinergic
Sweat glands

β
α
Genitals

Urinary bladder   Adrenal medulla

Cholinoceptors
Nicotinic receptors:
– All postganglionic, autonomic ganglia cells and dendrites
– Adrenal medulla
Muscarinic receptors:
– All target organs innervated by postganglionic parasympathetic nerve fibers (and sweat glands innervated by sympathetic fibers)

Adrenoceptors:
α   Usually excitatory (except in GI tract, where they are indirect relaxants)
β   Usually inhibitory (except in heart, where they are excitatory)
β_1 mainly in heart
β_2 in bronchi, urinary bladder, uterus, gastrointestinal tract, etc.
β_3 adipose tissue, smooth muscle

Postganglionic: Cholinergic   Preganglionic: Cholinergic   Postganglionic: Adrenergic

Fig. 4.1 The autonomic nervous system (ANS).
The ANS comprises a parasympathetic division and a sympathetic division. Parasympathetic preganglionic neurons arise in the cranial and sacral region of the spinal cord and are relatively long compared with the parasympathetic postganglionic neurons. Sympathetic preganglionic neurons arise in the thoracolumbar region of the spinal cord and are relatively short compared to sympathetic postganglionic neurons. The parasympathetic ganglia are small, numerous, and located on or near the effector organs. Both pre- and postganglionic parasympathetic neurons release acetylcholine (ACh) as their neurotransmitter substance. Within the ganglia, ACh activates nicotinic cholinergic receptors on the postganglionic neurons. At the effector organs, ACh acts on muscarinic cholinergic receptors. The sympathetic ganglia are located in a chain bilaterally along the spinal cord (paravertebral) or in the mesentery of the abdomen (prevertebral). Sympathetic preganglionic neurons also release ACh to activate nicotinic receptors on the postganglionic neurons, but the postganglionic neurons release norepinephrine to affect α and β adrenoceptors. The exception to this is sweat glands which are innervated by sympathetic fibers that release ACh from postganglionic neurons.

Foundations

Embryology of the Adrenal Gland

The adrenal cortex, which comprises 80% of the adrenal gland, is derived from mesothelium; the adrenal medulla, which comprises 20%, is derived from neural crest cells as are the neurons of the sympathetic nervous system. The adrenal medulla is innervated by preganglionic sympathetic nerves and is pharmacologically similar to a sympathetic ganglion. However, because the chromaffin cells of the adrenal medulla lack axons, the adrenal medulla responds to preganglionic secretion of acetylcholine by secreting the hormones EPI (and norepinephrine to a lesser extent) into the bloodstream.

Clinical Correlation

Quadriplegia

Quadriplegia is caused by spinal cord injury at the level of the cervical spine. A ventilator may be required if the injury involves C3–C5, as these spinal nerves control the diaphragm (via the phrenic nerve), which is the major muscle that allows us to breathe. However, quadriplegic patients can survive because the cranial nerves (ANS preganglionic parasympathetic nerves) remain intact and can coordinate vital bodily functions despite the patient's having no voluntary control from below the level of injury.

Chapter 5 covers cholinergic agents and Chapter 6 covers adrenergic agents in detail.

4.1.2 Somatic Nervous System

Efferent neurons of the SNS innervate skeletal muscle and are responsible for voluntary movements. The axons of these efferent neurons originate in the spinal cord and synapse directly on skeletal muscle.

Drugs that block nicotinic cholinergic receptors on skeletal muscle are covered in the section on "Depolarizing and Nondepolarizing Neuromuscular Blockers of Acetylcholine" in Chapter 5.

The efferent neurons of the parasympathetic, sympathetic, and somatic nervous systems are shown schematically in ▶ Fig. 4.1.

4.1.3 Enteric Nervous System

Enteric neurons include the submucosal and myenteric plexuses in the gastrointestinal (GI) tract. This system possesses all the elements necessary for the short reflex regulation of GI functions (i.e., modification of motility and secretory activity by afferent and efferent nerves entirely within the GI tract). It is able to do this without modulation from the ANS, with the exception of the proximal esophagus and the external anal sphincter.

4.2 Neurotransmitters of the Autonomic and Somatic Nervous Systems

4.2.1 Acetylcholine

Synthesis. The neurotransmitter acetylcholine is synthesized in the nerve terminal from acetate, derived from acetyl coenzyme A, and choline. This reaction is catalyzed by the enzyme choline acetyltransferase. The uptake of choline is the rate-limiting step in acetylcholine synthesis (▶ Fig. 4.3).

Storage and release. Acetylcholine is stored within vesicles in nerve terminals. An action potential causes Ca^{2+} influx through voltage-gated channels and the subsequent release of acetylcholine into the synaptic cleft.

Degradation. The breakdown of acetylcholine to acetic acid and choline is rapid and occurs via the enzyme acetylcholinesterase. This enzyme is located in neuronal membranes and red blood cells. Pseudocholinesterases (nonspecific) or butyrylcholinesterases, which are more widely distributed, can also hydrolyze acetylcholine.

Site of neurotransmission. Acetylcholine is the neurotransmitter released from the following types of neurons:
- Preganglionic neurons that innervate all autonomic (parasympathetic and sympathetic) ganglia.
- Postganglionic parasympathetic neurons.
- Somatic motor neurons that innervate the neuromuscular junction.

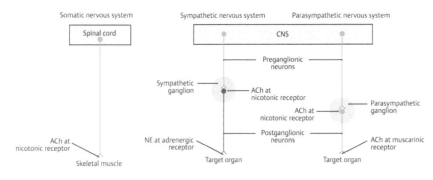

Fig. 4.2 Efferent neurons of the parasympathetic, sympathetic, and somatic nervous systems.
Somatic nervous system: Acetylcholine released from motor neurons activates nicotinic receptors on skeletal muscle to produce muscle contraction. Sympathetic nervous system: Preganglionic neurons release acetylcholine to activate nicotinic receptors on postganglionic neurons. The postganglionic neurons release norepinephrine to affect α and β adrenoceptors. The exception to this is sweat glands which are innervated by sympathetic fibers that release acetylcholine from postganglionic neurons.
Parasympathetic nervous system: Both pre- and postganglionic parasympathetic neurons release acetylcholine as their neurotransmitter substance. Within the ganglia, acetylcholine activates nicotinic cholinergic receptors on the postganglionic neurons. At the target organs, acetylcholine acts on muscarinic cholinergic receptors. ACh, acetylcholine; CNS, central nervous system; NE, norepinephrine; EPI, epinephrine.

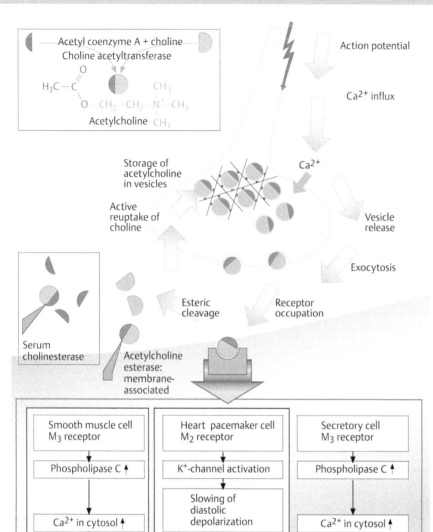

Fig. 4.3 Acetylcholine: synthesis, release, effects, and degradation.

Acetylcholine is synthesized from acetyl coenzyme A and choline by a reaction catalyzed by choline acetyltransferase. Acetylcholine is stored in vesicles in the axoplasm of presynaptic nerve terminals. These vesicles are anchored to a cytoskeletal network by the protein synapsin, thus allowing for the accumulation of vesicles near the presynaptic membrane while preventing fusion with the membrane. An action potential causes Ca^{2+} influx into the axoplasm through voltage-gated channels. Ca^{2+} then activates protein kinases that phosphorylate synapsin. This causes the vesicles to become free, fuse with the membrane, and release acetylcholine into the synaptic gap. Acetylcholine binds to receptors on the postsynaptic membrane and exerts its effects through muscarinic receptors. The signal transduction pathways and effects of the M_2 and M_3 subtypes of muscarinic receptors are illustrated. The action of acetylcholine is terminated by its rapid hydrolysis by acetylcholinesterase and serum cholinesterase followed by reuptake of the choline component into the axoplasm.

- Neurons that innervate the adrenal medulla.
- Postganglionic neurons that innervate sweat glands.

Foundations

Neuronal Communication

Nerve cells communicate with each other through the release of neurotransmitters from the presynaptic nerve terminal. The sequence of events that leads to the response of a postsynaptic neuron or effector organ is as follows:
- Presynaptic action potential.
- Influx of Ca^{2+} into the nerve terminal.
- Release of the neurotransmitter from the presynaptic terminal.
- Neurotransmitter binds to the postsynaptic receptor.
- Transduction of the message to the ion channel.
- Integration of signals from various inputs.
- Postsynaptic response.

Foundations

Coenzyme A

Pantothenic acid (vitamin B_5) is a precursor of coenzyme A (CoA). CoA participates in fatty acid synthesis and oxidation, as well as the oxidation of pyruvate in the citric acid cycle. A molecule of CoA that has an acetyl group is acetyl CoA. Acetate derived from acetyl CoA combines with choline to form the neurotransmitter acetylcholine.

4.2.2 Norepinephrine and Epinephrine

Synthesis

- Norepinephrine is synthesized in nerve terminals. Tyrosine is converted to dopa by tyrosine hydroxylase (rate-limiting step). Dopa is converted to dopamine by dopa decarboxylase and then dopamine is converted to norepinephrine by dopamine-β-hydroxylase (▶ Fig. 4.4a).

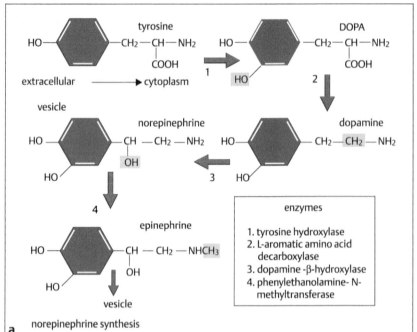

a norepinephrine synthesis

enzymes

1. tyrosine hydroxylase
2. L-aromatic amino acid decarboxylase
3. dopamine -β-hydroxylase
4. phenylethanolamine- N-methyltransferase

Fig. 4.4 Synthesis and termination of norepinephrine and adrenergic neurotransmission. (a) The synthetic pathway for dopamine, norepinephrine, and epinephrine is illustrated. (b) Post-ganglionic sympathetic nerve terminals possess varicosities that enable them to lie in close proximity to effector organs. Norepinephrine (NE) synthesis and storage in vesicles occurs in these varicosities. An action potential at the nerve terminal causes the influx of Ca^{2+} and the subsequent release of NE into the synaptic cleft. NE then binds to adrenergic receptors on effector organs, exerting a physiological effect. Note that NE has little effect on the β_2-adrenergic receptors, whereas epinephrine, synthesized in the adrenal medulla, acts at all adrenergic receptors. Approximately 70% of NE is taken back up into the presynaptic nerve terminal and repackaged in vesicles or is inactivated by monoamine oxidase (MAO). In the heart, NE is inactivated by MAO or catechol-O-methyltransferase (COMT).

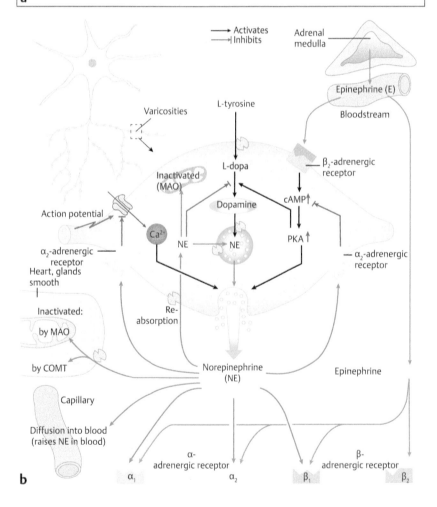

- EPI (and a lesser amount of norepinephrine) is synthesized in the adrenal medulla. A cytoplasmic enzyme in the adrenal medulla (phenylethanolamine-N-methyltransferase) transfers a methyl group to norepinephrine to form EPI.

Storage and Release

- Norepinephrine is stored in vesicles within nerve terminals. An action potential at the nerve terminal causes the influx of Ca^{2+} through voltage-gated channels and the subsequent release of norepinephrine into the synaptic cleft (▶ Fig. 4.4b).
- EPI (80%) and norepinephrine (20%) are released from the adrenal medulla following sympathetic stimulation (via acetylcholine).

Degradation

Termination of action is primarily by reuptake (60–90%) into the nerve terminal. Secondary degradation is by monoamine oxidase (MAO) and catechol-O-methyltransferase (COMT).

Site of Neurotransmission

- Norepinephrine is the neurotransmitter released from post-ganglionic sympathetic neurons (except sweat glands which release acetylcholine).

Foundations

Ascorbic Acid Redox Reactions

Ascorbic acid (vitamin C) is involved in many processes in the body, such as collagen and bile acid synthesis, activation of neuroendocrine hormones (e.g., gastrin, corticotropin-releasing hormone, and thyrotropin-releasing hormone), iron absorption, and detoxification (via stimulation of cytochrome P-450 enzymes in the liver). Ascorbic acid is oxidized to dehydroascorbic acid via an extremely reactive intermediate, semidehydro-L-ascorbate. The hydrogen ions that are liberated in this oxidation are able to act as donors in hydroxylation reactions throughout the body (which accounts for some of its effects). One such reaction where this occurs is when ascorbic acid acts as a cofactor for dopamine-β-hydroxylase in the synthesis of norepinephrine and EPI.

4.3 Neurotransmitter Receptors

There are two broad categories of neurotransmitter receptors in the ANS: cholinergic and adrenergic receptors. The cholinergic receptors can be further broken down into two types: nicotinic and muscarinic receptors.

4.3.1 Cholinergic Receptors

Nicotinic Receptors

Nicotinic receptors are ligand-gated ion channels composed of five protein subunits that combine to form a functional receptor and ion pore. Ligand binding induces Na^+ conductance. The two major subtypes are the muscle type and the neuronal type, and they each have different subunit compositions:

- The muscle type is composed of α_1, β_1, δ, and ϵ or γ subunits in a 2:1:1:1 ratio in adults.
- The neuronal subtypes are homomeric or heteromeric combinations of 12 different nicotinic receptor subunits: α_2 to α_{10} and β_2 to β_4.

Location and Function

- Autonomic ganglia. Acetylcholine released from both sympathetic and parasympathetic preganglionic neurons activates nicotinic receptors on postsynaptic neurons.
- Neuromuscular junction of somatic nerves and skeletal muscle. Acetylcholine released from motor neurons activates nicotinic receptors to produce muscle contraction.
- Adrenal medulla. Acetylcholine released from sympathetic preganglionic neurons causes release of EPI into the bloodstream.

4.3.2 Muscarinic Receptors

Muscarinic receptors are brain GPCRs (see section 2.2.1), which transduce receptor activation by acetylcholine into various intracellular changes. There are five main subtypes of muscarinic receptors. Three primary ones (M_1 to M_3) will be considered here.

Location and Function

- M_1 receptors are found in the central nervous system (CNS). These mediate synaptic transmission.

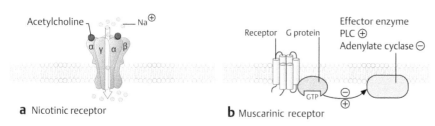

a Nicotinic receptor **b** Muscarinic receptor

Fig. 4.5 Acetylcholine receptors.
(a) The nicotinic receptor consists of five protein subunits. Binding of acetylcholine to the two α subunits results in a conformational change, allowing the central pore to open and for the influx of Na^+ ions into the cell. (b) The muscarinic receptor is coupled to intracellular G proteins which may then transduce excitatory effects via phospholipase C or inhibitory/excitatory effects via adenylate cyclase. G proteins may also interact directly with ion channels in the cell membrane (not illustrated).

- M_2 receptors are found in the heart. These decrease heart rate and force of contraction.
- M_3 receptors are found in smooth muscle and glands. These usually increase glandular secretions and may activate or relax smooth muscle (see ▶ Fig. 4.6).

Signal Transduction Mechanism

- M_1 and M_3 couple to G_q: G_q activates phospholipase which increases diacylglycerol (DAG) and inositol triphosphate (IP_3) (see page 23).
- M_2 couples to G_i: G_i inhibits cyclic adenosine monophosphate (see page 23).

Cholinergic nicotinic and muscarinic receptors are illustrated in ▶ Fig. 4.5.

4.3.3 Adrenergic Receptors

Adrenergic receptors are GPCRs. There are two main subtypes of adrenergic receptors: α and β.

Location and Function

- $α_1$ receptors are found on vascular smooth muscle. Activation leads to vasoconstriction.

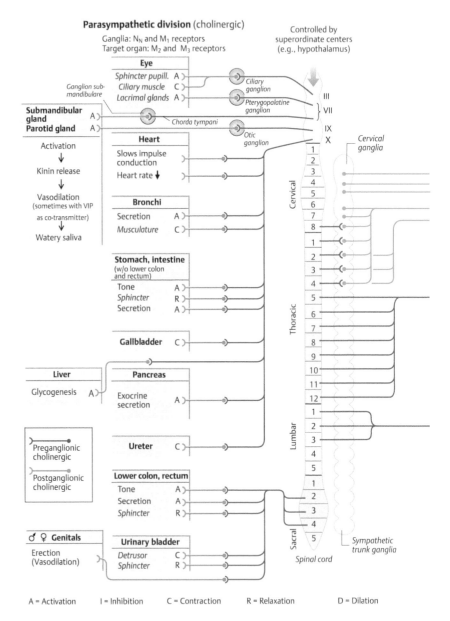

Fig. 4.6 Physiological responses of the autonomic nervous system.
The effects of parasympathetic and sympathetic stimulation on organs throughout the body are shown. Many organs are innervated by both systems, with each having a different effect; however, an exception to this is blood vessels, which only receive innervation by sympathetic postganglionic neurons. cAMP, cyclic adenosine monophosphate; CNS, central nervous system; DAG, diacylglycerol; IP_3, inositol triphosphate; VIP, vasoactive intestinal polypeptide.

- α_2 receptors are autoreceptors at presynaptic terminals of sympathetic neurons. Activation leads to inhibition of neurotransmitter release.
- β_1 receptors are found in cardiac muscle. Activation leads to increased heart rate, conduction, and force of contraction.
- β_2 receptors are found in the lung. Activation leads to bronchodilation.
- β_3 receptors are found in adipose tissue and smooth muscle. Activation leads to lipolysis and smooth muscle relaxation.

Signal Transduction Mechanism

- α_1 receptors couple to G_q.
- α_2 receptors couple to G_i.
- β receptors couple to G_s (see section 2.2.2).

▶ Table 4.2 provides a summary of ANS receptors.

II

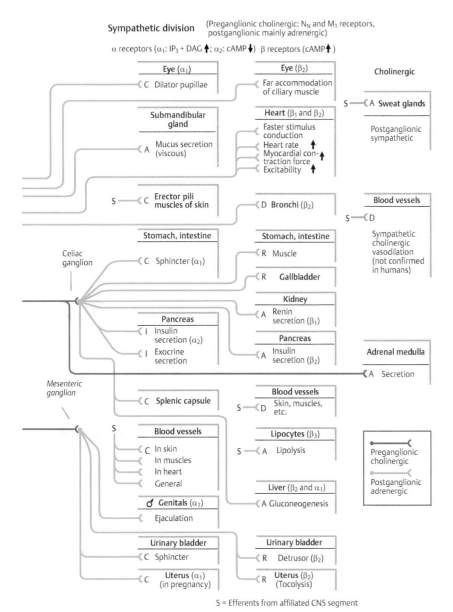

S = Efferents from affiliated CNS segment

Table 4.2 Autonomic nervous system receptors

Major types of ANS receptors	Receptor subclassification	Location of receptor	Neurotransmitter acting on the receptor	Signal transduction mechanism
Cholinergic receptors	Nicotinic	Autonomic ganglia Neuromuscular junction of somatic nerves and skeletal muscle Adrenal medulla	ACh	Ligand-gated channel that opens upon ACh binding
	Muscarinic	M_1: CNS M_2: Heart M_3: Smooth muscle[a] and glands	ACh	M_1 and M_3: G_q leading to $\uparrow$ IP_3 and DAG M_2: G_i leading to $\downarrow$ cAMP
Adrenergic receptors	α	α_1: vascular smooth muscle α_2: Autoreceptors at presynaptic terminals of sympathetic neurons	EPI and NE	α_1: G_q leading to $\uparrow$ IP_3 and DAG α_2: G_i leading to $\downarrow$ cAMP
	β	β_1: cardiac muscle β_2: lung β_3: adipose tissue and some smooth muscle	EPI and NE	β receptors: G_s leading to $\uparrow$ cAMP

[a]Effects on smooth muscle are the most important in terms of autonomic responses.

Abbreviations: ACh, acetylcholine; cAMP, cyclic adenosine monophosphate; CNS, central nervous system; DAG, diacylglycerol; EPI, epinephrine; IP_3, inositol triphosphate; NE, norepinephrine.

4.4 Physiologic Responses of the Autonomic Nervous System

Drugs that act on the ANS alter the physiological responses of the endogenous system. Understanding the normal sympathetic or parasympathetic responses of the various organs is important to understanding the actions of drugs that affect the ANS. Most organs receive dual innervation from both the sympathetic and parasympathetic divisions, which generally have opposing effects (▶ Fig. 4.6).

Clinical Correlation

Disorders of CNS Autonomic Control

Disorders involving central autonomic control may manifest as hyperactivity (e.g., hypertension and arrhythmias) or as autonomic failure (e.g., orthostatic hypotension, impotence, or GI tract dysmotility). In general, autonomic hyperactivity tends to occur acutely, whereas autonomic failure is more typical of chronic neurodegenerative disease (e.g., multiple sclerosis).

5 Cholinergic Agents

Summary

Cholinergic agonist drugs are termed **parasympathomimetics** or **cholinomimetics,** as they mimic the effects of the neurotransmitter acetylcholine in the parasympathetic nervous system. They can be either direct- or indirect-acting. Direct-acting parasympathomimetics bind directly to cholinergic receptors. These drugs include methacholine, carbachol, bethanechol, pilocarpine, and cevimeline. Varenicline is a direct-acting partial agonist at the nicotinic receptor. Indirect-acting parasympathomimetics inhibit the enzyme acetylcholinesterase (AChE), thereby increasing the concentration of acetylcholine in the synaptic cleft. These are further subdivided into reversible and irreversible agents. Reversible agents include physostigmine, neostigmine, pyridostigmine, edrophonium, donepezil, rivastigmine, and galantamine. Irreversible agents include the organophosphate insecticides parathion and isoflurophate. Cholinergic antagonists selectively block neuronal nicotinic receptors, muscle nicotinic receptors, or muscarinic receptors. Drugs that block peripheral neuronal nicotinic receptors are termed **ganglionic blocking agents** and are only used experimentally. Agents that block nicotinic receptors on skeletal muscle can be depolarizing or nondepolarizing. Succinylcholine is a depolarizing blocker that persistently activates the receptors, leading to receptor desensitization and thereby blocking the effects of acetylcholine. Nondepolarizing blockers include curare, vecuronium, and all other "curoniums." They are antagonists at muscle nicotinic receptors and thus block the effects of acetylcholine without depolarization. Muscarinic receptor antagonists differ mainly in their relative activities in the central nervous system and peripheral nervous system and include atropine, scopolamine, homatropine, cyclopentolate, ipratropium, benztropine, and glycopyrrolate.

Keywords: parasympathomimetics, anticholinesterases, parasympatholytics, nicotinic antagonists, muscarinic antagonists

5.1 Cholinergic Agonists

Cholinergic agonist drugs are termed **parasympathomimetics** or **cholinomimetics,** as they mimic the effects of the neurotransmitter acetylcholine (▶ Fig. 5.1) in the parasympathetic nervous system. They can be either direct or indirect acting.

- Direct-acting parasympathomimetics bind directly to cholinergic receptors.

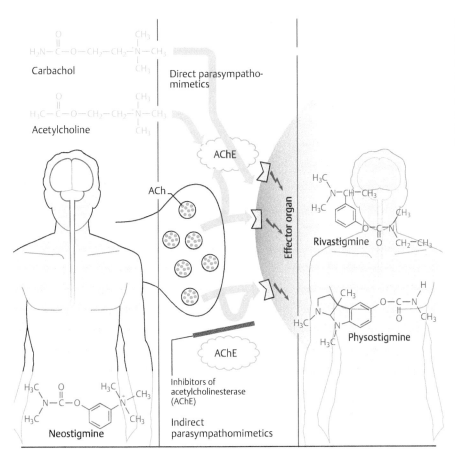

Fig. 5.1 Direct and indirect parasympathomimetics.
Direct parasympathomimetic (e.g., carbachol) mimics the effects of acetylcholine (ACh) at effector organs but is not hydrolyzed by acetylcholinesterase (AChE), allowing for its therapeutic use. Indirect parasympathomimetics (e.g., neostigmine, rivastigmine, and physostigmine) inhibit AChE, thus raising the concentration of ACh at cholinergic receptors.

- Indirect-acting parasympathomimetics inhibit the enzyme AChE, thereby increasing the concentration of acetylcholine in the synaptic cleft. These are further subdivided into reversible and irreversible agents.

▶ Table 5.1 summarizes the effects of acetylcholine activation in the parasympathetic system and therefore the effects of parasympathomimetic drugs.

5.1.1 Direct-Acting Parasympathomimetics

Direct-acting parasympathomimetics are chemical analogues of acetylcholine; therefore, they have actions similar to acetylcholine (see ▶ Fig. 5.1). They differ in their degree of selectivity for nicotinic versus muscarinic receptors. These agents are less susceptible to degradation by AChEs and serum esterases than acetylcholine.

General Properties

Side Effects

General side effects of direct-acting parasympathomimetics include salivation, lacrimation, urination, diarrhea, vomiting, bronchorrhea, bronchospasm, and bradycardia.

Contraindications

- Peptic ulcers (due to increased gastric acid production).
- Asthma (due to bronchoconstriction).
- Cardiac disease (due to decreased heart rate and velocity of conduction).
- Parkinson disease (worsened tremors).

Methacholine

Methacholine is acetyl-β-methylcholine. The methyl group endows selectivity for muscarinic receptors and decreases the rate of metabolism by cholinesterases.

Mechanism of Action

Strong muscarinic (little nicotinic) action.

Table 5.1 Effects of acetylcholine activation in the parasympathetic system and the effects of parasympathomimetic drugs

System/parameter	Effects
Cardiovascular system	↓ heart rate and velocity of conduction ↓ blood pressure Vasodilation of arterioles
Respiratory system	↑ bronchoconstriction
Gastrointestinal tract	↑ gastrointestinal motility and peristalsis
Urinary tract	↑ contraction of ureter and bladder smooth muscle Relaxation of the sphincter
Eye	↑ contraction of ciliary muscle and iris
Secretions	↑ salivation ↑ lacrimation ↑ gastrointestinal secretions ↑ bronchial secretions ↑ sweating

Pharmacokinetics

Partially susceptible to ester hydrolysis.

Uses

- Diagnosis of asthma (by inducing bronchial hypersensitivity).

Side Effects

- Light-headedness, itching, headache.

Carbachol

Carbachol is carbamoylcholine. Substitution of the acetyl group by carbamoyl endows resistance to cholinesterases.

Mechanism of Action

Muscarinic and nicotinic agonist.

Pharmacokinetics

Not susceptible to ester hydrolysis by serum esterases or AChE.

Uses

- Used as a miotic to treat glaucoma if pilocarpine is ineffective, to induce miosis during ophthalmic surgery, and to reduce intraocular pressure after cataract surgery.

Side Effects

- Few side effects at ophthalmologic doses.

Clinical Correlation

Primary Open-Angle Glaucoma

Glaucoma refers to a group of eye diseases that cause damage to the optic nerve. Primary open-angle glaucoma is the most common form of glaucoma. In this case, drainage of the aqueous humor is prevented due to blockage of the drainage channels between the cornea and the iris. The resultant buildup of aqueous humor raises intraocular pressure, causing damage to the optic nerve. The symptoms include the gradual loss of peripheral vision which progresses to tunnel vision. Drug treatment is aimed at reducing intraocular pressure by decreasing the production of aqueous humor (e.g., β-blockers [timolol], α-agonists [apra-clonidine]), and/or increasing the drainage of the aqueous humor (e.g., latanoprost, pilocarpine).

Bethanechol

It is carbamoyl-β-methylcholine, having both the methyl group of methacholine, giving it selectivity for muscarinic receptors, and the carbamoyl group of carbachol, leading to resistance to metabolism by cholinesterases.

Mechanism of Action

Strong muscarinic (little nicotinic) action.

Pharmacokinetics

- Not susceptible to ester hydrolysis by serum esterases or AChE.

Uses

- Treatment for urinary retention (stimulates the smooth muscle of the bladder).
- Used to increase gastrointestinal tract (GI) motility postoperatively and for gastric atony following bilateral vagotomy (stimulates the smooth muscle of the GI tract).

Notes

Bethanechol should not be used for urinary retention or to increase GI motility if there is a mechanical obstruction.

Side Effects

General side effects of cholinergic stimulation include decreased blood pressure, bronchospasm, nausea, abdominal pain, diarrhea, sweating, and flushing

Clinical Correlation

Sjögren's syndrome

Sjögren's syndrome is an autoimmune disease causing keratoconjunctivitis sicca (diminished tear production) and xerostomia (dry mouth). It is also associated with rheumatoid arthritis (in 50% of cases) and lupus. Lymphocytes and plasma cells infiltrate secretory glands and cause injury. Diminished tear production causes dry, itchy, gritty eyes, while diminished saliva production makes swallowing difficult and increases the likelihood of development of dental caries. Rheumatoid arthritis causes joint pain, swelling, and stiffness. Treatment for dry eyes involves the use of artificial tears. Dry mouth may be relieved by artificial saliva, taking frequent sips of water, and chewing gum to stimulate saliva flow. If this is insufficient, pilocarpine may be used to stimulate saliva production. Nonsteroidal antiinflammatory drugs (NSAIDs) are used for rheumatoid arthritis. Other drugs that may be useful include hydroxychloroquine (an antimalarial drug) and immunosuppressants (e.g., methotrexate and cyclosporine).

Pilocarpine

It is an alkaloid muscarinic agonist.

Mechanism of Action

Strong muscarinic action.

Pharmacokinetics

- Crosses the blood–brain barrier.
- Not susceptible to ester hydrolysis by serum esterases or AChE.

Uses

- Glaucoma.
- Sjögren's syndrome (to increase the secretion of saliva).

Side Effects

- Same as for bethanechol.

Cevimeline

It is a quinuclidine derivative of acetylcholine.

Mechanism of Action

Muscarinic agonist with selectivity for the M_3 subtype of muscarinic receptor which is found on epithelial cells of salivary and lacrimal glands.

Uses

- Sjögren's syndrome (to increase the secretion of saliva).

Side Effects

- Same as for bethanechol.

Varenicline

It is a partial agonist at the $\alpha_4\beta_2$ subtype of nicotinic receptor.

Mechanism of Action

Varenicline causes partial activation of $\alpha_4\beta_2$ receptors while simultaneously blocking the effects of nicotine. Its action to partially activate the receptor is thought to decrease the tobacco user's craving for nicotine. The drug will also prevent nicotine from activating the receptor if the patient relapses and consumes a tobacco product.

Uses

- Cessation of tobacco use.

Side Effects

- Nausea is common.
- Headache, difficulty sleeping, nightmares.
- Psychiatric symptoms such as changes in mood or thoughts.

5.1.2 Indirect-Acting Parasympathomimetics (Anticholinesterases)

Indirect-acting parasympathomimetics inhibit AChE, thereby increasing concentrations of acetylcholine and enhancing cholinergic function (▶ Fig. 5.1). The effects are the same as those seen following activation of nicotinic and muscarinic receptors.

General Properties

Side Effects

All of the side effects seen with direct-acting parasympathomimetics (e.g., salivation, lacrimation, urination, diarrhea, vomiting, bronchorrhea, bronchospasm, and bradycardia) plus muscle weakness, cramps, convulsions, coma, and cardiovascular and respiratory failure, caused by the increased nicotinic component.

Physostigmine

Mechanism of Action

Physostigmine is a reversible blocker of AChE.

Pharmacokinetics

- Can enter the CNS.
- Slowly hydrolyzed by AChE.
- Effects last 4 to 6 hours.

Uses

- Atropine poisoning.
- Glaucoma.
- Myasthenia gravis (rarely).

Neostigmine

Mechanism of Action

Neostigmine is a reversible blocker of AChE.

Pharmacokinetics

- Excluded from the CNS because it is polar.
- Slowly hydrolyzed by AChE.
- Effects last 4 to 6 hours.

Uses

- Myasthenia gravis.
- Reverses the effects of nondepolarizing (competitive) muscle relaxants.

Pyridostigmine

Mechanism of Action

Reversible blocker of AChE.

Pharmacokinetics

- Slowly hydrolyzed by AChE.
- Effects last 4 to 8 hours.

Uses

- Treatment of myasthenia gravis, especially in patients who have become tolerant to neostigmine.
- Reverses the effects of nondepolarizing (competitive) muscle relaxants.

Clinical Correlation

Myasthenia Gravis

It is an autoimmune disease in which there are too few functioning acetylcholine receptors at the neuromuscular junction. Patients with this condition often present in young adulthood with muscle fatigue that may progress to permanent muscle weakness. Often the eye muscles are the first to be affected causing ptosis (drooping of the eyelids) and diplopia (double vision). It is treated with neostigmine or similar agents to improve muscle contraction and muscle strength. Corticosteroids, such as hydrocortisone, or immunosuppressant drugs, such as azathioprine or cyclosporine, may also be given to inhibit the immune system.

Edrophonium

Mechanism of Action

Edrophonium is a reversible blocker of AChE.

Pharmacokinetics

- Rapidly reversible binding to AChE.
- Short-acting (10 to 20 minutes).
- Given intravenously or intramuscularly.

Uses

- Useful in diagnosis of myasthenia gravis.
- Reverses the effects of nondepolarizing (competitive) muscle relaxants.

Clinical Correlation

Edrophonium (Tensilon) Test

Edrophonium may be used to diagnose myasthenia gravis. In a patient with myasthenia gravis, an injection of edrophonium will result in a sudden and short-lived (5–10 min) improvement in muscle strength.

Donepezil, Rivastigmine, and Galantamine

Mechanism of Action

These agents are centrally acting, reversible blockers of AChE.

Uses

Mild to moderate Alzheimer disease (see Chapter 14).

Side Effects

Nausea, vomiting, and diarrhea.

Parathion and Isoflurophate

Mechanism of Action

These agents are irreversible blockers of AChE.

Pharmacokinetics

- Covalently bind to ester site on AChE.
- Very slowly released from AChE by hydrolysis (hence "irreversible").
- Removed from AChE by oxime reactivators, such as pralidoxime (2-PAM), along with atropine (to prevent muscarinic effects).

Uses

- Primarily used as an insecticide.
- Sometimes used topically to treat glaucoma.
- Component of nerve gas for biological warfare.

5.2 Cholinergic Antagonists

Drugs may selectively block neuronal nicotinic receptors, muscle nicotinic receptors, or muscarinic receptors. Drugs that block peripheral neuronal nicotinic receptors are termed *ganglionic blocking agents* and are only used experimentally. Agents that block nicotinic receptors on skeletal muscle can be depolarizing or nondepolarizing. Depolarizing blockers persistently activate the receptors, leading to receptor desensitization and thereby blocking the effects of acetylcholine. Nondepolarizing blockers are antagonists at muscle nicotinic receptors and thus block the effects of acetylcholine without depolarization. Muscarinic receptor antagonists differ mainly in their relative activities in the CNS and PNS.

5.2.1 Nicotinic Receptor Antagonists: Ganglionic Blocking Agents

Hexamethonium and Trimethaphan

Mechanism of Action

These agents block the nicotinic receptors of both sympathetic and parasympathetic ganglia, but they are not effective at the nicotinic receptor of skeletal muscle. These agents are no longer available for clinical use.

5.2.2 Nicotinic Receptor Antagonists: Depolarizing Neuromuscular Blockers of Acetylcholine

Succinylcholine

Mechanism of Action

Succinylcholine persistently activates nicotinic receptors, leading to initial target stimulation followed by persistent desensitization (▶ Fig. 5.2).

Pharmacokinetics

Neuromuscular blockade appears within 1 minute of injection and lasts up to 30 minutes.

Uses

Succinylcholine is used to produce skeletal muscle relaxation during surgery.

Side Effects

- Muscle pain—postoperative, due to muscle stimulation.
- Increased intraocular pressure—transient.
- Hyperkalemia (high plasma K^+)—muscle depolarization opens K^+ channels, K^+ enters bloodstream.

5.2.3 Nicotinic Receptor Antagonists: Nondepolarizing Neuromuscular Blockers of Acetylcholine

Curare and Vecuronium (and All Other "Curoniums")

Mechanism of Action

These agents act as competitive antagonists at nicotinic receptors, thus blocking the effects of acetylcholine without depolarization.

Pharmacokinetics

- Given intravenously.
- These drugs vary in duration of action by 1 to 3 hours.

Uses

Curare, vecuronium, and related drugs are used to produce skeletal muscle relaxation during surgery.

Side Effects

- Respiratory paralysis at toxic doses.

5.2.4 Muscarinic Receptor Antagonists

- Muscarinic receptor antagonists are active at muscarinic receptors throughout the body and as such have low organ specificity (▶ Fig. 5.3).

Atropine

Mechanism of Action

Atropine is a competitive antagonist at muscarinic receptors.

Pharmacokinetics

- Orally absorbed.
- Readily enters the CNS and therefore has both PNS and CNS actions.

Uses

Preanesthetic agent (when reductions of bronchial secretions are necessary).

Side Effects

- Typical anticholinergic effects are dry mouth, mydriasis (excessive dilation of the pupil), cycloplegia (paralysis of the ciliary muscle of the eye), constipation, difficulty in urination, and decreased sweating. There is little direct effect on blood

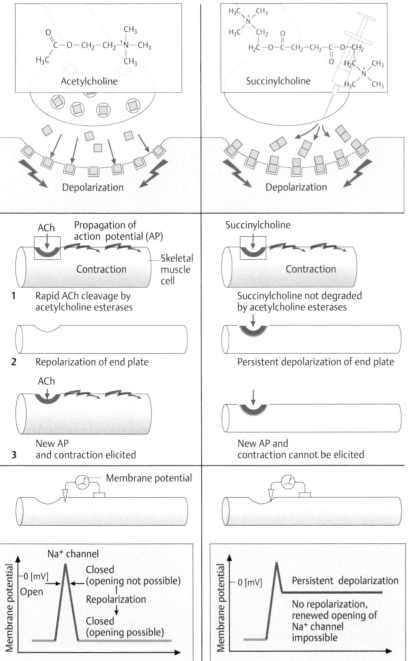

Fig. 5.2 Action of the depolarizing neuromuscular blocking agent succinylcholine. Succinylcholine is structurally like a double acetylcholine (ACh) molecule, and as such it can act as an agonist at motor end plate nicotinic receptors. However, it is unlike ACh in that it is not hydrolyzed by acetylcholinesterase, but rather is degraded more slowly by plasma cholinesterase. This allows it to accumulate in the synaptic cleft and cause persistent depolarization of the motor end plate, which is accompanied by the persistent contraction of skeletal muscle fibers.

pressure. Larger doses will increase the heart rate and speed conduction of impulses through the atrioventricular node.

• Very toxic in children.

Contraindications

• Glaucoma.

Scopolamine

Mechanism of Action

Scopolamine is a competitive antagonist at muscarinic receptors.

Uses

• Motion sickness.

Side Effects

• Same anticholinergic side effects as atropine but may cause more sedation.

Homatropine, Cyclopentolate, and Ipratropium

Mechanism of Action

These agents are synthetic atropine analogues that act as competitive antagonists at muscarinic receptors.

Pharmacokinetics

• Fewer CNS effects than atropine.

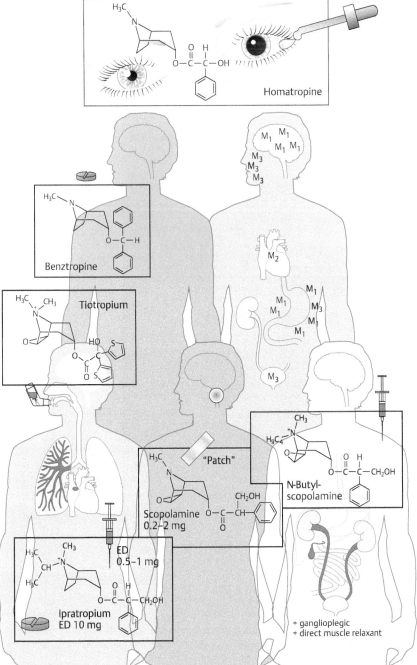

Fig. 5.3 Muscarinic receptor antagonists.
These agents act on all muscarinic receptors and have low organ selectivity. The mode of administration is therefore important for targeted treatment, as it determines distribution (as indicated by the shading) and organ concentration (indicated in *red*). E_D, effective dose.

Uses

- Dry eyes substitutes (homatropine and cyclopentolate).
- Bronchodilation in asthma (ipratropium).

Side Effects

- Mydriasis (excessive dilation of the pupil) and cycloplegia (paralysis of the ciliary muscle of the eye).

Benztropine

Mechanism of Action

Benztropine is a competitive antagonist at muscarinic receptors.

Pharmacokinetics

- Stronger CNS effects than atropine but less PNS action.

Uses

- Parkinson disease.

Side Effects

- Same anticholinergic side effects as atropine.

Glycopyrrolate

Mechanism of Action

Glycopyrrolate is a competitive antagonist at muscarinic receptors. It has fewer CNS effects than atropine (as it cannot cross the blood–brain barrier) but similar actions in the PNS, resulting in blockage of vagal inputs to the heart and decreased secretions.

Pharmacokinetics

Glycopyrrolate is a quaternary ammonium compound that does not cross the blood–brain barrier.

Uses

- Adjunctive agent in anesthesia (to reduce bronchial secretions).

Side Effects

- Same anticholinergic side effects as atropine.

▶ Table 5.2 summarizes the cholinergic antagonists and their mechanism of action.

Table 5.2 Summary of cholinergic antagonists

Drug(s)	Mechanism
Nicotinic antagonists	
Ganglionic blocking agents: Hexamethonium and trimethaphan	These agents block the following receptors: • Nicotinic receptors of pre- and postganglionic parasympathetic ganglia • Nicotinic receptors of preganglionic sympathetic ganglia Note. Not effective at the NMJ
Depolarizing neuromuscular blocker: Succinylcholine	Desensitization of nicotinic receptors at the NMJ
Nondepolarizing neuromuscular blockers: curare and vecuronium (and all other "curoniums")	Competitive antagonists of ACh at nicotinic receptors of the NMJ
Muscarinic antagonists	
Atropine, scopolamine, homatropine, cyclopentolate, ipratropium, benztropine, and glycopyrrolate	Competitive antagonists of ACh at muscarinic receptors

Abbreviations: ACh, acetylcholine; NMJ, neuromuscular junction.

Clinical Correlation

Botulinus Toxin

Botulinus toxin is a neurotoxin produced by *Clostridium botulinum*. It is highly potent and can be lethal in very small amounts. It works by preventing the release of acetylcholine at the neuromuscular junction, thereby causing paralysis of muscles. In its purified form (Botox), this paralysis of muscles is temporary (3 to 4 months) and is used cosmetically to soften the appearance of wrinkles. It is also used therapeutically in the treatment of cervical dystonia (a neuromuscular disorder of the head and neck), severe hyperhidrosis (excessive sweating), achalasia (failure of the lower esophageal sphincter to relax), migraine, and other conditions.

6 Adrenergic Agents

Summary

Drugs that mimic or enhance the actions of norepinephrine or epinephrine in adrenergic neurotransmission are termed *sympathomimetics*, including the endogenous catecholamines, synthetic catecholamines, and directly and indirectly acting synthetic sympathomimetics.

Drugs that inhibit adrenergic function are termed *sympatholytics*, including the adrenergic receptor antagonists and drugs that deplete catecholamines. Norepinephrine can stimulate all of the subtypes of adrenergic receptors, but its actions on α_1 receptors predominate. Epinephrine stimulates all of the adrenergic receptor subtypes. Dopamine, a precursor in the formation of norepinephrine and epinephrine, acts on dopamine receptors and on α_1- and β_1-adrenergic receptors in the peripheral autonomic nervous system. Synthetic catecholamines include isoproterenol, which acts on β receptors with no α action, and dobutamine, a direct-acting, selective β_1-adrenergic receptor agonist. Noncatecholamine sympathomimetics may exert effects by direct or indirect actions. Direct sympathomimetics act to stimulate α- or β-adrenergic receptors. Phenylephrine, metaraminol, tetrahydrozoline, oxymetazoline, xylometazoline, and naphazoline are direct-acting α-adrenergic receptor agonists. Clonidine is a selective α_2-agonist. Metaproterenol, terbutaline, albuterol, formoterol, and salmeterol are direct-acting β_2-adrenergic receptor agonists. Mirabegron is a direct-acting β_3-adrenergic receptor agonist. Mixed-acting sympathomimetics include amphetamine, methamphetamine, and ephedrine. These agents act as agonists at adrenergic receptors, cause the release of endogenous norepinephrine and inhibit its reuptake. Sympatholytics include the α-blockers phenoxybenzamine and phentolamine. Prazosin, terazosin, and doxazosin are selective blockers of α_1 receptors. Propranolol, nadolol, and timolol are nonselective β-receptor antagonists (block both β_1- and β_2-adrenergic receptors). Acebutolol, atenolol, esmolol, and metoprolol are cardioselective β_1-adrenergic receptor antagonists. Drugs that deplete catecholamines include reserpine and guanethidine.

Keywords: sympathomimetics, sympatholytics, alpha blockers, beta blockers

6.1 Catecholamine Sympathomimetics

6.1.1 Endogenous Catecholamines

Norepinephrine

Norepinephrine is the primary neurotransmitter released from the postganglionic neurons of the sympathetic nervous system. Its metabolism is discussed in section 4.2.2.

Mechanism of Action

Norepinephrine can stimulate all of the subtypes of adrenergic receptors, but its actions on α_1 receptors predominate. This is mainly observed as an increase in blood pressure.

Effects

- Arterioles in the skin and mucosa, as well as splanchnic, renal, and coronary vascular beds are directly constricted (α_1 and α_2) (▶ Fig. 6.1). As a result, total peripheral resistance (TPR) and diastolic and systolic blood pressure (BP) increase. Increased BP activates baroreceptors to reflexly decrease sympathetic tone and to increase vagal activity (see **box**).
- The direct effect on β_1-adrenergic receptors of the heart is to increase heart rate, force of contractions, and conduction velocity. This is offset by this reflex vagal slowing of the heart rate (▶ Fig. 6.2).
- Glycogenolysis occurs in the liver and skeletal muscle (β_2) and lipolysis occurs in adipose tissue (β_3). This is illustrated in ▶ Fig. 6.3.

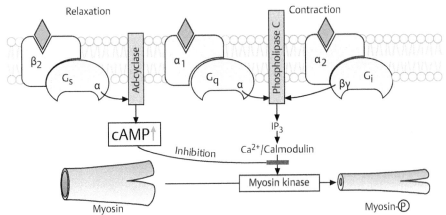

Fig. 6.1 Effects of catecholamines on vascular smooth muscle.
Differences in signal transduction are responsible for the opposing effects of α- and β-adrenergic receptor activation by epinephrine or norepinephrine. Binding to α_1 causes stimulation of phospholipase C (PLC) and inositol triphosphate (IP$_3$) and the release of Ca^{2+}. Ca^{2+} and calmodulin then activate the enzyme myosin kinase which phosphorylates myosin, leading to vasoconstriction. Binding to α_2 adrenergic receptors also activates PLC via different G protein subunit. Binding to β_2 adrenergic receptors activates adenylate cyclase which increases cyclic adenosine monophosphate (cAMP) production intracellularly. Myosin kinase is inhibited by cAMP, leading to vasodilation.

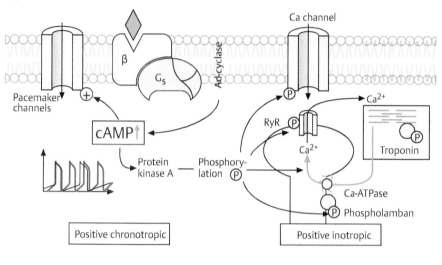

Fig. 6.2 Cardiac effects of catecholamines. Stimulation of β receptors in cardiac muscle increases cyclic adenosine monophosphate (cAMP), which then opens "pacemaker" channels. This hastens diastolic depolarization and reduces the threshold for action potential generation, resulting in an increase in conduction velocity, and thus increased heart rate. cAMP also activates protein kinase A which phosphorylates various Ca^{2+} transport proteins, leading to more Ca^{2+} entering the cell and more Ca^{2+} being released from the sarcoplasmic reticulum. This results in greater contraction of heart muscle. The necessary accompanying increased rate of heart muscle relaxation is caused by the phosphorylation of troponin and phospholamban.

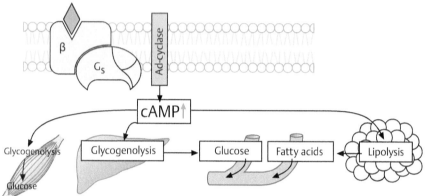

Fig. 6.3 Metabolic effects of catecholamines. Stimulation of β receptors increases cyclic adenosine monophosphate (cAMP). This causes glycogenolysis in the liver and skeletal muscle, with glucose being released into the bloodstream. Lipolysis occurs in adipose tissue, causing the hydrolysis of triglycerides to fatty acids (and glycerol). These fatty acids are also released into the bloodstream.

Clinical Correlation

Baroreceptor Reflex

The baroreceptor reflex allows the body to compensate rapidly for changes in arterial pressure. It is mediated by receptors sensitive to mechanical stretch that are located in the carotid sinuses and in the walls of the aortic arch. The carotid sinus baroreceptors respond to both increases and decreases in arterial pressure; aortic arch baroreceptors only respond to increases in arterial pressure. Decreased arterial pressure causes carotid sinus baroreceptors to experience a reduced amount of stretch. This decreases the rate of action potential firing of the glossopharyngeal nerve (cranial nerve [CN] IX), which innervates the carotid sinus. Impulses from CN IX are then relayed to the vasomotor center in the medulla oblongata which increases sympathetic outflow. This results in increased heart rate, contractility, and stroke volume. This also results in venoconstriction that reduces the capacitance of veins thus increasing preload and cardiac output (via the Frank–Starling mechanism) and vasoconstriction of arterioles.

Epinephrine

Epinephrine is also discussed in section 4.2.2.

Mechanism of Action

Epinephrine stimulates all of the adrenergic receptor subtypes (▶ Fig. 6.4).

Pharmacokinetics

- Given by intravenous (IV) infusion as it has poor enteral absorbability (▶ Fig. 6.5).

Effects

- With small doses or with slow infusion, vasodilation occurs (skeletal muscle) and diastolic BP decreases (β₂ effect).
- With larger doses, vasoconstriction (skin and splanchnics) occurs and TPR is increased (α effect) (▶ Fig. 6.1).
- The direct effect on β₁ receptors of the heart is the same as for norepinephrine: increased heart rate, force of contraction, and velocity of conduction. These effects combine to increase cardiac output. At large doses, it causes reflex vagal slowing of the heart and decreased cardiac output despite these direct effects (▶ Fig. 6.2).

Uses

- Often added to local anesthetic preparations to produce local vasoconstriction which decreases local bleeding and increases the duration of action of the anesthetic.

• Used clinically to treat anaphylaxis (parenterally) and bronchospasm (subcutaneously); also used for minor bleeding (topically).

Dopamine

Dopamine is a precursor in the formation of norepinephrine and epinephrine in the peripheral nervous system.

Mechanism of Action

Dopamine acts on dopamine receptors and on α_1- and β_1-adrenergic receptors (▶ Fig. 6.6) in the peripheral autonomic nervous system.

Effects

• Increases BP and heart rate (β_1 effect).
• In the central nervous system (CNS), it acts as a neurotransmitter (see Chapter 7).

Pharmacokinetics

• Given by IV infusion as it is not orally effective.

Uses

• Can be given to boost cardiac output in shock or heart failure.

6.1.2 Synthetic Catecholamines

Isoproterenol

Mechanism of Action

Isoproterenol acts directly on all subtypes of β-adrenergic receptors with no α action.

Effects

• Increases heart rate, force of contraction, and cardiac output (direct β_1 effects).
• Vasodilation, resulting in decreased diastolic BP and decreased TPR (β_2 effects).

Uses

• No longer used clinically.
• Used experimentally as a ß-agonist.

Dobutamine

Mechanism of Action

Dobutamine is a direct-acting, selective β_1-adrenergic receptor agonist.

Pharmacokinetics

• Given by IV infusion.

Effects

• Increases contractility and heart rate (contractility > heart rate).

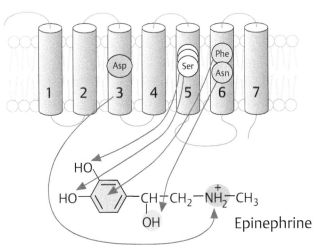

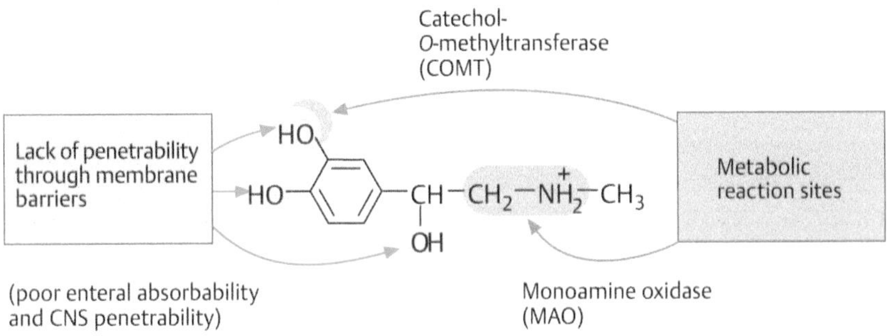

β₂ Adrenergic Receptor

Fig. 6.4 Interaction between epinephrine and the β₂-adrenergic receptor.
Epinephrine and other adrenergic receptor agonists typically share a phenylethylamine structure. The hydroxyl group on the side chain (*pink*) has an affinity to both α and β receptors. Substitution on the amino group (*blue*) decreases the affinity to α but increases the affinity to β receptors. Increasing the bulk of this amino substitute favors the β₂ receptor. Both hydroxyl groups on the aromatic ring (*purple*) also contribute to affinity. If these hydroxyl groups are at positions 3 and 4, the ligand will have a greater affinity to α receptors, but if they are at positions 3 and 5, they will have greater affinity to β receptors.

Catechol-O-methyltransferase (COMT)

Lack of penetrability through membrane barriers

Metabolic reaction sites

(poor enteral absorbability and CNS penetration)

Monoamine oxidase (MAO)

Fig. 6.5 Structure–activity relationship of epinephrine.
Epinephrine and other catecholamines have poor lipophilicity and therefore have poor absorbability and penetrability through lipid membranes. This is caused by the hydroxyl group; thus, deletion of one or more of the hydroxyl groups will improve penetrability. Substances without one or more of the aromatic hydroxyl groups will have increased indirect sympathomimetic activity. A change in the position of one or more of the aromatic hydroxyl groups or their substitution prevents inactivation by catechol-O-methyltransferase (COMT). Introduction of a small alkyl residue on the carbon atom adjacent to the amino group prevents the breakdown of epinephrine by monoamine oxidase (MAO).

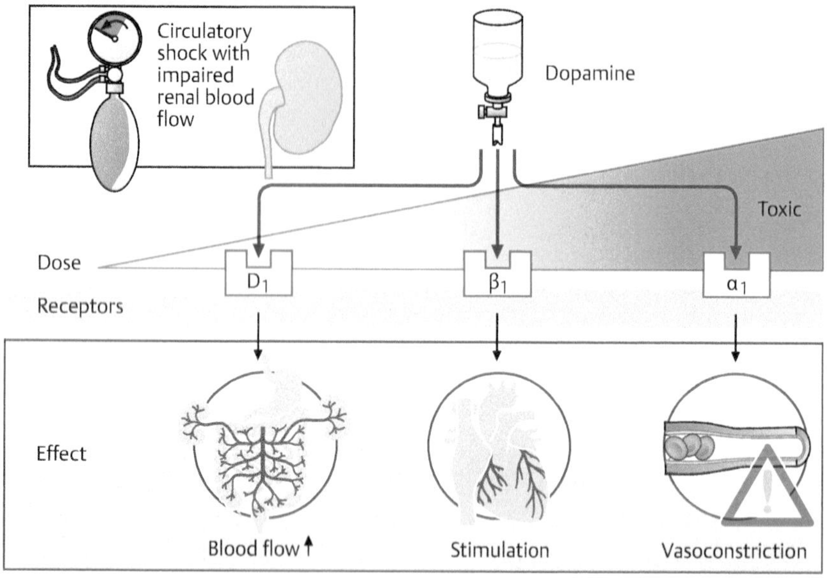

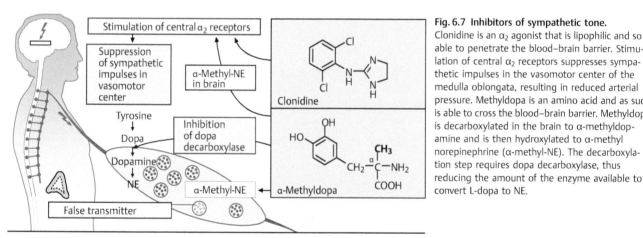

Fig. 6.6 Dopamine as a therapeutic agent.
Dopamine can be given as an infusion to treat circulatory shock with impaired renal blood flow. In this case, binding to the D_1 receptor causes dilation of the renal and splanchnic arteries, thus increasing renal blood flow and reducing cardiac afterload. At higher doses, dopamine will stimulate β_1 receptors, resulting in cardiac stimulation, and at progressively higher doses, it will also stimulate α_1 receptors. This will produce vasoconstriction, which would be undesirable in this case.

Fig. 6.7 Inhibitors of sympathetic tone.
Clonidine is an α_2 agonist that is lipophilic and so is able to penetrate the blood–brain barrier. Stimulation of central α_2 receptors suppresses sympathetic impulses in the vasomotor center of the medulla oblongata, resulting in reduced arterial pressure. Methyldopa is an amino acid and as such is able to cross the blood–brain barrier. Methyldopa is decarboxylated in the brain to α-methyldopamine and is then hydroxylated to α-methyl norepinephrine (α-methyl-NE). The decarboxylation step requires dopa decarboxylase, thus reducing the amount of the enzyme available to convert L-dopa to NE.

Uses

- Severe congestive heart failure.

6.2 Noncatecholamine Sympathomimetics

Noncatecholamine sympathomimetics may exert effects by direct or indirect actions. Direct sympathomimetics act to stimulate α- or β-adrenergic receptors. Indirect sympathomimetics may release stored norepinephrine from nerve terminals or may block reuptake mechanisms (many do both).

6.2.1 Direct-acting Sympathomimetics

Phenylephrine, Metaraminol, Tetrahydrozoline, Oxymetazoline, Xylometazoline, Naphazoline, and Pseudoephedrine

Mechanism of Action

These agents are direct-acting α-adrenergic receptor agonists.

Effects

- Produce vasoconstriction and increase BP.

Uses

- Phenylephrine and metaraminol may be used to restore blood pressure during spinal or general anesthesia, in hypotensive emergencies, or after overdose of an antihypertensive medication.
- Phenylephrine is also used either systemically or topically as a nasal decongestant and conjunctival vasoconstrictor.
- Tetrahydrozoline, oxymetazoline, xylometazoline, naphazoline, and pseudoephedrine are nonprescription sympathomimetics used topically as nasal decongestants and conjunctival vasoconstrictors.

Clonidine

Mechanism of Action

Clonidine is a selective α_2 agonist (▶ Fig. 6.7).

Effects

- Acts in the CNS to decrease sympathetic outflow to periphery.

Uses

- Hypertension.

Metaproterenol, Terbutaline, Albuterol, Formoterol, and Salmeterol

Mechanism of Action

These agents are direct-acting β$_2$-adrenergic receptor agonists.

Pharmacokinetics

- Metaproterenol, terbutaline, and albuterol are short-acting ß$_2$-agonist bronchodilators (SABAs) administered 3-4 times per day.
- Formoterol and salmeterol are long-acting ß$_2$-agonist (LABAs) bronchodilators given 2 times per day.

Effects

- Bronchodilation.
- Tachycardia.
- Restlessness.

Uses

- Asthma and chronic obstructive pulmonary disease (see Chapter 26).

Mirabegron

Mechanism of Action

Direct-acting β$_3$-adrenergic receptor agonist.

Effects

- β$_3$ receptors are expressed in the detrusor muscle of the bladder.
- Activation of these receptors produces relaxation of the detrusor muscle.

Uses

- Improves the symptoms of urge urinary incontinence caused by overactive bladder.

6.2.2 Mixed-acting Sympathomimetic

Ephedrine

Mechanism of Action

Ephedrine acts as an agonist at adrenergic receptors and causes the release of endogenous norepinephrine.

Pharmacokinetics

- Orally effective.

Effects

- Increases BP, heart rate, and contractility.
- Bronchodilation.
- Mydriasis without cycloplegia.
- Nasal decongestion.
- Also acts as a stimulant in the CNS.

Uses

- Its only approved use is in the reversal of hypotension during anesthesia.
- Previously used as a nasal decongestant, but this was discontinued due to CNS stimulatory actions.
- Found in ma huang and other dietary supplements.

Adverse Effects

- Increased risk of stroke, myocardial infarction, and sudden cardiac death.

6.2.3 Indirect-acting Sympathomimetics

Amphetamine and Methamphetamine

Mechanism of Action

These agents cause the release of endogenous norepinephrine and inhibit its reuptake.

Pharmacokinetics

- Orally effective.

Effects

- Increase BP, heart rate, and contractility.
- Bronchodilation.
- Mydriasis without cycloplegia.
- CNS stimulants.

Uses

- Attention deficit hyperactivity disorder (amphetamine) (see section 18.11).
- Drug of abuse (methamphetamine).

Tolerance

- Readily develops to the CNS stimulant effects, appetite suppression, and mood elevation.

Tyramine

Mechanism of Action

Tyramine causes the release of norepinephrine from sympathetic nerve terminals.

Effects

- Increases BP.

Uses

- No therapeutic uses.

Drug interactions

Tyramine may precipitate hypertensive crisis when ingested with monoamine oxidase inhibitors (see section 13.2.2).

6.3 Drugs Inhibiting Sympathetic Function (Sympatholytics)

6.3.1 α-Blockers

Phenoxybenzamine and Phentolamine

Mechanism of Action

These agents are antagonists at both α_1 and α_2 receptors.
- Phenoxybenzamine is an irreversible, noncompetitive antagonist.
- Phentolamine is a competitive antagonist.

Effects

These agents block vasoconstriction caused by sympathetic nerve stimulation or sympathomimetic drugs, producing a fall in BP.

Uses

- Used during treatment of pheochromocytoma to prevent the effects of epinephrine released from tumor.

Side Effects

- Postural (orthostatic) hypotension, reflex tachycardia, miosis, nasal stuffiness, and inhibited ejaculation.

Clinical Correlation

Pheochromocytoma

Pheochromocytoma is a rare, benign tumor of the adrenal medulla (90% unilateral) that produces catecholamines. Signs and symptoms include hypertension, cardiomyopathy, weight loss, hyperglycemia, and periods of crisis lasting ~15 minutes, characterized by fear, headache, palpitations, sweating, nausea, tremor, and pallor. Treatment involves reduction of BP with phenoxybenzamine and propranolol, followed by surgery to remove the tumor.

Prazosin, Terazosin, and Doxazosin

Mechanism of Action

These agents are selective blockers of α_1 receptors.

Uses

- Hypertension.

Side Effects

- Benign prostatic hypertrophy.

Note: The first dose may produce a precipitous hypotensive effect.

6.3.2 β-Blockers

Propranolol, Nadolol, and Timolol

Mechanism of Action

These agents are nonselective β receptor antagonists (block both β_1- and β_2-adrenergic receptors).

Uses

- Hypertension, angina, and cardiac arrhythmias. They are also used to reduce the incidence of myocardial reinfarction (▶ Fig. 6.8).
- Glaucoma.
- Treatment of the peripheral effects of hyperthyroidism.
- Prophylactic agents for migraine headache.

Side Effects

- Hypotension, bradycardia, increased airway resistance, decreased response to hypoglycemia, and fatigue.

Note: Use with caution in patients with heart disease, asthma, or diabetes (may mask the tachycardic sign of hypoglycemia in diabetics taking insulin).

Acebutolol, Atenolol, Esmolol, and Metoprolol

Mechanism of Action

These agents are cardioselective β_1-adrenergic receptor antagonists (50 times more potent for β_1).

Effects

These agents are designed to have less effect on bronchial smooth muscle than the nonselective agents (▶ Fig. 6.9).

Labetalol

Mechanism of Action

Labetalol is an α_1 antagonist, a nonselective β-antagonist, and a weak β_2-adrenergic receptor agonist.

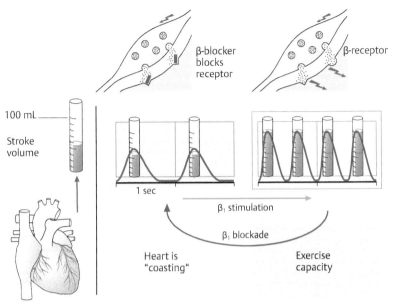

Fig. 6.8 Beta blockers: effect on cardiac function.
Beta blockers antagonize epinephrine and norepinephrine at β receptors. They reduce cardiac work to its base ("coasting") level and ensure that it cannot be stimulated above this level. As a consequence of this reduced cardiac work, oxygen consumption in cardiac muscle is reduced. Beta blockers also reduce heart rate and blood pressure and protect the failing heart against excessive sympathetic stimulation. However, exercise capacity is reduced because the heart cannot respond in the normal way to β_1 stimulation.

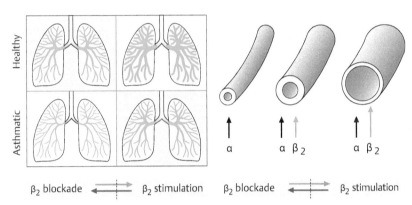

Fig. 6.9 Beta blockers: effect on bronchial and vascular tone.
Beta blockers cause bronchoconstriction in healthy individuals. In asthmatic patients, β blockers may cause bronchospasm, leading to acute respiratory distress. Beta blockers also cause partial vasoconstriction of blood vessels as β_2-mediated vasodilation is blocked, but α-mediated vascular tone is maintained.

Uses

- Used to treat hypertension and clonidine withdrawal syndrome.

Side Effects

- Postural (orthostatic) hypotension (α) as well as β side effects listed above.

6.3.3 Drugs that Deplete Catecholamines

Reserpine

Mechanism of Action

Reserpine prevents the storage and reuptake of norepinephrine thus causing neuronal depletion of norepinephrine. It also depletes stores of epinephrine, dopamine, and serotonin (▸ Fig. 6.10).

Effects

CNS effects include sedation.

Uses

- Hypertension.

Guanethidine

Mechanism of Action

Guanethidine blocks action potential propagation at fine terminals and acts like reserpine to deplete norepinephrine (▸ Fig. 6.10). It must be taken up by nerve endings; thus, the effect is blocked by reuptake inhibitors (tricyclic antidepressants and cocaine).

Uses

Hypertension (rarely used).

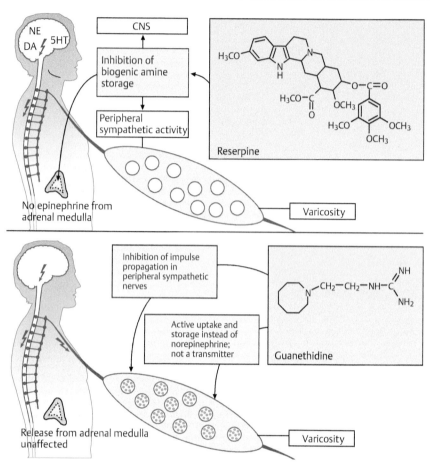

Fig. 6.10 Inhibitors of sympathetic tone. Reserpine prevents norepinephrine (NE) storage and causes the depletion of NE, dopamine, and serotonin by inhibiting a membrane transporter in storage vesicles. Free NE can then be degraded by monoamine oxidase. No epinephrine is released from the adrenal medulla. Guanethidine is taken up by the vesicular amine transporters and stored instead of NE, but it does not function as NE. It also blocks action potentials by stabilizing the axonal membrane. CNS, central nervous system; DA, dopamine; 5HT, 5-hydroxytryptamine.

Table 6.1 Interactions of drugs with adrenergic receptors

Drug	Receptor affected
Agonists	
Norepinephrine	α_1, α_2, β_1, β_2
Epinephrine	α_1, α_2, β_1, β_2, β_3
Dopamine	α_1, β_1
Isoproterenol	β_1, β_2
Phenylephrine	α_1
Clonidine	α_2
Albuterol terbutaline	β_2
Antagonists	
Phentolamine, phenoxybenzamine	α_1, α_2
Propranolol, nadolol, and timolol	β_1, β_2
Prazosin	α_1
Yohimbine	α_2
Atenolol, metoprolol	β_1

▶ Table 6.1 Summarizes the receptor activation of adrenergic agonists and antagonists.

Unit II Review Questions

1. Atropine blocks the action of
   A. Dopamine.
   B. Norepinephrine.
   C. Serotonin.
   D. Acetylcholine.
   E. Histamine.

2. Drugs that possess antimuscarinic activity are contraindicated in patients with
   A. Glaucoma.
   B. Diarrhea.
   C. Hypertension.
   D. Gout.

3. A 52-year-old woman became angry with her spouse and ingested a bottle of pesticide containing parathion, an organophosphate compound. She was brought to the emergency room within 30 minutes. A nasogastric lavage was performed immediately. The patient's symptoms progressed to include miosis, diaphoresis, salivation, lacrimation, defecation, and bronchorrhea. Which of the following drug pairs would comprise part of the treatment for this poisoning episode?
   A. Atropine and pralidoxime.
   B. Nitroglycerin and hydrochlorothiazide.
   C. Phenylephrine and isoproterenol.
   D. Propranolol and theophylline.
   E. Tubocurarine and lidocaine.

For questions **4** to **8**, refer to the pathway for catecholamine synthesis that follows. **A** to **D** represent the enzymes involved in the steps of that pathway.

A B C D

Tyrosine → Dopa → Dopamine → Norepinephrine → Epinephrine

4. Dopa decarboxylase catalyzes which step in the pathway above?

5. Dopamine-β-hydroxylase catalyzes which step in the above pathway?

6. Tyrosine hydroxylase catalyzes which step in the above pathway?

7. Phenylethanolamine-N-methyltransferase (PMNT) catalyzes which step in the above pathway?

8. Which is the rate-limiting step in catecholamine synthesis?

9. Direct inhibition of norepinephrine release is accomplished via
   A. α_1-adrenergic receptor stimulation.
   B. α_2-adrenergic receptor stimulation.
   C. β_1-adrenergic receptor stimulation.
   D. β_2-adrenergic receptor stimulation.

10. Antihypertensive action of clonidine in the CNS occurs via
    A. Activation of α_1-adrenergic receptors.
    B. Activation of α_2-adrenergic receptors.
    C. Activation of β_1-adrenergic receptors.
    D. Activation of β_2-adrenergic receptors.
    E. Activation of muscarinic receptors.

11. Which of the following blocks the blood pressure effects of norepinephrine but does not interfere with the presynaptic actions of norepinephrine to modulate its own release?
    A. Dopamine.
    B. Terbutaline.
    C. Prazosin.
    D. Pindolol.

12. A 54-year-old man with benign prostatic hypertrophy is experiencing uncontrollable leakage of small amounts of urine. Drug treatment to reduce prostatic hypertrophy is initiated, but it will take several weeks to alleviate the overflow incontinence. Which of the following agents will act directly in the bladder to decrease outflow obstruction and increase urinary flow rates so that a more rapid therapeutic response may be obtained?
    A. Clonidine.
    B. Epinephrine.
    C. Doxazosin.
    D. Pyridostigmine.
    E. Yohimbine.

13. An alternative approach to that taken in question 12 may be to activate the postganglionic parasympathetic responses of the bladder. Which of the following drugs would have this effect?
    A. Atropine.
    B. Bethanechol.
    C. Succinylcholine.
    D. Trimethaphan.
    E. Tubocurarine.

The following information refers to questions **14** to **17**.
In a dog anesthetized with pentobarbital, recording electrodes are placed on
I. Carotid sinus baroreceptor nerve fibers.
II. Splanchnic (sympathetic preganglionic) nerve fibers.
III. Inferior cardiac (sympathetic postganglionic) nerve fibers.
IV. Vagal (parasympathetic preganglionic) nerve fibers.

Answer choices A to E show the changes (if any) in firing rates that would be expected to occur at nerves I to IV following the administration of phenylephrine after the series of drugs listed in questions 14 to 17. Presume that sufficient time for the actions of the premedicating agents has been allowed and that phenylephrine is then given intravenously.

	I	II	III	IV
A.	⇔	⇔	⇔	⇔
B.	⇑	⇓	⇓	⇑
C.	⇔	⇓	⇓	⇑
D.	⇓	⇑	⇑	⇓
E.	⇑	⇓	⇔	⇑

Key: ⇑ = increase of nerve activity; ⇓ = decrease of nerve activity; ⇔ = no change in neural firing.

14. Propranolol and atropine; then phenylephrine.

15. Propranolol, atropine, and reserpine; then phenylephrine.

16. Propranolol, atropine, reserpine, and hexamethonium; then phenylephrine.

17. Propranolol, atropine, reserpine, hexamethonium, and phenoxybenzamine; then phenylephrine.

18. Which of the following blocks the release of a neurotransmitter?
   A. Succinylcholine.
   B. Cocaine.
   C. Botulinum toxin.
   D. Muscarine.
   E. Atropine.

19. Which of the following is hydrolyzed by acetylcholinesterase?
   A. Acetylcholine.
   B. Succinylcholine.
   C. Tubocurarine.
   D. Epinephrine.

20. Which of the following drugs will potentiate the cardiovascular actions of intravenously administered norepinephrine but block the cardiovascular actions of intravenously administered tyramine?
   A. A selective β_1-adrenergic antagonist (e.g., metoprolol).
   B. A nonselective β_1-adrenergic antagonist (e.g., propranolol).
   C. An α_1-adrenergic antagonist (e.g., phentolamine).
   D. A monoamine oxidase inhibitor (e.g., pargyline).
   E. An inhibitor of neuronal monoamine uptake (e.g., cocaine).

21. What is usually the most important mechanism by which the action of norepinephrine is terminated after norepinephrine is released by nerve stimulation?
   A. Reuptake into sympathetic nerves.
   B. Metabolism by monoamine oxidase.
   C. Metabolism by catechol-0-methyltransferase.
   D. Diffusion into surrounding tissue.
   E. Diffusion into blood.

22. A blocker muscarinic cholinergic with no central nervous system (CNS) effect is
   A. Scopolamine.
   B. Hexamethonium.
   C. Glycopyrrolate.
   D. Atropine.
   E. Succinylcholine.

23. A depolarizing neuromuscular blocking agent selective for neuromuscular-type receptors is
   A. Curare.
   B. Hexamethonium.
   C. Scopolamine.
   D. Atropine.
   E. Succinylcholine.

24. Which of the following drugs will potentiate the cardiac effects of norepinephrine?
   A. Propranolol.
   B. Metoprolol.
   C. Amphetamine.
   D. Succinylcholine.

25. Muscarine produces all the effects of acetylcholine at the
   A. Sympathetic ganglia.
   B. Neuromuscular junction.
   C. Parasympathetic ganglia.
   D. Postganglionic parasympathetic neuroeffector junctions.

26. Increased force of contraction of the left ventricle results from
   A. α_1-adrenergic receptor stimulation.
   B. α_2-adrenergic receptor stimulation.
   C. β_1-adrenergic receptor stimulation.
   D. β_2-adrenergic receptor stimulation.
   E. Muscarinic receptor stimulation.

27. Relaxation of bronchial smooth muscle results from
   A. α_1-adrenergic receptor stimulation.
   B. α_2-adrenergic receptor stimulation.
   C. β_1-adrenergic receptor stimulation.
   D. β_2-adrenergic receptor stimulation.
   E. Muscarinic receptor stimulation.

28. A 54-year-old man with benign prostatic hypertrophy is experiencing uncontrollable leakage of small amounts of urine. Drug treatment to reduce the prostatic hypertrophy is initiated, but it will take several weeks to alleviate the overflow incontinence. Which of the following will activate the postganglionic parasympathetic responses of the bladder directly to decrease outflow obstruction and increase urine flow rates so that a more rapid therapeutic response may be obtained?
   A. Atropine.
   B. Bethanechol.
   C. Succinylcholine.
   D. Trimethaphan.
   E. Tubocurarine.

29. A 52-year-old woman became angry with her spouse and ingested a bottle of pesticide containing parathion, an organophosphate compound. She was brought to the emergency room within 30 minutes. A nasogastric lavage was performed immediately. The patient's symptoms progressed to include miosis, diaphoresis, salivation, lacrimation, defecation, and bronchorrhea. These symptoms are due to an excess of which of the following neurotransmitters?
   A. Acetylcholine.
   B. Epinephrine.
   C. Muscarine.
   D. Norepinephrine.
   E. Serotonin.

30. A 32-year-old woman has experienced progressive ptosis of her left eyelid over the last several years, which now blocks her vision. She has no other complaints or problems. The curtain and lid twitch signs and bilateral ophthalmoplegia on upgaze are observed on examination. A diagnosis of myasthenia gravis is confirmed by a test that involves injecting a drug with which of the following mechanisms of action?

A. Atropine analogue.
B. Cholinesterase inhibitor.
C. Ganglionic blocking agent.
D. Reuptake inhibitor.
E. Sympathomimetic.

31. β-blockers may worsen symptoms in patients with which of the following diseases?

A. Asthma.
B. Diarrhea.
C. Hypertension.
D. Gout.
E. Incontinence.

Unit II Answers and Explanations

1. D. Atropine is a muscarinic cholinergic receptor antagonist. Of the listed agents, acetylcholine is the only one that is an agonist at cholinergic receptors. Thus, atropine blocks the actions of acetylcholine at the muscarinic subtype of cholinergic receptor.

A. Dopamine is an agonist at dopaminergic receptors.

B. Norepinephrine is an agonist at adrenergic receptors.

C. Serotonin is an agonist at serotonin receptors.

E. Histamine is an agonist at histamine receptors.

2. A. Antimuscarinic anticholinergics may worsen glaucoma and are therefore contraindicated in patients with this condition.

B. Antimuscarinic anticholinergics tend to produce constipation, an effect that would be helpful in diarrhea, therefore it is not contraindicated for this condition.

C and D. Antimuscarinic anticholinergics have little or no effect on blood pressure and gout.

3. A. Treatment for organophosphate poisoning involves giving atropine to block the muscarinic effects plus pralidoxime to reactivate acetylcholinesterase thereby permitting acetylcholine degradation.

B. Nitroglycerine is a venodilator and hydrochlorothiazide is a thiazide diuretic. Neither are indicated for organophosphate poisoning.

C. Phenylephrine is a direct-acting α-adrenergic receptor agonist. Isoproterenol is a β_1- and β_2-adrenergic receptor agonist. Neither are indicated for organophosphate poisoning.

D. Propranolol is a nonselective β-adrenergic receptor antagonist. Theophylline is a drug used in asthma therapy that acts in many different ways, including being a β receptor agonist. Neither are indicated for organophosphate poisoning.

E. Tubocurarine is a nondepolarizing neuromuscular nicotinic receptor antagonist. Lidocaine is a local anesthetic agent.

4. B. Dopa decarboxylase catalyzes the conversion of dopa to dopamine.

5. C. Dopamine-β-hydroxylase catalyzes the conversion of dopamine to norepinephrine.

6. A. Tyrosine hydroxylase catalyzes the conversion of tyrosine to dopa.

7. D. Phenylethanolamine-N-methyltransferase (PMNT) catalyzes the conversion of norepinephrine to epinephrine.

8. A. The rate-limiting step in catecholamine synthesis is conversion of tyrosine to dopa by tyrosine hydroxylase.

9. B. Activation of α_2 receptors located on presynaptic terminals of sympathetic neurons inhibits the release of norepinephrine (▶ Table 4.2).

A. Stimulation of α_1 receptors causes vasoconstriction.

C. Stimulation of β_1 receptors increases heart rate, force, and velocity of contraction.

D. Stimulation of β_2 receptors causes bronchodilation.

10. B. Clonidine is a selective α_2 agonist that acts in the CNS to decrease sympathetic outflow to the periphery. This decreased sympathetic tone leads to decreased blood pressure by lowering total peripheral resistance.

11. C. Norepinephrine increases blood pressure by activation of α_1 receptors thereby producing vasoconstriction. Its release is regulated by presynaptic α_2 receptors. Prazosin is an α_1 receptor antagonist that blocks the blood pressure effects of norepinephrine but does not interfere with its presynaptic actions.

A. Dopamine increases blood pressure by acting on α_1 receptors to produce vasoconstriction.

B. Terbutaline is a β_2 receptor agonist used as a bronchodilator that produces minimal effects on blood pressure.

D. Pindolol is a nonselective β-adrenergic receptor antagonist.

12. C. Urinary outflow is regulated by norepinephrine acting on α_1-adrenergic receptors on the bladder sphincter causing contraction. Doxazosin is an antagonist at α_1-adrenergic receptors and will, therefore, cause dilation of the bladder sphincter, decreasing outflow obstruction, and increasing urine flow rates.

A. Clonidine is a selective α_2 agonist that acts in the CNS to decrease sympathetic outflow to the periphery. This decreased sympathetic tone leads to decreased BP by lowering total peripheral resistance. It does not decrease outflow obstruction and increase urinary flow rates.

B. Epinephrine stimulates α_1, α_2 and β_2 adrenoceptors and so would contribute to the contraction of the bladder sphincter, not lessen it (via α_1 effects).

D. Pyridostigmine is an indirect-acting parasympathomimetic that inhibits acetylcholinesterase, thereby increasing concentrations of acetylcholine, and enhancing cholinergic function. It does not decrease outflow obstruction or increase urinary flow rates.

E. Yohimbine is an α_2 receptor antagonist. It has no important clinical use.

13. B. Bethanechol is a direct-acting parasympathomimetic at muscarinic receptors on the bladder sphincter and detrusor muscle. Activation of these receptors will cause relaxation of the sphincter and contraction of the detrusor muscle that expels urine, thus increasing urinary flow.

A. Atropine is a muscarinic cholinergic receptor antagonist which would have the opposite effects to bethanechol.

C. Succinylcholine is a nicotinic receptor antagonist at the neuromuscular junction.

D. Trimethaphan blocks nicotinic receptors of both sympathetic and parasympathetic ganglia.

14. B. Propranolol is a nonselective β-adrenergic receptor antagonist. Atropine is a muscarinic cholinergic receptor antagonist. These agents are given to prevent reflex changes in cardiac output in response to phenylephrine. Phenylephrine will increase BP by direct activation of α_1-adrenergic receptors. This will increase the baroreceptor firing rate (I) and activate the baroreceptor reflex, leading to decreased sympathetic outflow (II, III) and increased parasympathetic outflow (IV).

15. B. The addition of reserpine, which prevents storage and causes depletion of neuronal norepinephrine, will have no effect on the response to phenylephrine, which acts directly on α_1-adrenergic receptors.

16. E. Hexamethonium is a ganglionic blocking agent that blocks nicotinic receptors of both sympathetic and parasympathetic ganglia, so there will be no change in postganglionic sympathetic nerve activity.

17. A. Phenoxybenzamine is an irreversible noncompetitive antagonist at both α_1- and α_2-adrenergic receptors. It will thus prevent phenylephrine from having any effect.

18. C. Botulinum toxin, which is produced by Clostridium botulinum, works by preventing the release of the neurotransmitter acetylcholine at the neuromuscular junction.

A. Succinylcholine is a depolarizing neuromuscular blocking agent that persistently activates nicotinic receptors.

B. Cocaine is a dopamine and norepinephrine reuptake inhibitor.

D. Muscarine is a muscarinic cholinergic receptor agonist.

E. Atropine is a muscarinic cholinergic receptor antagonist.

19. A. Acetylcholine is rapidly hydrolyzed by acetylcholinesterase.

B. Succinylcholine is resistant to hydrolysis by acetylcholinesterase. It is degraded more slowly by plasma cholinesterase.

C, D. Neither tubocurarine nor epinephrine is a substrate for acetylcholinesterase.

20. E. Cocaine, a catecholamine reuptake inhibitor, will potentiate the actions of norepinephrine by increasing its lifetime in the synapse and will block the actions of tyramine by preventing its uptake, which is required for it to exert its effects.

A-C. Metoprolol, propranolol, and phentolamine are all antagonists to norepinephrine at their respective receptors.

D. Monoamine oxidase inhibitors, e.g., pargyline, will potentiate norepinephrine by inhibiting its degradation. However, these agents also block the catabolism of tyramine and so they also potentiate its cardiovascular actions.

21. A. Termination of norepinephrine action is mainly by specific reuptake mechanisms into sympathetic nerves.

B and C. Metabolism by monoamine oxidase or catechol-0-methyltransferase occurs secondary to reuptake.

D and E. Some diffusion of norepinephrine into surrounding tissue and blood occurs but this is minor.

22. C. Glycopyrrolate is a muscarinic cholinergic receptor antagonist that is unable to cross the blood-brain barrier (quaternary ammonium compound) and therefore does not act in the CNS.

A. Scopolamine is a competitive antagonist at muscarinic receptors that has CNS effects.

B. Hexamethonium blocks nicotinic receptors of both sympathetic and parasympathetic ganglia.

D. Atropine is a muscarinic cholinergic receptor antagonist that has CNS effects.

E. Succinylcholine is a nicotinic receptor antagonist at the neuromuscular junction.

23. E. Succinylcholine is a nicotinic receptor antagonist at the neuromuscular junction. It acts by persistently activating these nicotinic receptors, leading to initial target stimulation followed by persistent desensitization.

A. Curare is a non-depolarizing neuromuscular blocking agent.

B. Hexamethonium blocks nicotinic receptors of both sympathetic and parasympathetic ganglia.

C. Scopolamine is a muscarinic cholinergic receptor antagonist.

D. Atropine is a muscarinic cholinergic receptor antagonist.

24. C. Amphetamine is a mixed-acting sympathomimetic that includes among its actions inhibition of the reuptake of released norepinephrine.

A and B. Propranolol is a nonselective β1-adrenergic antagonist and metoprolol is a selective β1-adrenergic antagonist. Both of these agents will inhibit the actions of norepinephrine at β1 receptors in the heart.

D. Succinylcholine is a nicotinic receptor antagonist at the neuromuscular junction that has no effect on norepinephrine.

25. D. Muscarinic cholinergic receptors are located on postganglionic parasympathetic neurons. These receptors are activated by acetylcholine and muscarine.

A, B, and C. The cholinergic receptors at sympathetic ganglia, parasympathetic ganglia, and the neuromuscular junction are nicotinic receptors, which are not activated by muscarine.

26. C. The β1 subtype of adrenergic receptors predominates on cardiac muscle. Activation of these receptors increases heart rate, force of contraction, and velocity of conduction.

A. α1 receptors predominate on vascular smooth muscle where activation leads to vasoconstriction.

B. α_2 receptors are located on sympathetic preganglionic terminals. Activation inhibits the release of norepinephrine.

D. β_2 receptors are located mainly in the lungs and their activation causes bronchodilation.

E. Activation of muscarinic receptors in the heart has negative inotropic, chronotropic, and dromotropic effects.

27. D. The β_2 subtype of adrenergic receptors predominates on bronchial smooth muscle. Activation of these receptors leads to relaxation of the smooth muscle (bronchodilation).

A. $\alpha 1$ receptors predominate on vascular smooth muscle where activation leads to vasoconstriction.

B. α_2 receptors are located on sympathetic preganglionic terminals. Activation inhibits the release of norepinephrine.

C. The $\beta 1$ subtype of adrenergic receptors predominates on cardiac muscle. Activation of these receptors increases heart rate, force of contraction, and velocity of conduction.

E. In the lung, activation of muscarinic receptors produces vasoconstriction.

28. B. Bethanechol is a direct-acting parasympathomimetic at muscarinic receptors on the bladder sphincter and detrusor muscle. Activation of these receptors will cause relaxation of the sphincter and contraction of the detrusor muscle that expels urine, thus increasing urinary flow.

A. Atropine is a muscarinic cholinergic receptor antagonist which would have the opposite effects to bethanechol.

C. Succinylcholine is a nicotinic receptor antagonist at the neuromuscular junction.

D. Trimethaphan blocks nicotinic receptors of both sympathetic and parasympathetic ganglia.

29. A. Parathion is an indirect-acting parasympathomimetic which inhibits acetylcholinesterase, thereby increasing concentrations of acetylcholine and enhancing cholinergic function.

B. Epinephrine will activate all of the physiologic responses of the sympathetic division of the autonomic nervous system.

C. Muscarine will activate all of the physiologic responses of the parasympathetic division of the autonomic nervous system shown that are mediated by muscarinic receptors.

D. Norepinephrine will activate all of the physiologic responses of the sympathetic division of the autonomic nervous system except those mediated by β_2 or β_3 receptors.

E. Serotonin will activate receptors in the CNS, gastrointestinal tract, and on vascular smooth muscle.

30. B. Myasthenia gravis is an autoimmune disease in which autoantibodies bind to nicotinic receptors at the neuromuscular junction rendering them unable to bind acetylcholine. The short-acting cholinesterase inhibitor edrophonium will improve muscle strength in untreated myasthenia gravis by increasing concentrations of acetylcholine and enhancing cholinergic function and is therefore used for diagnosis of the condition.

31. A. β_2-adrenergic receptors on airway smooth muscle mediate bronchodilation. Blocking these receptors with a β-blocker could worsen the symptoms of asthma.

B–D. β-adrenergic receptors do not have a significant role in these disorders and β-blockers would not worsen them.

Unit III

Drugs Acting on the Central Nervous System

By Edwin C. Johnson

III

7 Neuropharmacological Principles

Summary

Understanding the general physiologic and pharmacologic features of the central nervous system (CNS) is essential to understanding CNS pharmacology. Most neuropharmacological drugs act on ion channels, neurotransmitter receptors, or neurotransmitter uptake mechanisms in the brain. The major CNS neurotransmitters are dopamine, norepinephrine, serotonin, acetylcholine, glutamate, aspartate, gamma-aminobutyric acid (GABA), and glycine. Neuropeptide neurotransmitters (comprising 3–100 amino acids) are found in much lower concentrations than amino acid and amine transmitters. Important neuropeptide receptors at which recent CNS-acting drugs are based include: angiotensin, bradykinin, melatonin, opioids, orexin, and tachykinin receptors. Neuropeptide receptors with drugs in discovery or development stages include corticotropin-releasing factor receptors, melanocortin receptors, and tachykinin receptors.

Keywords: synaptic transmission, neurotransmitter, receptors

7.1 Neuropharmacological Principles

Understanding the general physiologic and pharmacologic features of the CNS is essential to understanding the pharmacotherapy of CNS diseases. Since altered function of neurons in the brain underlies essentially all diseases of the CNS, most neuropharmacological drugs act on ion channels, neurotransmitter receptors, or neurotransmitter uptake mechanisms in the brain.

7.2 General Features of Central Neurotransmitters

Nearly all drugs that act on the CNS, except perhaps general anesthetics and ethanol, have specific effects on certain neurotransmitter systems, some of which have been discussed in the previous unit. They can be classified according to their action at a given synapse as excitatory (generally depolarizing), inhibitory (generally hyperpolarizing), or modulatory (conditional). Modulatory actions explain why a given neurotransmitter does not necessarily produce the same effect at all sites; for example, norepinephrine relaxes bronchial smooth muscle but increases contraction of the heart.

Clinical Correlation

Synaptic Plasticity

Neurons are not static, and, in addition to the primary responses to drugs, they undergo several longer-term synaptic changes in response to drugs. These changes may include receptor downregulation, receptor upregulation, and changes in intracellular signal transduction processes. At present, synaptic plasticity is not exploited as a mechanism of drug action, but it is a definite result of drug use, especially long-term use, and may contribute to the clinical development of tolerance and dependence.

7.3 Specific Central Neurotransmitters

This section discusses neurotransmitters that specifically act on the CNS. The effects of these and other CNS neurotransmitters, as well as their receptors, are summarized in ▶ Fig. 7.1.

7.3.1 Dopamine

Dopamine is also discussed in Chapter 6.1, Catecholamine Sympathomimetics.

Receptors

There are five types of dopamine receptors located on postsynaptic cells and as autoreceptors on dopamine neurons. Termed D_1 to D_5, these are G protein-coupled receptors (GPCRs) (▶ Fig. 7.2).

Pathways and Functions

The major relevant functions of dopamine are correlated with the three major dopaminergic tracts in the brain (▶ Fig. 7.4).

- *Nigrostriatal:* Dopamine-containing neurons in the substantia nigra project to the striatum (caudate and putamen). This tract is concerned with initiation and execution of movement. The loss of neurons in the substantia nigra is observed when motor symptoms of Parkinson disease have developed.
- *Mesolimbic-mesocortical:* Dopamine-containing neurons in the ventral tegmental area project to the nucleus accumbens (mesolimbic) and prefrontal cortex (mesocortical). These tracts are involved in emotions and the organization of thoughts; they are implicated in schizophrenia and addictive disorders.
- *Tuberoinfundibular:* Dopamine-containing neurons in the arcuate nucleus of the hypothalamus project to the portal vessels of the infundibulum or pituitary stalk, where dopamine inhibits prolactin secretion. Dopamine receptor antagonists can, therefore, cause mild hyperprolactinemia.

Clinical Correlation

Parkinson Disease

Parkinson disease is a chronic, progressive, age-related neurodegenerative disease resulting from the loss of dopamine-containing neurons in the substantia nigra. Symptoms usually start between 60 and 70 years of age and include a "pill-rolling" tremor, rigidity (limbs resist extension throughout movement), and bradykinesia (slow execution of movement and speech), resulting in a masklike face and shuffling gait. There are many drug treatment options for Parkinson disease. Levodopa is a dopamine precursor that is converted to dopamine in the brain by dopa decarboxylase. Levodopa is often used in combination with carbidopa, a drug that prevents the peripheral conversion of levodopa to dopamine by inhibiting dopa decarboxylase. Dopamine agonists (e.g., bromocriptine) mimic the effects of

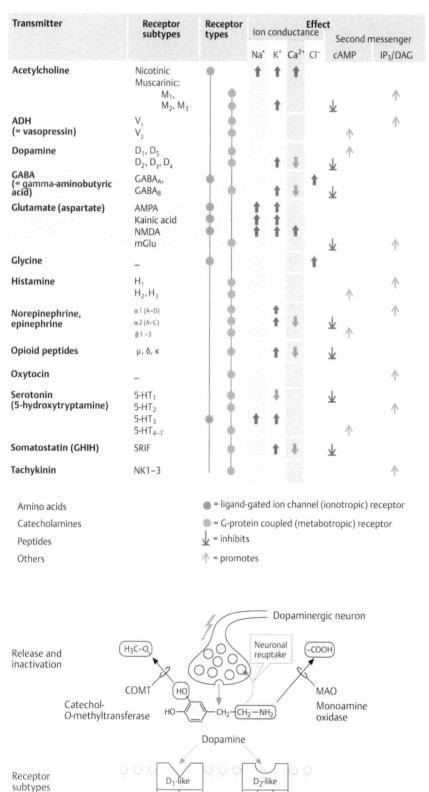

Fig. 7.1 Neurotransmitters in the central nervous system.
Most receptors for neurotransmitters in the central nervous system are metabotropic (G-protein mediated), and the effects seen are due to differences in ion conductance and signal transduction via second messengers. ADH, antidiuretic hormone; AMPA, α-amino-3-hydroxy-5-methyl-4-isoxazolepropionic acid; ATP, adenosine triphosphate; cAMP, cyclic adenosine monophosphate; DAG, diacylglycerol; IP$_3$, inositol 1,4,5-triphosphate; mGlu, metabotropic glutamic acid; NMDA, N-methyl-D-aspartate; PIP, phosphatidylinositol 4-phosphate; GHIH, growth hormone inhibiting hormone; SRIF, somatotropin release-inhibiting factor.

Legend:
- ● = ligand-gated ion channel (ionotropic) receptor
- ● = G-protein coupled (metabotropic) receptor
- ↓ = inhibits
- ↑ = promotes

Categories: Amino acids, Catecholamines, Peptides, Others

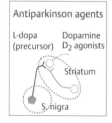
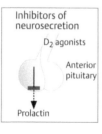
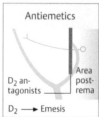
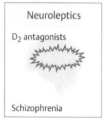

Release and inactivation — Dopaminergic neuron; Neuronal reuptake; H$_3$C–O; –COOH; COMT Catechol-O-methyltransferase; MAO Monoamine oxidase; Dopamine

Receptor subtypes — D$_1$-like: D$_1$, D$_5$; D$_2$-like: D$_2$, D$_3$, D$_4$

Drugs:
- Antiparkinson agents: L-dopa (precursor), Dopamine D$_2$ agonists; Striatum; S. nigra
- Inhibitors of neurosecretion: D$_2$ agonists; Anterior pituitary; Prolactin
- Antiemetics: D$_2$ antagonists; Area postrema; D$_2$ → Emesis
- Neuroleptics: D$_2$ antagonists; Schizophrenia

Fig. 7.2 Dopamine release, inactivation, and pharmacological uses.
Dopamine is released from dopaminergic neurons following an action potential. It then binds to two major types of receptors: D$_1$-like (subtypes D$_1$ and D$_5$), which increase cyclic adenosine monophosphate (cAMP), and D$_2$-like (subtypes D$_2$, D$_3$, and D$_4$), which decrease cAMP, so the differing effects of dopamine binding depend on signal transduction. Dopamine's action is terminated by reuptake into neurons, where it is stored in vesicles for reuse, or it is degraded by catechol-O-methyltransferase (COMT) or monoamine oxidase (MAO). D$_2$ agonists are used to treat Parkinson disease and to inhibit prolactin release, whereas D$_2$ antagonists are used as antiemetics and in the treatment of schizophrenia.

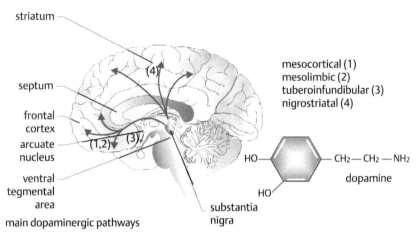

striatum

septum

frontal cortex

arcuate nucleus

ventral tegmental area

substantia nigra

main dopaminergic pathways

mesocortical (1)
mesolimbic (2)
tuberoinfundibular (3)
nigrostriatal (4)

dopamine

Fig. 7.3 Dopaminergic pathways in the brain.
(1) The mesocortical pathway projects from the ventral tegmental area (VTA) to the frontal cortex. (2) The mesolimbic system also originates in the VTA. It projects to several parts of the limbic system including the amygdala, frontal and cingulate cortex, nucleus accumbens olfactory tubercle and septum. (3) The tuberoinfundibular pathway is a short projection from the arcuate nucleus of the hypothalamus to the pituitary gland. (4) The nigrostriatal pathway projects from the substantia nigra to the putamen and caudate in the striatum.

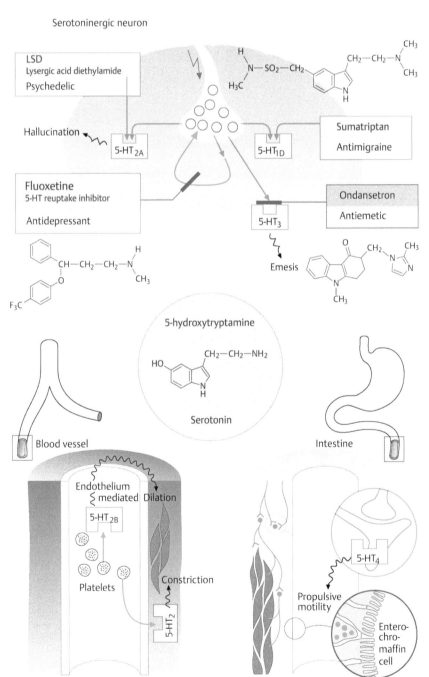

Serotoninergic neuron

LSD
Lysergic acid diethylamide
Psychedelic

Hallucination

Fluoxetine
5-HT reuptake inhibitor
Antidepressant

$5-HT_{2A}$

$5-HT_{1D}$

Sumatriptan
Antimigraine

Ondansetron
Antiemetic

$5-HT_3$

Emesis

5-hydroxytryptamine

Serotonin

Blood vessel

Intestine

Endothelium mediated Dilation

$5-HT_{2B}$

Platelets

Constriction

$5-HT_2$

Propulsive motility

$5-HT_4$

Entero-chromaffin cell

Fig. 7.4 Serotonin actions as influenced by drugs.
The effects of serotonin are complex because of the number of receptor subtypes and the differing, and sometimes opposing, effects at each subtype. In blood vessels, for example, serotonin acts on 5-hydroxytryptamine type 2 ($5-HT_2$) receptors to produce vasoconstriction, but it can also act via $5-HT_{2B}$ receptors to cause the release of vaso-relaxant mediators from vascular endothelium, resulting in vasodilation. In the bowel, serotonin acts on $5-HT_4$ receptors to increase gut motility. Serotonin is involved in many aspects of brain functioning, and as such, many of its central actions are affected by drugs. Serotonin agonists are used to treat migraine and are used recreationally as psychedelic drugs. Fluoxetine, which blocks serotonin reuptake, is used as an antidepressant. All the 5HT receptors are GPCRs except $5HT_3$, which is a ligand-gated cation channel. Ondansetron is an antagonist at the $5-HT_3$ receptor and is used to treat emesis induced by cytotoxic drugs.

dopamine in the brain. Catechol-O-methyltransferase (COMT) inhibitors (e.g., entacapone) are used to prevent the peripheral breakdown of levodopa. Monoamine oxidase B (MAO-B) inhibitors (e.g., selegiline) prevent the breakdown of dopamine in the brain. Anticholinergic drugs (e.g., benztropine) may be given as an adjunct for the tremor (see Chapter 14).

7.3.2 Norepinephrine

Norepinephrine is also discussed in sections 4.2.2 and 6.1.1.

Pathways

The largest norepinephrine-containing nucleus in the brain is the locus coeruleus of the caudal pons (▶ Fig. 7.5). Ascending and descending fibers from the locus coeruleus are part of the reticular activating system, which is responsible for behavioral arousal and levels of awareness. It is also involved in mood and cognitive processes.

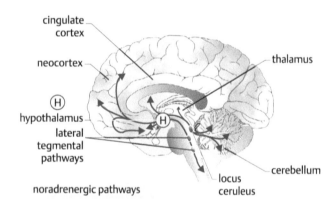

Fig. 7.5 Noradrenergic pathways in the brain.
The cell bodies of noradrenergic (norepinephrine)-containing neurons in the brain originate in the midbrain. Projections from cells in the locus coeruleus diverge to innervate thalamus, cortex, and cerebellum. Cell bodies in the lateral tegmentum innervate the hypothalamus, limbic system, and spinal cord.

Functions

Norepinephrine may be involved in depression, anxiety, and panic disorders.

7.3.3 Serotonin

Serotonin (5-hydroxytryptamine [5-HT]) is also discussed in Chapter 32.

Synthesis

Serotonin is synthesized from tryptophan by tryptophan hydroxylase and metabolized by oxidative deamination via monoamine oxidase.

Receptors

Serotonin receptors are located both pre- and postsynaptically. Major groups 5-HT$_1$ to 5-HT$_7$ have been identified, and there are further subtypes. They are all GPCRs except 5-HT$_3$, which is a ligand-gated ion channel.

Pathways

Cell bodies are located in the raphe nuclei of the brainstem. Descending systems innervate all spinal cord levels. Ascending systems innervate the cerebellum, substantia nigra, limbic system, and cortex (▶ Fig. 7.7).

Functions

Ascending systems are involved in the promotion of sleep, in determining mood, and in mental illness (through interactions in limbic areas). Descending 5-HT systems may be involved in modulating pain perception. ▶ Fig. 7.5 illustrates some of the actions of serotonin and how various pharmacological agents influence serotonin levels to produce their effects.

7.3.4 Acetylcholine

This neurotransmitter was discussed in section 4.2.1 in relation to its action in the peripheral nervous system, but acetylcholine also has an important role as a neurotransmitter in the CNS.

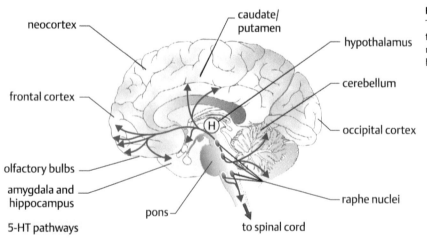

Fig. 7.6 Serotonergic pathways in the brain.
The cell bodies of serotonin-containing neurons in the brain originate in the raphe nuclei of the midbrain and send widespread projections to higher and lower centers.

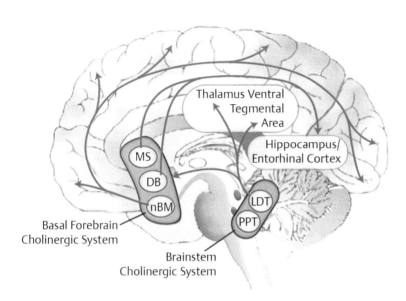

Fig. 7.7 Cholinergic pathways in the CNS.
There are two major acetylcholinergic projection systems in the brain, the magnocellular basal forebrain cholinergic system and the brainstem cholinergic system. The magnocellular basal forebrain cholinergic system includes the medial septal nucleus (MS), the vertical and horizontal limbs of the diagonal band of Broca (DB), and the nucleus basalis magnocellularis (nBM). The horizontal limb of the DB and nBM has extensive diffuse projections to neocortex as well as projections to basolateral amygdala and olfactory bulb (these latter two are not shown here). The MS and vertical limb of the DB project to hippocampus and entorhinal cortices. The brainstem cholinergic system includes the pedunculopontine tegmental nucleus (PPT) and laterodorsal pontine tegmentum (LDT) and projects predominantly to the thalamus but also to the basal forebrain region.

III

Receptors

Both nicotinic (ligand-gated cation channels) and muscarinic (GPCRs) receptors are found in the brain, but 95% of acetylcholine receptors in the brain are muscarinic. Acetylcholine may have excitatory or inhibitory actions in the brain.

Pathways

There are three acetylcholinergic projection systems in the brain (▶ Fig. 7.7). One major projection from the nucleus basalis of Meynert projects throughout the cortex. Another projection has cell bodies in the pedunculopontine nucleus and projects to the thalamus. The third are interneurons residing in the basal ganglia.

Functions

The result of loss of cholinergic neurons depends on the site. A global loss throughout the cortex results in senile dementia of the Alzheimer type, degeneration of acetylcholine neurons in the lateral horn of the spinal cord results in amyotrophic lateral sclerosis (ALS), and degeneration of cholinergic and GABA neurons in the striatum results in Huntington disease.

Clinical Correlation

Huntington Disease

Huntington disease is a rare autosomal dominant neurodegenerative disorder that usually starts in middle age. Its onset is insidious, but the course of the disease progresses with chorea (involuntary, continuous jerky movements), personality change, dementia, and death. There is no cure or any treatment to prevent progression of this disease.

7.3.5 Glutamate and Aspartate

Amino acids are the major transmitters in the CNS in terms of percentage of synapses at which they are transmitters.

Synthesis

Glutamate and aspartate are synthesized from glucose and other precursors by several routes.

Receptors

Glutamate acts on glutamate receptors in the brain. There are two types of glutamate receptors: ionotropic and metabotropic.

Ionotropic Glutamate Receptors

There are three types of cationic ionotropic glutamate receptors; they are classified according to the amino acid that is most potent at that receptor.

- *N-methyl-D-aspartate* (*NMDA*) receptors are heterodimers or heterotrimers of GluN1, GluN2A, GluN2B, GluN2C, GluN2D, GluN3A, and GluN3B subunits.
- *α-amino-3-hydroxy-5-methyl-4-isoxazolepropionic* (*AMPA*) receptors are homomers or heteromers of GluA1, GluA2, GluA3, and GluA4 subunits.
- *Kainate* receptors are homomers of GluK1, GluK2, or GluK3 subunits.

These receptors are said to be "excitotoxic," as their prolonged activation increases the entry of cations, including Ca^{2+}, into the cell leading to depolarization. The AMPA receptors are the primary excitatory postsynaptic receptors in the CNS. High intracellular Ca^{2+} levels trigger a cascade of events leading to neurotoxicity.

Metabotropic Glutamate Receptors

These are G protein-coupled glutamate receptors, including mGlu1, 2, 3, 4, 5, 6, 7, and 8.

Pathways

Essentially all of the excitatory pathways in the CNS are glutamatergic (▶ Fig. 7.3).

Functions

Glutamate are powerful excitatory amino acid transmitters. Excessive activation of the ionotropic receptors (particularly NMDA and AMPA) may lead to excitotoxicity.

Foundations

Fate of GABA

Free GABA can be transaminated by GABA aminotransferase (GABA-T) to form succinic semialdehyde (only if α-ketoglutarate is the acceptor of the amine group). Succinic semialdehyde is oxidized to succinic acid by succinic semialdehyde dehydrogenase (SSADH) to reenter the Krebs cycle. This transforms α-ketoglutarate into glutamate. GABA can be packaged into synaptic vesicles for release and is picked up by glial cells. GABA-T transaminates to glutamate. Glial cells lack GAD, so glutamate is transformed by glutamine synthetase to glutamine before being transported back to the nerve ending (▶ Fig. 7.7). Glutaminase converts glutamine back to glutamate. GABA-T and SSADH are attached to mitochondria. Glutaminase, glutamic acid decarboxylase (GAD), and glutamine synthetase are cytoplasmic. GAD occurs only in neurons, glutamine synthetase only in glia, and glutaminase in both.

Foundations

Krebs Cycle

The Krebs cycle (also known as the citric acid cycle/tricarboxylic acid cycle) is one of the metabolic pathways involved in the conversion of carbohydrates, fats, and proteins into carbon dioxide, water, and adenosine triphosphate (ATP) in aerobic organisms. Throughout the cycle, many compounds are produced that are the precursors for other substances needed in the body.

7.3.6 GABA

Synthesis

Glucose is probably the principal in vivo source of GABA. There is a GABA "shunt" of the Krebs cycle whereby α-ketoglutarate is transaminated to glutamic acid by GABA-T. Glutamic acid is decarboxylated by GAD to GABA. This process converts glutamate, the principal excitatory neurotransmitter, into the principal inhibitory neurotransmitter, GABA. There is 200 to 1000 times more GABA in the brain than dopamine, norepinephrine, serotonin, or acetylcholine.

Receptors

- $GABA_A$ receptors are postsynaptically located, multisubunit, ligand-gated ion channels. Activation leads to opening of a Cl⁻ channel and synaptic inhibition.
- $GABA_B$ receptors are GPCRs located on presynaptic terminals. Activation results in decreased release of GABA and other neurotransmitters from the terminal on which these receptors are located.

Pathways

- GABA is the neurotransmitter of inhibitory interneurons found throughout the cerebral and cerebellar cortices and spinal cord.
- It is also found in neurons projecting from the globus pallidus and substantia nigra to the thalamus and from the striatum to the globus pallidus and substantia nigra (▶ Fig. 7.8).

Functions

GABA accounts for most of the direct inhibitory action in the brain. It is also involved in inhibitory motor control in the spinal cord and is thus directly responsible for the regulation of muscle tone. Drugs that enhance GABA-mediated neurotransmission (e.g., benzodiazepines and barbiturates) are used as anxiolytic, sedative, and anticonvulsant drugs.

7.3.7 Glycine

Synthesis

Glycine is formed from serine by the enzyme serine hydroxymethyltransferase.

Pathways

Glycine is released by the inhibitory interneurons that are activated by Ia muscle afferents.

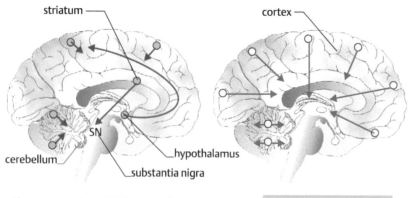

striatum
cortex
cerebellum
SN
hypothalamus
substantia nigra

pathways   ○→ GABAergic pathway   ○→ glutamate pathway

Fig. 7.8 GABAergic and glutamatergic pathways in the central nervous system.
Gamma-aminobutyric acid is found in inhibitory interneurons throughout the cerebral and cerebellar cortices. It is also found in neurons projecting from the striatum to the substantia nigra. Excitatory glutamatergic pathways project from the cortex and hippocampus to other parts of the brain.

Receptors

Glycine binds to glycine receptors. These receptors can be blocked by strychnine. There is also a glycine binding site on the NR1 subunit of NMDA receptors; glycine is coreleased with glutamate at excitatory synapses.

Functions

- Inhibitory motor control in the spinal cord as well as the inferior and superior colliculi.
- At postsynaptic excitatory membranes, glycine (and serine) acts as a coagonist of NMDA receptors.

▶ Table 7.1 provides a summary of the CNS neurotransmitters.

7.3.8 Neuropeptides

Neuropeptide neurotransmitters (comprising 3–100 amino acids) are found in much lower concentrations than amino acid and amine transmitters. They are formed by cleavage of larger molecules and are frequently colocalized with other peptides or with amino acid or amine transmitters. They have no reuptake mechanisms and are generally broken down by peptidases. Neuropeptides are frequently colocalized in, and coreleased from, neurons that also contain one of the smaller molecule neurotransmitters mentioned above.

Important neuropeptide receptors at which recent CNS-acting drugs are based include the following:
- Angiotensin receptors: AT_1, AT_2.
- Bradykinin receptors: B_1, B_2.
- Melatonin receptors: MT_1, MT_2.
- Opioid receptors: See Chapter 13.
- Orexin receptors: OX_1 and OX_2.

Neuropeptide receptors with drugs in discovery or development stages are as follows:
- Corticotropin-releasing factor receptors: CRF_1, CRF_2.
- Melanocortin receptors: MC_1 to MC_5.
- Tachykinin receptors: NK_1, NK_2, NK_3.

Table 7.1 Summary of central neurotransmitters

CNS neurotransmitter	Classification	Receptors	Signal transduction	Functions	Diseases/disorders
Dopamine	Modulatory	D_1–D_5	G protein-coupled receptors	Initiation and execution of movement; Emotions and organization of thought; Inhibition of prolactin	Parkinson disease, schizophrenia, and affective disorders
Norepinephrine	Modulatory	Adrenergic receptors: alpha 1 (A, B, C), alpha 2 (A, B, C) and beta 1, 2, 3	G protein-coupled receptors	Behavioral arousal and levels of awareness	Depression, anxiety, and panic disorders
Serotonin	Modulatory	$5\text{-}HT_1$ to $5\text{-}HT_7$	Most are G protein-coupled receptors; $5\text{-}HT_3$ is a ligand-gated ion channel	Ascending systems: promotion of sleep, in determining mood, and in mental illness; Descending 5-HT systems: modulating pain perception	Depression, emesis
Acetylcholine	Modulatory	95% are muscarinic (M1–M5), but there are nicotinic (alpha1–10, beta 1, 2, 4, 5) receptors	Muscarinic receptors are G protein-coupled; Nicotinic receptors are ligand-gated ion channels	Primarily in interneurons	Alzheimer disease, amyotrophic lateral sclerosis, Huntington disease
Glutamate	Excitatory	Ionotropic glutamate receptors and metabotropic glutamate receptors; *NMDA: NR1, NR2A, B, C, and D, NR3*; • AMPA: GluR1, 2, 3, and 4; • Kainate: GluR5, 6, and 7; KA1, KA2; • mGlu1–8	Ligand-gated ion channels; G protein-coupled	Major excitatory neurotransmitter in CNS	Epilepsy, schizophrenia
GABA	Inhibitory	$GABA_A$, $GABA_B$	Ligand-gated ion channels; G protein-coupled	Most inhibitory action in the CNS; Inhibitory motor control in the spinal cord; Regulation of muscle tone	Huntington disease
Glycine	Inhibitory	Glycine receptors	Ligand-gated ion channels	Inhibitory motor control in the spinal cord	

Abbreviations: AMPA, α-amino-3-hydroxy-5-methyl-4-isoxazolepropionic; CNS, central nervous system; GABA, gamma-aminobutyric acid; 5-HT, 5-hydroxytryptamine; NMDA, N-methyl-D-aspartate.

Table 7.2 Drug-sensitive sites in synaptic transmission

Site	Example	Therapeutic use
Electrically excitable ion channels (includes voltage-dependent Na^+, K^+, and Ca^{2+} channels)	Na^+ channels blocked by local anesthetics	Pain reduction
Chemically regulated ion channels (includes ligand-gated channels that are nicotinic, cholinergic, glutamate, and $GABA_A$ receptors)	Benzodiazepines increase Cl^- conductance of the $GABA_A$ receptor	Treatment of anxiety
Presynaptic synthetic pathways	Levodopa to increase dopamine levels	Parkinson disease
Transmitter reuptake mechanisms in neurons and glia	SSRIs	Treatment of depression
Extracellular and glial degradative enzymes	Acetylcholinesterase inhibitors block acetylcholine hydrolysis	Alzheimer disease
G protein-coupled membrane receptors (include norepinephrine, dopamine, serotonin, muscarinic cholinergic, $GABA_B$, and neuropeptide receptors)	Morphine	Pain reduction

Abbreviations: GABA, gamma-aminobutyric acid; SSRI, selective serotonin reuptake inhibitor.

▸ Table 7.2 lists some common drug-sensitive sites in synaptic transmission. The drugs and the conditions for which they are given are discussed in more detail in the following chapters in this unit.

8 Anesthetic Drugs

Summary

Surgical anesthesia is achieved through the combined use of general anesthetics, local anesthetics, muscle relaxants, and other agents. The major anesthetic gases include the halogenated hydrocarbons (halothane, isoflurane, desflurane, and sevoflurane), nitrous oxide, and the noble gas xenon. Propofol is an intravenous (IV) anesthetic agent used for general anesthesia and anesthetic induction. Ketamine is a "dissociative anesthetic" that is used for induction and maintenance of general anesthesia. The barbiturates thiopental, thiamylal, and methohexital are used for induction of anesthesia. The benzodiazepines diazepam, midazolam, and lorazepam are used as anesthetic premedications to produce sedation and amnesia. Etomidate is an IV anesthetic with minimal cardiovascular adverse effects and could be an agent of use for patients with cardiovascular issues. The neuromuscular blocking agents complement the efficacy of anesthesia by enhancing muscle relaxation and reducing the dose needed of other anesthetic agents. These agents include the depolarizing agents such as succinylcholine and nondepolarizing agents such as pancuronium. Local anesthetics produce a lack of sensation in a localized area of the body. These include lidocaine, articaine, and bupivacaine, which are amides, and benzocaine, procaine, and tetracaine, which are esters.

Keywords: local anesthetics, inhalation agents, intravenous anesthetics, surgical anesthesia, MAC

8.1 Anesthetic Drugs

Anesthesia is defined as the lack of sensation. Surgical anesthesia is achieved through the combined use of general anesthetics, local anesthetics, muscle relaxants, and other agents. The ideal general anesthetic agent(s) would produce unconsciousness, analgesia, amnesia, and muscle relaxation with no untoward side effects or toxicities (▶ Fig. 8.1).

Anesthetics developed to date are not ideal and are typically administered in combination with numerous other preoperative and postoperative medications, known as "adjuncts to anesthesia," in order to achieve the desired effects (see ▶ Table 8.1). The pharmacology of these adjuncts has been discussed in detail in other chapters, as cited in the table. This chapter covers inhalation agents, IV agents, and local anesthetics.

8.2 Inhalation Agents

The major anesthetic gases include several halogenated hydrocarbons (halothane, isoflurane, desflurane, and sevoflurane), nitrous oxide, and recently the noble gas xenon. These agents act in the brain to produce surgical anesthesia, but the precise mechanism of action for these agents and specific receptors with which these agents interact are not known. The pharmacokinetics of these agents is unique because they are administered as gases and exert their pharmacologic effects in gaseous form. Thus, the important factor for determining the level of anesthetic effect is the partial pressure or tension of the anesthetic gas. The standard for anesthetic dosing is the minimal alveolar concentration (MAC), which is the alveolar concentration, expressed as a percentage of inspired gas, at which 50% of the patients fail to respond to a noxious stimulus. The MAC also determines the relative potency of a given anesthetic gas. Recovery from anesthesia of inhaled anesthetics is principally through exhalation-induced elimination; agents with the lowest blood-to-tissue ratio are eliminated most rapidly.

Table 8.1 Adjuncts to anesthetics

Desired effect	Drugs used (intravenously)	Example(s)
Induction of anesthesia	Propofol or ultra-short-acting barbiturate	Propofol, ketamine, and methohexital
Muscle relaxation	Depolarizing and nondepolarizing neuromuscular blocking agents	Succinylcholine, pancuronium
Analgesia	Short-acting, intravenous opiates	Fentanyl, morphine
Amnesia	Short-acting benzodiazepines (doses given are higher than anxiolytic doses)	Diazepam, midazolam, and lorazepam
Autonomic stabilization	Anticholinergic drugs, antiadrenergic drugs	Atropine and glycopyrrolate, esmolol

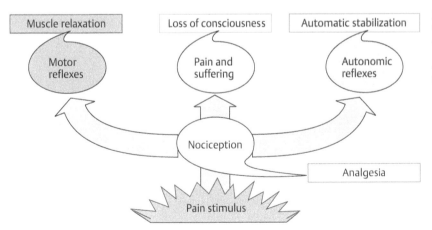

Fig. 8.1 Goals of surgical anesthesia. Commonly used agents as adjuncts to the general anesthetics include drugs that more selectively produce muscle relaxation, analgesia, loss of consciousness, amnesia, and autonomic stabilization.

8.2.1 Factors Influencing the Rate of Induction of Inhalation Anesthesia

▶ Table 8.2 discusses the factors influencing the rate of induction of inhalation anesthesia.

Effects

- All of the inhalation agents produce unconsciousness, amnesia, and analgesia. Most of these also decrease blood pressure, depress respiration, and increase intracranial pressure (with the exception of nitrous oxide and xenon). The relative analgesic and muscle relaxant effects and side effects are summarized in ▶ Table 8.3.
- The use of halogenated agents has been associated with rare cases of hyperkalemia and malignant hyperthermia, both of which require aggressive treatment.

Clinical Correlation

Malignant Hyperthermia

Malignant hyperthermia is a serious and rare complication of anesthesia with any volatile anesthetic but most commonly seen with halothane; it is believed to be a genetic, autosomal dominant disorder caused by a mutation of the ryanodine receptor type 1. The anesthetic produces a substantial increase in skeletal muscle oxidative metabolism, which consumes oxygen and causes a buildup of carbon dioxide. The body also loses its capacity to regulate the rapidly rising temperature (e.g., 1 °C/5 minutes). This can lead to circulatory collapse and death. Signs include muscular rigidity with accompanying acidosis, increased oxygen consumption, hypercapnia (increased carbon dioxide), tachycardia, and hyperthermia. Malignant hyperthermia may be treatable if dantrolene, a drug that reduces muscular contraction through blocking the ryanodine receptor and the hypermetabolic state, is given promptly as well as cessation of volatile anesthetic administration.

Table 8.2 Factors influencing the rate of induction of inhalation anesthesia

Factor	Explanation
Concentration of gas in inspired air	The higher the concentration of anesthetic in inspired air, the more rapid the increase in tension of anesthetic in the blood and therefore in the brain. In addition, administering an inhaled bolus of the agent can result in attaining the MAC more rapidly.
Ventilation rate and depth	Increased ventilation rate and depth lead to an increase in fresh gas in the alveoli and a higher alveolar concentration which lead to an increased rate of induction of anesthesia.
Blood solubility	The solubility of an anesthetic agent in the blood is a very important factor in determining the rate of induction of inhalation anesthesia. The blood:gas partition coefficient is the ratio of the concentration of anesthetic in the blood to the concentration of anesthetic gas at equilibrium. Note that anesthetic molecules that are dissolved in the blood are not exerting a partial pressure and therefore not contributing to anesthesia. Thus, an agent that has high blood solubility will show a slower increase in anesthetic tension and, therefore, a slower induction rate. Agents that are not very soluble in blood will have a much higher rate of induction of general anesthesia. Halothane has the highest blood:gas partition coefficient, followed by isoflurane, sevoflurane, and nitrous oxide, with desflurane having the lowest.
Blood flow	Uptake of anesthetic into tissues is dependent on blood flow to those tissues, so highly perfused organs (e.g., the brain) will see a more rapid rise in anesthetic tension.
Tissue solubility	In general, anesthetic gases are soluble in fatty tissues; therefore, the rate of rise of anesthetic tension in adipose tissue is slower than in lean tissues, such as the brain.[a]
Second gas	Adding a second anesthetic gas will result in a more rapid increase in alveolar concentration of both agents through a mass action effect.

[a]The brain is a lean, well-perfused organ; therefore, the rate of rise of anesthetic tension in the brain is rapid.

Table 8.3 Summary of analgesia, muscle relaxation, and side effects of inhalation agents

Agent	Analgesia	Muscle relaxation	Agent-specific side effects
Halothane	+ +	+	Sensitizes myocardium to catecholamines increasing possibility of arrhythmias and hepatotoxicity
Isoflurane	+ +	+ +	Decreased blood pressure can cause respiratory depression and tachycardia
Desflurane	+ +	+ +	May cause cough and laryngospasm, as it is an irritant to the upper respiratory tract; reduced blood pressure can result in respiratory depression tachycardia
Sevoflurane	+ +	+ +	None of note
Nitrous oxide	+ + + +	No effect	Contraindicated in cases of occluded middle ear and pneumothorax, as air pockets in the body may expand as larger amounts of nitrous oxide replace nitrogen
Xenon	+ + + + +	+ +	Interacts with rubber so must not be used with rubber instruments. Causes some respiratory depression and concomitant adverse events

8.2.2 Halogenated Hydrocarbons (Halothane, Isoflurane, Desflurane, Sevoflurane)

Uses

- All have modest to moderate analgesic and muscle relaxing properties.
- Sevoflurane is typically chosen for inhalation induction and maintenance.

Side Effects

- Most can cause respiratory depression, although halothane does not increase heart rate.
- Halothane (and isoflurane to some extent) increases cerebral blood flow and should be avoided in neurosurgery. In addition, prolonged use can cause hepatitis.

8.2.3 Nitrous Oxide

Uses

- Nitrous oxide is a good analgesic (produces superior analgesia than halogenated agents without decreases in blood pressure or depressed respiration).
- It does not produce surgical levels of anesthesia except with very high doses when oxygenation is inadequate, particularly because of its high MAC. It is, therefore, not used alone as an anesthetic agent but can be used as the sole agent for analgesia. It is frequently combined with one of the other anesthetic agents.

Side Effects

- It is always administered with 30 to 35% oxygen, as it can cause diffusion hypoxia.
- Long-term exposure to trace concentrations may cause pernicious anemia through bone marrow impairment and an increased incidence of spontaneous abortions.

Clinical Correlation

Diffusion Hypoxia with Nitrous Oxide

When nitrous oxide administration is terminated at the end of anesthesia, the concentration of nitrous oxide in the alveoli is lower than the blood. Consequently, it diffuses along this concentration gradient and enters into the lungs, displacing oxygen and nitrogen in the process. This causes a temporary diffusion hypoxia (lack of oxygen). To counteract this, patients are given 100% oxygen until the nitrous oxide is removed from the lungs by expiration.

8.2.4 Xenon

Properties

Lowest blood:gas partition coefficient results in fastest induction and recovery. With a moderate MAC, xenon can be more adequately combined with oxygen while maintaining anesthesia. It has quite strong analgesic properties. In addition, minimal or no reduction in blood pressure results in a better maintenance of arterial pressure; there is also evidence of neuroprotection with its use. Xenon interacts with rubber and cannot be used with any rubber instruments, and its cost is relatively high.

8.3 Intravenous Anesthetic Agents

8.3.1 Propofol

Mechanism of Action

The mechanism of action of propofol is not completely understood, but it is thought to work by enhancing gamma-aminobutyric acid (GABA)-mediated neuronal inhibition (via $GABA_A$ receptors) and possibly glycine-mediated inhibition, and it also blocks Na^+ channels (▶ Fig. 8.2).

Pharmacokinetics

- Given IV.
- Metabolized very rapidly by the liver and other organs.
- Rapid induction of anesthesia and recovery with little residual after effects due to this rapid metabolism.

Uses

- General anesthesia and anesthetic induction.
- Most effective choice for pulmonary intervention procedures.

Note: Propofol is a poor analgesic, so it must be supplemented with an analgesic.

Side Effects

- Of the induction agents, propofol has an overall cardiovascular depression resulting in a decrease in arterial and venous blood pressure (hypotension) and reduced heart rate and cardiac output. In addition, it causes strong pulmonary depression as well as inhibition of baroreceptors.
- Under rare situations with high propofol doses and/or long administration, "propofol infusion syndrome" can occur, resulting in severe bradycardia leading to asystole; and often it is associated with tissue damage in muscle or liver.

8.3.2 Ketamine

This is a "dissociative anesthetic" similar to the street drug phencyclidine (angel dust). Dissociative anesthetics make the patient feel dissociated from the environment and psychotic.

Mechanism of Action

The mechanism of action of ketamine is thought to be primarily through blocking excitatory N-methyl-D-aspartate receptor ion channels. This block is also believed to underlie its dissociative properties.

III

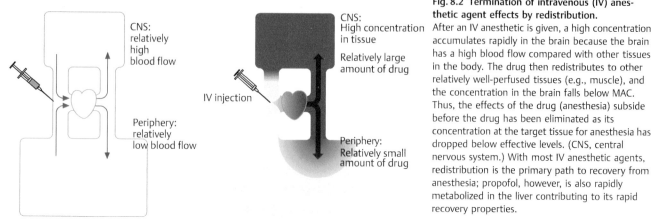

1. Initial situation

CNS: relatively high blood flow

Periphery: relatively low blood flow

IV injection

CNS: High concentration in tissue

Relatively large amount of drug

Periphery: Relatively small amount of drug

2. Preferential accumulation of drug in brain

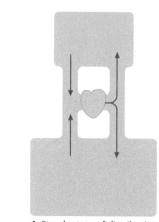

3. Redistribution

CNS: Decrease in tissue concentration

Periphery: Further increase in tissue concentration

4. Steady state of distribution

Fig. 8.2 Termination of intravenous (IV) anesthetic agent effects by redistribution. After an IV anesthetic is given, a high concentration accumulates rapidly in the brain because the brain has a high blood flow compared with other tissues in the body. The drug then redistributes to other relatively well-perfused tissues (e.g., muscle), and the concentration in the brain falls below MAC. Thus, the effects of the drug (anesthesia) subside before the drug has been eliminated as its concentration at the target tissue for anesthesia has dropped below effective levels. (CNS, central nervous system.) With most IV anesthetic agents, redistribution is the primary path to recovery from anesthesia; propofol, however, is also rapidly metabolized in the liver contributing to its rapid recovery properties.

Uses

- Induction and maintenance of general anesthesia particularly in emergency room surgery where positive cardiovascular properties are desired; it is not widely used due to side effects. In addition, ketamine is the agent of choice for some pediatric surgical procedures.

Effects

At anesthetic doses, it produces catatonia, analgesia, and amnesia.

Side Effects

- Disorientation and hallucinations.

8.3.3 Barbiturates (Thiopental, Thiamylal, and Methohexital)

These principally act through activating GABA-mediated neuronal inhibition.

Pharmacokinetics

- Unconsciousness occurs within the circulation time from arm to brain and is then maintained with an inhalation agent. Thiopental particularly has a slightly faster onset of action with IV bolus administration than propofol.
- Termination of central nervous system (CNS) action of the barbiturate is by redistribution of drug from the brain to other tissues (▶ Fig. 8.2) as well as by hepatic metabolism. These mechanisms are much slower than with propofol which can lead to a long-lasting hangover effect. Methohexital is metabolized markedly faster than thiopental.

Uses

- Induction of anesthesia.

Side Effects

- Respiratory and cardiovascular depression.

8.3.4 Benzodiazepines

These drugs are discussed in detail in Chapter 9.

Diazepam, Midazolam, and Lorazepam

Pharmacokinetics

- Given IV.

Uses

These agents are used as anesthetic premedications to produce sedation and amnesia.

8.3.5 Etomidate

Etomidate has minimal cardiovascular adverse effects and could be an agent of use for patients with cardiovascular issues. It is an imidazole and is thought to act by potentiation of GABA receptors. In addition, etomidate blocks the activity of CYP11B1 and 11-β-hydroxylase resulting in a drop in plasma levels of adrenal steroids; this is a very potent effect and prevents the use of etomidate in infusions. Nonetheless, the properties of etomidate often allow it to be the agent of choice in bolus injections for minor procedures including intubations and other emergency room procedures.

8.4 Neuromuscular Blocking Agents

These are discussed in section 5.2. As supplementary anesthetic agents, these drugs complement the efficacy of anesthesia by enhancing muscle relaxation and reducing the dose needed of other anesthetic agents. They can be particularly useful for endotracheal intubation. Two classes of agents are used: depolarizing agents (e.g., succinylcholine) and nondepolarizing agents (e.g., pancuronium). A peripheral nerve stimulator is often used to monitor the state of neuromuscular blockade; in the case of preparation for intubation, ulnar nerve response is monitored. Train-of-four fade is widely used in the operating room with the nerve stimulator where four stimuli at 2 Hz are administered, and loss of response to the fourth stimulus indicates approximate 80% neuromuscular blockade.

8.5 Local Anesthetics

Clinical Correlation

Vasoconstrictors in Local Anesthetics

Epinephrine is added to local anesthetic solutions to produce vasoconstriction at the site of injection. This decreases systemic absorption and prolongs the duration of action. Epinephrine should be used with caution in patients with cardiac disease, high blood pressure, hyperthyroidism, and other vascular diseases. Epinephrine is absolutely contraindicated in digital or penile blocks and around the nose or ears, as the ischemia produced may lead to gangrene.

Clinical Correlation

Facial Palsy with Dental Injections

The parotid salivary gland lies laterally to the ramus of the mandible and encloses the five branches of the facial nerve (cranial nerve VII). It is a wedge-shaped structure that wraps around the posterior border of the ramus. If a dentist is inaccurate when giving an inferior alveolar nerve block, some of the local anesthetic may penetrate the capsule of the parotid gland, causing anesthesia of the facial nerve. Symptoms include a drooping mouth and inability to blink on the affected side. The patient's affected eye should be taped closed to prevent drying and contamination with airborne debris until anesthesia subsides and the symptoms resolve.

Local anesthetics act directly on nerve axons to reversibly block nerve conduction. They produce a lack of sensation in the area innervated by those nerve fibers. The methods by which local anesthetics can be administered are outlined in ▶ Table 8.4.

8.5.1 Lidocaine, Articaine, and Bupivacaine (Amides); Benzocaine, Procaine, and Tetracaine (Esters)

Mechanism of Action

Local anesthetics exist in two forms in the body: as an uncharged base and as a charged acid. Only the uncharged base

Table 8.4 Methods of local anesthesia administration

Methods of local anesthetic administration	Technique	Clinical situation
Topical	Applied to skin or mucous membranes	Typically used prior to injection of anesthetics to make the procedure less painful. Also used prior to eye surgery and endoscopy
Infiltration	Inject dilute solution and let it diffuse (e.g., subcutaneous or submucosal)	Very common in dentistry to anesthetize most teeth
Nerve block	Inject close to the nerve trunk, proximal to the intended area of anesthesia	Very common in dentistry to anesthetize mandibular teeth. Can be useful in cases where pain sensation to a limb needs to be blocked (e.g., following femur fracture)
Spinal (intrathecal)	Inject anesthetic in the subarachnoid space	Chronic pain or surgery
Epidural	Inject within the vertebral canal but outside the dura	Very commonly used in labor and delivery

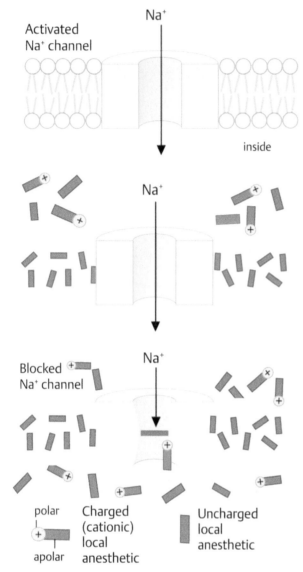

Fig. 8.3 Effects of local anesthetics.
Local anesthetics block the inner gate of the Na⁺ channels in nerve cells, preventing Na⁺ influx and action potential initiation and propagation. Charged (cationic) local anesthetic is thought to block the sodium channel by becoming incorporated into the phospholipid membrane or channel protein. Uncharged local anesthetic may also become incorporated into the apolar region of the channel protein. CNS, central nervous system.

can cross nerve membranes. However, once inside the axon, the charged form is active. Local anesthetics interfere with the propagation of action potentials in nerve axons by blocking Na⁺ channels from the cytoplasmic side of the channel (▶ Fig. 8.3).

Pharmacokinetics

- Local anesthetics differ mainly in their rate of onset and duration of action (▶ Table 8.5).

Table 8.5 Rate of onset and duration of action of some common local anesthetic agents

Local anesthetic agent	Rate of onset	Duration of actionᵃ
Amide local anesthetics: hepatic elimination leads to longer half-life/ duration of action		
Lidocaine	Intermediate	Intermediate
Articaine	Slow	Intermediate
Bupivacaine	Slow	Long
Ropivacaine	Slow	Long
Ester local anesthetics: very brief half-life due to plasma metabolism to soluble metabolites which leads to low potential for toxicity		
Procaine	Very slow	Short
Tetracaine	Slow	Long
Benzocaine	Intermediate	Intermediate

ᵃThe duration of action is prolonged when combined with epinephrine.

- Termination of action at the site of injection is by diffusion of the active drug into the systemic circulation followed by metabolism. Ester local anesthetics are inactivated primarily by hydrolysis via esterases in plasma and the liver. Amide local anesthetics are metabolized primarily by the liver.
- Local anesthetic can also be administered topically for ocular and dermal applications.

Clinical Correlation

Sensitivity of Different Nerve Fibers to Block

There are variations in sensitivity of different types of nerve fibers to block by local anesthetics. Smaller-diameter, unmyelinated nerve fibers are more sensitive than larger-diameter, myelinated fibers. Thus, there is a definite order in which sensation is blocked. Pain fibers are smallest and blocked first, followed by sensations of cold, warmth, touch, and deep pressure. Proprioceptive and motor fibers are blocked last.

Side Effects

The toxic effects of local anesthetics are dependent on the amount of drug that gains entry into the systemic circulation.

- *CNS effects:* These include stimulation, restlessness, and tremor that may lead to clonic convulsions. This is followed by depression and death due to respiratory failure. Direct systemic injection may lead directly to death.
- *Cardiac effects:* Direct effects on the myocardium include decreased electrical excitability, decreased conduction rate, and a negative inotropic effect. Sudden cardiac death may occur.
- *Hypersensitivity:* This is rare, but it can cause dermatitis, asthma attacks, or fatal anaphylactic reactions. Allergy is more frequent with esters.

9 Anxiolytic and Sedative-Hypnotic Drugs

Summary

Central nervous system (CNS) depressants are used to relieve anxiety (anxiolytic), produce sedation (sedative), or induce sleep (hypnotic). They are also anticonvulsants, centrally acting muscle relaxants, and drugs that produce amnesia. Physical and psychological dependence develops with prolonged use of these agents. There are many benzodiazepines in use, varying mainly in potency and pharmacokinetics. The benzodiazepines (i.e., diazepam, midazolam, temazepam, triazolam, flurazepam, clonazepam, clobazam, clorazepate, estazolam, oxazepam, lorazepam, alprazolam, and chlordiazepoxide) potentiate the actions of gamma-aminobutyric acid (GABA) by increasing the flow of Cl^- ions through the $GABA_A$ receptor. Another drug used for the treatment of anxiety disorders is the $5HT1_A$ agonist buspirone. Flumazenil is a relatively specific competitive antagonist at benzodiazepine receptors used to treat overdose or poisoning with benzodiazepines. The nonbenzodiazepine benzodiazepine receptor agonists include eszopiclone, zaleplon, and zolpidem. These agents are structurally unrelated to the benzodiazepines but bind to a specific subclass of benzodiazepine receptor found in the brain. They are used exclusively to treat insomnia. The barbiturates (i.e., thiopental, phenobarbital, thiamylal, methohexital, amobarbital, pentobarbital, and secobarbital) facilitate the action of GABA and also have direct GABA-like effects. They are mainly used for induction of anesthesia and treatment of epilepsy. Benzodiazepines have a higher therapeutic index than barbiturates. Doxylamine and diphenhydramine are H_1 antihistamines that are able to penetrate into the CNS, causing sedation. Ramelteon and tasimelteon are melatonin receptor agonists used for insomnia. Suvorexant is an antagonist of the orexin receptors that are involved in wakefulness.

Keywords: anxiety, insomnia, benzodiazepines, barbiturate, buspirone

9.1 Anxiolytic and Sedative-Hypnotic Drugs

CNS depressants are used to relieve anxiety (anxiolytic), produce sedation (sedative), or induce sleep (hypnotic). They are also anticonvulsants, centrally acting muscle relaxants, and drugs that produce amnesia. Physical and psychological dependence develops with prolonged use of these agents.

9.2 Anxiety Disorders

There are a number of anxiety disorders as recognized by the Diagnostic and Statistical Manual of Mental Disorders, Fifth Edition (DSM-5) and the International Classification of Diseases. These include: separation anxiety disorder, selective mutism, specific phobia, social anxiety disorder (social phobia), panic disorder, panic attack specifier, agoraphobia, generalized anxiety disorder, substance/medication-induced anxiety disorder, anxiety disorder due to another medical condition, other specified anxiety disorder, and unspecified anxiety disorder.

9.2.1 Treatment Strategies

The first line of drug treatment, following cognitive behavioral therapy (CBT), are the selective serotonin reuptake inhibitor (SSRI) and serotonin and norepinephrine reuptake inhibitor (SNRI) antidepressants (e.g., fluoxetine, citalopram, escitalopram; see ▶ Table 10.2). While these agents take weeks before efficacy is seen, they are well-tolerated and do not cause sedating side effects. The SSRIs and SNRIs are discussed in Chapter 10.2, Antidepressants and Drugs for Bipolar Disorders. Prior to the introduction of these drugs, the benzodiazepines were the mainstay of anxiety treatment. They are still used for certain patients with anxiety, especially to address acute symptoms while an SSRI or SNRI takes effect. They are not recommended for long-term treatment of anxiety. Similarly, benzodiazepines or nonbenzodiazepine benzodiazepine receptor agonists can be used to treat insomnia, but long-term use is not recommended. Benzodiazepines are also used for selected patients with epilepsy (see Chapter 11), as antispasmodics (see Chapter 14), for anesthetic induction (see Chapter 8), and to alleviate the symptoms of withdrawal from alcohol or barbiturates (Chapter 15).

9.3 Benzodiazepines

There are many benzodiazepines in use, varying mainly in potency and pharmacokinetics (i.e., onset and duration of action). Depending on these properties, specific agents are used to treat insomnia, anxiety, epilepsy, and spasticity and for anesthetic induction. Generally, there is a very good correlation between pharmacokinetics and pharmacodynamic efficacy. There is a clear understanding of their mechanism of action at the $GABA_A$ receptor (▶ Fig. 9.1). Because of this strong pharmacokinetics–pharmacodynamics relationship, benzodiazepines can be divided into four subgroups (see ▶ Table 9.1). However, increasing plasma levels above optimal exposures do correspond to an increasing central depression; this is likely due to tolerance.

The pharmacokinetic properties of the benzodiazepines are critical for good efficacy. For example, stable, steady plasma levels can result in a long-lasting anxiolytic effect. On the other hand, for the treatment of sleep disorders, rapid elimination can be useful to help with sleep initiation but to prevent interference with sleep patterns.

9.3.1 Diazepam, Midazolam, Temazepam, Triazolam, Flurazepam, Clonazepam, Oxazepam, Lorazepam, Alprazolam, and Chlordiazepoxide

Mechanism of Action

The benzodiazepines potentiate the actions of GABA by increasing the flow of Cl^- ions through the $GABA_A$ receptor (▶ Fig. 9.1). Many benzodiazepines have active metabolites; the most common is desmethyldiazepam which has an extremely long half-life particularly in the elderly (up to 200 h).

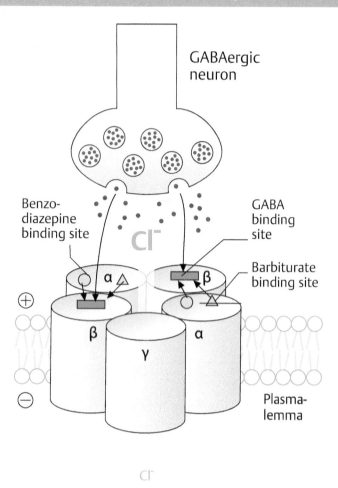

Fig. 9.1 Mechanism of action of benzodiazepines and barbiturates.
Gamma-aminobutyric acid (GABA) is the main inhibitory neurotransmitter in the central nervous system (CNS). When GABA is released from GABAergic neurons, it binds to the β subunit of the pentameric GABA receptor, leading to opening of the chlorine channel, Cl⁻ influx, neuronal hyperpolarization, and decreased excitability. Benzodiazepines bind to the α subunits of the $GABA_A$ receptor, enhancing the binding and the effects of GABA. Barbiturates also bind to the α subunits of the $GABA_A$ receptor. They increase the length of time that the chlorine channel is open when acted upon by GABA.

Effects

Benzodiazepines act almost exclusively in the CNS. The only peripheral effects are coronary vasodilation after certain benzodiazepines are injected intravenously (IV) and neuromuscular block after very high doses.

Note: Benzodiazepines have a higher therapeutic index than barbiturates. This is because benzodiazepines act by facilitating the effects of endogenous GABA, whereas barbiturates facilitate the effects of endogenous GABA and have direct GABA-like effects, thus producing more, and potentially excessive, CNS depression.

- Diazepam has a direct muscle relaxant effect in addition to CNS actions.
- Alprazolam has an additional antidepressant effect.
- Triazolam may result in rebound anxiety following cessation of administration.

Table 9.1 Summary of benzodiazepine uses

Benzodiazepine agent	Use(s)	Metabolism
Very short duration of action: 1–7 h		
Midazolam	Anesthetic induction	Half-life of 3 h. Prolonged in neonates and renal failure
Triazolam	Insomnia	Half-life of 2–3 h
Short duration of action: 8–24 h		
Alprazolam	Anxiolysis, panic disorders	Metabolized by CYP3A4. Significant drug–drug interactions with CYP3A4 inhibitors (antifungals, cimetidine)
Lorazepam	Anxiolysis, insomnia, anesthetic induction, status epilepticus	Drug–drug interactions can impair elimination, particularly antifungals. Metabolized by O-glucuronidation: less risk for accumulation particularly in elderly
Oxazepam	Anxiolysis, alcohol withdrawal	Metabolite of diazepam. Metabolized by O-glucuronidation: less risk for accumulation particularly in elderly
Intermediate duration of action: 24–48 h		
Clonazepam	Panic disorders, enhances efficacy of antipsychotics while reducing extrapyramidal symptoms, anticonvulsant	Half-life of parent compound is >30 h. Minimal drug–drug interactions.
Estazolam	Insomnia	Metabolized to low activity metabolites within 24 h
Temazepam	Insomnia	Metabolized to inactive metabolites within 24 h
Long duration of action: longer than 48 h		
Chlordiazepoxide	Anxiolysis, alcohol withdrawal	From 1950s. Metabolized to desmethyl chlordiazepoxide and demoxepam which have very long half-lives, particularly in the elderly. Prolonged accumulation with repeated dosing
Clobazam	Lennox–Gastaut syndrome, adjunct for epilepsy	Metabolized by CYP3A4. Active metabolite N-desmethylclobazam has 80-h half-life
Clorazepate	Anxiolysis, alcohol withdrawal, partial seizures	Metabolized in liver to active metabolite nordiazepam with half-life of 2 days. Main drug interaction is potentiation of other CNS depressants
Diazepam	Anxiolysis, anticonvulsant, alcohol withdrawal, muscle spasms, sedation	Second benzodiazepine. Hepatic metabolism principally by CYP3A4. Active metabolites: desmethyldiazepam, temazepam, and oxazepam with half-lives of up to 100 h
Flurazepam	Insomnia	Rapidly metabolized to active metabolites with long half-lives
Prazepam	Anxiolysis	Plasma levels are steady avoiding peaks. Elimination is reduced in the elderly and with hepatic failure

Uses

▶ Table 9.1 lists the primary use for each of the benzodiazepine drugs, which is related to their duration of action.

Side Effects

- Incoordination, dizziness, drowsiness, and decreased cognitive function.
- Fatal overdose can occur when combined with ethanol.

9.3.2 Flumazenil

Mechanism of Action

Flumazenil is a relatively specific competitive antagonist at benzodiazepine receptors.

Uses

- Overdose or poisoning with benzodiazepines.

9.4 Nonbenzodiazepine Benzodiazepine Receptor Agonists

9.4.1 Eszopiclone, Zaleplon, and Zolpidem

Mechanism of Action

These agents are structurally unrelated to the benzodiazepines but bind to a specific subclass of benzodiazepine receptor found in the brain. They have poor muscle-relaxing or anticonvulsant activity (▶ Table 9.2).

Table 9.2 Nonbenzodiazepine drugs for insomnia

Drug name	Mechanism	Comment
Eszopiclone	GABA$_A$ receptor positive allosteric modulator	A cyclopyrrolone, with moderate half-life
Zaleplon	GABA$_A$ receptor alpha1 subunit positive allosteric modulator	Nonbenzodiazepine, short-acting sedative
Zolpidem	GABA$_A$ receptor alpha1 subunit positive allosteric modulator	Somnambulation and next day drowsiness may occur
Suvorexant	Orexin 1 receptor antagonist and orexin 2 receptor antagonist	Novel mechanism, avoiding the dependence of benzodiazepines. Efficacy is limited to insomnia
Ramelteon, tasimelteon	Melatonin MT1 agonist and melatonin MT2 agonist	Nonbenzodiazepines for insomnia. Act on melatonin receptors to maintain the sleep-wake cycle
Melatonin	Melatonin receptor agonist	Available over the counter. Acts like endogenous melatonin to maintain sleep-wake cycle
Doxepin	Histamine H1 receptor antagonist; histamine H2 receptor antagonist; muscarinic receptor antagonist	A tricyclic antidepressant approved as a sleep aid, nonbenzodiazepine

Uses

They are used exclusively to treat insomnia.

Tolerance, Dependence, and Withdrawal

- Tolerance develops to the effects of these agents.
- Physical dependence can occur.
- Withdrawal symptoms are generally opposite to the effects of the drugs: anxiety, insomnia, and convulsions in severe withdrawal.

9.5 Barbiturates

9.5.1 Thiopental, Phenobarbital, Thiamylal, Methohexital, Amobarbital, Pentobarbital, and Secobarbital

Barbiturates as drugs of abuse are discussed in section 15.8.

Mechanism of Action

Barbiturates increase the chloride conductance of the GABA$_A$ receptor by facilitating the action of GABA. They also have direct GABA-like effects (see ▶ Fig. 9.1).

Pharmacokinetics

- Barbiturates have a low therapeutic index, so overdose (accidental or deliberate) is a problem with these agents (see note in Benzodiazepine section). They are also used recreationally and have substantial abuse potential.
- Rapid onset of pharmacodynamic efficacy.
- These agents induce cytochrome P-450 microsomal enzyme activity, which increases the rate of their own metabolism, as well as other drugs metabolized by this system.
- They also induce δ-aminolevulinic acid (δ-ALA) synthetase, the rate-limiting step in heme biosynthesis. Thus, barbiturates are contraindicated in patients with acute intermittent porphyria, porphyria variegata, or a positive family history of these porphyrias (see call-out box in section 3.3).

Uses

▶ Table 9.3 summarizes the use of each of the barbiturate drugs.

Table 9.3 Summary of barbiturate uses

Barbiturate drug	Duration of action	Use(s)
Thiopental Methohexital Thiamylal	Ultra-short-acting	Anesthetic induction
Amobarbital Pentobarbital Secobarbital	Intermediate[a]	Insomnia, only in clinical setting
Phenobarbital	Long	Anticonvulsant, only in clinical setting

[a]Intermediate-acting drugs are more prone to abuse.

Side Effects

- Incoordination, dizziness, drowsiness, and decreased cognitive function occur with intensity proportional to potency and dose.
- Fatal overdose may occur by suppression of the neurogenic and hypoxic drive for respiration.

9.6 Other Drugs for the Treatment of Anxiety Disorders and Insomnia

9.6.1 Ethanol

Ethanol is discussed in detail in section 15.4.

Mechanism of Action

The mechanism of action is unknown.

Uses

Ethanol is the most widely used sedative-hypnotic. It is also used as a solvent, germicide, and intravenously as a treatment of ethylene glycol or methanol poisoning.

9.6.2 5HT1$_A$ Agonist: Buspirone

Mechanism of Action

Buspirone is a selective 5-hydroxytryptamine type 1A (5-HT$_{1A}$) receptor agonist.

Pharmacokinetics

Buspirone has a selective anxiolytic action with a slow therapeutic onset (action may be delayed up to 2 weeks).

Uses

Buspirone is used in the treatment of anxiety.

Note: Buspirone does not potentiate the effects of ethanol or other CNS depressants; thus, it is useful for treating anxiety in alcoholics.

Side Effects

Headache, dizziness, and nervousness.

9.6.3 Doxylamine and Diphenhydramine

Mechanism of Action

Doxylamine and diphenhydramine are H$_1$ antihistamines that are able to penetrate into the CNS causing sedation.

Use

Insomnia.

Side effects

Drowsiness, dry mouth, headache, and increased appetite.

9.6.4 Ramelteon

Mechanism of Action

Ramelteon is a melatonin receptor agonist (both MT1 and MT2 receptors).

Pharmacokinetics

Metabolized by CYP-1A2 and 3A4 in the liver, thus has drug–drug interaction potential. The major metabolite is also active resulting in longer and higher exposures.

Uses

Insomnia.

Side Effects

Dizziness, drowsiness, and decreased alertness.

Contraindications

Ramelteon is contraindicated in combination with fluvoxamine, a strong CYP-1A2 inhibitor that can dramatically increase the plasma half-life and C$_{max}$ of ramelteon.

9.6.5 Suvorexant

Mechanism of Action

Suvorexant is an antagonist of the orexin receptors (OX1 and OX2) that are involved in wakefulness.

Use

Insomnia.

Side Effects

Sleep disturbances, abnormal dreams, suicide ideation, long-term negative effects on wakefulness.

9.6.6 Beta-adrenergic Receptor Antagonists

Beta-adrenergic receptor antagonists, such as propranolol, have been used for the acute treatment of anxiety, particularly in the presence of somatic or autonomic symptoms.

Uses

Restricted to anxiety patient not responding to benzodiazepine treatment and with autonomic symptoms.

Side-Effects

Nausea, diarrhea, bronchospasm, bradycardia, hypotension, heart failure, sexual dysfunction.

10 Antidepressants and Drugs for Bipolar Disorders

Summary

Antidepressants and bipolar disease drugs are used to treat affective disorders which include major depression, bipolar disease I, and bipolar disease II. First-generation antidepressant drugs include the tricyclic antidepressants (amitriptyline, nortriptyline, imipramine, desipramine) and the monoamine oxidase inhibitors (MAOIs, tranylcypromine, phenelzine, isocarboxazid). Second-generation antidepressant drugs include bupropion, mirtazapine, fluoxetine, reboxetine, duloxetine, amoxapine, maprotiline, and trazadone. Third-generation antidepressants are paroxetine, sertraline, fluvoxamine, citalopram, and venlafaxine. Lithium salts are used to treat bipolar disorders.

Keywords: trycyclics, SSRIs (selective serotonin reuptake inhibitor), SNRIs (serotonin and norepinephrine inhibitor), mania, depression

10.1 Introduction

Antidepressants and bipolar disease drugs are used to treat affective disorders. These include major depression, bipolar disease I, and bipolar disease II. These disorders may be bipolar (cycling back and forth between mania and depression) or unipolar (mania or depression only). ▶ Table 10.1 lists the symptoms of depression and mania.

Antidepressant drugs block the reuptake of the biogenic monoamines, norepinephrine, and serotonin and also have other actions. Their selectivity for different uptake mechanisms varies and is summarized in ▶ Table 10.2. While the efficacy of first-generation antidepressants, such as amitriptyline, has not been surpassed, the more selective agents are now the primary drugs of choice. Patients with major depressive disorder respond slowly to the treatment. Typically, those responding to first-line treatment respond in weeks to a month or longer. Many patients do not respond to first- or second-line treatment. The United States and international guidelines recommend the use of selective serotonin reuptake inhibitors (SSRIs) as first-line treatment. Since there is little demonstrated difference in efficacy across the range of antidepressants, the selection of an appropriate medication is largely made based on the potential for adverse side effects, drug–drug interactions, and patient-specific concerns including CYP450 interactions. Typically, treatment begins with an SSRI, serotonin and norepinephrine reuptake inhibitor (SNRI), bupropion, or mirtazapine. MAOIs are only administered to patients that do not respond to first- and second-line treatment.

Approximately two-thirds of patients with major depressive disorder respond to any given therapy; however, the remaining patients do not respond to pharmacotherapy, particularly those patients with symptoms such as sleeplessness and avolition.

Table 10.1 Symptoms of depression and mania

Affective disorders	Symptoms
MDD	Intense sadness, despair, and disinterest in regular activities. These symptoms continue for at least 2 weeks. Also associated with fatigue, musculoskeletal complaints, sleep disorders, feeling of worthlessness, and loss of joy in living. Most likely after 32 years of age, and more common in women
Bipolar I disorder	Described at one full manic episode with abnormally elevated mood, feelings of grandiosity, decreased sleep, increased talkativeness, and increased activity or agitation; these symptoms occur nearly every day for at least 1 week. This may be followed or preceded by hypomanic or major depressive symptoms. In addition, these must differentiate from schizophrenia-like symptoms
Bipolar II disorder	One or more MDD episodes and at least one hypomanic (not full mania) episode

Abbreviation: MDD, major depressive disorder.

Table 10.2 Antidepressant agents

Antidepressant agent	Mechanism of action	Uses	Comments
Citalopram	SSRI	MDD, anxiety disorder, OCD	Racemic mixture, the R form is a weak CYP450 2D6 inhibitor and H_1 inhibitor
Escitalopram	SSRI	MDD, generalized anxiety disorder, OCD, panic disorder, social phobia	S enantiomer of citalopram. It is more selective.

(Continued)

Table 10.2 (*Continued*)

Antidepressant agent	Mechanism of action	Uses	Comments
Bupropion		MDD	
Venlafaxine	SNRI. More potent at serotonin reuptake inhibition	MDD, generalized anxiety disorder, panic disorder, social phobia	Metabolized by CYP450 2D6 into a form that has more NET inhibition. Metabolite is "desvenlafaxine" and is also marketed separately
Fluoxetine	SSRI	MDD	
Paroxetine	SSRI, mild M_1 inhibitor, and weak norepinephrine uptake inhibitor	MDD, generalized anxiety disorder, OCD, panic disorder, post-traumatic stress disorder, social phobia	Strong inhibitor of CYP450 2D6
Fluvoxamine	SSRI also acts on sigma$_1$ receptors	MDD, OCD, social phobia	Inhibits CYP450 1A2 and 3A4
Duloxetine	SNRI	MDD, generalized anxiety disorder, OCD, many pain-related indications	Inhibitor of CYP450 2D6
Reboxetine	NRI	MDD, ADHD	Substrate of CYP450 3A4. One of the safest antidepressant drugs

(Continued)

Table 10.2 (*Continued*)

Antidepressant agent	Mechanism of action	Uses	Comments
Vortioxetine	5-HT$_{1a}$ receptor agonist; 5-HT$_{1b}$ receptor partial agonist; 5-HT$_{1d}$ receptor antagonist; 5-HT$_3$ receptor antagonist; 5-HT$_7$ receptor antagonist; serotonin transporter inhibitor	MDD, ADHD	Reduced sexual dysfunction relative to other antidepressants
Mirtazapine	α$_2$ adrenoceptor antagonist, 5-HT$_{2A}$ receptor antagonist; 5-HT$_3$ receptor antagonist and H$_1$ receptor antagonist	MDD, also has antiemetic properties	Similar structural backbone to antipsychotics

Abbreviations: ADHD, attention deficit hyperactivity disorder; MDD, major depressive disorder; OCD, obsessive-compulsive disorder; SNRI, Serotonin and norepinephrine reuptake inhibitor; SSRI, selective serotonin reuptake inhibitor; NRI, norepinephrine reuptake inhibitor.

10.2 First-Generation Antidepressant Drugs

10.2.1 Tricyclic Antidepressants (Amitriptyline, Nortriptyline, Imipramine, and Desipramine)

Tricyclic antidepressants are structurally related to phenothiazines (antipsychotic drugs; see Chapter 12) but have different pharmacological effects (▶ Fig. 10.1).

Mechanism of Action

These agents block the reuptake of the biogenic monoamines, norepinephrine, and serotonin. They also interact with several receptor types, including muscarinic (M$_1$), histaminic (H$_1$), and adrenergic (α$_1$) receptors.
- Desipramine is the most potent inhibitor of norepinephrine reuptake. It is 1000 times less potent on serotonin reuptake.
- Amitriptyline blocks both norepinephrine and serotonin reuptake equally.
- Tricyclics also block muscarinic, serotonergic, histaminic, and α-adrenergic receptors. These actions are thought to be related to their side effects.

Uses

Treatment for major depressive disorder, but not used as first-line therapy.

Effects

- Acute effects include drowsiness and decreased blood pressure, but sustained use will cause an elevation of mood.
- Suppression of rapid eye movement (REM) sleep.
- Sleep promotion.

Side Effects

- *Anticholinergic:* dry mouth, blurred vision, urinary retention, and constipation.
- *Antiadrenergic:* orthostatic hypotension and delayed cardiac conduction.
- Weight gain.
- Mania, confusion, and delirium.
- Overdose potential can be lethal, thus not recommended for potential suicide patients.

Clinical Correlation

Acute Poisoning with Tricyclic Antidepressants

Accidental and deliberate overdose of tricyclic antidepressants occurs frequently and constitutes a serious medical emergency that may result in death. Signs may include excitement, seizures, coma with depressed respiration, hypoxia, hypothermia, and hypotension. Anticholinergic effects are also evident. Because no antagonists are available, treatment includes supportive measures in an intensive care unit setting. These adverse effects have greatly reduced the use of this class of agents.

Drug Interactions

When tricyclic antidepressants are taken with other drugs, their effects or side effects can be potentiated.
- When they are taken with alcohol, this leads to additive sedation.
- When taken with other anticholinergic drugs, additive anticholinergic effects occur.

93

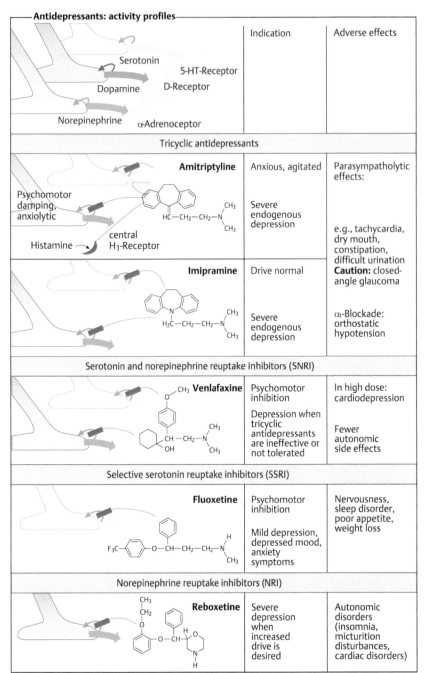

Antidepressants: activity profiles

	Indication	Adverse effects
Serotonin — 5-HT-Receptor		
Dopamine — D-Receptor		
Norepinephrine — α-Adrenoceptor		
Tricyclic antidepressants		
Amitriptyline	Anxious, agitated	Parasympatholytic effects:
Psychomotor damping, anxiolytic	Severe endogenous depression	
Histamine — central H₁-Receptor		e.g., tachycardia, dry mouth, constipation, difficult urination
Imipramine	Drive normal	**Caution:** closed-angle glaucoma
	Severe endogenous depression	α₁-Blockade: orthostatic hypotension
Serotonin and norepinephrine reuptake inhibitors (SNRI)		
Venlafaxine	Psychomotor inhibition	In high dose: cardiodepression
	Depression when tricyclic antidepressants are ineffective or not tolerated	Fewer autonomic side effects
Selective serotonin reuptake inhibitors (SSRI)		
Fluoxetine	Psychomotor inhibition	Nervousness, sleep disorder, poor appetite, weight loss
	Mild depression, depressed mood, anxiety symptoms	
Norepinephrine reuptake inhibitors (NRI)		
Reboxetine	Severe depression when increased drive is desired	Autonomic disorders (insomnia, micturition disturbances, cardiac disorders)

Fig. 10.1 Antidepressants.
Activity profiles of selected first-generation antidepressants (tricyclic antidepressants) and third-generation antidepressants (selective serotonin and norepinephrine reuptake inhibitors, selective serotonin reuptake inhibitors, and selective norepinephrine reuptake inhibitors), including the neurotransmitter affected, indications, and adverse effects.

- When they are taken with MAOIs, severe central nervous system (CNS) toxicity can occur, but this is rare.
- Overdose can be lethal, thus not recommended for potential suicide patients.

10.2.2 Monoamine Oxidase Inhibitors (Tranylcypromine, Phenelzine, and Isocarboxazid)

Mechanism of Action

MAOIs inhibit both monoamine oxidase A and B (MAO-A and MAO-B).

Clinical Correlation

Hypertensive Crisis with Monoamine Oxidase Inhibitors

Hypertensive crisis may occur within hours of ingestion of tyramine-containing foods, including cheese, certain meats (liver and fermented or cured meats), cured or pickled fish, overripe fruits and vegetables, Chianti wine, and some beers. Hypertensive crisis is characterized by headache, palpitation, neck pain or stiffness, nausea, vomiting, sweating (sometimes with fever or cold, clammy skin), photophobia, tachycardia or bradycardia, constricting chest pain, and dilated pupils. Potentially fatal intracranial bleeding may result from this crisis.

Patients should avoid tyramine-containing foods while taking MAOIs and for 2 weeks after treatment with MAOIs is discontinued to avoid precipitating this condition. If hypertensive crisis does occur, then treatment is with intravenous (IV) phentolamine (a nonselective α antagonist agent).

Pharmacokinetics

- Phenelzine and isocarboxazid are "suicide" inhibitors of the enzyme. This means that once an MAO molecule binds to one of these drugs, its activity cannot be restored. Restoration of MAO activity depends on synthesis of new enzyme molecules. The exception to this is tranylcypromine, which is reversible.
- MAOIs interfere with hepatic metabolism of many drugs and are not selective for MAO-A or MAO-B.
- The effects of MAOIs take 2 to 3 weeks to become apparent.

Uses

MAOIs are used to treat major depressive disorder, but are not used as first-line therapy because of the reduced safety and toxicity profile.

Effects

- Cardiovascular system: postural (orthostatic) hypotension.
- Suppression of REM sleep.

Side Effects

- Hepatotoxicity and CNS stimulation.

Note: Acute poisoning causes agitation, hallucinations, hyperreflexia, and convulsions. Treatment is by maintaining vital functions in the hospital setting for approximately 1 week.

Drug Interactions

- MAOIs interact with sympathomimetic drugs, leading to hypertensive crisis.
- MAOIs taken with meperidine (an opioid analgesic) can lead to fever, delirium, and hypertension.

10.3 Second-Generation Antidepressant Drugs

Second-generation antidepressant drugs were developed to eliminate some of the troublesome side effects seen with tricyclic antidepressants, such as cardiac manifestations, orthostatic hypotension, drowsiness, overdose risk, and weight gain.

10.3.1 Fluoxetine, Paroxetine, Sertraline, Fluvoxamine, Citalopram, and Venlafaxine

Mechanisms of Action

- Fluoxetine (see also ▶ Fig. 7.4), paroxetine, sertraline, fluvoxamine, and citalopram are SSRIs.
- Venlafaxine affects serotonin and norepinephrine reuptake and weakly inhibits dopamine reuptake.

Pharmacokinetics

- Completely absorbed from the gastrointestinal (GI) tract and extensively metabolized in the liver.
- Eliminated in the urine and feces.
- The therapeutic effect takes 10 to 14 days to develop.
- Long half-life (days).

Uses

- Depression.
- Obsessive-compulsive disorder (fluvoxamine and fluoxetine).
- Anxiety.

Side Effects

Fewer anticholinergic and sedative effects are seen than with tricyclics (they do not interfere with cardiac conduction or cause orthostatic hypotension). Side effects do include the following:
- Headache, tremor, insomnia, diarrhea, and nausea. Diarrhea and nausea diminish or resolve over time.
- They also stimulate the CNS, with agitation as the most frequent adverse effect.
- Psychotic reactions may be exacerbated in depressed schizophrenics.
- Liver enzymes are inhibited by fluoxetine and paroxetine but not affected by sertraline.
- Sexual dysfunction and anorgasmia occur in both men and women.
- Generally less weight gain than seen with other classes. Altered sleep.
- Akathisia (a movement disorder characterized by motor restlessness).

10.4 Third-Generation Antidepressant Drugs

Third-generation antidepressants may be safer than tricyclics in overdose situations. SSRIs are not as effective in treating severe depression as first- or second-generation agents.

10.4.1 Bupropion, Mirtazapine, Fluoxetine, Reboxetine, Duloxetine, Amoxapine, Maprotiline, and Trazadone

Mechanism of Action

These agents are pharmacologically similar to tricyclics. They may act as SNRIs as well as at some serotonin and adrenergic receptors (see ▶ Table 10.2). The prevailing hypothesis for the mechanism of action of these agents has been through modulating the synaptic concentrations of monoamines (particularly serotonin and norepinephrine) or through blocking the pre- or postsynaptic receptors for these neuromodulators. However, there is a substantial delay of minimally several weeks between onset of therapy and clinically meaningful onset of efficacy. This delay strongly suggests that the mechanism of action is more complicated than a direct effect on neurotransmitter systems; the prevailing hypotheses include downstream effects on neurotrophin mechanisms, particularly brain derived neurotropic factor (BDNF), and changes in synaptic architecture.

Uses

Major depressive disorder.

Effects

- Anticholinergic: dry mouth, blurred vision, urinary retention, and constipation.
- Antiadrenergic: postural (orthostatic) hypotension and delayed cardiac conduction.
- Antihistaminergic: sedation.
- Weight gain.

Side Effects

This generation of antidepressants generally has fewer side effects than tricyclic antidepressants. Exceptions include:
- Bupropion: seizures and cardiac arrhythmias.
- Amoxapine: extrapyramidal side effects.
- Maprotiline: rashes and seizures.

10.5 Bipolar I Disorder and Bipolar II Disorder Drugs

10.5.1 Lithium Salts

Lithium is an alkali metal ion used to treat mania, manic-depressive illness, and unipolar depression. It has no effects on healthy individuals unless toxic levels are reached. With bipolar I disorder (acute mania), 70 to 80% of patients improve when given lithium.

Clinical Correlation

Serotonin Syndrome

Acute intoxication with third-generation antidepressants can cause serotonin syndrome when given with MAOIs. The effects of the syndrome include hyperthermia, rigidity, myoclonus (quick, involuntary muscle jerks), confusion, delirium, and coma.

Mechanism of Action

The mechanism of action for lithium salts is unknown.

Pharmacokinetics

- Completely absorbed from the GI tract.
- Eliminated in the urine.
- Narrow therapeutic index, so frequent monitoring of serum or urine levels is required to prevent toxicity. This is performed daily during treatment of acute mania.
- There is a lag of 10 to 14 days before treatment becomes effective.

Uses

- Bipolar I disorder.
- Bipolar II disorder.
- Major depressive disorder.

Side Effects

- Neurologic effects can range from mild side effects such as tremor to muscle twitches or fasciculations, ataxia, and confusion. Severe side effects such as seizures, hallucinations, and delirium may also occur.
- Cardiac effects: fattened or inverted T waves (benign), arrhythmias, and sudden death.
- Polydipsia (excessive thirst) and polyuria (excessive urination) are seen, possibly from the inhibition of antidiuretic hormone by lithium. This may be disturbing to the patient. Mild polyuria usually occurs early in treatment. Polyuria appearing late may indicate impaired renal function.
- Nephrogenic diabetes insipidus (see Chapter 19).
- Thyroid enlargement.

Note: Acute intoxication is characterized by nausea, vomiting, profuse diarrhea, tremor, coma, and convulsions. Treatment is supportive.

10.6 Obsessive-Compulsive Disorder

Obsessive-compulsive disorder is characterized by obsessive thoughts and compulsive behaviors. Obsessions are unwanted thoughts that run repeatedly through the patient's mind. Compulsions are irresistible urges to perform ritualistic behaviors (See ▶ Table 10.2).

10.6.1 Clomipramine, Fluvoxamine, and Fluoxetine

- Clomipramine is a tricyclic antidepressant agent.
- Fluvoxamine and fluoxetine are SSRIs.

Treatment with these drugs may take up to 10 weeks for a full response. About half of all patients treated with these drugs respond favorably.

11 Anticonvulsant Drugs

Summary

Phenobarbital is the oldest anticonvulsant in use. Phenytoin is effective in many types of epilepsies. Carbamazepine has excellent tolerability and efficacy that make it the drug of choice particularly for focal seizures. It is also used for generalized tonic-clonic seizures, complex partial seizures, and trigeminal neuralgia. Primidone is similar to phenobarbital. Valproic acid is the most widely used and most effective drug for generalized idiopathic seizures and tonic-clonic seizures. For absence seizures, especially of the myoclonic types that are difficult to treat with other drugs, it appears to have an equivalent effect as ethosuximide. For patients with partial seizures that have not responded sufficiently, lacosamide may be utilized. Benzodiazepines are used only as combination therapy (clonazepam and clobazam primarily). Ethosuximide is effective only in absence seizures, so it is the drug of choice for this condition. Gabapentin is used for treatment only of partial, focal seizures typically as an adjunctive (in United States) to other drugs. It is also used for postherpetic neuralgia and restless leg syndrome. Felbamate is approved for monotherapy but serious idiosyncratic toxicity limits its use to second- or third-line therapy for partial seizures and Lennox–Gastaut syndrome in children. Lamotrigine is used for monotherapy and adjunctive therapy for focal seizures and generalized tonic-clonic seizures in adults. Topiramate is used as monotherapy in patients 10 years of age and older with partial focal or primary generalized tonic-clonic seizures and as adjunctive therapy in partial seizures. Levetiracetam, rufinamide, tiagabine, vigabatrin, and zonisamide are other drugs available for specific patients.

Keywords: generalized seizures, partial seizures, absence seizures, anticonvulsants, antiepileptics

11.1 Epilepsy and Seizures

The term *epilepsy* is a collective designation for a group of chronic central nervous system (CNS) disorders characterized by recurrent abnormal discharges of CNS neurons. The abnormal discharge may be limited to a focal area or may encompass diffuse areas of the brain. Although the abnormal discharge itself may have no clinical manifestations, such a discharge often leads to a seizure. The epileptic seizure takes many forms, ranging from brief cessations of responsiveness without loss of consciousness to convulsions with accompanying loss of consciousness. ▶ Table 11.1 describes the different seizure types.

Misdiagnosis or improper drug selection generally makes epilepsy worse, so it is critical that the correct seizure disorder is identified and treated with the most efficacious drug. If the drug of choice fails to control the seizures, then a follow-up agent is used.

11.2 Antiepileptic Agents

11.2.1 Phenobarbital

It is the oldest continuously used anticonvulsant, in use since 1912.

Table 11.1 Types of seizures

	Seizure type	Features
Partial seizures (focal, local)	Simple	Motor, somatosensory, autonomic, or psychic symptoms, with loss of consciousness
	Complex	Impaired consciousness at the outset, simple partial seizure followed by impaired consciousness
Generalized seizures (convulsive or nonconvulsive)	Absence typical	Sudden brief lapses of consciousness with loss of posture
	Atypical	Typical form plus brief motor activity or loss of muscle tone
	Myoclonic	Isolated jerking movements
	Clonic	Repetitive jerking movements without muscle rigidity
	Tonic	Muscle rigidity without jerking movements
	Tonic-clonic	Muscle rigidity followed by rhythmic jerking movements
	Atonic	Loss of muscle tone

Note: Partial seizures can evolve to generalized tonic-clonic type.

Mechanism of Action

Phenobarbital is a long-acting barbiturate that potentiates and mimics gamma-aminobutyric acid (GABA; see Chapter 9). It increases the threshold for action potential firing and inhibits the spread of activity from the focus (▶ Fig. 11.1).

Pharmacokinetics

- Effective orally with excellent oral bioavailability.
- Primarily hepatic metabolism, secondary renal elimination.
- Induces hepatic enzymes which limits its use in combination therapy.
- Extremely long half-life up to 100 hours.

Uses

- Generalized tonic-clonic epilepsy.
- Partial and focal seizures.
- Status epilepticus with parenteral solution.
- Prophylaxis or treatment of febrile convulsions.

The side effects limit its use as first-line therapy, but its low cost results in its continued use, especially in developing countries.

Side Effects

- Sedation (tolerance develops), impaired concentration and mood changes.
- Rashes are seen in 1 to 2% of patients. These may be scarlatiniform or morbilliform and are symptomatic of allergic reaction.
- Nystagmus (a rapid, involuntary, oscillatory motion of the eyeball) and ataxia (the inability to coordinate voluntary muscular movement) at excessive doses.
- Long-term effects on bone density.
- Teratogenicity risk results in pregnancy warning.

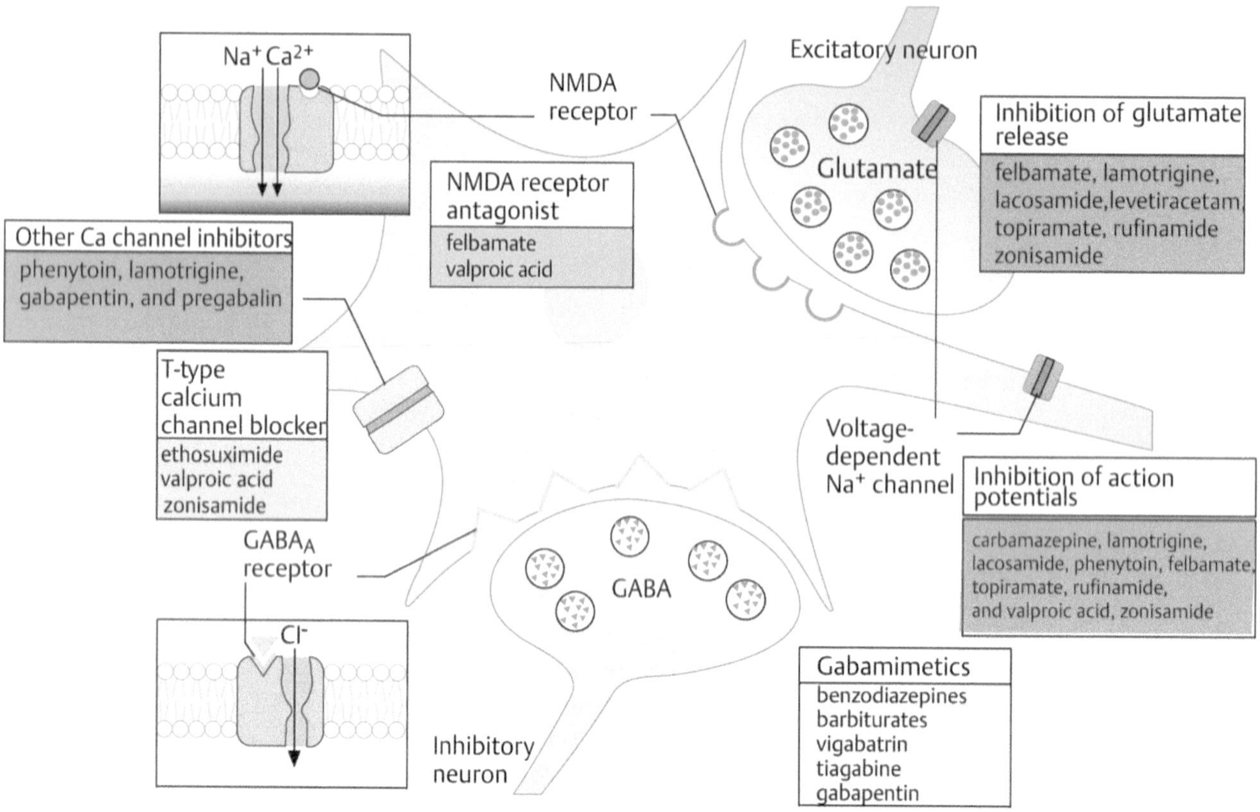

Fig. 11.1 Neuronal sites of action of antiepileptics.
Antiepileptic drugs act at many neuronal sites to inhibit excitation of the neuron. Gamma-aminobutyric acid (GABA) mimetics enhance the inhibitory effects of GABA at the GABA$_A$ receptor/Cl$^-$ channel. Other antiepileptics block voltage-dependent Na$^+$ channels, which can inhibit the release of the excitatory neurotransmitter glutamate, or they can act on the neurons themselves to inhibit action potentials. Other drugs block the N-methyl-D-aspartate (NMDA) glutamate receptor, T-type Ca^{2+} channels, or N-type Ca^{2+} channels.

Respiratory depression is not seen with this long-acting barbiturate given orally, but it may be observed after IV injection.

Drug Interactions

- Phenobarbital induces hepatic microsomal enzymes; it thus reduces the plasma concentration of drugs that are metabolized by these enzymes including warfarin, oral contraceptives, carbamazepine, and some antibiotics.
- Additive effects are seen when phenobarbital is taken with other CNS depressants.
- Valproic acid increases phenobarbital blood levels by inhibiting cytochrome P-450 enzymes.

11.2.2 Phenytoin

Mechanism of Action

Phenytoin limits the repetitive firing of action potentials in brain neurons by binding to the inactive state of voltage-activated Na$^+$ channels, slowing the rate of recovery from inactivation (▶ Fig. 11.1). This results in a reduction in high-frequency firing of action potentials during a seizure. In use since 1938.

Pharmacokinetics

- Slow, unpredictable absorption.
- Ninety percent bound to plasma proteins.
- Metabolized in liver by CYP 2C9 (major) and CYP 2C19 to inactive metabolites. The metabolism of phenytoin is dose dependent. At higher doses the rate of metabolism saturates, resulting in zero-order pharmacokinetics. This warrants careful dosing and monitoring.

Uses

- Effective in many types of epilepsies including focal seizure and generalized tonic-clonic epilepsy.
- Not effective in generalized absence myoclonic or atonic seizures.
- Previously it was the most widely used anticonvulsant, but safer and better pharmacokinetic properties of newer drugs have reduced its use.
- Trigeminal neuralgia.

Clinical Correlation

Status Epilepticus

Status epilepticus is the term used to describe prolonged seizures (usually lasting 30 minutes or more) or multiple seizures that occur without recovery of consciousness. Status epilepticus constitutes a medical emergency, as the longer the seizures continue the higher is the risk of death or brain damage. Treatment involves maintaining the patient's airway and giving oxygen, a bolus of glucose (as the brain is a huge consumer of glucose), and intravenous (IV) or rectal diazepam to terminate the seizure. IV diazepam is given in the form of an emulsion to prevent thrombophlebitis (inflammation of a vein due to a blood clot).

Side Effects

Phenytoin is relatively safe, but the following side effects may occur.

- Gingival hyperplasia is the most common side effect in children (20% of patients). Infections are minimized by good oral hygiene.
- Less sedating than phenobarbital. Cognitive impairment.
- CNS depression: nystagmus, ataxia, vertigo, and diplopia are observed at high drug dose exposures.
- Hyperglycemia, osteomalacia, lymphadenopathy, rashes (Stevens–Johnson syndrome [erythema multiforme bullosum]), and hematological reactions (leukopenia, megaloblastic anemia, thrombocytopenia, agranulocytosis, and aplastic anemia). These are allergic reactions that require cessation of therapy.
- Hirsutism.
- Fetal abnormalities.
- Cardiovascular collapse can occur after IV phenytoin.

Drug Interactions

- Metabolism of phenytoin can be increased or decreased by agents that can induce or inhibit cytochrome P-450 enzymes. Drugs including fluoxetine, fluvoxamine, and azole antifungal agents can adversely alter the exposure of phenytoin.
- Phenytoin induces hepatic microsomal enzymes; it thus reduces the plasma concentration of drugs that are metabolized by these enzymes, including warfarin, oral contraceptives, carbamazepine, and some antibiotics.
- Drugs that bind to plasma proteins will displace phenytoin including valproate, which could result in toxicity. Combination therapy should be appropriately monitored.

11.2.3 Carbamazepine

Mechanism of Action

Carbamazepine, similar to phenytoin, limits the repetitive firing of action potentials by slowing the rate of recovery of voltage-activated Na+ channels from inactivation (▶ Fig. 11.1).

Pharmacokinetics

- Good oral bioavailability.
- Absorption is slow and erratic.
- Metabolized in liver, primarily by CYP 3A4 into an active metabolite cabamezepine-10,11 epoxide.
- Inducer of hepatic enzymes.
- An extended release formulation has better tolerability.

Uses

- Excellent tolerability and efficacy make it the drug of choice particularly for focal seizures.
- Generalized tonic-clonic seizures.
- Complex partial seizures.
- Trigeminal neuralgia.

Note: Carbamazepine is ineffective for absence seizures.

Side Effects

- Gastrointestinal (GI) upset.
- Vertigo, diplopia, and blurred vision.
- Hematological disorders: aplastic anemia, thrombocytopenia (low platelet count), agranulocytosis (failure of bone marrow to produce white blood cells), and leukopenia (low white blood cell count).
- Hypersensitivity.

Drug Interactions

- Metabolism of carbamazepine can be increased or decreased by agents that can induce or inhibit cytochrome P-450 enzymes. It may accumulate when used with agents that inhibit CYP 3A4 including erythromycin, fluoxetine, and grapefruit juice.
- Carbamazepine induces hepatic microsomal enzymes; it thus reduces the plasma concentration of drugs that are metabolized by these enzymes, including warfarin, oral contraceptives, some antibiotics, and even carbamazepine itself.

11.2.4 Oxcarbazepine

Mechanism of Action

Oxcarbazepine is structurally similar to carbamazepine. Similar to phenytoin, it limits the repetitive firing of action potentials by slowing the rate of recovery of voltage-activated Na+ channels from inactivation (▶ Fig. 11.1).

Pharmacokinetics

- Good oral bioavailability.
- Absorption is slow and erratic.
- Metabolized in liver into the primary active metabolite 10-hydroxycarbazepine.
- An extended release formulation has better tolerability.

Uses

- In focal seizures as monotherapy or an adjunct.

III

Side Effects

- Gastrointestinal (GI) upset.
- Vertigo, diplopia, and blurred vision.
- Hyponatremia.

Drug Interactions

- Unlike carbamazepine, does not interact with warfarin and antibiotics.
- May affect bioavailability of contraceptives.

Clinical Correlation

Febrile Convulsions

Febrile seizures (seizures associated with elevated body temperature) are the most common type in children, affecting 2 to 5% of patients between the ages of 6 months and 5 years, with the peak incidence at 18 months. These seizures are not associated with trauma, infection, metabolic disturbances, or a history of seizures, and most of these last less than 10 minutes. More serious illnesses must be ruled out, but treatment of simple febrile seizures with anticonvulsants is generally not recommended, as the potential drug toxicities associated with these medications outweigh the relatively minor risks associated with the convulsions. There is also no need to specifically cool the child in a cooling bath or to administer an antipyretic drug, such as acetaminophen, to reduce the fever. Most febrile convulsions will stop on their own after a few minutes.

11.2.5 Primidone

Mechanism of Action

Mechanism is similar to that of phenobarbital.

Pharmacokinetics

- Primidone is metabolized in the liver to phenobarbital (approximately 25%) and phenylethylmalonamide (PEMA).
- Half-life is 10 to 15 hours but reduced in the presence of enzyme inducers.

Uses

- Complex partial seizures (primidone is more effective than phenobarbital).
- Focal seizures, generalized tonic-clonic seizures, and simple partial seizures.
- Frequently combined with phenytoin in refractory cases.
- Essential tremors.

Side Effects

- Rashes, leukopenia, thrombocytopenia, and systemic lupus erythematosus.
- CNS depressant effects like those observed with phenobarbital (sedation, ataxia).

- Primidone-specific adverse event of acute toxic reaction leading to dizziness, sedation, ataxia, and emesis. This risk limits its use and requires careful dose escalations and monitoring.

Drug Interactions

Drug interactions are the same as for phenobarbital.

11.2.6 Valproic Acid

Mechanism of Action

Valproic acid increases Na^+ channel inactivation, increases GABA-mediated synaptic inhibition, and inhibits T-type Ca^{2+} channel activation (▸ Fig. 11.1). Its anticonvulsant action continues after the drug has been withdrawn.

Pharmacokinetics

- Ninety percent bound to plasma proteins. Excellent oral bioavailability, but when coadministered with phenytoin competition for protein binding affects the free fraction.
- Plasma half-life is 13 to 16 hours, but reduced by drug interactions.
- Metabolized by the cytochrome P-450 enzymes, but it does not induce these enzymes.

Uses

- Most widely used and most effective for generalized idiopathic seizures and tonic-clonic seizures. With generalized epilepsy, it is the drug of first choice.
- Absence seizures, especially of the myoclonic types that are difficult to treat with other drugs. It appears to have an equivalent effect as ethosuximide for absence seizures but has greater cognitive impairment.
- Combination therapy in the treatment of generalized tonic-clonic seizures and for complex partial seizures.

Side Effects

- Alopecia (reversible) in 5% of patients.
- Transient GI effects (nausea, vomiting, and anorexia) in 16% of patients. Reduced in the extended release formulation.
- CNS: mild behavioral effects, ataxia, and tremor; not a CNS depressant. Serious CNS effects in the elderly, including parkinsonism, dementia, and atrophy of the brain.
- Hepatic and pancreatic failure has been reported. It is rare but potentially life threatening.
- Highest risk of teratogenicity as compared to any other anticonvulsant, thus there is risk during pregnancy.

Note: Valproic acid should not be used in pregnancy, as it has been shown to be teratogenic in animals.

Drug Interactions

- Valproic acid increases blood levels of phenobarbital and primidone by inhibiting their metabolism.
- Valproic acid lowers phenytoin levels.

11.2.7 Lacosamide

Mechanism of Action

Lacosamide is believed to act by modulating the activity of voltage-gated sodium channels by slowing the inactivation phase. There is some evidence that it may also modulate neuronal plasticity. It is generally well-tolerated.

Use

For partial seizures in patients that have not responded sufficiently to other antiepileptic drugs (AEDs).

Pharmacokinetics

- Long half-life of 13 hours.
- Minimal protein binding.
- Minimal interactions with CYP P-450.
- No evidence of drug–drug interactions.

Side Effects

- Dizziness and vertigo.
- Nausea.
- Headache.

11.2.8 Benzodiazepines

Mechanism of Action

Benzodiazepines augment the action of GABA at $GABA_A$ receptors, which are ligand-gated chloride ion channels (▶ Fig. 9.1 and ▶ Fig. 11.2).

Uses

- Used only as combination therapy (clobazam).
- Chronic treatment of epilepsy (clonazepam and clorazepate).

- Status epilepticus (lorazepam or diazepam IV).
- Atonic and akinetic seizures, especially as adjuncts.
- Absence seizures, but not preferred because of CNS depression.

Note: Benzodiazepines do not prevent generalized tonic-clonic seizures.

Side Effects

- Sedation is the most common side effect.
- Ataxia.
- Behavioral problems such as aggression, anxiety, and restlessness.
- Amnesia.
- Seizures following abrupt withdrawal.

11.2.9 Ethosuximide

Mechanism of Action

The mechanism of action for ethosuximide is believed to be through blocking of T-type calcium channels, but it does enhance CNS inhibition.

Uses

Ethosuximide is effective only in absence seizures. It is the drug of choice for this condition.

Side Effects

- GI irritation: nausea, vomiting, and anorexia (a lack or loss of appetite for food).
- CNS depression: drowsiness, lethargy, euphoria, dizziness, headache, and hiccups.
- Rashes: urticaria (hives) and Stevens–Johnson syndrome (rare).
- Blood dyscrasias (an abnormal condition of the blood) (rare).

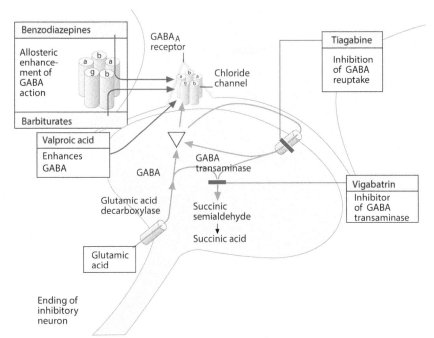

Fig. 11.2 Sites of action of antiepileptics in GABAergic synapse.
Many antiepileptic drugs act on GABA in a number of ways. Some drugs act presynaptically to increase the production of GABA or to reduce its degradation. Others act to inhibit the reuptake of GABA from the synaptic cleft. Benzodiazepines and barbiturates act on the $GABA_A$ receptor to enhance the effects of GABA.

11.2.10 Gabapentin

Mechanism of Action

The mechanism of action for gabapentin is believed to be through its binding to the $\alpha_2\delta$ subunit of N-type voltage-gated calcium channels; such binding could reduce neurotransmitter release during high firing rates. Gabapentin is chemically related to GABA but is not an agonist at GABA receptors. It may enhance GABA release.

Pharmacokinetics

- Low and variability bioavailability.
- No appreciable metabolism, renal elimination.
- Half-life is 5 to 7 hours.

Uses

- For treatment only of partial, focal seizures typically as an adjunctive (in the United States) to other drugs. Approved for monotherapy in Europe.
- Postherpetic neuralgia.
- Restless leg syndrome (extended release formulation).

Side Effects

- Sedation, dizziness, ataxia, nystagmus, and tremor.
- Weight gain.
- Myoclonus.
- Emotional conditions in children.
- Cognitive impairment in elderly.

Note: Gabapentin should be used with caution in children because it may produce adverse psychiatric symptoms, such as thought disorders and hostility.

Drug Interactions

This agent does not alter serum concentration of other anticonvulsants.

11.2.11 Pregabalin

Mechanism of Action

The mechanism of action for pregabalin is similar to gabapentin. Although it is chemically similar to GABA, it is not an agonist at GABA receptors. Its actions may be through its binding to the $\alpha_2\delta$ subunit of N-type voltage-gated calcium channels, thus reducing neurotransmitter release during high firing rates.

Pharmacokinetics

- High bioavailability.
- No appreciable metabolism, renal elimination.
- Half-life is 5 to 7 hours.

Uses

- As an adjunct for partial seizures not fully controlled by a single medication.
- Neuropathic pain due to diabetic peripheral neuropathy, spinal cord injury, or postherpetic neuralgia.
- Fibromyalgia.

Side Effects

- Sedation, dizziness, ataxia, nystagmus, and tremor.
- Weight gain.
- Myoclonus.
- Cognitive impairment in elderly.

Drug Interactions

This agent does not alter serum concentration of other anticonvulsants.

11.2.12 Felbamate

Mechanism of Action

Unclear mechanisms, but includes inhibition of *N*-methyl-D-aspartate (NMDA) channels, inhibition of sodium channels, and enhancement of GABA receptors.

Pharmacokinetics

- Good oral bioavailability, long plasma half-life of 20 to 24 hours.

Uses

- Approved for monotherapy but serious idiosyncratic toxicity limits its use to second- or third-line therapy.
- Partial seizures.
- Lennox–Gastaut syndrome in children.

Side Effects

- CNS: insomnia and headache.
- GI: anorexia, vomiting, and nausea.
- Allergic reactions: hematological and dermatological reactions.
- Acute aplastic anemia (potentially lethal), 1 in 5,000 to 8,000.
- Acute liver failure (approx. 1 in 50,000).

Drug Interactions

Felbamate may alter concentrations of other anticonvulsants by inducing CYP3A4. Inhibitor of CYP 2C19, CYP1A2.

11.2.13 Lamotrigine

Mechanism of Action

Lamotrigine inhibits voltage-dependent Na$^+$ channels but is effective in absence seizures and likely has additional mechanisms.

Uses

- Monotherapy and adjunctive therapy for focal seizures and generalized tonic-clonic seizures in adults.
- Apparently synergistic effects with valproate with good efficacy.
- Lennox–Gastaut syndrome in both children and adults.

Side Effects

Approximately 1 in 1,000 people experience severe and potentially life-threatening skin rashes. These are rarely fatal, but children are at higher risk. This can be reduced by slowly increasing the dose.

Substantially lower rate of sedation and cognitive impairment as compared to other anticonvulsants.

Lowest teratogenicity risk, thus may be indicated during pregnancy.

11.2.14 Topiramate

Mechanisms of Action

- Inhibits voltage-dependent Na$^+$ channels.
- Potentiates the action of GABA by a unique mechanism, different from that of the benzodiazepines or barbiturates.
- Blocks excitatory amino acid (AMPA/kainate) receptors.

Uses

- Monotherapy in patients 10 years of age and older with partial focal or primary generalized tonic-clonic seizures. Because of adverse events, it is not a drug of first choice. Recommended with comorbidities of headache and obesity.
- Adjunctive therapy in partial seizures.

Side Effects

- Mainly involves CNS depression: fatigue, dizziness, ataxia, and decreased cognition.
- Less tolerated than lamotrigine.
- Kidney stones.
- Paresthesia.
- Hypersensitivity.
- Increased birth defects including cleft palate.

11.2.15 Tiagabine

Mechanism of Action

Tiagabine is a GABA reuptake inhibitor (▶ Fig. 11.2).

Uses

- Adjunctive therapy in focal seizures only.

Side Effects

- CNS depression: fatigue, dizziness, ataxia, and decreased cognition.
- May exacerbate absence and myoclonic seizures.

11.2.16 Vigabatrin

Mechanism of Action

Irreversibly binds to and thus inhibits the activity of GABA transaminase (see ▶ Fig. 11.2).

Use

Primarily used for add-on therapy after other therapeutics have failed.

Side Effects

- CNS: sedation, headache, agitation.
- GI: adverse events include GI pain, constipation, and emesis.

Pharmacokinetics

- Good bioavailability.
- Half-life is 8 to 12 hours.
- Renal elimination without metabolism.

11.2.17 Rufinamide

Mechanism of Action

While not clearly understood, there is some evidence of sodium channel inhibition by enhancing channel inactivation, thus limiting repetitive firing of neurons.

Use

As adjunctive therapy in children and adults with Lennox–Gastaut syndrome.

Side Effects

- CNS: headache, dizziness, fatigue, somnolence.
- Nausea.
- Shortened QT interval. Rufinamide is contraindicated in patients with familial short QT syndrome.

Pharmacokinetics

- Good bioavailability.
- Non-CYP-mediated metabolism.
- Renal excretion.
- Half-life is 6 to 10 hours.

11.2.18 Levetiracetam

Mechanism of Action

The mechanism of action for levetiracetam is believed to be through binding the synaptic vesicle protein SV2A.

Uses

- Therapy of focal seizures and generalized tonic-clonic seizures. Approved for monotherapy in Europe, but not in the United States.

Side Effects

- Mainly involve CNS depression: fatigue, dizziness, ataxia, and decreased cognition.
- Relatively well-tolerated and there are no drug–drug interactions.

11.2.19 Zonisamide

Mechanism of Action

Zonisamide prolongs Na^+ channel inactivation and inhibits T-type Ca^{2+} current.

Uses

- Adjunctive therapy in partial seizures.

Side Effects

- Mainly involve CNS depression: fatigue, dizziness, ataxia, and decreased cognition.

▶ Table 11.2 summarizes the drug(s) of choice for each seizure disorder, as well as alternative drugs.

Table 11.2 Summary of antiepileptic drugs

Seizure disorder	Drug(s) of choice	Alternative drugs
Partial, including secondarily generalized	Carbamazepine or phenytoin	Lamotrigine or levetiracetam or topiramate or valproic acid
Typical absence	Ethosuximide	Valproic acid
Atypical absence	Valproic acid	Combination of valproic acid and ethosuximide or lamotrigine
Myoclonic	Valproic acid	Lamotrigine or topiramate
Clonic or tonic	Valproic acid	Phenytoin
Tonic-clonic	Carbamazepine or phenytoin or valproic acid	Lamotrigine or topiramate
Atonic/akinetic	Valproic acid	Clonazepam or phenytoin
Recurrent febrile	Diazepam	Phenobarbital
Status epilepticus	Lorazepam or diazepam, followed by phenytoin	Phenytoin or phenobarbital

12 Antipsychotic Drugs

Summary

Antipsychotic drugs are used to treat schizophrenia and other psychoses. The two major groups of antipsychotic medications are the classical neuroleptic antipsychotics and the second-generation agents that are also known as atypical agents. The primary therapeutic receptor mechanism of action for the classical neuroleptic antipsychotics is thought to be related to their ability to block the action of excess dopamine at the D_2 subtype of dopamine receptor on postsynaptic neurons in the dopaminergic mesolimbic-mesocortical pathways in the brain. The second-generation antipsychotic drugs possess $5\text{-}HT_2$ as well as D_2 antagonist properties. These drugs have fewer extrapyramidal side effects (EPSE). The typical antipsychotics include perphenazine, fluphenazine, chlorpromazine, thioridazine, thiothixene, haloperidol, pimozide, and loxapine. The atypical antipsychotics include clozapine, olanzapine, quetiapine, paliperidone, risperidone, ziprasidone, iloperidone, pimavanserin, and aripiprazole.

Keywords: psychosis, schizophrenia, antipsychotics, atypical antipsychotics

12.1 Antipsychotic Drugs

Antipsychotic drugs ameliorate the positive symptoms and, to a lesser extent, the negative symptoms of schizophrenia. They are also used to treat psychosis accompanying other disorders such as bipolar disorder I and schizoaffective disorders. They may also be useful to treat the behavioral and psychiatric symptoms associated with dementia and personality disorders. In addition, these agents are used as antiemetics and for a variety of other disorders, such as chronic multiple tics, neurogenic pain, Huntington disease, ballismus, infantile autism, and intractable hiccups. The two major groups of antipsychotic medications are the classical neuroleptic antipsychotics and the second-generation agents that are also known as atypical agents. These two groups differ in the receptors that they block, the symptoms of schizophrenia that they alleviate, and their side effects. The classical neuroleptics were identified in animal studies by their cataleptic effects which were known to translate to antipsychotic efficacy in the clinic. The second-generation agents did not induce catalepsy and were thus termed "atypical" antipsychotics. The "atypical" moniker can be confusing because these drugs are quite effective in reversing psychosis. The lack of preclinical catalepsy has translated to reduced EPSEs, or extrapyramidal symptoms (EPS), in the clinic.

Historically, haloperidol has been the most widely used classical neuroleptic and is still employed clinically for treatment-resistant cases. Clozapine is recognized as the first second-generation (atypical) antipsychotic because of its greatly reduced EPSEs. It is highly effective for treating both the positive and negative symptoms of schizophrenia as well as some aspects of the cognitive deficits associated with schizophrenia. Its major disadvantage is that it can cause agranulocytosis, a severe blood disorder.

Clinical Correlation

Ballismus

It is a quite rare hyperkinetic disorder caused by damage, usually vascular, to the subthalamic nucleus, which is functionally related to the basal ganglia. This ultimately disinhibits neurons in the thalamus leading to excessive activity of the motor cortex. Ballismus is characterized by irregular, flinging movements of the limbs. Treatment, when necessary, involves the use of dopamine-blocking agents (e.g., pimozide, haloperidol, and chlorpromazine), even though dopamine has not been definitively linked to the disorder.

Foundations

Extrapyramidal System

The extrapyramidal system is the collective name for the neurons, tracts, and pathways that regulate and coordinate movement. Tracts of the extrapyramidal system mainly originate in the reticular formation of the pons and medulla and receive input from the cortex, basal ganglia, thalamus, and cerebellum. They then act upon cells of the ventral horn of the spinal cord. As they do not directly innervate motor neurons, the extrapyramidal system has a modulatory and regulatory function on movement, especially reflexes, postural control, and complex motor functions.

Clinical Correlation

Bipolar Disorders

Bipolar I disorder: Its diagnosis requires at least one manic episode. Most cases may be accompanied by depressive episodes.

Bipolar II disorder: Its diagnosis requires observation of at least one hypomanic occurrence and at least one of major depression. Hypomania refers to episodes less than full mania and is difficult to diagnose.

Cyclothymia: Cycles of hypomania interspersed with periods of depression. The depression is not to the level of major depressive disorder.

12.2 Features of Typical and Atypical Antipsychotic Agents

12.2.1 Mechanisms of Action

The primary therapeutic receptor mechanism of action for the classical neuroleptic antipsychotics is thought to be related to their ability to block the action of excess dopamine at the D_2 subtype of dopamine receptor on postsynaptic neurons in the dopaminergic mesolimbic-mesocortical pathways in the brain (see Chapter 7). Blockade of D_2 receptors in the nigrostriatal

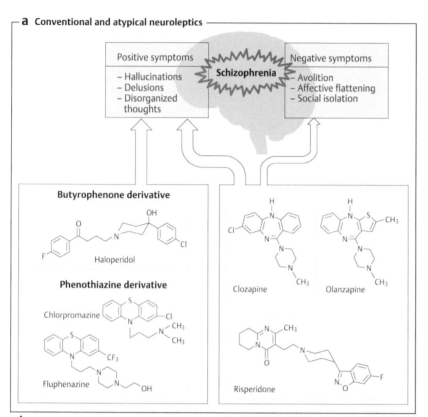

a Conventional and atypical neuroleptics

Fig. 12.1 Antipsychotics.
(a) Activity profiles of selected typical (*blue*) and atypical (*green*) antipsychotic agents. (b) Receptor affinity profiles of selected antipsychotic agents.

b Receptor affinity profile with reference to D_2 dopamine receptor

	D_2	M-ACh	a_1	H_1	$5\text{-}HT_{2A}$	$5\text{-}HT_{1A}$
Chlorpromazine	++	+	+++	++	+++	–
Fluphenazine	++	–	+	+	+	–
Haloperidol	++	+	+	+	+	–
Clozapine	++	+++	+++	+++	+++	–
Olanzapine	++	++	++	+++	+++	–
Risperidone	++	–	++	++	++	–
Ziprasidone	++	+	+	+	+++	!++!

The receptor affinities of each drug are compared in relation to its D_2 receptor affinity, arbitrarily set at (++); antagonistic effects, except for ziprasidone ($5\text{-}HT_{1A}$ agonism)

pathway is implicated in the EPSEs seen with these agents. Positron-emission tomography (PET) imaging of striatal dopamine receptors has shown that optimal antipsychotic efficacy is observed with at least 60% D_2 receptor occupancy; EPSE and movement disorders occur with 80% and greater D_2 occupancy. This indicates the optimal drug brain concentration range for efficacy and tolerability. This range is difficult to attain with antipsychotics which exhibit substantial brain concentration variability across the patient population.

- The second-generation antipsychotic drugs possess $5\text{-}HT_2$ as well as D_2 antagonist properties. These drugs have reduced activity in the nigrostriatal pathway, and thus fewer EPSEs.
- The atypical antipsychotic aripiprazole is unique in that it is a partial agonist at the D_2 receptor.

- Most of the antipsychotics also block M_1 muscarinic, H_1 histamine, and α_1-adrenergic receptors to varying degrees, which accounts for many of their side effects.

▶ Fig. 12.1 shows the relationship between striatal D_2 occupancy, efficacy, and extrapyramidal adverse effects.

12.2.2 Pharmacokinetics

- Erratic and unpredictable absorption from the gastrointestinal (GI) tract.
- Elimination half-life ranges from 20 to 40 hours.
- High therapeutic indices.
- Wide variations in plasma levels occur among individuals.
- Varied metabolic pathways by CYP enzymes.

12.2.3 Effects

- Neuroleptic/antipsychotic efficacy:
  - Hallucinations, delusions, and incoherent thoughts tend to decrease.
  - Spontaneous movement and complex behavior are suppressed, but spinal reflexes remain intact.
  - Reduced initiative, reduced interest in the environment, and reduced displays of emotion or affect.
  - Patients are easily aroused and can answer direct questions; intellectual function remains intact.
  - Psychotic patients become less agitated.
  - Withdrawn patients may become more responsive.
  - Aggression and impulsive behavior are decreased.
- Extrapyramidal (motor):
  - No motor incoordination at usual doses.
  - Spontaneous activity is diminished.
  - Catatonic signs are relieved, or rigidity is induced.
- *Antiemetic*: These prevent nausea and vomiting by blocking the effect of emetics that act on D_2 receptors in the chemoreceptor trigger zone (CTZ), an area of the medulla oblongata in the area postrema outside the blood–brain barrier that provides input to the vomiting control center (also in the medulla) to initiate vomiting.

12.2.4 Side Effects

- Extrapyramidal (motor):
  - Parkinsonism with bradykinesia, rigidity, and tremor may develop within 1 week to 1 month of initiation of antipsychotic drugs, typically when there is 80% or greater occupancy of corticostriatal D_2 receptors. Treated with anticholinergics (e.g., benztropine), amantadine (see Chapter 14), or by reducing the dose of antipsychotic.
  - Acute dystonia: This is sustained, often painful, muscular spasms in which the patient adopts a twisted posture. It occurs rarely with antipsychotic therapy and is treated with anticholinergic antiparkinsonian agents (e.g., benztropine), reducing antipsychotic dose, or using an alternative.
  - Akathisia: This is a strong subjective feeling of distress or discomfort; compelling need to be in constant movement that may start within the first 2 weeks of antipsychotic therapy. It must be distinguished from anxiety or agitation, but if these are ruled out, then the dose of antipsychotic should be lowered or changed.
  - Tardive dyskinesia (see Clinical Correlations Box).
- Autonomic nervous system:
  - Orthostatic (postural) hypotension, impotence, and failure to ejaculate.
  - Anticholinergic effects, including dry mouth, blurred vision, nasal stuffiness, urinary retention, palpitations, and toxic-confusional state at high doses.
- Endocrine:
  - Hyperprolactinemia (increased blood prolactin), which can result in amenorrhea (absence of a menstrual period), galactorrhea (spontaneous flow of milk from the breast, unassociated with lactation following childbirth), infertility, and impotence (inability to develop or maintain an erection).
  - Osteoporosis, likely related to hyperprolactinemia.
- Cardiovascular
  - Increased risk of QT prolongation with some antipsychotics, particularly thioridazine, mesoridazine, chlorpromazine, and haloperidol among the classic neuroleptics. In addition, iloperidone and ziprasidone carry this risk.
- Other:
  - Sedation.
  - Weight gain.
  - Agranulocytosis (acute low white blood cell count), primarily a concern with clozapine. Therapy may be continued with careful hematological monitoring.
  - Pigmentary degeneration of the retina (rare).
  - Neuroleptic malignant syndrome.
  - In the elderly, antipsychotics are prescribed for behavioral and psychological symptoms of dementia (BPSD) or neuropsychiatric symptoms of dementia. An increased mortality has been observed with many of the available antipsychotics in this patient population. As a result, the Food and Drug Administration (FDA) has put a black box warning on this class of drugs for this patient population.

Clinical Correlation

Tardive Dyskinesia

It is characterized by involuntary movements and appears only after months or years of treatment with antipsychotic agents. It is less common with atypical agents than typical agents. The involuntary movements consist of sucking and smacking of the lips, lateral jaw movements, and fly-catching dartings of the tongue. These movements disappear during sleep. Symptoms may persist indefinitely or will sometimes disappear (in weeks to years), especially in younger patients. This condition worsens on withdrawal of antipsychotics and with concomitant use of anticholinergic drugs. There is no adequate drug therapy, so it must be prevented.

Clinical Correlation

Neuroleptic Malignant Syndrome

Neuroleptic malignant syndrome (NMS) is a neurologic disorder that occurs as a result of an idiosyncratic reaction to neuroleptic (antipsychotic) drugs. It usually appears within the first 2 weeks of therapy and presents with fever, muscular rigidity, altered mental status, and autonomic dysfunction (e.g., arrhythmias and fluctuating blood pressure). NMS tends to occur more frequently with classical neuroleptic antipsychotics. The drug management of NMS depends on the symptoms but includes discontinuing the neuroleptic medication, antipyretic drugs (e.g., acetaminophen), dopamine agonists (e.g., bromocriptine), and muscle relaxants (e.g., dantrolene sodium). NMS can be fatal if not properly monitored, but the prognosis improves with early detection and treatment.

12.2.5 Tolerance, Dependence, and Withdrawal

- Tolerance develops to sedative effects.
- Some signs of dependence may occur.
- Withdrawal may include muscular discomfort and difficulty in sleeping.

12.2.6 Drug Interactions

- Antipsychotics may potentiate the sedative effects of central depressants and opioid analgesics.
- Antiparkinsonian agents should not be used routinely in combination with antipsychotics, as they confound EPSEs.

▶ Table 12.1 summarizes the effects of antipsychotic agents based on the receptors they block.

12.3 Typical Antipsychotics (Classical Neuroleptics)

12.3.1 Phenothiazines

Phenothiazine antipsychotics are divided into three chemical classes based on their side chain.

12.3.2 Perphenazine and fluphenazine (piperazine chain)

Uses

These agents are the most potent antipsychotics and antiemetics, but have the highest incidence of EPSEs.

Note: Typical antipsychotic agents alleviate some of the positive symptoms of schizophrenia (see box "Signs and Symptoms of Schizophrenia").

Table 12.1 Effects of antipsychotic agents based on receptors blocked

Receptor blocked	Effects
5-HT$_2$ receptors in the CNS	Antipsychotic
D$_2$ receptors in the mesolimbic-mesocortical pathway	Antipsychotic
D$_2$ receptors in the nigrostriatal pathway	Extrapyramidal (motor) side effects
D$_2$ receptors in the tuberoinfundibular pathway	Hyperprolactinemia (increased blood prolactin)
D$_2$ receptors in the chemoreceptor trigger zone	Antiemetic
M$_1$ muscarinic	Anticholinergic effects: dry mouth, blurred vision, nasal stuffiness, constipation, urinary retention, palpitations
α$_1$ adrenergic	Orthostatic (postural) hypotension, impotence, drowsiness and dizziness, failure to ejaculate
H$_1$ histamine	Sedation, metabolic syndrome and weight gain

Clinical Correlation

Signs and Symptoms of Schizophrenia

Schizophrenia is characterized by positive, negative, and cognitive signs and symptoms.

Positive: Delusions, hallucinations, agitation, disorganized speech, and disorganized behavior.

Negative: Flattened affect, alogia (lack of unprompted content in normal speech), avolition (lack of drive or motivation), anhedonia (inability to experience pleasure), catatonia, and social isolation.

Cognitive: Disorganized thinking, difficulty concentrating, and memory (particularly working memory) problems.

12.3.3 Chlorpromazine (aliphatic chain)

Uses

- Chlorpromazine has both antipsychotic and antiemetic efficacy, but adverse effects have made it obsolete in treating schizophrenia.
- Intractable hiccups (drug of choice).

12.3.4 Thioridazine (piperidine chain)

Uses

Thioridazine is the least potent antipsychotic agent and has the lowest incidence of EPSEs.

12.3.5 Thioxanthenes

Thiothixene

Use

Personality disorders (drug of choice).

12.3.6 Butyrophenones

Haloperidol

Uses

Haloperidol is used extensively, especially for initial stabilization of the psychotic patient.

Side Effects

It causes fewer adverse autonomic effects than phenothiazines; however, the induction of tardive dyskinesia and other EPSEs limits its chronic use.

Pimozide

Uses

This agent prevents the acute exacerbation of chronic schizophrenia and suppresses motor and vocal tics in Tourette's syndrome.

Table 12.2 Prominent differences between classical neuroleptics and second-generation antipsychotics

Antipsychotic agent	Receptor action	Symptom relief in schizophrenia	Extrapyramidal system side effects (motor disorders)	Metabolic disturbances (weight gain, diabetes, lipid abnormalities)	Agranulocytosis	QT interval prolongation
Typical	Primarily D_2 antagonists	Decrease positive symptoms	Greater tendency for EPSEs	None	None	Some risk
Atypical	$5\text{-}HT_{2A}$ and D_2 antagonists (aripiprazole is a D^2 partial agonist)	Decrease positive symptoms, some improvement in negative symptoms	Less tendency for EPSEs	Substantial risk	Risk particularly with clozapine	Some risk

Abbreviations: 5-HT, 5-hydroxytryptamine; EPSE, extrapyramidal side effects.

Clinical Correlation

Tourette's Syndrome

Tourette's syndrome (TS) is a neurological disorder with hallmark "tics," which are rapid, recurring involuntary movements and speech. The pathology underlying TS is not understood, but research is focused on basal ganglia and frontal cortex. Most patients do not require therapeutics to reduce tics. In more severe cases, antipsychotics have been employed to reduce these symptoms. Atypical antipsychotics have better tolerability for this indication.

Loxapine

Uses

This drug is indicated for the treatment of schizoaffective disorders because its major metabolite, amoxapine, is an antidepressant.

12.4 Atypical Antipsychotics (Second-Generation Agents)

12.4.1 Clozapine, Olanzapine, Quetiapine, Paliperidone, Risperidone, Ziprasidone, Iloperidone, Pimavanserin, and Aripiprazole

Atypical antipsychotics improve positive symptoms, alleviate negative symptoms to a lesser degree, and have minimal efficacy on cognitive symptoms of schizophrenia.

Uses

- Psychotic disorders (olanzapine, quetiapine, paliperidone, risperidone, ziprasidone, aripiprazole). Clozapine is reserved for the treatment of refractory severe psychosis.
- Bipolar disorder I (olanzapine, ziprasidone).
- Bipolar disorder II (quetiapine, risperidone, aripiprazole).
- Autism spectrum disorder (risperidone, aripiprazole).
- Psychosis associated with Parkinson disease (pimavanserin). Pimavanserin is a newly approved drug for this indication. It is primarily a $5HT_{2A}$ and $5HT_{2C}$ antagonist, with negligible activity at D_2, H_1, α_1, or M_1 receptors.

Side Effects

- Atypical agents tend to produce less extrapyramidal reactions and anticholinergic side effects than the typical agents. However, they tend to produce weight gain leading to type II diabetes, and can cause cardiac QT interval prolongation leading to cardiac arrhythmias.
- Clozapine may also cause agranulocytosis.

▶ Fig. 12.1 and ▶ Table 12.2 summarize the differences between typical and atypical antipsychotic drugs.

III

13 Opiate Receptor Agonists and Antagonists

Summary

Opioids or opiates interact with opiate receptors and are used mainly to treat pain. Opiate agonists include morphine, which is the standard for comparison among opioids. Many semisynthetic compounds, including heroin, hydromorphone, oxymorphone, oxycodone, and hydrocodone, are made by modifying the morphine molecule. Codeine and dihydrocodeine are prodrugs converted in the liver to morphine and hydromorphone. Meperidine is a synthetic opiate. Fentanyl is a meperidine analogue 80 times as potent as morphine. Sufentanil is a meperidine analogue 6,000 times as potent as morphine. These three drugs act in the same way as morphine at opiate receptors but have less antitussive and constipating actions. Methadone and levo-α-acetylmethadol (LAAM) are synthetic, long-acting opiate agonists with similar pharmacological effects as morphine. Loperamide is a morphine derivative with a very low brain penetration. Its activity is mainly confined to the gut where it is highly efficacious in reducing gastrointestinal (GI) motility. Pentazocine is a mixed opiate agonist-antagonist, a μ-receptor antagonist, and a δ- and κ-receptor agonist. Buprenorphine is a partial agonist at μ receptors. Naloxone, naltrexone, and nalmefene are opiate antagonists. Naloxegol is an opioid receptor antagonist with a polyethylene glycol chain added to prevent the drug from crossing the blood–brain barrier. Dextromethorphan is an opioid analogue that is available over the counter but has no analgesic or addictive properties. Tramadol is a weak opiate receptor agonist chemically unrelated to opioids. Ziconotide is a peptide blocker of neuronal N-type Ca^{2+} channels used for the management of severe chronic pain.

Keywords: opiates, opioids, opiate receptors, opiate antagonists, pain

13.1 Opiate Receptor Agonists and Antagonists

Opioids or opiates are a class of drugs with opium-like properties that interact with a set of specific membrane receptors, the opiate receptors. Opioids are used mainly to treat pain.

13.1.1 Pain Modulation

Pain can be modulated at several sites, from its point of origin and through the various synaptic junctions in the pain pathways (▶ Fig. 13.1). These pathways may correlate with both the perception of pain and the reaction to that sensation. Opioids act in the spinal cord to decrease the sensation of pain (spinal analgesia) and act at higher centers to both decrease the sensation of pain and increase the patient's ability to tolerate the pain (supraspinal analgesia).

13.1.2 Opiate Receptors

There are three major categories of opiate receptors: μ (mu), δ (delta), and κ (kappa) receptors. The actions of opioids in current use are interpreted with regard to their actions at μ, δ, and κ receptors, as shown in ▶ Table 13.1.

13.2 Opiate Agonists

13.2.1 Morphine and Related Compounds

Morphine is the standard for comparison among opioids. Many semisynthetic compounds are made by modifying the morphine molecule.
- Diacetylmorphine (heroin) is made by acetylation at the three and six carbon positions.
- Hydromorphone, oxymorphone, oxycodone, and hydrocodone are also made by altering the morphine molecule.

Mechanisms of Action

- Morphine and related compounds act at all opiate receptors, but with the highest affinity at μ receptors. Activation of μ receptors decreases the spontaneous activity of neurons in the gut and in the central nervous system (CNS).

Foundations

Pain Pathways

Pain is transmitted from the periphery by Aδ fibers, activated by noxious heat and mechanical stimuli, and by C fibers, which respond to intense mechanical, chemical, and thermal stimuli. The cell bodies of these nerve fibers are in the dorsal root ganglion. Centrally, they innervate cells in the dorsal horn of the cord. Most of the axons from these cells cross and relay this information to the brain in the spinothalamic tracts. Most of these fibers synapse below the level of the thalamus, but some do go on to the thalamus. The impulses are then relayed to the limbic system and cortex. There are also descending fibers involved in pain, mainly serotonergic fibers from the midbrain raphe nuclei.

- Morphine acts on areas known to be involved in respiration, pain perception, mood, and emotion.
- At the cellular level, all three subtypes of opiate receptors couple to G_i and G_o. Activation of these G proteins by opioid-binding to opiate receptors decreases cyclic adenosine monophosphate levels (cAMP), increases K^+ currents, and decreases Ca^{2+} currents. This results in hyperpolarization and decreased release of neurotransmitters (▶ Fig. 13.2).
- Morphine selectively inhibits the excitatory inputs to neurons involved in transmitting information about noxious stimuli without changing the responses to other types of stimuli.

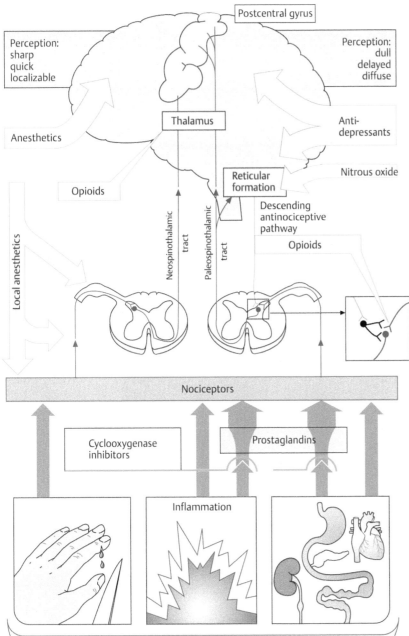

Fig. 13.1 Pain mechanisms and pathways.
Nociceptors detect painful stimuli and relay nociceptive impulses via Aδ fibers and C fibers to the brain. Impulses that are conveyed to specific areas of the postcentral gyrus produce short, sharp, well-localized pain, whereas impulses conveyed to more than one area of the cortex are perceived as dull, poorly localized pain. Drugs can act at multiple levels of the pain pathway to produce analgesia or alter the perception of pain.

III

Table 13.1 Actions mediated by opiate receptors

Opiate receptor	CNS location[a]	Action
μ	Dorsal horn of the spinal cord, nucleus of the solitary tract, periaqueductal gray region, thalamus, nucleus accumbens, amygdala, cerebral cortex	Supraspinal analgesia, respiratory depression, euphoria dependence
κ	Dorsal horn of the spinal cord, periaqueductal gray region, hypothalamus	Spinal analgesia Miosis (pupillary constriction) Sedation
δ	Pontine nucleus, nucleus accumbens, amygdala, cerebral cortex	Involved in affective behaviors (related to feelings or mental state)

Abbreviation: CNS, central nervous system.
[a]Opiate receptors are also found in the enteric nervous system, placenta, vas deferens, and immune system.

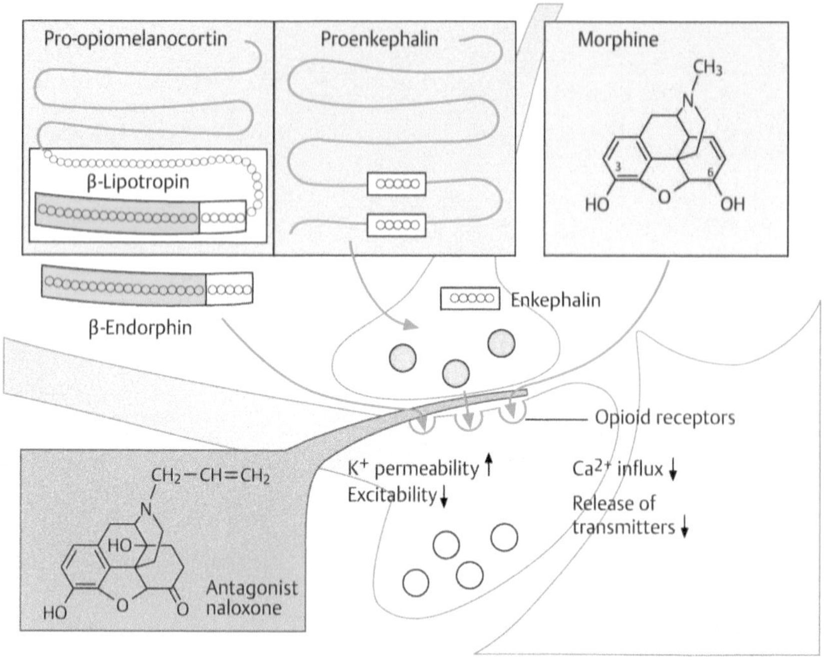

Fig. 13.2 Actions of endogenous and exogenous opioids at opiate receptors.
Endogenous opioids are all cleaved from the precursor peptides proenkephalin, pro-opiomelanocortin, and prodynorphin. Endogenous and exogenous opioids reduce neuronal excitability by increasing K^+ permeability leading to hyperpolarization of the neuronal membrane. Ca^{2+} influx into nerve terminals during excitation is also reduced causing decreased release of transmitter substances and decreased synaptic activity. Stimulant or depressant effects then occur depending on the transmitters and receptors affected.

Pharmacokinetics

- Morphine is readily absorbed from the GI tract, nasal mucosa, and lungs.
- Bioavailability of oral preparation ranges from 15 to 50% due to first-pass metabolism in the liver.
- Metabolized in the liver by glucuronide conjugation (▶ Fig. 13.3) to an active metabolite, morphine-6-glucuronide.
- Both morphine and morphine-6-glucuronide have very poor brain penetration, with brain:plasma ratio of nearly 1:10. This can result in an increased action on peripheral opioid receptors.
- Excreted as a glucuronide conjugate in the urine.
- Diacetylmorphine (heroin) is rapidly deacetylated in the liver to monoacetylmorphine, which is further deacetylated to morphine.

Foundations

Endogenous Opioids: Endorphins, Enkephalins, and Dynorphins

Endorphins, enkephalins, and dynorphins are endogenous neuropeptide neurotransmitters that are agonists at opiate receptors. Endorphins are found in the pituitary gland, whereas enkephalins and dynorphins are found throughout the nervous system and gut. Endorphins principally cause pain reduction, but they also produce euphoria, cause the release of sex hormones, and modulate appetite. The release of endorphins during prolonged/strenuous exercise results in the sense of euphoria and well-being accompanying exercise ("runner's high"). Enkephalins and dynorphins are also involved in the regulation and modulation of pain.

Effects

The effects of opioids are summarized in ▶ Table 13.2.

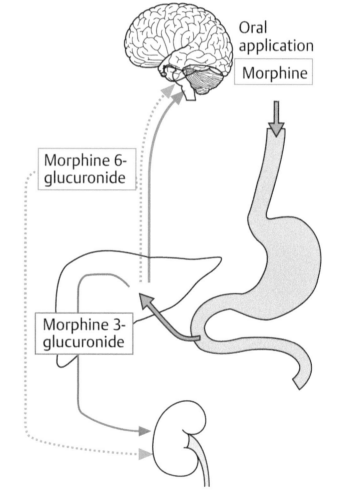

Fig. 13.3 Metabolism of morphine.
Morphine has a free hydroxyl group and is conjugated to glucuronic acid in the liver and excreted renally.

Table 13.2 Effects of morphine

System	Effects	Explanation/comment
CNS	Analgesia without loss of consciousness	Opioids are more selective for pain than other CNS drugs Other sensory modalities remain intact
	Respiratory depression	Direct inhibition of 5-HT$_{4A}$ receptors in the rhythm-generating respiratory neurons in the pre-Boetzinger complex of the brainstem
	Miosis	Excitation at the nucleus of the oculomotor nerve. This is pathognomonic of opiate intoxication (so-called pinpoint pupils)
	Euphoria	
	Antitussive (cough suppressant)	Inhibition of central cough reflex
	Nausea and vomiting	Opiates have a direct action on the chemoreceptor trigger zone in the medulla
	Warmth and drowsiness	
	Itchy nose	
Cardiovascular system	Peripheral vasodilation Inhibition of baroreceptor reflexes Orthostatic hypotension	There is little or no direct effect on the heart
GI system	Antidiarrheal, constipation	Decreased stomach motility, increased tone and nonpropulsive contractions in the small and large intestine, and increased tone of the anal sphincter
	Increased biliary tract pressure	

Abbreviations: CNS, central nervous system; GI, gastrointestinal.

Clinical Correlation

Abnormal Pupillary Reactions to Drugs

Many drugs cause miosis (constriction of the pupils), including opioids, antipsychotics (e.g., haloperidol), and parasympathomimetic cholinergic drugs (e.g., pilocarpine). Likewise, drugs can cause mydriasis (dilation of the pupils), including anticholinergics (e.g., atropine), hallucinogens (e.g., lysergic acid diethylamide [LSD]), cocaine, and some antidepressant drugs.

Uses

- Acute relief of pain (symptomatic treatment only).
- Chronic treatment of pain.
- Antitussives.
- Useful in diarrhea to produce constipation. Small amounts of opium tincture or paregoric are ingested. This effect is of

particular use following ileostomy or colostomy and in diarrhea and dysentery.

Side Effects

Nausea, vomiting, mental cloudiness, dysphoria, moderate to severe constipation, and increased biliary pressure. Opioid induced constipation (OIC) can be a severe AE in chronic opioid users. Note, loperamide is a morphine derivative with very limited brain penetration that is used to treat diarrhea.

Drug Interactions

Opioid action is potentiated by phenothiazines, monoamine oxidase inhibitors (MAOIs), and tricyclic antidepressants. Some phenothiazines will enhance the sedative effects of morphine while decreasing the analgesic effects.

Tolerance and Dependence

They are characteristics of the opioid drugs.

Contraindications

- It may not be advisable to use opioids in patients with head injury, as mental clouding, vomiting, and miosis may interfere with neurologic assessment of the patient.
- Caution must be used in patients with lung disease due to respiratory depression.

13.2.2 Codeine and Dihydrocodeine

Both prodrugs converted in the liver by CYP 2D6 to morphine (codeine) and hydromorphone (dihydrocodeine). CYP 2D6 is polymorphic in the human population; thus there can be a very wide exposure variability in the human population. In the population with active copies of CYP 2D6 there can be a resulting high exposure to the active metabolite. Codeine has a superior brain penetration to morphine, with 1:1 brain:plasma ratio. It can be converted by CYP2D6 in the brain. This can result in an increased action on central opioid receptors relative to morphine.

13.2.3 Meperidine, Fentanyl, Sufentanil

- Meperidine is a synthetic opiate.
- Fentanyl is a meperidine analogue 80 times as potent as morphine.
- Sufentanil is a meperidine analogue 6,000 times as potent as morphine.

Mechanism of Action

Meperidine acts in the same way as morphine, that is, as an agonist at opiate receptors.

Pharmacokinetics

- Meperidine has better bioavailability than morphine: 50% of absorbed meperidine escapes first-pass metabolism. Liver metabolism by CYP2B6, CYP3A4, and CYP2C19 results in several active and inactive metabolites. Normeperidine is neurotoxic with hallucinogenic and epileptogenic properties.

- Fentanyl has a rapid onset of action and has an extremely short half-life (several minutes). Typically given transdermally.

Effects

- Analgesia.
- May cause CNS excitement at toxic doses (unlike morphine).
- Respiratory depression.
- Cardiovascular: postural (orthostatic) hypotension but no significant effects.
- Smooth muscle: spasmogenic like morphine, but less intense in relation to its analgesia.

Note: Meperidine does not have antitussive or constipating actions.

Uses

- Analgesia.

Side Effects

The side effects are the same as for morphine, except there is less constipation. The metabolite normeperidine accumulates with repeated dosing. Normeperidine is not an analgesic, but it produces CNS excitation.

Drug Interactions

Meperidine may react with MAOIs, causing excitation, delirium, hyperpyrexia, convulsions, and severe respiratory depression.

13.2.4 Methadone and Levo-α-acetylmethadol (LAAM)

Mechanism of Action

These agents are synthetic, long-acting opiate agonists with similar pharmacological effects as morphine.

Pharmacokinetics

- Long half-life (1–1.5 days).

Uses

- Analgesia (equally as potent as morphine).
- Treatment of opioid withdrawal symptoms.

Side Effects

- Constipation and biliary spasm.

13.2.5 Oxycodone

Oxycodone is a potent and selective μ-opioid receptor agonist. It is metabolized through multiple pathways, primarily CYP3A4, followed by CYP2D6. The resulting metabolites are active, some with greater potency than the parent compound. The half-life of the parent is 3 to 6 hours with a moderately fast onset of action (less than 30 minutes). It is produced in many formulations, including extended release, and combination with various nonsteroidal anti-inflammatory drugs and acetaminophen.

13.2.6 Propoxyphene (Darvon)

Mechanism of Action

Propoxyphene is an agonist at opiate receptors.

Pharmacokinetics

It is not as potent or effective as codeine, but it does have less potential for dependence.

Uses

Previously used as an analgesic agent but has recently been removed from the market.

13.2.7 Loperamide

Loperamide is a morphine derivative with a substituent added to make the molecule a strong Pgp substrate. Consequently it has very low brain penetration and is essentially devoid of CNS activity of any kind. On the other hand, it is highly efficacious in reducing GI motility in diarrhea and has been shown to be effective in treating other GI disorders including inflammatory bowel disease and short bowel syndrome.

13.3 Mixed Opiate Agonist-Antagonists

13.3.1 Pentazocine

Mechanism of Action

Pentazocine is a μ-receptor antagonist and a δ- and κ-receptor agonist.

Effects

- Produces analgesia, sedation, and respiratory depression.
- May block the analgesia produced by morphine.

Uses

- Primarily used as an analgesic, but not effective against severe pain.

Side Effects

- Respiratory depression.
- May cause confusion and hallucinations.

Tolerance, Dependence, and Withdrawal

- Originally thought to have less potential for abuse and released for general use, but then drug abusers combined pentazocine and tripelennamine as a substitute for heroin. Talwin Nx (pentazocine and naloxone) includes naloxone to prevent intravenous (IV) use.
- May precipitate withdrawal symptoms in patients who have been receiving opioids.

13.3.2 Buprenorphine

Mechanism of Action

Buprenorphine is a partial agonist at μ receptors.

Pharmacokinetics

- Given intramuscularly, IV, or sublingually.

Uses

- Analgesia.

Side Effects

- Respiratory depression at high doses.

13.4 Opiate Antagonists

13.4.1 Naloxone, Naltrexone, and Nalmefene

Mechanism of Action

These antagonists bind with high affinity to all opiate receptors but have highest affinity for μ receptors. They act as competitive inhibitors.

Pharmacokinetics

- Naloxone and nalmefene are only effective IV, with nalmefene having a longer duration of action (10 hours versus 1 hour for naloxone).
- Naltrexone is effective orally.

Uses

- Naloxone and nalmefene are used to treat opioid poisoning.
- Naltrexone has been tested for treating drug and alcohol addictions.

Withdrawal

In patients dependent on opiates, antagonists will induce withdrawal symptoms.

13.4.2 Naloxegol

Mechanism of Action

Naloxegol is a selective μ antagonist with a polyethylene glycol chain added to prevent crossing the blood–brain barrier. This allows opioid agonists to reach their target in the CNS to have their desired analgesic effect; however, naloxegol is dose to plasma exposures to prevent the opioid agonists from binding to their target in the periphery, particularly μ opioid receptors in the GI tract. This allows opioid agonists to have their central analgesic effects while preventing peripherally opioid-induced constipation (OIC), which can be a very serious condition with chronic use of opioid analgesics. It is generally well-tolerated.

Pharmacokinetics

- Plasma half-life is about 4 hours.
- Mainly hepatic metabolism, mainly CYP3A4.

Use

For the treatment and prevention of OIC while taking opioid agonist analgesics.

Drug Interactions

Drugs inhibiting CYP3A4 (such as diltiazem or quinidine) can markedly increase exposure of naloxegol; use with such drugs should be avoided or dosing reduced.

Adverse Effects

- GI effects, including abdominal pain, diarrhea, nausea, and flatulence.

Clinical Correlation

Opioid Poisoning

Opioid poisoning may result from clinical use, abuse, or suicide attempt. Symptoms include coma, pinpoint pupils, and depressed respiration. Overdose is frequently accompanied by other drugs, which may confound the diagnosis and treatment. Treatment involves supporting ventilation and administering naloxone intravenously.

13.5 Related Compounds

13.5.1 Dextromethorphan

Dextromethorphan is an opioid analogue that is available over the counter but has no analgesic or addictive properties.

Mechanism of Action

- Unclear, but may involve μ and κ receptors.

Uses

- Antitussive.

13.5.2 Tramadol

Tramadol is chemically unrelated to opioids.

Mechanism of Action

Tramadol is a weak opiate receptor agonist. It also inhibits norepinephrine and 5-hydroxytryptamine (5-HT) reuptake. It is only partially inhibited by naloxone. It is equal to or less effective than codeine plus aspirin or codeine plus acetaminophen.

Uses

- Neuropathic pain.

Side Effects

• Constipation, nausea, vomiting, dizziness, and drowsiness.

13.5.3 Ziconotide

Ziconotide is not an opioid.

Mechanism of Action

Ziconotide is a peptide blocker of neuronal N-type Ca^{2+} channels.

Pharmacokinetics

• Given by intrathecal infusion.

Uses

• Management of severe chronic pain.

Side Effects

• Severe psychiatric symptoms, such as hallucinations, paranoia, and delirium. Drunk-like reactions also occur (e.g., dizziness, sleepiness, confusion, incoordination, and mental slowness). These symptoms take days or weeks to resolve after discontinuation.
• Bacterial meningitis.

▶ Table 13.3 provides a summary of the primary indications for the opioid analgesics.

Table 13.3 Primary indications for opioid analgesics

Opioid	Indications
Morphine and related compounds	Acute pain Chronic pain Cough (codeine)[a] Diarrhea
Meperidine and analogues	Analgesia Regional analgesia (fentanyl) Preanesthetic (fentanyl)
Methadone and LAAM	Opioid withdrawal
Pentazocine	Analgesia for moderate pain
Buprenorphine	Analgesia
Naloxone and nalmefene	Opioid poisoning
Dextromethorphan	Cough[a]
Tramadol	Neuropathic pain
Ziconotide	Severe chronic pain

Abbreviation: LAAM, levo-α-acetylmethadol.
[a]Opioids and related compounds are used for severe cough when nonopioid cough suppressants have failed.

14 Treatment of Neurodegenerative Diseases

Summary

Neurodegenerative diseases, particularly Alzheimer and Parkinson diseases, are caused by the progressive degeneration of specific parts of the central nervous system (CNS) and are primarily observed in the elderly population. At present, there are no treatments to slow the progression or any cure of these eventually fatal diseases. Symptomatic treatments for Parkinson disease, particularly dopamine replacements (e.g., L-dopa) or enhancements, have reasonable efficacy in early and mid-stages of the disease.

Parkinson disease motor symptoms result from loss of dopamine-containing neurons in the substantia nigra. Strategies to combat the dopamine deficiency include increasing dopamine precursor levels (levodopa and carbidopa), decreasing dopamine breakdown (entacapone, selegiline, and rasagiline), and administering dopamine receptor agonists (apomorphine, bromocriptine, pramipexole, and ropinirole).

Anticholinergic agents, such as trihexyphenidyl, benztropine, procyclidine, and diphenhydramine, are also used to treat Parkinson disease in early stages, in patients who are intolerant to levodopa, or as a supplement to levodopa.

Symptomatic treatments for Alzheimer disease include cholinesterase inhibitors and N-methyl-D-aspartate (NMDA) channel blockers. Donepezil, rivastigmine, and galantamine are centrally acting, reversible inhibitors of cholinesterase. Memantine is an NMDA receptor antagonist approved for symptomatic treatments of moderate to severe Alzheimer disease.

Spasticity and muscle spasms can result from lesions at various levels of the CNS. Baclofen is a gamma-aminobutyric acid type B ($GABA_B$) receptor agonist that acts in the spinal cord to hyperpolarize afferent nerve terminals and thus inhibit synaptic transmission. Diazepam enhances presynaptic inhibition in the spinal cord. Dantrolene acts directly on skeletal muscle to reduce skeletal muscle contractions.

Keywords: Parkinson, Alzheimer, spasticity, dopamine, acetylcholine

14.1 Treatment of Neurodegenerative Diseases

Neurodegenerative diseases particularly affect the elderly. As the population ages, this becomes an increasing problem. While there are a number of specific neurodegenerative diseases, the greatest number of patients have Alzheimer disease, characterized primarily by progressive memory decline. The second largest group of patients has Parkinson disease, characterized primarily by motor control deficits. At present there is no cure or any pharmacotherapies to slow the progression of these diseases, and these diseases are typically fatal. For Parkinson disease, there are a number of symptomatic treatments, such as L-dopa, that treat the dopamine deficiency and have reasonable efficacy, particularly early in the disease. For Alzheimer disease, there are two classes of pharmacotherapies, the cholinesterase inhibitors for the symptomatic treatment of all stages of the disease and memantine, an NMDA channel blocker, for the treatment of moderate to severe Alzheimer disease.

14.2 Parkinson Disease

14.2.1 Description

Parkinson disease is a chronic, progressive, age-related neurodegenerative disease where the motor symptoms result from loss of dopamine-containing neurons in the substantia nigra (▶ Fig. 14.1). This affects the complex release of excitatory and inhibitory neurotransmitters in the basal ganglia and subthalamic nucleus which culminates in excessive inhibition of the thalamus. Inhibition of the thalamus suppresses voluntary movement and accounts for the motor signs and symptoms of Parkinson disease with the following primary symptoms.

- Bradykinesia (slow initiation of movements) and decrease of spontaneous movements and at least one of the following.
  ○ Rigidity.
  ○ Tremor (typically 4–6 Hz at rest).
  ○ Postural disturbances occurring in later phases. Such disturbances are not specific to Parkinson disease and can be due to deficits in the cerebellum, vestibular, and sensory systems.
- Misdiagnosis of PD can be as high as 30% in the early stages. Typically, this is because of failure to recognize other Parkinson-like or Parkinson-plus disorders such as progressive supranuclear palsy, multiple system atrophy, corticobasal ganglionic degeneration, or Lewy body dementia (LBD).
- Parkinson disease dementia (PDD) is observed in at least 30% of Parkinson patients, where motor symptoms precede the development of dementia. In LBD, considered a different disease than Parkinson disease, development of cognitive impairment precedes or is coincident with the development of motor symptoms.

Clinical Correlation

Lewy Body Dementia

LBD is the third most common form of dementia after Alzheimer disease and vasculature dementia. While the cause of the disease is unknown, the hallmark is the deposition of alpha-synuclein protein (Lewy body proteins) that deposit throughout the cortex of the brain. LBD typically manifests with cognitive impairment and increasing difficulty in performing tasks, as well as memory problems and visual hallucinations. When this deposition occurs in the substantia nigra, dopamine stores become depleted, resulting in parkinsonian motor symptoms. There is no cure for this disease, so treatment aims to reduce symptoms by using cholinesterase inhibitors, levodopa, and antipsychotic (neuroleptic) drugs. A dangerous reaction known as neuroleptic malignant syndrome can occur frequently in patients taking antipsychotic (neuroleptic) drugs; therefore, such drugs are used cautiously and typically at low doses.

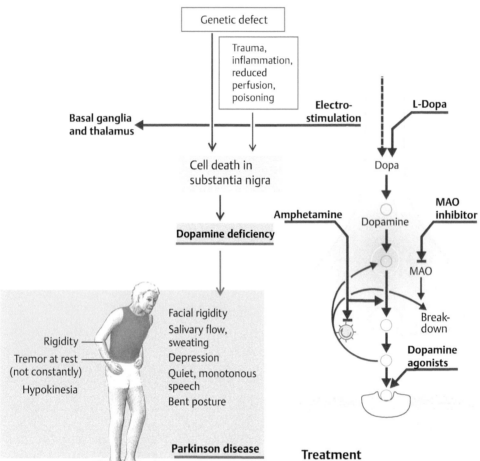

Fig. 14.1 Parkinson disease.
In Parkinson disease, till the time motor symptoms emerge, degeneration of up to 50% of dopaminergic neurons in the substantia nigra has already occurred. This results in less dopamine availability to neurons in the striatum. Ultimately, these changes result in excess inhibition of the thalamus (via gamma-aminobutyric acid) and are principally responsible for the motor symptoms of Parkinson disease. Treatment of the motor symptoms aims to increase the availability of dopamine in these neurons.

14.2.2 Nigrostriatal Tract and Motor Symptoms of Parkinson Disease

In a normal, healthy person, there is a balance between inhibitory dopamine components and excitatory acetylcholine (ACh) components in the nigrostriatal tract. In Parkinson disease, however, there is a deficiency of the dopamine component; therefore, the goal of therapy is to restore dopamine levels. Alternatively, the ACh component can be reduced with anticholinergics (▶ Fig. 14.2).

14.3 Antiparkinsonian Drugs

Present therapies for Parkinson disease only treat, primarily, the motor symptoms that are due to the degeneration of the nigral dopaminergic neurons. Multiple therapeutic approaches seek to compensate for the loss of dopamine release in this brain region. Dopamine cannot be given directly because it is rapidly metabolized in the periphery, has adverse side effects on the cardiovascular system, and does not effectively penetrate the CNS. Strategies to combat the dopamine deficiency include increasing dopamine precursor levels (levodopa and carbidopa), decreasing dopamine breakdown (entacapone, tolcapone, selegiline, and rasagiline), enhancing dopamine release (amantadine), and administering dopamine receptor agonists (apomorphine, bromocriptine, pramipexole, and ropinirole).

14.3.1 Levodopa

Mechanism of Action

Levodopa, or L-3,4-dihydroxyphenylalanine (L-dopa), is a precursor in dopamine synthesis. It is formed from L-tyrosine and is transformed to dopamine by aromatic L-amino acid decarboxylase (dopa decarboxylase). Levodopa itself is pharmacologically inert; its effects are a result of decarboxylation to dopamine (▶ Fig. 14.3).

Pharmacokinetics

- Levodopa is rapidly absorbed from the intestine by active transport. Administration with meals reduces absorption.
- It has a short plasma half-life of 1 to 3 hours.
- It undergoes peripheral decarboxylation.
- Small amounts enter the CNS.
- It is converted to dihydroxyphenylacetic acid and homovanillic acid, and is excreted in the urine.
- The optimal efficacy of levodopa is seen in the early stages of Parkinson disease. As the disease progresses, the duration of efficacy is shorter and excessive dopamine results in dyskinesias. At advanced stages of Parkinson disease, this dyskinesia can be difficult to tolerate and the efficacy of levodopa becomes very brief.

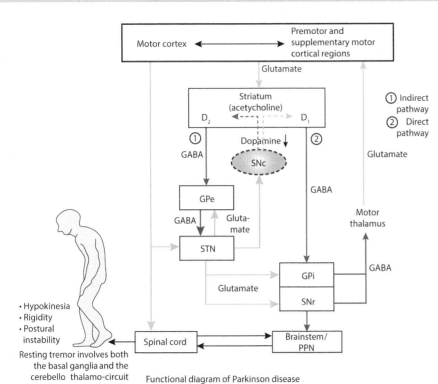

Fig. 14.2 Functional diagram of Parkinson disease.
Neurons projecting from the substantia nigra pars compacta (SNc) to the striatum release dopamine (DA) which normally interacts with excitatory D_1 and inhibitory D_2 receptors. In Parkinson disease, the degeneration of neurons in the SNc leads to a deficiency of dopamine released in the SNc. Through indirect (1) and direct (2) pathways, this leads to altered outputs from the internal globus pallidus (GPi) and substantia nigra pars reticulata (SNr) that control movements. Indirect pathway: (1) Reduced DA release in the striatum increases the activity of GABAergic neurons projecting to the external globus pallidus (GPe), decreasing the normal inhibitory action of the GPe projections to the subthalamic nucleus (STN). This leads to increased excitation from STN to the GPi and SNr. Direct pathway: (2) D_1 receptors normally excite neurons that maintain direct inhibitory control of the GPi and SNr. A decrease in DA release leads to decrease in the activity of the direct inhibitory pathway to GPi and SNr. As a result, both of these pathways contribute to increased drive to the GPi and SNr, abnormally increasing the inhibitory outputs to thalamus and spinal cord.

Functional diagram of Parkinson disease
(red= inhibition, green= activation, dotted lines= diminished activation/inhibition; the thickness of the arrows reflects the degree of activation/ inhibition) Obeso et al 2000

Foundations

Basal Ganglia

The basal ganglia are made up of the corpus striatum (which is composed of the caudate nucleus and putamen), globus pallidus, subthalamic nucleus, and substantia nigra. It functions to control movement in conjunction with the cerebellum and motor cortex (▶ Fig. 14.2).

Foundations

Control of Movements

The pyramidal and extrapyramidal motor systems are involved in the control of movement. The pyramidal system is involved in initiation and termination of movement. Disorders of the pyramidal system are characterized by paralysis, spasticity, and inability to easily initiate movements. The extrapyramidal motor system consists of the basal ganglia (caudate putamen, globus pallidus, subthalamic nuclei, and substantia nigra), with connections to the thalamus, cortex, reticular formation, and spinal cord (▶ Fig. 14.2). The extrapyramidal system integrates and coordinates impulses arising in the pyramidal system. Disorders of this system are characterized by dyskinesias.

Table 14.1 Effects of levodopa

System	Effects
CNS	Relieves bradykinesia and rigidity preferentially over relieving tremor. Secondary improvements are seen in posture, gait, ability to modify facial expression, speech, and handwriting. There is no relief of dementia
Cardiovascular system	Postural (orthostatic) hypotension and cardiac stimulation occur, although tolerance usually develops (mechanism unknown)
Endocrine system	Prolactin secretion is inhibited.[a] Growth hormone release may also be observed in healthy individuals but not in patients with Parkinson disease

Abbreviation: CNS, central nervous system.
[a]Dopamine is a prolactin-inhibiting hormone.

Effects

▶ Table 14.1 describes the effects of levodopa.

Side Effects

▶ Table 14.2 lists the side effects experienced by most patients who take levodopa.

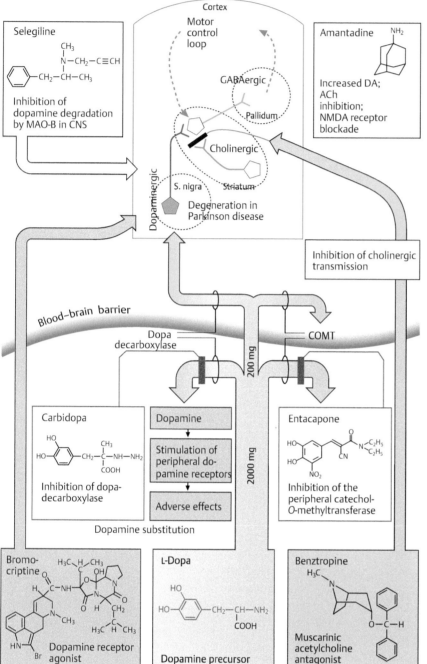

Fig. 14.3 Antiparkinsonian drugs.
The dopamine precursor levodopa (L-dopa) penetrates the blood–brain barrier (unlike dopamine), where it can directly replenish striatal dopamine levels. Carbidopa inhibits dopa decarboxylase and thus prevents the peripheral production of dopamine that can cause adverse effects (e.g., vomiting). Carbidopa cannot cross the blood–brain barrier; thus, central decarboxylation is unaffected. Bromocriptine is a dopamine agonist in the central nervous system (CNS). Entacapone is a catechol-*O*-methyltransferase (COMT) inhibitor that prevents the peripheral breakdown of levodopa, allowing more levodopa to be available for the CNS. Benztropine is a muscarinic receptor antagonist that blocks acetylcholine in the striatum and thereby counteracts excessive cholinergic activity that results from dopamine deficiency. Selegiline inhibits the degradation of dopamine by monoamine oxidase type B in the striatum. Amantadine increases DA release and has anticholinergic properties.

Drug Interactions

- Pyridoxine, a form of vitamin B_6 found in multivitamins, is a cofactor for dopa decarboxylase and may enhance the metabolism of levodopa.
- Antipsychotics antagonize dopamine receptors and thus antagonize the efficacy of levodopa. Therefore, these are contraindicated with levodopa.
- Reserpine is contraindicated because it depletes dopamine.
- Monoamine oxidase inhibitors (MAOIs) block dopamine breakdown and may exaggerate effects (hypertensive crisis and hyperpyrexia). MAOIs should be withdrawn at least 2 weeks prior to levodopa administration.
- Anticholinergics may slow gastric emptying.

Contraindications

Care must be exercised in patients with heart disease, cerebrovascular disease, or neurological disease.

14.3.2 Aromatic L-Amino Acid Decarboxylase Inhibitors: Carbidopa and Benserazide

Carbidopa is the only type available in the United States. Benserazide, which is available in Europe and Canada, has similar properties.

Table 14.2 Side effects of levodopa[a]

	Side effects
Short-term	Nausea and vomiting, cardiac arrhythmias
Long-term	As described above, dyskinesia develops as the disease progresses and overwhelms efficacy in advanced Parkinson disease. These are observed as abnormal movements such as tics, grimacing, head bobbing, and oscillatory movements of the limbs seen in 50% of patients within 2 to 4 months and in 80% of patients by 1 year. No tolerance develops to these effects, and they will worsen if the dose is not reduced
	Psychiatric disturbances (serious in 15% of patients) largely due to overaction of D_2 receptor pathways: hallucinations, paranoia, mania, insomnia, anxiety, nightmares, and depression
	False-positive test for ketoacidosis by the dipstick test due to the presence of levodopa metabolites
	Red-colored urine that changes to black on exposure to air or alkali

[a]All side effects are seen in the majority of patients. These are reversible and can be controlled by reducing the dose.

Mechanism of Action

These agents inhibit the peripheral production of dopamine from levodopa by inhibiting dopa decarboxylase. This allows more levodopa availability to the CNS (▶ Fig. 14.3).

Uses

Carbidopa and benserazide are usually administered with levodopa. They confer the following advantages:
- They allow for a dose reduction of levodopa and for a reduced number of doses.
- The effective dose is achieved more rapidly.
- A larger percentage of patients respond favorably.
- Pyridoxine interaction is avoided.

Side Effects

- No side effects are seen when these agents are given alone. All side effects are associated with the increased effect of levodopa.
- CNS side effects may appear more frequently or earlier in therapy.
- There are fewer peripheral side effects, such as nausea, vomiting, and cardiac effects.

14.3.3 Entacapone

Mechanism of Action

Entacapone is a selective and reversible inhibitor of catechol-*O*-methyltransferase (COMT), which is the enzyme responsible for the peripheral breakdown of levodopa. This allows more levodopa to be available in the CNS (▶ Fig. 14.3). It acts mainly in the periphery.

Uses

Adjunctive therapy to patients experiencing fluctuations in disability related to levodopa and dopa decarboxylase inhibitor combinations.

Side Effects

No adverse effects alone but enhanced adverse effects of levodopa.

Drug Interactions

May potentiate the actions of drugs metabolized by COMT (i.e., dopamine, epinephrine, and methyldopa).

14.3.4 Pramipexole, Ropinirole, Rotigotine, and Apomorphine

Mechanism of Action

These agents are dopamine agonists.

Uses

- Parkinson disease.
- Restless leg syndrome (pramipexole and ropinirole).
- Apomorphine is widely used in place of levodopa, particularly in Europe; however, it is not orally available and must be administered subcutaneously. Commonly it is administered via a pump.

Side Effects

- Same as levodopa.

14.3.5 Selegiline, Rasagiline, and Safinamide

Mechanism of Action

Selegiline, rasagiline, and safinamide are selective inhibitors of MAO-B, the enzyme involved in dopamine metabolism in the CNS (▶ Fig. 14.3).

Side Effects

These agents potentiate the effects of dopamine in the brain but do not potentiate the effects of catecholamines to produce a hypertensive crisis.

14.3.6 Trihexyphenidyl, Benztropine, Procyclidine, and Diphenhydramine

These anticholinergics were the primary agents prior to the introduction of levodopa.

Uses

- Useful in early stages, in patients who are intolerant to levodopa, or as a supplement to levodopa therapy.
- More effective in relieving tremor than either rigidity or bradykinesia.

Side Effects

- Cycloplegia, constipation, and urinary retention.
- CNS: confusion, delirium, and hallucinations.
- Paralysis of the ciliary muscle of the eye.

14.4 Alzheimer Disease

14.4.1 Description

Alzheimer disease is a progressive neurodegenerative disorder characterized by marked atrophy of the cerebral cortex. It is the most common cause of dementia. It produces the following signs and symptoms:

- Impairment of short-term memory.
- Impairment of cognition and language.
- Increasing difficulty in performing the activities of daily living or executive function.
- Personality changes, for example, anxiety, depression, aggression, psychosis, and social withdrawal. These symptoms are now classified as behavioral and psychiatric symptoms associated with dementia (BPSD).
- Immobility leading to death.

Clinical Correlation

The Mini-Mental State Exam (MMSE)

The MMSE is a clinician-administered pen and paper test to determine the stage of dementia. A normal person has a score of 30, while a score of 25 to 29 is considered mild cognitive impairment without a definitive diagnosis of Alzheimer disease or dementia.

Mild Alzheimer disease: MMSE 20 to 24. Family begins to notice cognitive or memory difficulties. Typical difficulties include problems coming up with the correct word, remembering names, misplacing objects, and difficulty planning and performing complicated tasks.

Moderate Alzheimer disease: MMSE 13 to 20. This is the longest lasting stage of this disease, typically lasting many years. The cognitive difficulties affect daily living and require greater external care. The patient confuses words, forgets events, including their personal history. Memory difficulties lead to behavioral difficulties, poor mood, and social withdrawal. Inability to live independently leads to increased frustration; patients often wander and get lost. Sleep, bladder, and bowel control can be disrupted.

Severe Alzheimer disease: MMSE less than 12. In this stage, patients no longer respond to the environment, cannot converse, and eventually cannot properly control their movements. Their personality is altered, memory and cognitive performance are greatly impaired, and substantial assistance is needed for most activities of daily living. Finally, patients become vulnerable to infections, such as pneumonia.

Cognitive and memory impairment in Alzheimer disease has been linked to the progressive loss of neurons and synapses, and the subsequent loss of cholinergic transmission within the cerebral cortex. In addition, amyloid-rich neuritic plaques and neurofibrillary tangles are observed in postmortem brains; these changes begin years before the onset of clinical symptoms. Other neurodegenerative processes may result from damage to neurons due to overstimulation by glutamate, particularly at NMDA receptors.

14.4.2 Alzheimer Disease Drugs

Presently there are two classes of drugs for the symptomatic treatment of this disease which lead to a mild improvement in cognitive deficits. However, the more debilitating psychiatric symptoms of the disease (i.e., BPSD) are not adequately treated.

Donepezil, Rivastigmine, and Galantamine

Mechanism of Action

These agents are centrally acting, reversible inhibitors of cholinesterase. They prevent the hydrolysis of ACh, thus increasing the concentration of ACh available to neurons.

Uses

Donepezil is approved for all stages of Alzheimer disease. Rivastigmine and galantamine are approved for treating cognition deficits in mild to moderate Alzheimer disease. All three have moderate effects on improving cognitive deficits.

Side Effects

Nausea, diarrhea, vomiting.

Memantine

Mechanism of Action

Memantine is an NMDA receptor antagonist. It is thought to act by reducing excessive activity of GABAergic interneurons and allow normal excitatory signaling.

Uses

Approved for symptomatic treatments of moderate to severe Alzheimer disease.

Side Effects

Confusion and dizziness.

14.5 Spasticity and Muscle Spasms

Spasticity and muscle spasms can result from lesions at various levels of the CNS. Dysfunction in the descending pathways controlling motor neurons results in hyperexcitability of the tonic stretch reflexes. The mechanisms by which drugs can affect skeletal muscle tone are illustrated in ▶ Fig. 14.4.

14.5.1 Baclofen

Mechanism of Action

Baclofen is a gamma-aminobutyric acid type B (GABA$_B$) receptor antagonist that acts in the spinal cord to hyperpolarize afferent nerve terminals and thus inhibit synaptic transmission.

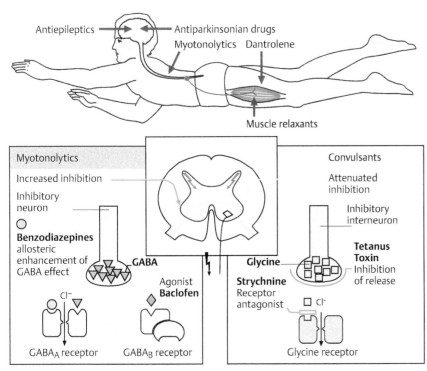

Fig. 14.4 Mechanisms influencing skeletal muscle tone.
Myotonolytics lower muscle tone by increasing the activity of intraspinal inhibitory neurons. Benzodiazepines augment the action of GABA at GABA$_A$ receptors, which are ligand-gated Cl$^-$ ion channels. Baclofen is an antagonist at GABA$_B$ receptors, which are G protein-coupled. Dantrolene acts on muscle cells to reduce Ca^{2+} release from the sarcoplasmic reticulum, causing muscle relaxation. Muscle relaxants themselves also act on muscle cells to cause relaxation. Antiepileptics and antiparkinsonian drugs act centrally to affect muscle tone. These agents are used to treat various spasticity disorders, as well as painful muscle spasms. Convulsants, such as tetanus toxin and strychnine, inhibit glycine, which is an interneuronal synaptic inhibitor. This allows impulses to propagate unchecked along the spinal cord, leading to convulsions.

Uses

- Treatment of spasticity in multiple sclerosis and spinal trauma.
- Cerebral palsy (given intrathecally).

Note: It is not used for stroke.

Side Effects

- Sedation, insomnia, dizziness, weakness, and ataxia.
- The threshold for seizures is decreased.

Withdrawal

- Causes hallucinations, anxiety, and tachycardia.

14.5.2 Diazepam

Mechanism of Action

Diazepam enhances presynaptic inhibition in the spinal cord.

Uses

- Spinal lesions.
- Some cases of cerebral palsy.

14.5.3 Tizanidine

Mechanism of Action

Tizanidine is an α_2-adrenergic receptor agonist that relieves spasticity by increasing presynaptic inhibition of motor neurons.

Uses

- Treatment of spasticity in multiple sclerosis and spinal trauma.

14.5.4 Dantrolene

Mechanism of Action

Dantrolene acts directly on skeletal muscle to apparently decrease Ca^{2+} release from the sarcoplasmic reticulum, thus reducing skeletal muscle contractions (▶ Fig. 14.5).

Uses

- Reduces spasticity in paraplegics and hemiplegics.
- Cerebral palsy (improvement seen in 50% of cases).

Side Effects

- Hepatotoxicity.
- Weakness.

Clinical Correlation

Muscular Dystrophy

Muscular dystrophy is a term used to describe a group of inherited muscle diseases. Each individual type of muscular dystrophy has its own genetic defect. The most common type of muscular dystrophy is due to a genetic defect that causes a mutation in dystrophin, part of a protein complex that conveys force from the Z disks to connective tissue on the surface of the fiber. Dystrophin mutations result in degeneration of muscle fibers with increasing muscle weakness. As the disease progresses, there will be muscular contractures with loss of mobility of joints. There is no cure for this group of diseases, but drugs are sometimes used to provide symptomatic relief or to slow its progression. Drugs that help with contractures include phenytoin, carbamazepine, and dantrolene. Prednisone, cyclosporin, and azathioprine may also be used to protect muscle cells from damage. Physical therapy is the mainstay of

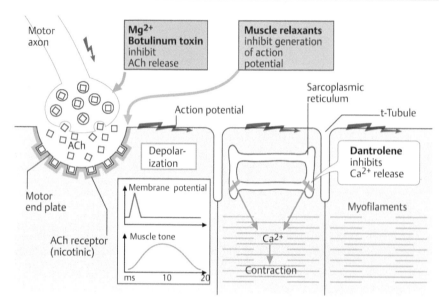

Fig. 14.5 Inhibition of neuromuscular transmission and electromechanical coupling.
Acetylcholine (ACh) is released from motor neurons upon stimulation. It then binds to nicotinic receptors in the motor end plate, causing it to depolarize and propagate an action potential to the surrounding sarcolemma. The sarcoplasmic reticulum then releases Ca^{2+} which causes myofilaments to contract. This electromechanical coupling can be inhibited at different stages. Mg^{2+} and botulinum toxin inhibit ACh release from motor neurons, muscle relaxants inhibit the generation of action potentials, and dantrolene inhibits Ca^{2+} release from the sarcoplasmic reticulum.

treatment for muscular dystrophy to try to preserve mobility. Surgery may be used for the relief of contractures.

14.6 Huntington Disease and Amyotrophic Lateral Sclerosis

14.6.1 Huntington Disease

Huntington disease (HD) is an autosomal dominant, progressive, neurodegenerative disorder that affects movement control, emotion, and cognition. Age of onset is usually in the 30 s to 40 s, with initial signs including agitation, dysthymia, minor problems with voluntary control, poor coordination, and early signs of cognitive deficits, including executive function. With age, these problems become more pronounced, developing into choreas, or involuntary jerking movements, eventually resulting in difficulty walking, speaking, and swallowing along with more severe cognitive and mood dysfunction. The disease is fatal within 15 to 20 years of symptom onset.

There are no curative agents or agents that can slow the progression of HD. Tetrabenazine and reserpine may be used to reduce the choreiform movements in patients with HD. Other CNS-active agents may be used to treat depression, anxiety, paranoia, or psychosis in these patients.

Tetrabenazine and Reserpine

Mechanism of Action

HD is characterized by a loss of GABAergic neurons in the striatum (see ▶ Fig. 14.1). However, the inhibitory dopamine input from the substantia nigra is preserved. Tetrabenazine and reserpine deplete monoamine neurotransmitters, including dopamine, thus decreasing the dopamine inhibition of the remaining GABA neurons.

Side Effects

- Anxiety.
- Depression.
- Hypotension.
- Insomnia.
- Nausea.

14.6.2 Amyotrophic Lateral Sclerosis

Amyotrophic lateral sclerosis (ALS), also known as Lou Gehrig disease, is an autosomal dominant genetic disease characterized by a progressive degeneration of motoneurons. Symptoms include the loss of movement control, speech, the ability to eat, and, eventually, the ability to control the diaphragm, which leads to death. There are no curative treatments for ALS. Riluzole and edaravone provide a modest slowing of the progression of the disease and a relief of symptoms.

Riluzole

Mechanism of Action

The precise mechanism is unknown but may inhibit presynaptic glutamate release and block postsynaptic glutamate effects, thus reducing neurotoxicity.

Side Effects

- Nausea.
- Dizziness.
- Elevated liver enzymes.

Edaravone

Mechanism of Action

Free radical scavenger that may reduce oxidative stress.

Pharmacokinetics

Given intravenously daily for two weeks followed by two weeks drug free.

Side Effects

- Headache.
- Abnormal gait.

III

15 Drugs of Abuse

Summary

Numerous central nervous system (CNS)-active drugs are subject to licit and illicit nonmedical use which can lead to addiction and dependence. Prescription and illicit preparations of opiates may be abused. Methadone and buprenorphine are used to manage opiate abuse. Naltrexone will not relieve withdrawal but can improve compliance. Alcohol is the most widely abused drug. Withdrawal symptoms will be mild to moderate in 80 to 85% of patients and more severe in 15 to 20% of patients. Drugs to manage alcoholism include naltrexone, acamprosate, and disulfiram. Benzodiazepines are also subject to abuse. Flumazenil is a benzodiazepine-site negative modulator with a short plasma half-life that can be used to treat benzodiazepine overdose. Barbiturates produce intoxication similar to benzodiazepines, but their effects are not blocked by flumazenil. Methaqualone is a former prescription medication with pharmacology similar to barbiturates that is now synthesized and sold illicitly. Caffeine is a stimulant that may lead to dependence in the form of a throbbing, diffuse headache. Amphetamines and cocaine commonly produce dependence and an extremely intense drug craving. Psychedelic hallucinogens include d-lysergic acid diethylamide (LSD), psilocybin, and mescaline. Deliriant hallucinogens include phencyclidine and ketamine. The main psychoactive ingredient in marijuana and hashish is tetrahydrocannabinol (THC). Tolerance develops to the effects of THC; physical dependence does not occur. Nicotine produces psychological dependence with intense craving. Treatments include nicotine replacement therapy, varenicline, and bupropion. A variety of inhalants including nitrous oxide, gasoline, volatile solvents, and aerosols are subject to abuse. Gamma-hydroxybutyrate (GHB) is a gamma-aminobutyric acid receptor agonist that is abused.

Keywords: opiates, CNS depressants, CNS stimulants, hallucinogens, marijuana, tobacco

Table 15.1 Definition of terms

Term	Definition
Drug abuse	The use, usually by self-administration, of any drug in a manner that deviates from the approved medical or social patterns within a culture
Drug misuse	Inappropriate use of a drug
Compulsive drug use or compulsive drug abuse	Continued self-administration of a drug despite the fact that the user may be suffering adverse social or medical consequences. In compulsive drug use, the user feels the drug is needed for his or her well-being. There is a continuum of compulsive drug use, from a simple desire to have more drug to a craving and preoccupation with procurement of the drug
Drug addiction[a]	According to the World Health Organization, drug addiction is a behavioral pattern of drug use that is characterized by overwhelming involvement with the use of a drug and overwhelming involvement with securing a supply. Along with this, there is a high tendency to relapse after withdrawal. There is some overlap in the definitions of compulsive use and addiction, and it is not always clear when compulsive use becomes addiction
Tolerance	Decreased responsiveness to a drug with repeated or continued dosing. Cross-tolerance may occur between drugs or between drug classes
Dependence	Continued use of that drug is required to prevent withdrawal
Withdrawal	Withdrawal may consist of physical and/or psychological signs and symptoms that occur upon abstinence from a drug

[a]There is a difference between addiction and dependence. It is possible for a person to exhibit signs of dependence following withdrawal of a drug, yet not crave the drug.

15.1 Introduction to Drugs of Abuse

Nonmedical use of drugs includes experimental use, in which a person tries a drug out of curiosity; recreational use, when moderate amounts are used to get "high," sedated, or hallucinate; and situational use, when drugs are used in specific circumstances, for example, amphetamines to stay alert. Sometimes these patterns can lead to more frequent use and dependence. Some key terms related to drugs of abuse are defined in ▶ Table 15.1.

15.2 Opioids

The pharmacology of these agents is discussed in Chapter 13. See ▶ Table 15.1 and ▶ Table 15.2.

Table 15.2 Opioid withdrawal symptoms[a]

Early symptoms (10–12 h after withdrawal)	Rhinorrhea (runny nose), perspiration, lacrimation (secretion of tears), and yawning
Intermediate symptoms (18–24 h after withdrawal)	Mydriasis, piloerection, anorexia, and muscular tremors
Peak symptoms (36–72 h after withdrawal)	Restlessness, hot flashes alternating with chills, an increase in both blood pressure and heart rate, an increase in the rate and depth of respiration, fever of 1 °C or more, nausea, retching, vomiting, and diarrhea

[a]Withdrawal from an opioid is generally not life threatening, although it is almost unbearable. The intensity of the withdrawal symptoms will be in proportion to the amount of drug being used and the duration of the abuse. Withdrawal will be more intense and of a shorter duration after use or abuse of more potent, shorter-acting agents. Likewise, it will be less intense but more prolonged with less potent, longer-acting agents.

15.2.1 Morphine, Diamorphine (Heroin), Codeine, Meperidine, and Methadone

Effects

The effects of opioids on performance include mental clouding, faulty judgment, and a reduced ability to concentrate. Physical signs of abuse include miosis (pupillary constriction), depression, and apathy.

Tolerance, Dependence, and Withdrawal

Tolerance, dependence, and withdrawal are characteristics of opioid use.
• Pain relief may be less effective as tolerance develops, even after a single dose. Tolerance develops more slowly to meperidine than morphine.

15.3 Drugs to Manage Opioid Use

(See Chapter 13 for details of these agents.)

15.3.1 Methadone

A synthetic μ opioid agonist. Used as replacement therapy for opioid addiction in a controlled setting (typically specialty opioid abuse clinics) in order to stabilize the patient in an asymptomatic state and control withdrawal.

15.3.2 Buprenorphine

A partial μ opioid receptor agonist; the partial agonism can reduce opioid agonist effect. Increasing doses will never reach full agonism. The drug reduces the reinforcing effects of opioid use. Care should be taken to avoid abuse of agents such at benzodiazepines that may result in enhancement of respiratory depression. Because of poor oral bioavailability, it is formulated as a sublingual tablet. Can induce immediate withdrawal.

15.3.3 Naltrexone

A μ opioid receptor antagonist with long plasma half-life. As an antagonist, it will not relieve withdrawal. Naltrexone is administered to patients after they are free of opioid use for one week. An extended release injectable formulation can improve compliance.

Clinical Correlation

Detoxification

Detoxification is the same for all drugs that produce physical dependence. It involves substituting a longer-acting, orally effective, pharmacologically equivalent drug for the abused drug. The patient is stabilized on the substitute, and then it is gradually withdrawn. There is a high recidivism rate among drug abusers. At present, there are many psychotherapeutic programs after detoxification, but these programs have success rates varying from 10% to perhaps a maximum of 50%.

15.4 Alcohol

15.4.1 Ethanol Toxicology

Alcohol is rapidly absorbed from the gastrointestinal (GI) tract after oral administration. Its acute effects appear within minutes of ingestion. Ethanol is metabolized in the liver, primarily by alcohol dehydrogenase to acetaldehyde, then by acetaldehyde dehydrogenase to acetate. This metabolism follows zero-order kinetics, which means that a constant amount of ethanol is metabolized per unit of time. The implication of this is that as more ethanol is ingested, the degree of intoxication increases rapidly, as well as the time for the blood level to drop to a non-intoxicating level.

Effects

Effects are listed ▶ Table 15.3.

Table 15.3 Effects of acute and chronic intoxication with ethanol

System/tissue	Effects
Acute intoxication	
CNS	Progressive CNS depression is correlated in time with blood concentrations of ethanol and may include vision and judgment impairments, decreased inhibitions, and muscular incoordination, progressing to staggering gait, slurred speech, and possible coma and death at higher doses
GI system	Increased salivary and gastric secretions, direct irritation to gastric and buccal mucosa, emesis due to a central effect on the chemoreceptor trigger zone, and irritation of the gastric mucosa. Prolonged use also leads to decreased absorption of folates
Other	Suppression of antidiuretic hormone (vasopressin) secretion Increased adrenocorticotropin hormone, cortisol, and catecholamine secretion Diuresis due to decreased antidiuretic hormone release Increased consumption of fluids Hypothermia
Chronic intoxication	
CNS	Wernicke syndrome, Korsakoff psychosis, cerebral atrophy, cerebellar atrophy, and alcoholic polyneuropathy
GI system	Peptic ulcers, esophagitis, gastritis, pancreatitis, and malnutrition
Liver	Steatosis, hepatitis, and cirrhosis (▶ Fig. 15.1 and ▶ Fig. 15.2)
Muscle	Cardiomyopathy and skeletal muscle myopathy
Fetus	Fetal alcohol syndrome
Other	Face: puffy cheeks and nose flushed, eyes: bloodshot, palmar erythema, rhinophyma, acne rosacea, and spider nevi

Abbreviations: CNS, central nervous system; GI, gastrointestinal.

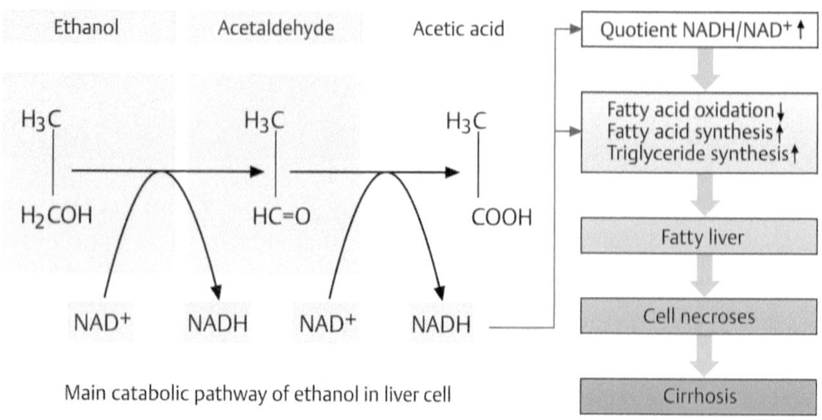

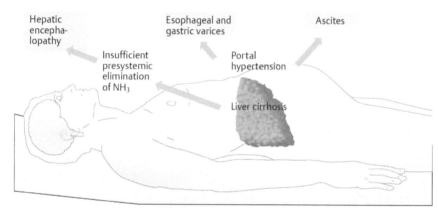

Fig. 15.1 Alcohol catabolism and effects of excess alcohol on the liver.
In hepatocytes, ethanol is broken down into acetic acid via acetaldehyde. This process utilizes the oxidized form of nicotinamide adenine dinucleotide (NAD⁺), so the requirement for this increases. If alcohol intake is chronic, hepatocytes initially undergo fatty degeneration that is reversible; however, if it continues, cirrhosis occurs as hepatocytes die and are replaced by connective tissue. NADH, reduced form of nicotinamide adenine dinucleotide.

Fig. 15.2 Liver cirrhosis.
Liver cirrhosis occurs when hepatocytes die and are replaced by connective tissue. Hepatic blood flow is impaired, causing portal hypertension, which in turn causes ascites and the formation of varices. The normal functioning of the liver is reduced, including the elimination of toxins, which then build up and affect the functioning of the brain.

Clinical Correlation

Fetal Alcohol Syndrome

Fetal alcohol syndrome is the term used to describe a spectrum of disorders that can occur in a fetus if a woman drinks alcohol when she is pregnant. It includes the following: abnormal facial features, growth deficiencies, vision or hearing deficits, and mental disabilities, such as difficulty in learning, memory problems, poor attention span, and poor communication skills.

Tolerance, Dependence, and Withdrawal

Withdrawal symptoms in chronic users of alcohol include tremor, sweating, anxiety, irritability, nausea, vomiting, and insomnia. These symptoms will be mild to moderate in 80 to 85% of patients and more severe in 15 to 20% of patients. Severe withdrawal condition, known as delirium tremens, is seen in ~ 1% of the cases.

- Benzodiazepines are cross-tolerant with alcohol and will alleviate the withdrawal symptoms, but they do not have the same stimulating effects on the central nervous system (CNS) as alcohol.
- For serious complications or delirium tremens, replace fluids and electrolytes and treat symptoms. Treat arrhythmias with lidocaine or procainamide, severe tremor with propranolol, and hallucinations and paranoia with a phenothiazine or haloperidol.

Clinical Correlation

Delirium Tremens

Delirium tremens is a disorder that occurs as a result of alcohol withdrawal (onset ~72 hours after the last drink). Signs include increased pulse, reduced blood pressure, tremors, fits and visual or tactile hallucinations. Treatment is with diazepam.

15.5 Drugs to Manage Alcoholism

Acute intoxication rarely requires treatment. Management includes supporting ventilation, maintaining temperature, and correcting dehydration, acidosis, or electrolyte imbalance. Gastric lavage (stomach pumping) is rarely necessary. Chronic intoxication may be treated with the agents listed below.

15.5.1 Naltrexone

Mechanism of Action

Naltrexone is an opioid antagonist similar to naloxone but with greater bioavailability and longer duration of action. It apparently blocks the ability of alcohol to activate dopaminergic reward pathways.

Uses

First-line therapy to maintain alcohol abstinence.

Pharmacokinetics

Orally active, but also available in once-monthly injectable, extended-release form. The injectable long-release formulation was developed because of poor compliance with oral naltrexone.

Side Effects

Nausea and liver damage (in high dosages).

Contraindications

Liver failure or acute hepatitis.

15.5.2 Acamprosate

Mechanism of Action

Their mechanism is unclear.

Uses

Acamprosate is approved for first-line prevention of relapse to alcoholism. Most effect is seen in patients desiring complete abstinence. Concomitant use of disulfiram appears to increase the effectiveness of acamprosate. Efficacy does not reach full levels until a week of dosing.

Pharmacokinetics

Renally eliminated and does not affect levels of opioids or other analgesics.

Side Effects

• Diarrhea.

15.5.3 Disulfiram (Antabuse)

Mechanism of Action

Disulfiram is an inhibitor of aldehyde dehydrogenase. If alcohol is taken in the presence of disulfiram, blood acetaldehyde levels increase, producing flushing, dyspnea (shortness of breath), nausea, thirst, chest pain, and palpitations. The effects are intended to be unpleasant so as to discourage alcohol ingestion; however, they can be serious and even life threatening.

Note: Patients must be informed to avoid alcohol, or their life may be in danger. This includes avoiding sauces, cough syrups, and liquid cold medicines that contain alcohol.

Uses

Approved as second-line treatment for alcohol abuse.

15.6 Toxicology of Other Alcohols

15.6.1 Methanol

Metabolism

Methanol is metabolized to formaldehyde by alcohol dehydrogenase. This occurs at about one-fifth of the rate of ethanol. It is then further metabolized to formic acid.

Effects

• Metabolic acidosis and organ damage.
• Methanol can cause blindness by damaging the optic nerve.

Clinical Correlation

Alcoholism and Vitamin Deficiencies

Alcoholics frequently develop vitamin deficiencies, especially thiamine and niacin. Thiamine (vitamin B_1) is essential for carbohydrate metabolism and is a modulator of neurotransmitter activity. Niacin (vitamin B_3) is a component of nicotinamide adenine dinucleotide, nicotinamide adenine dinucleotide phosphate (NADP), and the reduced form of NADP (NADPH). It is also the cofactor for numerous dehydrogenases. The reason that alcoholics develop such vitamin deficiencies is multifactorial and includes poor nutrition and the role that alcohol plays in the ability of the body to absorb, metabolize, and store vitamins. Vitamin replacement therefore plays a role in the management of alcoholism.

Treatment

This involves suppressing methanol metabolism by administering ethanol and giving bicarbonate to correct the acidosis. Fomepizole, which is a synthetic parenteral alcohol dehydrogenase inhibitor, may also be used. It prevents the initial metabolism of methanol (and ethylene glycol) to toxic metabolites.

15.6.2 Ethylene Glycol

Metabolism

Ethylene glycol is metabolized to oxalic acid, causing systemic acidosis.

Toxic Effects

Metabolic acidosis and organ damage.

Treatment

The same as for methanol poisoning.

15.7 Benzodiazepines

Benzodiazepines are also discussed in Chapter 9.

15.7.1 Diazepam, Midazolam, Temazepam, Triazolam, Flurazepam, Clonazepam, Oxazepam, Lorazepam, and Alprazolam

Intoxication

Intoxication with benzodiazepines produces progressive CNS depression with increasing dose. They may be fatal at high doses due to respiratory depression and cerebral hypoxia.

Tolerance, Dependence, and Withdrawal

- Tolerance develops to the effects of benzodiazepines.
- Physical dependence can occur.
- Withdrawal symptoms are generally opposite the effects of the drugs: anxiety, insomnia, and convulsions (in severe withdrawal). They can be minimized by slowly decreasing the dose to wean the patient from the drug.
- Flumazenil is a benzodiazepine-site negative modulator with a short plasma half-life; it can be used to support withdrawal and increase the level of consciousness. Adverse events include convulsions and use must be avoided with epileptic patients.

15.8 Barbiturates

Barbiturates are also discussed in Chapter 9.

15.8.1 Thiopental, Phenobarbital, Thiamylal, Methohexital, Amobarbital, Pentobarbital, and Secobarbital

Intoxication

Same as for benzodiazepines.

Tolerance, Dependence, and Withdrawal

- Tolerance develops to their sedative and hypnotic effects. No tolerance develops to the anticonvulsant actions of barbiturates.
- True physical dependence occurs.
- Moderate withdrawal consists of rebound increases in rapid eye movement (REM) sleep, insomnia, and anxiety. Seizures and delirium can occur in patients taking high doses for long periods. These patients should be withdrawn slowly to avoid these serious complications.

15.9 Quaaludes

15.9.1 Methaqualone

Methaqualone is a former prescription medication that is now synthesized and sold illicitly. It is a CNS depressant with pharmacology similar to barbiturates.

Intoxication

Same as for benzodiazepines.

Tolerance, Dependence, and Withdrawal

The symptoms and treatments are the same as for barbiturates.

15.10 Stimulants

15.10.1 Caffeine

Mechanisms of Action

Caffeine inhibits cyclic nucleotide phosphodiesterases, increases cellular Ca^{2+}, and is an antagonist at central adenosine receptors.

Effects

Caffeine decreases fatigue, increases arousal, and improves performance, but it produces insomnia, and may have a disruptive effect and worsen performance at very high doses.

Tolerance, Dependence, and Withdrawal

- No tolerance develops to caffeine.
- A throbbing, diffuse headache is the most common symptom of caffeine dependence.
- Symptoms of withdrawal may include nausea, lethargy, and headache.

15.10.2 Amphetamines and Cocaine

Effects

Mechanism of Action

These agents are indirect-acting sympathomimetics (see Chapter 6). They cause the release of endogenous norepinephrine and inhibit its reuptake.
- CNS actions include euphoria, decreased fatigue, alleviation of sleepiness, and decreased appetite. Amphetamines and cocaine may also increase libido and talkativeness. Restlessness may occur, and the heart rate may increase.
- After prolonged self-administration (a "run") with amphetamines, prolonged sleep, apathy, and depression are common.
- Sympathetic effects may be absent in chronic users.
- Chronic toxicity produces anxiety and confusion, leading to paranoia and psychosis, which is indistinguishable from schizophrenia.

Uses

- Cocaine is sometimes used as a local anesthetic agent.
- Amphetamines are used for attention deficit/hyperactivity disorder (ADHD) and narcolepsy.

Intoxication

- Acute intoxication causes hyperpyrexia, convulsions, and shock. It may result in death. Treatment involves chlorpromazine, which will block many of the acute effects of amphetamines, and diazepam to control convulsions. Acidification of the urine will enhance excretion. Death can occur following acute cocaine use by convulsions or cardiac arrhythmias. Chlorpromazine can be used.
- Chronic intoxication may cause toxic syndrome. Signs and symptoms of toxic syndrome include visual, auditory, and tactile hallucinations; paranoia and changes in affect. Treatment for paranoid delusions and excitement involves dopamine antagonists (haloperidol). Acidification of the urine will facilitate excretion of amphetamines.

Clinical Correlation

Attention Deficit/Hyperactivity Disorder

ADHD is characterized by inattention and hyperactive-impulsive behavior. It is a chronic disorder that affects children but may persist in adulthood. Symptoms are usually evident before the child is 7 years old, with the relative amount of inattention or hyperactivity symptoms differing in each case. Attention deficit symptoms include difficulty in sustaining attention during activities, trouble organizing activities, making careless mistakes in schoolwork, lack of listening when spoken to directly, forgetfulness, and often losing things. Hyperactivity symptoms include fidgeting, squirming, inability to remain seated, inappropriate running or climbing, trouble playing quietly, excessive talking, and always being "on the go." ADHD is often accompanied by anxiety and depression, making the diagnosis more complicated. The cause of ADHD is unknown, although it is known to have a strong hereditary element. Maternal smoking, drug use, and exposure to toxins have been shown to increase the likelihood of having a child with ADHD. Treatment involves the use of stimulant medications, such as methylphenidate (Ritalin) and dextromethamphetamine. Nonstimulant medications, such as atomoxetine, are also used. Therapy plays an important role in the management of this condition.

Clinical Correlation

Narcolepsy

It is a chronic sleep disorder that is characterized by sudden attacks of sleep and overwhelming daytime drowsiness. There may also be cataplexy (sudden loss of muscle tone), sleep paralysis (temporary paralysis that occurs when asleep or upon waking), hallucinations, and autonomic behavior while sleeping (e.g., talking or performing tasks). People with narcolepsy often have restless nighttime sleep patterns. This condition tends to occur mainly in adolescents and young adults. Damage to hypocretin cells, which regulate wakefulness and the timing of REM sleep, has been implicated as a cause for narcolepsy. Treatment involves the use of stimulant drugs, such as modafinil and methylphenidate, to help people stay awake; antidepressants to alleviate cataplexy, hallucinations, and sleep paralysis; or sodium oxybate to combat cataplexy.

Tolerance, Dependence, and Withdrawal

- Marked tolerance develops to amphetamines but not to cocaine.
- Dependence is common and produces an extremely intense drug craving. Physical dependence is minor.
- Withdrawal may include prolonged sleep, laziness, fatigue, overeating, and, occasionally, depression. Craving may persist for years.

15.11 Hallucinogens

15.11.1 Psychedelic Hallucinogens

d-Lysergic Acid Diethylamide, Psilocybin, Mescaline and Other Tryptamines

These agents differ primarily in potency. d-Lysergic Acid Diethylamide (LSD) is an extremely potent synthetic ergoline.

Mechanism of Action

Their mechanism is unclear, but they are serotonin agonists, particularly of the (5-hydroxytryptamine) 5-HT$_2$ receptor (see ▶ Fig. 7.3).

Intoxication

Psychedelic hallucinogens may produce vivid visual hallucinations and profound changes in thought processes, with confusion alternating with seemingly vivid perceptions and foresight, but these depend greatly on the situation and the individual. Tachycardia, tachypnea, and hypertension can be present with abuse. Sedation can be helpful in managing adverse events.

Side Effects

- Paranoia, panic reaction, and overt psychosis.
- Synesthesia and "flashbacks" are unique features (seen in up to 15% of users).

Note: No deaths due to direct drug effects have been reported.

Treatment

Involves emotional support and antianxiety agents, phenothiazines, or barbiturates in doses to produce sleep.

Tolerance, Dependence, and Withdrawal

- Tolerance and cross-tolerance will occur.
- No dependence or withdrawal.

15.11.2 Deliriant Hallucinogens

Phencyclidine and Ketamine

Phencyclidine (PCP) and ketamine are frequently touted as pure tetrahydrocannabinol (THC, the active ingredient in marijuana), LSD, or mescaline. Chemically these agents are known as arylcyclohexylamines.

Intoxication

At low doses, intoxication resembles an acute confused state. At higher doses, serious neurologic, cardiovascular, and psychotic reactions occur.

Side Effects

They are mainly psychological and include changes in body image, apparent loss of contact from reality, disorganized thoughts, and apathy or catatonia. Individuals on PCP may exhibit bizarre and hostile behaviors. Use has declined because of unpleasant experiences. Long-term abuse is associated with severe chronic cystitis, cognitive dysfunction, and hepatic dysfunction.

Treatment

Treatment for overdosing involves maintenance of vital functions until the drug effects subside.

Tolerance, Dependence, and Withdrawal

- Tolerance may develop.
- There is no clear withdrawal syndrome.

15.12 Cannabis

15.12.1 Marijuana and Hashish

The main psychoactive ingredient is THC. Endogenous cannabinoid receptors have been discovered along with an endogenous ligand, anandamide.

Effects

- CNS effects: relaxation, sense of well-being, euphoria, and spontaneous laughter. Short-term memory and capacity to carry out goal-directed behavior are impaired, and there is also motor impairment. THC has variable effects on mood, emotion, and social feelings.
- Heart: tachycardia (paroxysmal atrial tachycardia) may occur.
- Respiratory system: the lungs are adversely affected by smoke.
- Reproductive system: changes in the menstrual cycle, decreased sperm count and motility, and increased number of abnormal sperm.
- Amotivational syndrome: no scientific evidence that such a syndrome occurs.

Uses

- Antiemetic in cancer chemotherapy patients.
- There is also preclinical and anecdotal evidence of analgesic effects.

Tolerance, Dependence, and Withdrawal

- Tolerance develops to the effects of THC.
- Physical dependence does not occur.
- A withdrawal syndrome has not been defined. Many individuals stop using marijuana at will with no craving.

Synthetic Cannabinoid Receptor Agonists

These are highly potent, synthetic cannabinoid CB1 and CB2 receptor agonists. Typically, they are added to plant material for smoking and sold as *black mamba, K2, clockwork orange*, etc. Nowadays they are found in e-cigarette use. Serious adverse events are observed including hallucinations, heart palpitations, vomiting, convulsions, and serious renal dysfunction.

15.13 Tobacco

15.13.1 Nicotine

Mechanism of Action

Nicotine mimics acetylcholine at nicotinic receptors. It also decreases the activity of the enzyme monoamine oxidase (MAO) in the brain, which increases dopamine levels.

Intoxication

Nicotine causes an alert pattern in the electroencephalogram. It decreases skeletal muscle tone, appetite, and irritability and has a mild euphorigenic effect.

Tolerance, Dependence, and Withdrawal

- Withdrawal is variable, but increased appetite and inability to concentrate may persist for months. Intense psychological craving to smoke persists for months to years after quitting smoking.

Treatment

- Nicotine replacement therapy: a variety of strategies are available for administering nicotine in place of smoking, including oral (gum or lozenge), transdermal (patches), and intranasal (spray).
- Varenicline, a partial agonist at the $\alpha_2\beta_4$ subtype of nicotinic acetylcholine receptors, stimulates the receptor to relieve cravings and withdrawal while simultaneously blocking nicotine binding, thus reducing the rewarding effect of smoking.
- Bupropion, an antidepressant drug that inhibits dopamine and norepinephrine reuptake, has some efficacy in nicotine addiction. A sustained release formulation of bupropion is available for treatment of tobacco dependence.

15.14 Inhalants

15.14.1 Nitrous Oxide, Gasoline, Volatile Solvents, and Aerosols

See page 77 for a further discussion of nitrous oxide.

Intoxication

- Acute toxicity may lead to respiratory arrest and cardiac arrhythmias.
- Direct administration of aerosol propellants has resulted in laryngospasm, airway freezing, and suffocation due to an occluded airway.
- Chronic toxicity varies depending on the solvent but is characterized by irreversible tissue damage. This irreversible tissue damage means that solvent abusers are the most difficult group to rehabilitate.

15.15 Gamma-hydroxybutyrate (GHB)

GHB is a $GABA_A$ receptor agonist that is abused for its euphoria, increase of sex drive, and sedation. It was originally developed commercially as an anesthetic agent. It is now known as a *club drug* or *date rape drug*. Toxicity includes headaches, ataxia, and agitation with more serious toxicity leading to tremor, seizures, and eventually coma. Management of toxicity involves treating the symptoms as there is no recognized pharmacological agent to reverse the effects.

III

Unit III Review Questions

1. The major 5-hydroxytryptamine (5-HT)-containing nuclei in the brain are located in the
   A. Intermediolateral column of the spinal cord.
   B. Thalamus.
   C. Red nucleus.
   D. Locus coeruleus.
   E. Raphe nuclei.

2. Which of the following changes will increase the rate of induction of surgical anesthesia with an inhalation agent if all other factors remain unchanged?
   A. Increased patient respiration.
   B. Increased tissue solubility of anesthetic.
   C. Increased weight of patient.
   D. Increased blood:gas solubility.

3. A patient has just undergone a procedure that required general anesthesia. In the recovery room, the patient's respiration rate and heart rate are noted to be gradually increasing. His blood pressure is 155/90 mm Hg, and his temperature, which was normal before the surgery, is 38 °C (100.4 °F). These symptoms could be indicative of a reaction to which drug combination?
   A. Morphine/diazepam.
   B. Halothane/succinylcholine.
   C. Halothane/nitrous oxide.
   D. Nitrous oxide/succinylcholine.
   E. Morphine/atropine.

4. Oxygen is administered to the patient in question 3, and measures are taken to reduce the patient's core temperature. In addition, intravenous administration of a drug is ordered. What is the purpose of this drug?
   A. To dilate peripheral vessels by a direct action on smooth muscle.
   B. To decrease respiration via an action in the brainstem.
   C. To block muscarinic cholinergic receptors.
   D. To provide sedation via depression of the central nervous system.
   E. To decrease Ca^{2+} release from the sarcoplasmic reticulum of skeletal muscle.

5. Local anesthetic agents block nerve conduction by
   A. Altering metabolism.
   B. Interfering with Na^+-K^+-ATPase.
   C. Increasing the resting membrane potential.
   D. Blocking Na^+ channels in the nerve membrane.
   E. Blocking $GABA_B$ receptors.

6. Which is usually lost first after the injection of a local anesthetic?
   A. Sense of touch.
   B. Sense of pressure.
   C. Sense of proprioception.
   D. Motor control.
   E. Sense of pain.

7. A 7-year-old boy who fell off his bike has a laceration on his right knee that requires sutures. Lidocaine hydrochloride as a 2% solution with epinephrine 1:100,000 is used for local infiltration anesthesia. What is the purpose of the inclusion of epinephrine?
   A. To produce vasoconstriction and increase the duration of action of the local anesthetic.
   B. To produce vasodilation and increase absorption of the local anesthetic into the circulation.
   C. To decrease the sensitivity of C fibers to the local anesthetic.
   D. To decrease the sensitivity of sympathetic nerve endings to the local anesthetic.
   E. To produce a higher degree of anesthesia in tissues supplied by end organs.

For questions 8 to 13, the following are the answer choices:
   A. Voltage-dependent ion channels.
   B. Ligand-gated ion channels.
   C. Presynaptic synthetic pathways.
   D. Transmitter reuptake mechanisms.
   E. Extracellular and glial degradative enzymes.
   F. G protein-coupled membrane receptors.

8. Which is the site of action for lidocaine?

9. Which is the site of action for GABA at $GABA_A$ receptors?

10. Which is the site of action for fluoxetine?

11. Which is the site of action for morphine?

12. Which is the site of action for levodopa?

13. Which is the site of action for galantamine?

14. Phenelzine and isocarboxazid are termed "suicide" inhibitors because they
   A. Are effective in preventing suicidal behavior.
   B. Are apparently irreversible inhibitors of MAO.
   C. Prevent hallucinations.
   D. Decrease monoamine levels in the brain.

15. An unconscious patient is admitted to the emergency room. She has ingested a combination of ethanol and diazepam. Which of the following might be appropriate therapy?
   A. Naloxone.
   B. Naltrexone.
   C. Fluphenazine.
   D. Flumazenil.
   E. Amphetamine.

16. An 18-year-old female patient has been experiencing severe abdominal pain for several days. This has been accompanied by occasional vomiting. The patient is anxious and appears confused. Blood pressure and heart rate are increased. Her urine is red in color. Porphobilinogen, δ-aminolevulinic acid, and porphyrins in urine are increased. How could administering a barbiturate to this patient exacerbate these symptoms?
   A. By producing incoordination.
   B. By producing insomnia.
   C. By inducing liver enzymes.
   D. By inducing vomiting.
   E. By interacting with ethanol.

III

17. A 45-year-old man with a history of alcoholism reports feeling constantly anxious. He says he is always on edge, is irritable, and has difficulty concentrating. Although he finds this tiring, he has not been sleeping well. Because of this patient's history, what would be the most desirable agent to use to treat anxiety?
    A. Buspirone.
    B. Phenobarbital.
    C. Fluphenazine.
    D. Diazepam.
    E. Amphetamine.

18. The selective serotonin reuptake inhibitors (e.g., fluoxetine) differ from the tricyclic antidepressants (e.g., amitriptyline) in that they
    A. Have an immediate onset of antidepressant action.
    B. Inhibit MAO.
    C. Have no effect on 5-hydroxytryptamine, or serotonin, pathways in the central nervous system.
    D. Are less likely to produce weight gain.

19. A 32-year-old man developed a decreased need for sleep, increased energy, elevated mood, and hyperactivity. He was diagnosed with a manic disorder, and treatment with an antimanic drug was initiated. After 2 weeks of treatment, the patient developed a mild hand tremor. What does the tremor indicate?
    A. Lithium toxicity.
    B. Lack of sleep.
    C. Fluoxetine toxicity.
    D. Chlorpromazine toxicity.
    E. Fatigue as a result of hyperactivity.

20. The therapeutic effects of lithium
    A. Are observed following the first dose.
    B. Are antagonized by the administration of chlorpromazine.
    C. Are observed in normal, nonmanic patients.
    D. Occur in 70 to 80% of manic patients.

21. You see an adolescent female patient in your office who is being treated for epilepsy. She has hirsutism, her lips are thickened, the mass of skin around her cheekbones is increased, and she has gingival hyperplasia. Which drug would be most likely to cause these effects?
    A. Phenytoin.
    B. Carbamazepine.
    C. Phenobarbital.
    D. Ethosuximide.
    E. Valproic acid.

22. Which of the following is very effective for the control of absence (petit mal) seizures?
    A. Phenobarbital.
    B. Phenytoin.
    C. Valproic acid.
    D. Carbamazepine.

23. Useful therapy for generalized tonic-clonic (grand mal) epilepsy includes
    A. Phenytoin.
    B. Ethosuximide.

C. Pentazocine.
D. Chlorpromazine.

24. A patient who has recently begun treatment for generalized tonic-clonic seizures complains of red, itchy skin. He also says he has been feeling as if he has the flu. His body temperature is 38 °C (100.4 °F). Upon examination, a multiforme erythematous maculopapular rash is observed on his arms and chest. Which of the following would be the most appropriate therapy?
    A. Discontinue the drug treatment immediately.
    B. Discontinue the drug treatment immediately, and initiate treatment with valproic acid.
    C. Discontinue the drug treatment immediately, and initiate treatment with ethosuximide.
    D. Prescribe hydrocortisone cream for the skin lesions.
    E. No action is needed, as the rash is common with anticonvulsant therapy.

25. A patient taking thioridazine has xerostomia (dry mouth), tachycardia, dry skin, and urinary hesitancy. In what capacity is thioridazine acting that brings about these effects?
    A. As an agonist at muscarinic receptors.
    B. As an antagonist at muscarinic receptors.
    C. As an agonist at dopamine receptors.
    D. As an antagonist at dopamine receptors.
    E. As a mixed agonist-antagonist at opioid receptors.

26. The therapeutic actions of an antipsychotic drug, such as chlorpromazine, are most likely due to its action as an
    A. Antagonist at dopamine receptors on cells receiving mesolimbic innervation.
    B. Antagonist at dopamine receptors on cells receiving nigrostriatal innervation.
    C. Antagonist of muscarinic receptors.
    D. Agonist at opioid receptors.
    E. Antagonist at adenosine receptors.

27. A 20-year-old male college student is brought to the clinic by his parents. He has recently stopped attending classes and has refused to answer his cell phone. When questioned, he says that he is afraid that he is being watched and that his classmates are out to get him. He doesn't want them to track him through his phone, but they can call him without using the phone. He has not been showering or eating regularly. Organic and substance abuse disorders are ruled out, and a diagnosis of schizophrenia is made. You must decide whether to treat him with haloperidol or thioridazine. Which statement correctly compares the effectiveness of the drugs and their propensity for producing acute extrapyramidal neurotoxicities?
    A. Haloperidol is more likely to be effective, but it is also more likely to produce extrapyramidal neurotoxicities.
    B. Thioridazine is more likely to be effective, but it is also more likely to produce extrapyramidal neurotoxicities.
    C. The likelihood of effective treatment is equal, but haloperidol is more likely to cause extrapyramidal neurotoxicities.
    D. The likelihood of effective treatment is equal, but thioridazine is more likely to cause extrapyramidal neurotoxicities.

E. The likelihood of effective treatment is equal; so is the likelihood of extrapyramidal neurotoxicities.

28. A patient undergoing chronic treatment for schizophrenia, first with a typical antipsychotic and then with an atypical agent, continues to experience episodes of paranoia and hallucinations. It is decided to use clozapine as therapy. Patients being treated with clozapine must have a baseline white blood cell count (WBC) and absolute neutrophil count (ANC) before initiation of treatment, as well as regular WBCs and ANCs during treatment and for at least 4 weeks after discontinuation of treatment. Which of the following may be caused by clozapine, thus necessitating these blood tests?
   A. Agranulocytosis.
   B. Weight gain.
   C. Orthostatic hypotension.
   D. Anticholinergic side effects.
   E. Neuroleptic malignant syndrome.

29. At 2 weeks of treatment with clozapine, the patient in question 28 has blood tests that reveal an elevated creatine kinase (CK) and white blood cell count (WBC). This could be associated with the development of which of the following?
   A. Akathisia.
   B. Acute dystonia.
   C. Tardive dyskinesia.
   D. Extrapyramidal symptoms.
   E. Neuroleptic malignant syndrome.

30. Drug-induced parkinsonism may occur during treatment with typical antipsychotic agents. The parkinsonian symptoms can be treated with
   A. Anticholinergic drugs.
   B. Levodopa.
   C. Chlorpromazine.
   D. Haloperidol.

31. κ (kappa) opiate receptors mediate
   A. Supraspinal analgesia.
   B. Respiratory depression.
   C. Euphoria.
   D. Dependence.
   E. Spinal analgesia.

32. Which of the following is converted to a metabolite that is capable of inducing stimulation of the CNS, especially in patients with renal failure?
   A. Acetaminophen.
   B. Meperidine.
   C. Pentazocine.
   D. Naloxone.
   E. Naltrexone.

33. A 23-year-old man fell from a roof and suffered a ruptured spleen. He has been in a methadone maintenance program for several months and is taking a regular large dose of methadone. Physical examination suggests abdominal bleeding. He is rushed to the operating room for an emergency splenectomy. The anesthesiologist uses sodium thiopental to induce anesthesia and halothane during the surgery. After 1 week, the patient is recovering and is now receiving the same daily dose of methadone he was taking before his accident. That night, pain from the incision keeps him awake, and the resident on duty administers a drug. Within a few minutes, the patient is nauseated, sweating, tremoring, and having intestinal cramps. He also has waves of gooseflesh and involuntary kicking movements of the legs. This is an expected result of administering which of the following drugs to this patient?
   A. Methadone.
   B. Codeine.
   C. Chloral hydrate.
   D. Pentazocine.
   E. Diazepam.

34. Methadone differs from morphine in that methadone
   A. Is not an effective analgesic.
   B. Produces a shorter and more tolerable abstinence syndrome than morphine.
   C. Is metabolized to morphine.
   D. Has a longer half-life.
   E. Is selective for κ opioid receptors.

35. A 27-year-old pregnant woman who has had no prenatal care was brought to the hospital in the final stages of labor. A healthy, full-term infant was delivered with no apparent complications. However, within 24 hours, the infant became irritable, cried constantly, and would not nurse. The mother admitted to recent heavy use of illegally obtained oxycodone. Given the history, what are the infant's symptoms most likely indicative of?
   A. Tolerance to oxycodone.
   B. Normal response at birth.
   C. Opiate withdrawal.
   D. Hunger.
   E. Bilirubinemia.

36. A 65-year-old male retired autoworker complains of tightness in his arms and legs, as well as difficulty walking and going down stairs. He is well nourished and shows no change in facial expressions during the examination. A mild resting tremor of his right hand is noted. Parkinson disease is diagnosed, and treatment is begun with a dopamine receptor agonist. What is the rationale of this therapy?
   A. To increase glucose production in skeletal muscle.
   B. To prevent the peripheral decarboxylation of dopamine.
   C. To activate dopamine receptors on interneurons in the motor cortex.
   D. To mimic the central actions of dopamine in the substantia nigra.
   E. To directly stimulate postsynaptic receptors within the striatum.

37. An alternative strategy to treat Parkinson disease is to inhibit the metabolism of endogenous dopamine. Which of the following drug combinations inhibit the breakdown of dopamine?
   A. Entacapone and selegiline.
   B. Levodopa and carbidopa.
   C. Dopa decarboxylase and MAO.
   D. Fluoxetine and sertraline.
   E. Bromocriptine and trihexyphenidyl.

38. Which of the following is a dopamine receptor agonist?
    A. Levodopa.
    B. Bromocriptine.
    C. Amantadine.
    D. Carbidopa.
    E. Benztropine.

39. In the treatment of Parkinson disease, which of the following is an alternative approach to increasing dopamine?
    A. Decrease the cholinergic component.
    B. Increase the cholinergic component.
    C. Decrease the noradrenergic component.
    D. Increase the noradrenergic component.
    E. Antagonize the serotonergic component.

40. For which of the following drugs are miosis, respiratory depression, and lack of bowel sounds the signs of acute intoxication?
    A. LSD.
    B. Amphetamine.
    C. Morphine.
    D. Methaqualone.

41. Liver damage may result from chronic abuse of
    A. LSD.
    B. Ethanol.
    C. Amphetamine.
    D. Cocaine.

42. Ethanol may have interactions with several other drugs. The interaction of ethanol with other CNS depressant drugs is characterized by
    A. An enhanced CNS depressant action.
    B. A decreased CNS depressant activity of the other drug.
    C. An increased gastric irritation.
    D. A decreased gastric irritation.
    E. There is no interaction.

43. A patient comes to you complaining of insomnia and nausea. Examination shows a coarse tremor of the extremities, oral temperature of 38.5 °C (101.3 °F), hyperactive deep tendon reflexes, and orthostatic hypotension. He admits a daily alcohol intake of at least a pint of whiskey and several cans of beer. During the examination, there is a short period of myoclonic jerking of the arms and legs. The patient then volunteers that he had been in jail all night, having been arrested for being drunk and disorderly, though he barely remembers the episode. He has had no drug or alcohol for ~ 18 hours. Before the patient can be treated, he slumps over, clutching his abdomen. Examination later in the hospital suggests a perforated duodenal ulcer with internal bleeding. The surgeon recommends immediate surgery. During recovery, the patient shows tremor, anxiety, agitation, and muscle twitches. A drug is given that suppresses these signs of alcohol withdrawal. What is the drug?
    A. A vitamin.
    B. An opiate receptor blocker.
    C. An acetaldehyde dehydrogenase inhibitor.
    D. A benzodiazepine receptor agonist.
    E. An antimicrobial.

44. Upon discharge, the patient in question 43 agrees to seek therapy for his alcohol addiction, including group therapy and a medication. The patient is given a wallet card listing the medication and is warned that, when taking this drug, exposure to alcohol in his diet, in over-the-counter medications, and in toiletries may produce sweating, flushing, headache, nausea, and vomiting. Which drug is prescribed?
    A. A vitamin.
    B. An opiate receptor blocker.
    C. An aldehyde dehydrogenase inhibitor.
    D. A benzodiazepine receptor agonist.
    E. An antimicrobial.

45. A heavy user of alcohol is in the hospital and scheduled to have his gallbladder removed. He was given pentobarbital to promote sleep the night before the operation. The nurse is surprised to find him still awake after she has doubled the usual dose. What is this an example of?
    A. Addiction.
    B. Physical dependence.
    C. Psychological dependence.
    D. Cross-tolerance.
    E. Synergism.

46. For which of the following drugs are ataxia and sedation the signs of acute intoxication?
    A. LSD.
    B. Amphetamine.
    C. Morphine.
    D. Methaqualone.

47. For which of the following drugs are decreased fatigue and increased talkativeness the signs of acute intoxication?
    A. LSD.
    B. Amphetamine.
    C. Morphine.
    D. Methaqualone.

48. Of the following drugs of abuse, which is most likely to produce the greatest degree of psychological dependence in the largest percentage of users?
    A. Cocaine.
    B. Codeine.
    C. Heroin.
    D. Methadone.
    E. Methaqualone.

49. For which of the following drugs are anxiety, paranoia, and hallucinations the signs of acute intoxication?
    A. LSD.
    B. Amphetamine.
    C. Morphine.
    D. Methaqualone.

50. Intoxication with which one of the following agents causes changes in body image, feelings of estrangement, negativism, and hostility?
    A. Barbiturates.
    B. Caffeine.
    C. Cocaine.
    D. Marijuana.
    E. Phencyclidine hydrochloride (PCP).

51. A 32-year-old woman has enrolled in a smoking cessation program at work. She has been smoking since she was a

teenager. She currently smokes a pack a day but has been unable to quit, despite several tries. Pharmacotherapies she is considering include the nicotine patch, varenicline, and bupropion. How does varenicline differ from the nicotine patch?

A. Varenicline is a nicotinic receptor antagonist that prevents nicotine from acting at its receptor and blocks the rewarding effects of nicotine.

B. Varenicline is a partial agonist that stimulates the receptor to relieve cravings and withdrawal while simultaneously blocking nicotine binding.

C. Varenicline is a nicotine analogue agonist that stimulates the receptor and acts as a replacement for the nicotine found in tobacco.

D. Varenicline is a selective serotonin reuptake inhibitor that acts as an antidepressant to prevent the negative mood experienced during withdrawal from nicotine.

E. Varenicline is a dopamine/norepinephrine reuptake inhibitor that acts to increase dopamine in the brain, leading to a decreased craving to smoke.

52. Strychnine poisoning leads to muscle cramps and increased sensitivity to sensory stimuli that may proceed to generalized muscle spasms. These actions are due to the blockade of

A. Cholinergic receptors in the brain.

B. Gamma-aminobutyric acid (GABA) receptors in the brain.

C. Substance P receptors in the spinal cord.

D. Glycine receptors in the spinal cord.

E. Nicotinic receptors on skeletal muscle.

53. Which of the following is an endogenous opioid peptide?

A. Substance P.

B. β-Endorphin.

C. Neuropeptide Y.

D. Pro-opiomelanocortin.

E. Opium.

54. Local anesthetics used to produce spinal anesthesia are eliminated primarily by

A. Hydrolysis catalyzed by esterases in the cerebrospinal fluid (CSF).

B. Local absorption into the bloodstream.

C. Metabolism in the choroid plexus.

D. Recirculation of the CSF with reabsorption in arachnoid granulations.

E. Uptake into neurons with subsequent metabolism by monoamine oxidase.

55. The short duration of anesthesia after intravenous administration of thiopental is due to

A. Renal excretion of thiopental.

B. Distribution of thiopental.

C. Acute tolerance.

D. Hepatic biotransformation.

E. Extensive protein binding.

56. Clinically significant expansion of encapsulated air spaces within the body occurs with

A. Halothane.

B. Enflurane.

C. Nitrous oxide.

D. Isoflurane.

57. Maintaining anesthesia at 1 minimal alveolar concentration (MAC) of halothane in one patient and at 1 MAC of enflurane in another means that

A. The partial pressure of both agents in the alveolar space will be identical.

B. The partial pressure of both agents in the brain will be identical.

C. Anesthesia will be "deeper" with the more potent agent.

D. The probability that either patient will move on skin incision is the same.

58. Which of the following is used in the operating room specifically to produce amnesia and sedation?

A. Ketamine.

B. Thiopental.

C. Diazepam.

D. Isoflurane.

E. Halothane.

59. Benzodiazepines facilitate gamma-aminobutyric acid (GABA) neurotransmission by

A. Acting as GABA type A (GABA$_A$) receptor agonists.

B. Inhibiting GABA-transaminase in glial cells and neurons.

C. Exerting an allosteric action at the GABA receptor chloride channel complex.

D. Blocking presynaptic inhibitory receptors to increase the release of GABA.

60. Benzodiazepines differ from the barbiturates in that the benzodiazepines

A. Have a lower therapeutic index than barbiturates.

B. Mimic the actions of gamma-aminobutyric acid (GABA) at the postsynaptic GABA receptor.

C. Do not produce dependence or withdrawal.

D. Have a greater therapeutic index than barbiturates.

61. Which medication causes an anxiolytic action mediated by a 5-hydroxytryptamine type 1A (5-HT$_{1A}$) serotonin receptor?

A. Diazepam.

B. Buspirone.

C. Pentobarbital.

D. Ethanol.

62. Which of the following has a selective "antidepressant-like" action in panic disorder?

A. Diazepam.

B. Oxazepam.

C. Alprazolam.

D. Phenobarbital.

E. Buspirone.

63. Which of the following blocks reuptake of biogenic amines into nerve endings?

A. Monoamine oxidase inhibitors (MAOIs).

B. Tricyclic antidepressants.

C. Benzodiazepines.

D. Opiates.

E. Ethanol.

64. Which one of the following agents is most efficacious in the treatment of obsessive-compulsive disorder?

A. Primidone.

B. Meprobamate.

C. Haloperidol.
D. Propranolol.
E. Fluoxetine.

65. The selective serotonin reuptake inhibitors (SSRIs) used to treat depression are superior to the tricyclic antidepressants in that the SSRIs
A. Have a side effect profile that is more acceptable to the patient.
B. Are effective at lower doses.
C. Are more efficacious in relieving depression.
D. Are less likely to produce sexual side effects.

66. Which of the following antidepressants is most likely to produce anticholinergic effects?
A. Amitriptyline.
B. Amoxapine.
C. Fluoxetine.
D. Sertaline.

67. Which of the following is effective in the treatment of status epilepticus?
A. Ethosuximide.
B. Valproic acid.
C. Carbamazepine.
D. Diazepam.

68. Which of the following drugs is metabolized to phenobarbital and phenylethylmalonamide?
A. Amobarbital.
B. Secobarbital.
C. Primidone.
D. Felbamate.
E. Valproate.

69. What is the site at which antipsychotic drugs reduce nausea and vomiting?
A. Dopaminergic neurons in the pars compacta of substantia nigra.
B. Caudate neurons innervated by substantia nigra neurons.
C. Neurons in the chemoreceptor trigger zone.
D. Pituitary cells.
E. Neurons in the limbic system and cortex innervated by dopaminergic neurons in the midbrain.

70. A Parkinson-like syndrome may result from
A. Amphetamine toxicity.
B. Psychoses, especially schizophrenia.
C. Anticholinergic agents.
D. Antipsychotic agents.

71. The chlorpromazine side effect that is least likely to be reduced by benztropine is
A. Akathisia.
B. Acute dystonia.
C. Oculogyric crisis.
D. Drug-induced parkinsonism.
E. Tardive dyskinesia.

72. Which of the following agents is used as a mixed agonist/antagonist at opiate receptors?
A. Propoxyphene.
B. Naltrexone.
C. Pentazocine.

D. Fentanyl.
E. Meperidine.

73. The mechanism underlying the respiratory depressant action of opiate agonists is
A. Marked sedation.
B. Decreased oxygen (O_2) consumption by the heart, decreasing cardiac work.
C. Inhibition of the respiratory center in the brainstem, decreasing responsiveness to carbon dioxide (CO_2) tension.
D. Direct stimulation of the chemoreceptor trigger zone of the medulla, decreasing responsiveness to CO_2 tension.
E. Increased tonicity of the alveoli.

74. The drug of choice for the treatment of respiratory depression due to an overdose of heroin is
A. Buprenorphine.
B. Methadone.
C. Naloxone.
D. Pentazocine.
E. Propoxyphene.

75. Prolonged use of opiates will result in
A. Tolerance.
B. Diarrhea.
C. Tooth decay.
D. Psychosis.
E. Halitosis.

76. Naloxone is included with oral preparations of pentazocine to
A. Block the constipating effects of pentazocine.
B. Prevent intravenous use by individuals dependent on opiates.
C. Enhance the absorption of pentazocine from the gastrointestinal tract.
D. Elevate the therapeutic index of pentazocine.
E. Increase the shelf life of pentazocine.

77. Which of the following drugs is the most suitable to be administered orally for the treatment of chronic pain?
A. Meperdine.
B. Morphine.
C. Pentazocine.
D. Naloxone.
E. Naltrexone.

78. Which of the following has the greatest analgesic efficacy?
A. Acetaminophen.
B. Meperdine.
C. Pentazocine.
D. Naloxone.
E. Naltrexone.

79. Methadone maintenance for the treatment of physical dependence on heroin is based on the fact that methadone
A. Is much less dependence-producing than heroin.
B. Withdrawal is more intense, prompting compliance.
C. Is an antagonist of opiate receptors.
D. Prevents withdrawal by acting as a replacement for heroin.

80. Which of the following causes dry mouth, reduced sweating, and tachycardia?
    A. Levodopa.
    B. Bromocriptine.
    C. Amantadine.
    D. Carbidopa.
    E. Benztropine.

81. Which of the following inhibits dopa decarboxylase only outside the central nervous system, thus decreasing the required dose of dopa in the treatment of parkinsonism?
    A. Carbidopa.
    B. Chlorpromazine.
    C. Pyridoxine.
    D. Benztropine.
    E. α-methyl dopa.

82. Which one of the following agents may be useful in the treatment of spinal spasticity?
    A. Amantadine.
    B. Dantrolene.
    C. Levodopa and carbidopa.
    D. Baclofen.
    E. Bromocritpine.

83. Which one of the following antiviral agents has proven to be useful for Parkinson disease therapy?
    A. Selegiline.
    B. Amantadine.
    C. Bromocritpine.
    D. Imipramine.
    E. Atropine.

84. The effectiveness of levodopa to relieve the dyskinesias of Parkinson disease is most likely due to
    A. An increase in dopaminergic neuronal transmission in the mesolimbic dopamine pathway.
    B. A decrease in dopaminergic neuronal transmission in the mesolimbic dopamine pathway.
    C. An increase in dopaminergic neuronal transmission in the nigrostriatal dopamine pathway.
    D. A decrease in dopaminergic neuronal transmission in the striatopallidal dopamine pathway.
    E. An increase in noradrenergic neuronal transmission in the locus caeruleus.

85. An anesthesiologist has a choice between two inhalation anesthetic agents. Agent A provides a very rapid rate of induction and recovery, whereas both induction and recovery are slower with agent B. How can this difference be explained?
    A. Agent A has a higher blood:gas partition coefficient.
    B. Agent A is more soluble in lipid.
    C. Agent A has a higher vapor pressure.
    D. Agent A has lower blood solubility.
    E. The minimal alveolar concentration for agent A is 1% and for agent B, 2%.

86. Local anesthetics are less efficacious in infected and inflamed tissue. What is the reason for this?
    A. The ionized form of the local anesthetic is more diffusible in inflamed tissues.

B. The ambient pH of infected tissue is lower due to increased concentrations of lactic acid.
C. The local anesthetic loses its affinity for the Na⁺ channel in infected tissue.
D. There are fewer Na⁺ channels in inflamed tissue.
E. Diffusion through inflamed tissue is slower.

87. A 46-year-old woman with a severe headache, blood pressure of 228/188 mm Hg, and temperature of 38.5 °C (101.3 °F) is seen in the emergency room. Laboratory values from a complete blood count, metabolic panel, and thyroid-stimulating hormone (TSH) test were all within normal limits. A computed tomography (CT) scan of the head showed no abnormalities or intracranial hemorrhages. A 12-lead electrocardiogram (EKG) showed a normal sinus rhythm. The patient states that she has been treated for depression for the past 10 years. She says her depression was severe at times until the doctors finally found the right medicine. She caught a cold a few days ago and has been using a menthol nasal spray, because she "is not supposed to take cold medicines." The spray bottle lists the contents as phenylephrine hydrochloride 1%; inactive ingredients: benzalkonium chloride, boric acid, camphor, eucalyptol, menthol, polysorbate 80, sodium borate, water. Which of the following antidepressant medications is she most likely taking?
    A. Chlorpromazine.
    B. Tranylcypromine.
    C. Chlordiazepoxide.
    D. Fluoxetine.
    E. Amitryptiline.

88. A married 28-year-old woman has been experiencing insomnia, decreased energy, decreased mood and sadness, a lack of interest in the activities of her children, and no interest in sexual activity with her husband. She is oriented but sad. She has had suicidal thoughts but has not taken any suicidal actions. She is diagnosed with a depressive disorder, and treatment is initiated. After 2 weeks of treatment, the patient reports that she experienced nausea and diarrhea during the first week of treatment, but that has gone away. Her mood has improved, and her social activities have increased. Although she says she loves her husband, and they have not been having serious arguments, she still has no interest in sexual activity. These effects are most likely seen following the administration of which of these agents?
    A. Lithium.
    B. Amphetamine.
    C. A selective serotonin reuptake inhibitor (SSRI).
    D. A tricyclic antidepressant.
    E. A mixed agonist-antagonist.

89. A child suffers from brief periods of staring with no recall of the event. An electroencephalogram shows a 3 Hz spike-and-wave pattern. Which of the following drugs might she be given initially?
    A. Ethosuximide.
    B. Phenytoin.
    C. Pentazocine.
    D. Chlorpromazine.

90. A 10-year-old girl is seen by the neurologist because she is having difficulties at school. During the day, the girl experiences brief losses of consciousness. An electroencephalogram (EEG) reveals a 3 Hz polyspike-and-wave pattern characteristic of absence epilepsy. A course of treatment with ethosuximide provides inadequate relief of her symptoms. What would be an appropriate alternative therapy for this patient?
A. Decrease the dose of ethosuximide.
B. Supplement the ethosuximide with phenobarbital.
C. Switch to phenytoin, and withdraw ethosuximide.
D. Switch to valproic acid, and withdraw ethosuximide.
E. Determine the blood levels of ethosuximide.

91. A 77-year-old man with lung cancer is being treated with morphine to alleviate pain. When morphine was started, the patient was also given a prescription for docusate. The purpose of the docusate is to lessen which side effect of morphine?
A. Constipation.
B. Nausea.
C. Respiratory depression.
D. Sedation.
E. Vomiting.

92. A female patient spends 4 weeks in the hospital with a severe case of peritonitis, a very painful condition. Meperidine (Demerol) is prescribed, 50 mg every 4 to 6 hours as needed. During the second week, the dosage is increased to 100 mg every 4 hours as needed. During the last week, the peritonitis clears up, the pain subsides, and the drug is discontinued. The patient shows symptoms that make her think she has a cold or flu. This is an example of which of the following?
A. Tolerance.
B. Physical dependence.
C. Psychological dependence.
D. Cross-tolerance.
E. Drug addiction.

93. In a patient with liver disease, it would be most appropriate to use which of the following local anesthetics?
A. Bupivacaine.
B. Lidocaine.
C. Articaine.
D. Procaine.

94. A patient has undergone a surgery with desflurane as the general anesthetic and succinylcholine to provide muscle relaxation. During recovery he exhibits increased expiration of carbon dioxide, tachycardia, and muscle rigidity. This is followed by a persistent increase in body temperature. In addition to cooling of the patient, the operating room pharmacist recommends administration of a drug that acts directly on skeletal muscle to decrease the release of calcium from the sarcoplasmic reticulum. Which of the following drugs is administered?
A. Skelaxin.
B. Diazepam.
C. Tizanidine.
D. Cyclobenzaprine.
E. Dantrolene.

Unit III Answers and Explanations

1. E. The cell bodies of the main groups of 5-HT-containing neurons are located in the raphe nuclei of the brainstem.

2. A. Because anesthetic induction with inhalation agents is via the lungs, increasing respiration will increase the rate of absorption and thus induction of anesthesia.

B. Increased tissue solubility will decrease the rate of induction.

C. The rate of anesthetic induction is generally independent of the patient's weight.

D. Increased blood gas solubility will decrease the rate of induction.

3. B. Malignant hyperthermia is a rare complication of anesthesia with any volatile anesthetic but, most commonly, with halothane, particularly when it is combined with a depolarizing neuromuscular blocking agent such as succinylcholine. During malignant hyperthermia, there is a substantial increase in skeletal muscle oxidative metabolism, which increases body temperature, consumes oxygen, and leads to a buildup of carbon dioxide.

4. E. Dantrolene is used as a treatment for malignant hyperthermia. This drug acts directly on skeletal muscle to decrease Ca^{2+} release from the sarcoplasmic reticulum. This in turn decreases muscle contraction, metabolism, and the generation of heat, thereby decreasing hyperthermia.

5. D. Local anesthetics prevent action potential propagation by blocking Na^+ channels in the nerve membrane from the cytoplasmic side of the channel.

A–C, E. Local anesthetics do not alter metabolism, interfere with ATPase, increase the resting membrane potential, or block $GABA_B$ receptors.

6. E. Smaller diameter unmyelinated nerve fibers are most sensitive to block by local anesthetics. Pain fibers are the smallest and so are blocked first.

A–D. The loss of the sense of pain is followed by the loss of sensations of cold, warmth, touch, and deep pressure. Proprioceptive and motor fibers are least sensitive.

7. A. Epinephrine is added to local anesthetic solutions to produce vasoconstriction at the site of injection. Termination of the action of a local anesthetic depends on its diffusion from the site of injection. Vasoconstriction decreases systemic absorption and prolongs the duration of action.

8. A. Lidocaine blocks voltage-dependent Na^+ channels from the cytoplasmic side of the channel.

9. B. GABA acts at $GABA_A$ receptors, which are ligand-gated ion channels. Activation leads to opening of the Cl^- channel and synaptic inhibition.

10. D. Fluoxetine is a serotonin-specific reuptake inhibitor (SSRI).

11. F. Morphine acts at opioid receptors (highest affinity for µ receptors), which are G protein-coupled receptors.

12. C. Levodopa is a precursor of dopamine synthesis. It is transformed to dopamine by aromatic amino acid decarboxylase.

13. E. Galantamine is a competitive cholinesterase inhibitor. By inhibiting cholinesterase, it increases the concentration of acetylcholine in the brain. It is used to treat the symptoms of Alzheimer disease.

14. B. "Suicide" inhibitors are so named because they bind irreversibly to the enzyme, in this case MAO, inactivating it. Restoration of enzymatic activity requires synthesis of new enzyme.

A, C. The term does not refer to prevention of suicidal behavior or hallucinations.

D. Phenelzine and isocarboxazid increase monoamine levels in the brain by inhibiting their breakdown by MAO.

15. D. Flumazenil is a relatively specific competitive benzodiazepine receptor antagonist useful in overdose or poisoning. Even in the presence of ethanol, blocking the effect of the benzodiazepine, diazepam may be sufficient to restore consciousness.

16. C. The symptoms are consistent with acute intermittent porphyria, a disorder of porphyrin metabolism. Barbiturates are potent inducers of liver enzymes and will further increase porphyrin synthesis and worsen the disease. Barbiturates are contraindicated in patients with acute intermittent porphyria, porphyria variegata, or a positive family history of these porphyrias.

17. A. Benzodiazepines and ethanol produce similar depressant effects on the CNS. Benzodiazepines are more likely to be abused by patients with a history of CNS depressant abuse. For this patient, an anxiolytic like buspirone that produces less sedation and has a lower propensity for mimicking or enhancing the effects of ethanol is preferable.

B. Phenobarbital is a barbiturate used for anesthetic induction, insomnia, and as an anticonvulsant. It is not used for anxiety and is prone to abuse.

C. Fluphenazine is an antipsychotic and an antiemetic drug. It is not used to treat anxiety.

E. Amphetamine is a stimulant drug that would keep the patient awake. Chronic use will lead to anxiety.

18. D. The SSRIs are less likely than the tricyclic antidepressants to produce weight gain.

A. None of the antidepressant drugs have an immediate onset of antidepressant action.

B, C. The SSRIs do not inhibit MAO, but they do inhibit 5-HT reuptake.

19. A. Lithium is an antimanic drug with a narrow therapeutic index. Tremor is an indicator of mild toxicity.

B–E. Under these circumstances, tremor does not indicate a lack of sleep, fluoxetine or chlorpromazine toxicity, or fatigue as a result of hyperactivity.

20. D. Lithium is effective in treating mania in 70 to 80% of patients.

A. The effects of lithium take 1 to 2 weeks to fully develop; they are not seen immediately following the first dose.

B. The effects of lithium are not antagonized by the antipsychotic drug chlorpromazine. On the contrary, antipsychotic drugs may be used to treat severe acute mania.

C. Lithium has no effects on nonmanic patients, unless toxic doses are ingested.

21. A. These are side effects of phenytoin.

B. Carbamazepine side effects include GI upset, hematological disorders, hypersensitivity, vertigo, diplopia, and blurred vision.

C. Phenobarbital side effects include sedation and rashes. Ataxia and nystagmus may also occur at excessive doses.

D. Ethosuximide side effects include GI upset, CNS depression, rashes (rarely Stevens–Johnson syndrome), and blood dyscrasias (rarely).

E. Valproic acid side effects include alopecia, GI upset, ataxia, tremor, and mild behavioral effects.

22. C. Of the drugs listed, valproic acid is the only one that is effective in absence seizures.

A. Phenobarbital is a barbiturate used to treat generalized tonic-clonic seizures, partial seizure, and febrile convulsions.

B. Phenytoin is effective for all types of seizures except absence and atonic seizures. It is also used for trigeminal neuralgia.

D. Carbamazepine is used to treat generalized tonic-clonic seizures, complex partial seizures, and trigeminal neuralgia.

23. A. Of the agents listed, phenytoin is the only one used for generalized tonic-clonic seizures.

B. Ethosuximide is the drug of choice for absence seizures.

C. Pentazocine is an opioid drug used to treat pain.

D. Chlorpromazine is an antipsychotic agent.

24. B. The patient is experiencing an allergic reaction to the drug, which may progress to Stevens–Johnson syndrome if the drug is not withdrawn. Of the drugs indicated for use in generalized tonic-clonic seizures, valproic acid is the least likely to lead to Stevens–Johnson syndrome.

25. B. The side effects are characteristic anticholinergic effects.

26. A. The therapeutic efficacy of typical antipsychotics is correlated with their ability to block the D_2 subtype of dopamine receptors. The mesolimbic pathway is the dopaminergic pathway involved in the modulation of behaviors related to schizophrenia.

B. The nigrostriatal dopaminergic pathway is involved in the control of movements and in therapy for Parkinson disease.

27. C. In general, the antipsychotic agents are similarly effective in treating schizophrenia. The likelihood of extrapyramidal side effects is greater with haloperidol than thioridazine.

28. A. WBC and ANC are measured prior to and during clozapine therapy to detect for bone marrow suppression by the drug and to prevent agranulocytosis.

29. E. Neuroleptic malignant syndrome is an idiosyncratic reaction to antipsychotic drugs that tends to occur more frequently with typical antipsychotics, but it can occur with atypical agents, such as clozapine. It presents with fever, muscular rigidity, altered mental status, and autonomic dysfunction (e.g., arrhythmias and fluctuating blood pressure), leading to elevated CK and WBCs.

30. A. Anticholinergic drugs such as benztropine can be used to treat drug-induced parkinsonism. Benztropine is a muscarinic receptor antagonist that blocks acetylcholine in the striatum and so counteracts excessive cholinergic activity that results from dopamine deficiency.

B. It would not make sense to treat drug-induced parkinsonism with levodopa to increase dopamine levels because the typical antipsychotics are dopamine antagonists and because this could worsen the symptoms of schizophrenia.

C, D. Chlorpromazine and haloperidol are typical antipsychotics that may induce Parkinson-like symptoms.

31. E. κ (kappa) opiate receptors are found mainly in the spinal cord where they modulate pain sensations.

A–D. The other choices are mediated by μ receptors.

32. B. Meperidine is a synthetic opiate agonist, especially at μ receptors. Of the drugs listed, it is the only one that can induce CNS stimulation.

A. Acetaminophen is an analgesic and antipyretic drug.

C. Pentazocine is a mixed opiate agonist-antagonist that is used as an analgesic.

D, E. Naloxone and naltrexone are opiate antagonists.

33. D. The patient's responses are typical signs of opiate withdrawal. Pentazocine is a mixed agonist-antagonist at opiate receptors that may precipitate opiate withdrawal in dependent individuals.

34. D. The half-life of methadone is ~ 24 hours compared with 4 hours for morphine. This allows once-daily dosing of methadone to prevent opiate withdrawal.

A. Methadone is an effective analgesic agent (equally potent as morphine).

B. The methadone abstinence syndrome is longer and may not be more tolerable than withdrawal from morphine.

C. Methadone is not metabolized to morphine.

E. Methadone is not selective for the κ receptor but acts at all three subtypes of opiate receptor.

35. C. Morphine-like opiate agonist ligands readily cross the placenta and may affect the fetus. In this case, the infant is most likely experiencing opiate withdrawal.

36. E. Parkinson disease results from a degeneration of the dopaminergic neurons in the substantia nigra that project to the striatum. One of the primary therapeutic approaches to Parkinson disease is to restore dopaminergic function, in this case with a dopamine agonist. While the cell bodies of dopamine neurons are in the substantia nigra, these neurons project to the striatum where dopamine is released.

37. A. Entacapone is a catechol-*O*-methyltransferase inhibitor, and selegiline is an MAO type B inhibitor.

38. B. Of the agents listed, the only one that is a dopamine receptor agonist is bromocriptine.

A. Levodopa is a precursor of dopamine synthesis. Levodopa is pharmacologically inert; its effects are a result of decarboxylation to dopamine.

C. Amantadine probably enhances dopamine release in the CNS.

D. Carbidopa inhibits the peripheral production of dopamine from L-dopa by inhibiting dopa decarboxylase.

E. Benztropine is a muscarinic receptor antagonist that blocks acetylcholine in the striatum and so counteracts excessive cholinergic activity that results from dopamine deficiency.

39. A. An alternative approach to restoring dopaminergic function in Parkinson disease is to decrease the cholinergic activity.

40. C. Miosis, respiratory depression, and lack of bowel sounds are the signs of acute intoxication with morphine.

41. B. Chronic use of ethanol, but not the other drugs listed, leads to progressive liver damage that increases with increased ethanol doses and duration of ethanol use.

A. Chronic abuse of LSD includes flashbacks and other psychological problems.

C, D. Chronic abuse of amphetamine causes anxiety and confusion, leading to paranoia and psychosis which is indistinguishable from schizophrenia.

42. A. Ethanol potentiates the sedative and motor incoordination effects of other drugs that cause CNS depression.

43. D. Benzodiazepines are cross-tolerant with alcohol and will alleviate withdrawal symptoms, but they do not have the same stimulating effects on the CNS as alcohol.

A, B, C, E. The other drugs do not suppress alcohol withdrawal.

44. C. Disulfiram, the drug prescribed in this case, is an inhibitor of aldehyde dehydrogenase. Ethanol is metabolized to acetaldehyde by alcohol dehydrogenase. Acetaldehyde is then metabolized to acetate by aldehyde dehydrogenase. Disulfiram inhibits aldehyde dehydrogenase, blocking the conversion of ethanol-derived acetaldehyde to acetate. In the presence of disulfiram,

acetaldehyde will accumulate and produce flushing, dyspnea, nausea, thirst, chest pain, and palpitation. The effects are intended to be unpleasant so as to discourage alcohol ingestion; however, they can be serious and even life threatening.

45. D. Users of ethanol develop tolerance to ethanol and cross-tolerance to other sedative hypnotic agents, such as benzodiazepines and barbiturates like pentobarbital.

46. D. Ataxia and sedation are the signs of acute intoxication with methaqualone.

47. B. Decreased fatigue and increased talkativeness are the signs of acute intoxication with amphetamines.

48. A. Psychological dependence consisting of craving and a desire to acquire more of the drug may occur with any of the agents listed, but cocaine has the greatest potential for producing such an effect.

49. A. Anxiety, paranoia, and hallucinations are the signs of acute intoxication with LSD.

50. E. The first two symptoms are characteristic following ingestion of PCP, with the latter two occurring in some individuals and more likely following ingestion of larger doses of the drug.

A–D. These symptoms are not typically associated with barbiturate, caffeine, cocaine, or marijuana use.

51. B. Varenicline is a partial agonist at the $\alpha_2\beta_4$ subtype of nicotinic acetylcholine receptors. It stimulates the receptor to relieve the cravings and withdrawal from nicotine while simultaneously blocking nicotine binding, thus reducing the rewarding effect if the patient does relapse to smoking.

52. D. Strychnine is used to kill rodents. It acts by blocking glycine receptors. Glycine is the major inhibitory neurotransmitter in the spinal cord, released by the inhibitory interneurons that are activated by Ia muscle afferents. Inhibition of glycine allows impulses to propagate unchecked along the spinal cord, leading to generalized muscle spasms.

53. B. The three types of endogenous opioid peptides are the endorphins, the enkephalins, and the dynorphins.

A. Substance P is a peptide composed of 11 amino acids that acts as a neurotransmitter for pain perception.

C. Neuropeptide Y is a peptide neurotransmitter composed of 36 amino acids that plays an important role in food intake.

D. Pro-opiomelanocortin is the precursor to several peptides, including β-endorphin, melanocyte-stimulating hormone (MSH), and adrenocorticotropic hormone (ACTH).

E. Opium is an opioid derived from poppy plants.

54. B. Termination of action at the site of injection is by diffusion of the active drug into the systemic circulation followed by metabolism by plasma esterases (ester local anesthetics) or liver microsomal enzymes (amide local anesthetics).

55. B. Intravenous thiopental rapidly enters the brain to produce sedation. Its effects are terminated by redistribution from the central nervous system to other tissues.

56. C. Nitrous oxide (N_2O) will diffuse into air spaces, and, because N_2O is larger than nitrogen (N_2), the air cavity will expand. If the walls surrounding the cavity are rigid, pressure rises instead of volume. Nitrous oxide is contraindicated in patients with air emboli, pneumothorax, acute intestinal obstruction, intracranial air (e.g., following a pneumoencephalogram), or pulmonary air cysts as expansion of these air-filled spaces could cause significant morbidity.

A, B, D. Halothane, enflurane, and isoflurane do not have this effect on air spaces.

57. D. The MAC is the standard for anesthetic dosing. One MAC of halothane exerts the same anesthetic effect as 1 MAC of enflurane. Thus, the probability that either patient will move on skin incision is the same.

A, B. The partial pressure of a gas that provides 1 MAC is different for different anesthetics; thus, the partial pressure for the different agents to provide 1 MAC will be different, not identical. Similarly, the partial pressure of the different agents in the brain will be different.

C. Anesthesia will not be "deeper" with either agent because they are both being given at 1 MAC, which is a standard depth of anesthesia.

58. C. Diazepam and other benzodiazepines are commonly used as an anesthetic to produce amnesia and sedation during surgical and diagnostic procedures.

A. Ketamine is a dissociative anesthetic that produces catatonia, analgesia, and amnesia.

B. Thiopental is a barbiturate used for induction of anesthesia.

D and E. Isoflurane and halothane are inhalation anesthetic agents that produce unconsciousness, amnesia, analgesia, and muscle relaxation.

59. C. Benzodiazepines bind to the $GABA_A$ receptor, at a site distinct from that to which GABA binds, and increase the chlorine (Cl^-) current produced by GABA.

A, B, D. They are not $GABA_A$ receptor agonists, do not inhibit GABA-transaminase, or block presynaptic inhibitory receptors.

60. D. The benzodiazepines are generally safer than the barbiturates; thus, they have a greater, not a lower (A), therapeutic index.

B. The ability of the benzodiazepines to depress activity in the central nervous system (CNS) is self-limited because they act by facilitating the effects of endogenous GABA. The barbiturates, in addition to facilitating the effects of GABA, exert direct GABA agonist-like effects to produce further CNS depression. The benzodiazepines potentiate but do not mimic the actions of GABA at the GABA type A ($GABA_A$) receptor.

C. Both the benzodiazepines and barbiturates produce dependence.

61. B. Buspirone is novel among the anxiolytics in that it acts at $5-HT_{1A}$ receptors rather than at gamma-aminobutyric acid type A ($GABA_A$) receptors.

A. Diazepam is a benzodiazepine that potentiates the actions of GABA by increasing the flow of chloride ions through the $GABA_A$ receptor.

C. Pentobarbital is a barbiturate that increases the chloride conductance of the $GABA_A$ receptor by facilitating the action of GABA and also by a direct action.

D. The mechanism of action of ethanol is unknown.

62. C. Alprazolam is unique among the benzodiazepines in that it has, in addition to anxiolytic effects, antidepressant actions.

A, B. Diazepam and oxazepam are benzodiazepines that have anxiolytic effects.

D. Phenobarbital is a barbiturate that acts as a hypnotic and anticonvulsant agent.

E. Buspirone is a $5-HT_{1A}$ receptor agonist that is used to treat anxiety.

63. B. The tricyclic antidepressants block the reuptake of the biogenic monoamines norepinephrine and serotonin.

A, C–E. The MAOIs, benzodiazepines, opiates, and ethanol do not have this effect.

64. E. The selective serotonin reuptake inhibitors (SSRIs) clomipramine, fluvoxamine, and fluoxetine are used to treat obsessive-compulsive disorder.

A. Primadone is an anticonvulsant drug that is active in its own right and is also metabolized to phenobarbital.

B. Meprobamate is an anxiolytic drug.

C. Haloperidol is an antipsychotic drug.

D. Propranolol is a nonselective β-adrenergic receptor blocker that is used to treat hypertension, effort-induced angina and certain arrythmias.

65. A. The main advantage of the SSRIs is that they produce fewer adverse side effects than the first-generation agents.

B. They are not effective at lower doses than tricyclic antidepressants.

C. They are not more effective than the tricyclics or monoamine oxidase inhibitors in relieving depression.

D. They are more likely than the tricyclics to produce sexual dysfunction and anorgasmia.

66. A. Amitriptyline is a first-generation tricyclic antidepressant and as such is more likely to produce anticholinergic side effects.

B. Amoxapine is pharmacologically very similar to tricyclic antidepressants. It is a second-generation antidepressant and so is less likely to produce anticholinergic side effects.

C and D. Fluoxetine and sertaline are third-generation selective serotonin reuptake inhibitors.

67. D. Benzodiazepines such as diazepam can be given intravenously to treat status epilepticus and terminate the seizure.

A. Ethosuximide is the drug of choice for absence seizures.

B. Valproic acid is useful alone for the treatment of absence seizures. It is also used for generalized tonic-clonic seizures and complex partial seizures in combination with other agents.

C. Carbamazepine is used to treat generalized tonic-clonic seizures, complex partial seizures and trigeminal neuralgia.

68. C. Primidone is metabolized to phenobarbital and phenylethylmalonamide.

69. C. The antipsychotic drug chlorpromazine is effective in treating nausea and vomiting by blocking receptors in the chemoreceptor trigger zone.

70. D. Extrapyramidal symptoms, including Parkinson-like rigidity and tremor, can be produced by the typical antipsychotic agents.

A–C. These side effects are less likely with anticholinergic agents and are not related to amphetamine toxicity and psychoses such as schizophrenia.

71. E. The list includes adverse reactions that may be observed during antipsychotic therapy with chlorpromazine. All except tardive dyskinesia can be reduced by benztropine, the anticholinergic antiparkinson agent. There is no adequate treatment for tardive dyskinesia, so it must be prevented by judicious use of the drug.

72. C. Opiate receptor ligands include agonists, partial agonists, antagonists, and the mixed agonist-antagonist pentazocine, which is a δ- and κ-receptor agonist and a μ-receptor antagonist.

A. Propoxyphene is an agonist at opiate receptors.

B. Naltrexone is a competitive antagonist at opioid receptors.

D. and E. Fentanyl and meperidine are synthetic opiate agonists, especially at μ receptors.

73. C. Opiate agonists decrease respiration by a direct effect on the brainstem to decrease the sensitivity to CO_2, thus decreasing respiratory drive. Respiratory depression is usually the cause of death in opiate overdose cases.

A, B, D, and E. Opiate agonists are not associated with marked sedation or decreased O_2 consumption, decreased responsiveness to CO_2 tension via stimulation of the medulla's chemoreceptor trigger zone, or increased tonicity of the alveoli.

74. C. Naloxone is an opiate receptor antagonist that, following intravenous injection, rapidly reverses the effects of opiate agonists such as heroin.

A. Buprenorphine is a partial agonist at μ receptors.

B. Methadone is a synthetic, long-acting opiate agonists with similar pharmacological effects to morphine.

D. Pentazocine is a δ- and κ-receptor agonist and a μ-receptor antagonist.

E. Propoxyphene is an agonist at opiate receptors.

75. A. Of the processes listed, tolerance is the only one that is directly attributable to long-term opiate use.

76. B. Illicit use of the pentazocine/naloxone combination by intravenous injection will block the effects of pentazocine and may induce a withdrawal reaction. Naloxone is poorly absorbed orally and therefore will not block pentazocine if they are taken via this route.

77. B. Even though the bioavailability of oral morphine is in the range of 15 to 50%, a sufficient amount reaches the systemic circulation so that it is an orally effective agent.

A, C. Meperidine and pentazocine are not recommended for chronic use.

D, E. Naloxone and naltrexone are opiate antagonists and therefore have no analgesic effects.

78. B. Of the drugs listed, meperidine is the most effective and can relieve severe pain.

A. Acetaminophen is useful to treat mild to moderate pain and fever.

C. Pentazocine, a mixed agonist-antagonist, is somewhat more effective in producing pain relief.

D, E. Naloxone and naltrexone are opiate antagonists and therefore have no analgesic effects.

79. D. Methadone is an opiate agonist. As such, it acts as a substitute for heroin and prevents withdrawal.

A. On its own, methadone will produce dependence.

B. Withdrawal from methadone is characterized by less intense but more prolonged symptoms.

80. E. The symptoms listed are typical anticholinergic effects. Of the agents listed, benztropine is a muscarinic cholinergic receptor antagonist and would produce such effects.

A. Levodopa is a precursor of dopamine synthesis. Levodopa is pharmacologically inert, its effects are a result of decarboxylation to dopamine. Side effects include nausea, vomiting, and cardiac arrhythmias.

B. Bromocriptine is a dopamine receptor agonist. Side effects include nausea, vomiting, and cardiac arrhythmias.

C. Amantadine probably enhances dopamine release in the CNS. Side effects include restlessness, irritability, insomnia, headache, delirium, nausea, and diarrhea.

D. Carbidopa inhibits the peripheral production of dopamine from L-dopa by inhibiting dopa decarboxylase. No side effects are associated with this drug when used alone. All side effects are as a result of the concomitant use of levodopa (nausea, vomiting, and cardiac arrhythmias).

81. A. Of the agents listed, carbidopa is a peripherally acting dopa decarboxylase inhibitor.

B. Chlorpromazine is an antipsychotic and antiemetic agent.

C. Pyridoxine is a form of vitamin B_6. It acts as a cofactor for dopa decarboxylase and so may enhance the metabolism of levodopa.

D. Benztropine is a muscarinic receptor antagonist which blocks acetylcholine in the striatum and so counteracts excessive cholinergic activity that results from dopamine deficiency.

E. α-methyl dopa is a competitive inhibitor dopa decarboxylase that converts L-dopa to dopamine.

82. D. Baclofen is a gamma-aminobutyric acid type B ($GABA_B$) receptor agonist. $GABA_B$ receptors are G protein-coupled receptors located on the terminals of motor neurons in the spinal cord. Activation of the $GABA_B$ receptor increases conductance of K^+ channels, inhibits adenylate cyclase, and inhibits Ca^{2+} influx. This leads to hyperpolarization of the nerve terminals, decreased neurotransmitter release, and inhibition of both monosynaptic and polysynaptic reflexes at the spinal level. By decreasing α motoneuron and interneuron activity, baclofen reduces muscle tone in spasticity.

A, E. Amantadine and bromocriptine act on the dopamine system in the brain and are used to treat Parkinson disease.

B. Dantrolene acts directly on skeletal muscle to apparently decrease calcium release from the sarcoplasmic reticulum, thus reducing skeletal muscle contractions.

C. Levodopa and carbidopa are antiparkinsonian drugs.

83. B. Amantadine is an antiviral agent that has a therapeutic effect in Parkinson disease, presumably by increasing dopamine release.

A. Selegiline is a type B monoamine oxidase inhibitor (MAOI).

C. Bromocriptine is a dopamine agonist.

D. Imipramine is an MAOI that is used to treat major depression.

E. Atropine is a muscarinic cholinergic receptor blocker.

84. C. Because the deficit in Parkinson disease is a loss of dopaminergic neurons, one approach to treatment involves replacing this deficit by increasing dopamine. The neurons that are affected in Parkinson disease are located in the substantia nigra and project to the striatum; thus, the nigrostriatal pathway is involved.

85. D. Induction with an inhalation anesthetic is more rapid if the agent has low blood solubility.

A. A higher blood:gas partition coefficient would indicate greater solubility in blood and slower induction.

B, C, E. None of the other choices would increase the rate of induction.

86. B. Local anesthetics are weak bases, with pK_a slightly higher than physiological pH. Only the uncharged form can cross nerve membranes. However, once inside the nerve axon, it is the charged form that is active. As the pH decreases, the fraction of the drug in the charged protonated form will increase, decreasing diffusion across the nerve membrane.

87. B. Monoamine oxidase inhibitors such as tranylcypromine interfere with the metabolism of many drugs. In the case of sympathomimetic amines like phenylephrine, this can lead to increased drug levels and increased sympathomimetic effects.

88. C. Decreased sexual function expressed as a decreased libido and anorgasmia is a common side effect of SSRIs in both women and men. Other common side effects are headache, tremor, insomnia, diarrhea, and nausea.

A, B, D, E. Lithium, amphetamines, tricyclic antidepressants, and mixed agonists-antagonists are not associated with these side effects.

89. A. These are signs and symptoms of absence seizures. Of the drugs listed, the only agent indicated for absence seizures is ethosuximide.

B. Pheynytoin is effective for all types of seizures except absence and atonic seizures. It is also used for trigeminal neuralgia.

C. Pentazocine is an opioid drug used to treat pain.

D. Chlorpromazine is an antipsychotic and antiemetic agent.

90. D. These are signs and symptoms of absence seizures. An alternative to ethosuximide for absence seizures is valproic acid.

A. Decreasing the dose would further decrease the effectiveness of the therapy.

B, C. Phenobarbital and phenytoin are not effective in absence seizures.

E. Taking blood levels is unnecessary as the clinical response is inadequate.

91. A. Constipation is a common effect of morphine. Docusate is a laxative given to lessen the constipation.

B–E. Docusate is not prescribed for nausea, vomiting, respiratory depression, or sedation.

92. B. The patient has developed a physical dependence on meperidine. The symptoms can be lessened by gradual withdrawal from the drug.

93. D. Procaine is an ester local anesthetic that is metabolized in the plasma to soluble metabolites. This leads to a low potential for toxicity.

A, B and C are amide local anesthetics that are metabolized in the liver. In a patient with liver disease, lack of hepatic elimination could lead to increased local anesthetic levels and the blood leading to toxicity due to decreased metabolism.

94. E. The patient is experiencing symptoms of malignant hyperthermia, a serious and rare complication of anesthesia. Dantrolene reduces muscular contraction and the hypermetabolic state by blocking the ryanodine receptor.

A. Skelaxin is the trade name for metaxalone. It is a centrally-acting skeletal muscle relaxant that may be used for relief of acute muscle spasms.

B. Diazepam is a benzodiazepine that enhances presynaptic inhibition in the spinal cord and may be used to treat spasticity due to spinal lesions or cerebral palsy.

C. Tizanidine is an α_2-adrenergic receptor agonist that relieves spasticity by increasing presynaptic inhibition of motor neurons. It may be used to treat spasticity in multiple sclerosis and spinal trauma.

D. Cyclobenzaprine is a centrally acting skeletal muscle relaxant that may be used for relief of acute muscle spasms.

Unit IV

Drugs Acting on the Endocrine and Reproductive Systems

By T. Sean Vasaitis

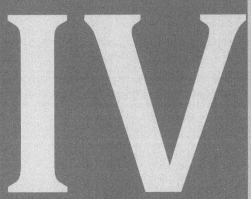

16 Drugs Used in the Treatment of Hypothalamic, Pituitary, Thyroid, and Adrenal Disorders

Summary

The hypothalamus and pituitary gland produce and release hormones that control the function of multiple target organs, including other endocrine glands. Somatotropin is a recombinant form of growth hormone. Octreotide, pasireotide, and lanreotide are cyclic peptide analogues of the active portion of somatostatin. Pegvisomant is a receptor antagonist that blocks the effects of growth hormone. Corticorelin is a bovine corticotropin-releasing hormone that acts like the natural hormone. Cosyntropin is a synthetic form of adrenocorticotropic hormone. Leuprolide, goserelin, triptorelin, nafarelin, and histrelin are gonadotropin-releasing hormone agonists. Ganirelix, degarelix, and cetrorelix are gonadotropin-releasing hormone antagonists. Protirelin is a synthetic thyroid-stimulating hormone. Protirelin and thyrotropin act like the natural hormones. The thyroid hormones are thyroxine (T$_4$) and triiodothyronine (T$_3$). Levothyroxine, a synthetic form of T$_4$, is the drug of choice for replacement therapy. Propylthiouracil and methimazole inhibit thyroid hormone synthesis. Radioiodine accumulates in the thyroid gland and destroys parenchymal cells. Iodine inhibits thyroid hormone release. Teriparatide is a synthetic polypeptide parathyroid hormone analogue. Cinacalcet and etelcalcetide decrease parathyroid hormone secretion. *Vitamin D* refers to cholecalciferol (vitamin D$_3$) and ergocalciferol (vitamin D$_2$). Estrogens include estradiol, Premarin, ethinyl estradiol, and mestranol. The bisphosphonates alendronate, etidronate, ibandronate, pamidronate, risedronate, tiludronate, and zoledronate are exogenous regulators of bone metabolism used for prevention and treatment of osteoporosis. The adrenocortical steroids include glucocorticoids, mineralocorticoids, and androgens. Hydrocortisone (cortisol), prednisone, methylprednisolone, triamcinolone, dexamethasone, betamethasone, beclomethasone, and fluocinonide are synthetic glucocorticoids that act like the endogenous hormones. Fludrocortisone is a synthetic corticosteroid that has much greater mineralocorticoid than glucocorticoid activity.

Keywords: adrenal insufficiency, thyroid hormone, glucocorticoids, growth hormone, calcium, hypothalamic-pituitary axis

16.1 Introduction to Drugs Used in the Treatment of Hypothalamic, Pituitary, Thyroid, and Adrenal Disorders

The hypothalamus and pituitary gland produce and release hormones that control the function of multiple target organs, including other endocrine glands. This system thus provides a bridge between the nervous and endocrine systems. Both neural inputs and hormonal signals (e.g., negative feedback) modulate hypothalamic activity, which in turn regulates pituitary function and subsequent function of target endocrine organs.

The hypothalamic and pituitary hormones, and their related drugs, are discussed in relation to the hormones and target organs that they modulate.

▶ Table 16.1 lists the second messengers used by the hormones discussed in this unit.

16.2 Pituitary Hormones

The pituitary gland is divided into the anterior and posterior pituitary. Anterior pituitary hormones are secreted or inhibited in response to the action of releasing hormones or inhibiting hormones from the hypothalamus. Posterior pituitary hormones are synthesized in the hypothalamus, stored in the posterior pituitary, and secreted in response to direct neural stimulation (▶ Fig. 16.1). ▶ Table 16.2 summarizes the hormonal cascade from the hypothalamus to target organs or the posterior pituitary.

Foundations

Hormone Receptors

Hormones that are hydrophilic cannot penetrate the plasma membrane; they, therefore, interact with membrane receptors and exert their effects via second messenger molecules such as cyclic adenosine monophosphate (cAMP), phospholipase C, and Ca^{2+}. Examples of hydrophilic hormones are insulin and adrenocorticotropic hormone (ACTH). Conversely, lipophilic hormones (e.g., cortisol and estrogen) are able to pass through the cell membrane and interact with receptors in the cytoplasm or nucleus. In this case, receptor binding alters the gene transcription of proteins to exert the hormones' physiological effects.

Table 16.1 Second messengers used by hormones

Hormones	Second messenger
CRH, ACTH, LH, FSH, TSH, PTH, calcitonin, glucagon, ADH (V$_2$ receptors), hCG	↑ cyclic AMP
Prolactin	↓ cyclic AMP
GRH, GnRH, TRH, ADH (V$_1$ receptors), oxytocin	DAG and IP$_3$
Cortisol, aldosterone, testosterone, estrogen, progesterone, calcitriol (vitamin D), thyroid hormones (T$_3$ and T$_4$)	Steroid mechanism
NO	Cyclic GMP
Insulin and IGF-1	Tyrosine kinase

Abbreviations: ACTH, adrenocorticotropic hormone; ADH, antidiuretic hormone; AMP, adenosine monophosphate; CRH, corticotropin-releasing hormone; DAG, diacylglycerol; FSH, follicle-stimulating hormone; GRH, growth hormone-releasing hormone; GMP, guanosine monophosphate; GnRH, gonadotropin-releasing hormone; hCG, human chorionic gonadotropin; IGF-1, insulin-like growth factor; IP$_3$, inositol triphosphate; LH, luteinizing hormone; NO, nitric oxide; PTH, parathyroid hormone (dopamine); TRH, thyrotropin-releasing hormone; TSH, thyroid-stimulating hormone.

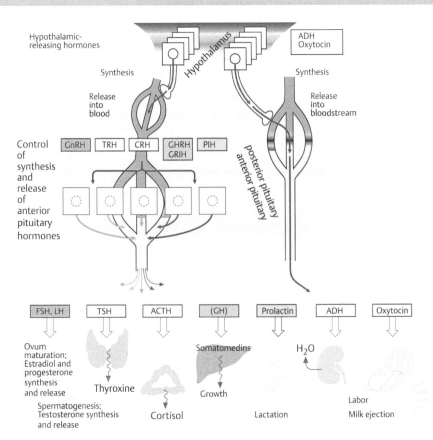

Fig. 16.1 Hypothalamic and pituitary hormones. Hormones released from the hypothalamus stimulate or inhibit the release of hormones from the anterior pituitary. The pituitary hormones then travel to target tissues, where they exert their physiological effects. Posterior pituitary hormones are synthesized in the hypothalamus and stored in the posterior pituitary until release is stimulated by an action potential. These hormones then travel in the blood to their target tissues. ACTH, adrenocorticotropic hormone; ADH, antidiuretic hormone; CRH, corticotropin-releasing hormone; FSH, follicle-stimulating hormone; GH, growth hormone; GnRH, gonadotropin-releasing hormone; GRH, growth hormone-releasing hormone; GRIH, growth hormone-inhibiting hormone (somatostatin); LH, luteinizing hormone; PIH, prolactin inhibiting hormone (dopamine); TRH, thyrotropin-releasing hormone; TSH, thyroid-stimulating hormone.

Table 16.2 Hypothalamic and pituitary hormones and their target organs

Hypothalamic hormone	Anterior pituitary hormone	Target organ(s)
GRH	↑ GH	Liver, skeletal muscle, and bone
Somatostatin	↓ GH	Liver, GI tract, and pancreas
CRH	ACTH	Adrenal cortex
GnRH	LH and FSH	Gonads
TRH	TSH	Thyroid gland
PIH (dopamine)	Prolactin	Mammary glands and gonads
Posterior pituitary hormones		
Oxytocin		Uterine and other smooth muscle
ADH (vasopressin)		Kidney tubules (mainly); also vascular smooth muscle, liver, and anterior pituitary gland

Abbreviations: ACTH, adrenocorticotropic hormone; ADH, antidiuretic hormone; CRH, corticotropin-releasing hormone; FSH, follicle-stimulating hormone; GH, growth hormone; GRH, growth hormone-releasing hormone; GI, gastrointestinal; GnRH, gonadotropin-releasing hormone; LH, luteinizing hormone; PIH, prolactin-inhibiting hormone; TRH, thyrotropin-releasing hormone; TSH, thyroid-stimulating hormone.

16.2.1 Growth Hormone

Hypothalamic Regulation

Growth hormone (GH) release from the anterior pituitary is controlled by following two hormones released from the hypothalamus:

- GH-releasing hormone (GHRH) that increases the synthesis and secretion of GH.
- Somatostatin (GH release-inhibiting hormone [GRIH]) that decreases the sensitivity of the anterior pituitary to GHRH, thus decreasing levels of GH.

Foundations

Negative Feedback

Negative feedback is a phenomenon when the output of a pathway inhibits the input to a pathway. This physiological phenomenon is particularly evident in the endocrine system and is an important mechanism in homeostasis.

Foundations

Growth Hormone Receptors

The receptors for GH are found in peripheral tissues and belong to the class 1 cytokine receptor superfamily. These are receptor-associated tyrosine kinase receptors that, upon binding of GH, dimerize and activate the Janus kinase-signal transducer and activator of transcription (JAK–STAT) pathway. The JAK–STAT pathway is a signaling alternative to the second messenger systems. Its activation ultimately causes deoxyribonucleic acid (DNA) transcription within the cell.

Effects

See ▶ Table 16.3.

Table 16.3 Effects of growth hormone (GH) and somatomedins[a]

Effects mediated by GH	Effects mediated by somatomedins
↑ somatomedin synthesis[a]	Protein synthesis resulting in the following effects:
↑ gluconeogenesis	↑ muscle mass
↑ lipolysis	↑ cartilage growth (this causes linear growth)
↑ protein synthesis	↑ growth of the internal organs
↑ amino acid uptake in the gut	
↓ insulin (causing ↓ glucose uptake into cells)	

[a]Somatomedins are insulin-like growth factors that are intermediaries for some GH actions. Many of the actions of GH occur in association with cortisol.

Factors Affecting Growth Hormone Secretion

The major stimuli for GH secretion are deep sleep, hypoglycemia, stress, GHRH, and metabolites (e.g., amino acids and free fatty acids). Secondary stimuli include exercise, glucagon, antidiuretic hormone (ADH), opioids, and pyrogens (fever-inducing substances). GH secretion is inhibited by hyperglycemia and cortisol secretion.

Growth Hormone and Nitrogen Balance

GH creates a positive nitrogen balance in the body. This is mainly due to an increased rate of lipolysis which provides the energy the body needs while sparing proteins and glucose. Diseases in which there is a negative nitrogen balance, such as acquired immunodeficiency syndrome (AIDS), cachexia (loss of lean body mass that cannot be corrected with increased calorific intake), trauma, and severe burns, can be treated with GH to improve lean body mass and wound healing.

Growth at Epiphyseal Plates

The epiphyseal plates consist of hyaline cartilage at the end of long bones. Chondrocytes in the epiphyseal plates are constantly undergoing mitosis throughout childhood and adolescence that ceases in adulthood. The older cells (at the diaphysis end) are then ossified by osteoblasts. This progressive laying down of bone leads to longitudinal growth. GH acts to increase the mitosis of chondrocytes in the epiphyseal plates.

Carpal Tunnel Syndrome

Carpal tunnel syndrome is a condition caused by compression of the median nerve within the carpal tunnel of the wrist. It may be caused by anything that produces soft-tissue swelling such as pregnancy and rheumatoid arthritis. Symptoms include burning pain, tingling, and numbness in the hand, especially in the thumb, index finger, middle finger, and radial half of the ring finger but not in the little finger. This pain may be relieved by placing the hand in cold water or by patients "shaking out" their hands. There may also be muscle weakness and wasting. Treatment includes wrist splints, nonsteroidal anti-inflammatory drugs (NSAIDs), and corticosteroids (hydrocortisone). Surgical decompression may be necessary if other treatments are ineffective.

Vasoactive Intestinal Peptide

Vasoactive intestinal peptide (VIP) is a neurocrine peptide secreted by neurons in the mucosa and smooth muscle of the gastrointestinal (GI) tract in response to distention of the stomach and small intestines and vagal activity. It acts to reduce lower esophageal sphincter tone, relax the proximal muscles of the stomach, allowing for entrance of food ("receptive relaxation"), and increase water and electrolyte secretion in intestine.

Disorders

- Deficiency of GH causes short stature with normal body proportions.
- Excess GH leads to gigantism in children and acromegaly in adults.

Somatotropin

Mechanism of Action

Somatotropin is a recombinant form of GH.

Uses

- To treat GH deficiencies in children prior to epiphyseal plate closure (complete ossification).

Side Effects

- Peripheral edema.
- Localized muscle pain and weakness.
- Carpal tunnel syndrome.

Contraindications

- Closed epiphyses.
- Active neoplasia.

Octreotide, Pasireotide, and Lanreotide

Mechanism of Action

These agents are cyclic peptide analogues of the biologically active portion of somatostatin.

Effects

- These agents mimic the actions of somatostatin to inhibit GH secretion from the anterior pituitary.
- They also inhibit GH secretion from tumors.

Uses

- Acromegaly.
- Carcinoid syndrome and VIP-secreting tumors (octreotide).
- Cushing disease (pasireotide).

Side Effects

GI side effects, including nausea, diarrhea, and steatorrhea (excess fat in stools), are seen in a majority of patients with acromegaly who are treated with octreotide. Cholelithiasis (gallstones) is observed in one-third of patients with use of octreotide for 6 months or more. Hyperglycemia is noted in case of all three agents. Pasireotide may cause hypocortisolism.

Pegvisomant

Mechanism of Action

Pegvisomant is a GH receptor antagonist that blocks the effects of endogenous GH.

Uses

For treatment of acromegaly in patients unresponsive to surgery, radiation, or octreotide.

16.2.2 Adrenocorticotropic Hormone

Hypothalamic Regulation

Corticotropin-releasing hormone (CRH) from the hypothalamus stimulates the release of ACTH from the anterior pituitary.

Effects

The primary target of ACTH is the MC_2 subtype of melanocortin receptor, a G protein-coupled receptor expressed primarily by cells of the adrenal cortex. The MC_2 receptor activates G_s to increase intracellular levels of cAMP that stimulates the synthesis of corticosteroids, including glucocorticoids, mineralocorticoids, and androgens.

Disorders

- ACTH deficiency causes secondary adrenal insufficiency. This is characterized by fatigue, weakness, anorexia, nausea, and vomiting.
- ACTH excess leads to Cushing syndrome.

Corticorelin

Mechanism of Action

Corticorelin is bovine CRH that acts like the natural human hormone.

Uses

Corticorelin is used to differentiate pituitary ACTH-dependent Cushing disease from ectopic ACTH-secreting tumors (Cushing syndrome). Patients with Cushing disease show normal to increased plasma ACTH and cortisol response, whereas ectopic tumors do not.

Adrenocorticotropic Hormone and Cosyntropin

Mechanism of Action

Cosyntropin is a synthetic peptide consisting of the first 24 amino acids of ACTH. It acts like the natural hormone and is used for similar purposes.

Uses

This agent is used for the differential diagnosis of primary versus secondary adrenal insufficiency. If there is primary adrenal insufficiency, there will be no response to ACTH; however, if there is secondary adrenal insufficiency due to inadequate ACTH release from the pituitary, administered ACTH will increase plasma glucocorticoids.

16.2.3 Gonadotropins (Follicle-stimulating Hormone and Luteinizing Hormone)

Hypothalamic Regulation

Gonadotropin-releasing hormone (GnRH) released from the hypothalamus stimulates the release of luteinizing hormone (LH) and follicle-stimulating hormone (FSH) from the anterior pituitary.

Effects

- In men, LH stimulates testosterone production by the Leydig cells of the testes. FSH stimulates the Sertoli cells and is critical for maturation of spermatozoa.
- In women, LH stimulates estrogen and progesterone production by the ovaries. FSH stimulates the development of the ovarian follicle (▶ Fig. 16.2).

Clinical Correlation

Cushing Syndrome

Cushing syndrome is a group of signs and symptoms that occur due to high levels of cortisol in the blood. It can be caused by corticosteroid (and ACTH) administration, pituitary adenomas, adrenal gland adenomas/carcinomas, and by excessive intake of alcohol. Signs and symptoms typically include weight gain, particularly to the trunk, with sparing of the limbs; moon face (or moon facies); "buffalo hump" (due to fat deposition on the back); purple striae, especially on the abdomen; sweating; thin skin; and hirsutism. Treatment depends on the cause.

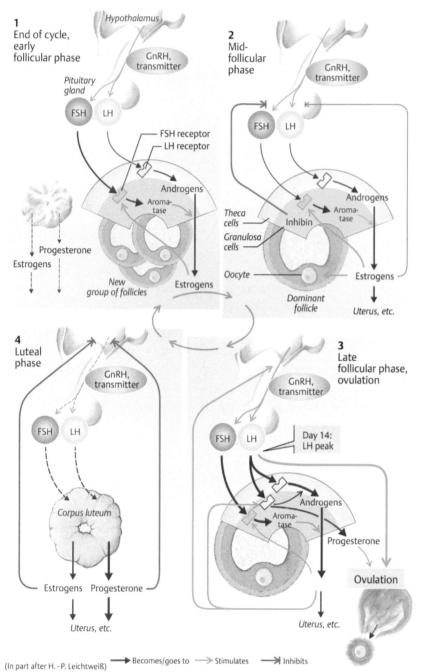

1 End of cycle, early follicular phase

Hypothalamus

GnRH, transmitter

Pituitary gland

FSH LH

FSH receptor
LH receptor

Androgens
Aroma-tase

Progesterone

Estrogens

New group of follicles

Estrogens

2 Mid-follicular phase

GnRH, transmitter

FSH LH

Androgens
Aroma-tase

Theca cells
Granulosa cells

Inhibin

Oocyte

Estrogens

Dominant follicle

Uterus, etc.

4 Luteal phase

GnRH, transmitter

FSH LH

Corpus luteum

Estrogens Progesterone

Uterus, etc.

3 Late follicular phase, ovulation

GnRH, transmitter

FSH LH

Day 14: LH peak

Androgens
Aroma-tase

Progesterone

Ovulation

Uterus, etc.

(In part after H. - P. Leichtweiß) ━━▶ Becomes/goes to ──▷ Stimulates ━━⊣ Inhibits

Fig. 16.2 Hormonal control of the menstrual cycle.
Follicle-stimulating hormone (FSH) and luteinizing hormone (LH) act in the follicular phase to cause follicular growth, estrogen production (causing the selection of a dominant follicle in which the ovum develops), progesterone production (which is primarily responsible for endometrial thickening), and ovulation. Estrogens and progesterone produced in the luteal phase induce endometrial thickening necessary for implantation of the ovum. If this does not occur, feedback inhibition of FSH and LH triggers menstruation.

Clinical Correlation

Primary and Secondary Adrenal Insufficiency

Primary adrenal insufficiency occurs when there is impairment or destruction of the adrenal glands. The cause of this may be idiopathic (unknown) or it may be due to autoimmune disease (e.g., Addison's disease), adrenal hyperplasia, or adenoma. Secondary adrenal insufficiency occurs when there is inadequate ACTH secretion from the pituitary to stimulate adrenal hormone production.

Foundations

Menstrual Cycle

The menstrual cycle varies in length from 21 to 35 days. The first half of the cycle is the follicular phase, which begins with menstruation. Following menstruation, in the early follicular phase, FSH induces the production of ~ 20 follicles. Small amounts of LH are also secreted. Both FSH and LH stimulate enzymes that catalyze the production of androgens that are needed for estrogen synthesis. Estrogens released from follicles cause upregulation of FSH receptors, so the follicle with the highest estrogen content is most sensitive to FSH. This follicle becomes the dominant (Graafian) follicle in which an ovum develops. The remaining follicles containing oocytes undergo atresia. In the mid follicular phase, the follicular cells also start to produce progesterone that causes progressive thickening of the endometrium. In the late follicular phase, increased quantities of FSH and LH are secreted once again. This causes more androgen and estrogen production, which positively feeds back to the hypothalamus, causing an increase in LH. This rapid rise in LH concentration (LH surge) induces ovulation. Just after ovulation, the basal body temperature rises and stays elevated until the end of the cycle. The second half of the cycle is known as the luteal phase. LH, FSH, and estrogen transform the follicle into a corpus luteum, which secretes large quantities of progesterone, causing further endometrial thickening. If fertilization of the ovum has not occurred, estrogen and progesterone now inhibit FSH and LH both directly and via negative feedback on the hypothalamus and anterior pituitary. This causes a marked drop in plasma estrogen and progesterone concentration, causing constriction of endometrial blood vessels and discharge of the endometrium (menses).

Leuprolide, Goserelin, Triptorelin, Nafarelin, and Histrelin

Mechanism of Action

These agents are GnRH agonist analogues. Chronic treatment with one of these agents produces desensitization of the normal response to GnRH. After an initial surge of LH and FSH, the secretion of these hormones decreases.

Pharmacokinetics

These agents are administered subcutaneously, intramuscularly in depot form, or inhaled intranasally.

Uses

- Endometriosis in women.
- Prostatic carcinoma in men.
- Central precocious puberty.
- Preoperative treatment of anemia due to uterine fibroids (leuprolide).
- Ovarian suppression in premenopausal breast cancer (off-label use).

Side Effects

These agents may cause bone loss through a prolonged hypoestrogenic state.

Ganirelix, Degarelix, and Cetrorelix

Mechanism of Action

Ganirelix, degarelix, and cetrorelix are competitive antagonists of GnRH.

Uses

Ganirelix and cetrorelix are used to suppress the LH surge and prevent premature follicular luteinization in ovarian-stimulation protocols. Degarelix is used to reduce testicular androgen production in advanced prostate cancer.

Human Chorionic Gonadotropin and Human Menopausal Gonadotropin

Human chorionic gonadotropin (hCG) and human menopausal gonadotropin (hMG) are discussed further in the ovulatory agents section in Chapter 17.

Mechanism of Action

Both hCG and hMG mimic the effects of gonadotropins.

Pharmacokinetics

Administered parenterally.

Uses

Used to promote fertility.

16.2.4 Thyroid-stimulating Hormone (Thyrotropin)

Hypothalamic Control

Thyrotropin-releasing hormone (TRH) is a tripeptide released from the hypothalamus that stimulates thyroid-stimulating hormone (TSH) synthesis and release in the anterior pituitary.

Effects

TSH stimulates the release of thyroid hormones via several mechanisms (see ▸ Table 16.4).

Clinical Correlation

Endometriosis

It is a condition in which endometrial tissue that normally lines the uterus grows outside the uterus. The displaced endometrial tissue (or "implants") responds to FSH and LH during the menstrual cycle as normal endometrial tissue does, causing thickening and then breakdown and bleeding. Surrounding tissue eventually becomes inflamed leading to fibrosis. Symptoms include dysmenorrhea (painful periods); pain during intercourse, bowel movements, or urination; and infertility (usually due to obstruction of the fallopian tubes by scar tissue). Treatment involves the use of NSAIDs for pain, contraceptive hormones to control endometrial buildup, GnRH agonists and antagonists to block the production of FSH and LH, and aromatase inhibitors that block estrogen production. Surgery may be required to remove endometrial implants or hysterectomy in cases of severe endometriosis.

IV

Table 16.4 How thyroid-stimulating hormone (TSH) increases the release of thyroid hormones

↑ sensitivity of TSH receptors to TSH

↑ thyroglobulin synthesis

↑ thyroid peroxidase and glucose oxidase levels which increase the iodination of thyroglobulin

↑ activity of the iodide pump

↑ Na^+–K^+–ATPase activity which increases the capacity for iodide intake

↑ T_3 formation relative to T_4 under acute increases in metabolic demand

Clinical Correlation

Ovarian Hyperstimulation Syndrome

This syndrome occurs when gonadotropins, such as hCG, are given to stimulate ovulation. In ~10 to 25% of patients who are given these drugs parenterally, the ovaries are overstimulated and fluid leaks from them into the belly and chest following ovulation. Most of the time this produces mild symptoms, such as nausea, vomiting, diarrhea, mild abdominal pain, bloating, and weight gain. However, in a small percentage of cases, these symptoms can be more severe, and there may be additional symptoms, such as shortness of breath (dyspnea), blood clots, electrolyte disturbance, and kidney failure. No treatment may be required in case of mild symptoms, but hospitalization for fluid replacement and management of any serious complications may be necessary for severe cases.

Foundations

Origins of the Thyroid Gland

The thyroid gland is formed from the pharyngeal arches. During embryonic development, it descends from the foramen cecum of the forming tongue, through the thyroglossal duct, until it reaches its final location in the neck, surrounding the trachea.

Disorders

- TSH deficiency causes secondary hypothyroidism. Symptoms generally mimic those of primary hypothyroidism but are less severe.
- Excess TSH secretion is characterized by goiter and hyperthyroidism.

Protirelin and Thyrotropin

Mechanism of Action

Protirelin is a synthetic peptide identical to TSH. Protirelin acts like the natural hormone.

Uses

- Diagnosis of hypothyroid states (protirelin).
- Given intramuscularly to stimulate iodine 131 (I^{131}) uptake in the treatment of metastatic thyroid carcinoma, but its diagnostic use has largely been replaced by TRH.

16.2.5   Prolactin

Hypothalamic Regulation

Hypothalamic regulation of prolactin secretion is primarily inhibitory. Dopamine (prolactin-inhibiting hormone [PIH]) released from the hypothalamus binds to the D_2 subtype of dopamine receptor in the anterior pituitary, which is coupled to G_i and leads to inhibition of adenylate cyclase. This, in turn, causes tonic inhibition of the release of prolactin from the anterior pituitary.

Effects

Prolactin stimulates the mammary glands to produce milk in the postpartum period.

Disorders

Loss of PIH after hypothalamic destruction is associated with hypersecretion of prolactin. This causes amenorrhea or galactorrhea. Drug-induced hyperprolactinemia also occurs with dopamine antagonists, whereas dopamine agonists may be used to treat some types of hyperprolactinemia.

Cabergoline and Bromocriptine

Mechanism of Action

Cabergoline and bromocriptine are dopamine (PIH) analogue agonists at the D_2 dopamine receptor.

Pharmacokinetics

Cabergoline has a much longer duration of action (7–14 days) compared with bromocriptine (1–2 days).

Uses

- To treat prolactin-secreting adenomas.
- To treat amenorrhea or galactorrhea.
- For suppression of physiological lactation.

16.2.6   Antidiuretic Hormone and Oxytocin

ADH (or vasopressin) and oxytocin are synthesized in the hypothalamus and are transported to the posterior pituitary, where they are stored. Both are peptide hormones consisting of nine amino acids. They differ only in the amino acids at positions 3 and 8, and both have a short half-life (15–30 minutes) once released into the systemic circulation. Due to their chemical similarities, ADH has slight oxytocic activity, and oxytocin has slight antidiuretic activity. However, oxytocin has no vasoconstricting activity.

See Chapter 17 for a further discussion of oxytocin and Chapter 19 for a discussion of ADH.

Table 16.5 Drugs affecting hypothalamic and pituitary hormones

Drug	Mechanism
Agonists	
Octreotide, lanreotide	Somatostatin analogues
Somatotropin	GH analogue
Corticorelin	CRH analogue
ACTH, cosyntropin	ACTH analogue
hCG, hMG	Mimics gonadotropins
Protirelin, thyrotropin	TSH analogues
Cabergoline, bromocriptine	Dopamine (PIH) analogues
Antagonists	
Pegvisomant	GH receptor antagonist
Ganirelix, cetrorelix	Competitive inhibitors of GnRH

Abbreviations: ACTH, adrenocorticotropic hormone; CRH, corticotropin-releasing hormone; GH, growth hormone; GnRH, gonadotropin-releasing hormone; hCG, human chorionic gonadotropin; hMG, human menopausal gonadotropin; PIH, prolactin-inhibiting hormone; TSH, thyroid-stimulating hormone.

Foundations

Stimuli for ADH Synthesis and Secretion

ADH is synthesized and released in response to increased plasma osmolality (detected by hypothalamic osmoreceptors), such as dehydration; decreased plasma volume (detected by peripheral mechanoreceptors), such as hemorrhage (hypovolemia); and decreased blood pressure (detected by baroreceptors). Its release is most sensitive to plasma osmolality, yet larger quantities of ADH are released in response to changes in blood pressure and blood volume.

▶ Table 16.5 summarizes the drugs affecting hypothalamic and pituitary hormone levels.

16.3 Thyroid Hormones

The natural thyroid hormones produced by the thyroid gland are thyroxine (T_4) and triiodothyronine (T_3). The mechanism of their release and degradation is shown in ▶ Fig. 16.3.

Foundations

Thyroid Hormone Synthesis

The follicles of the thyroid gland synthesize and store thyroglobulin (TG), a glycoprotein with tyrosine residues. These tyrosine residues are conjugated with iodine (from dietary sources), under the influence of the enzyme thyroid peroxidase, to form monoiodotyrosine (MIT) or diiodotyrosine (DIT). These then undergo a coupling reaction, while still attached to TG, to produce T_3 (MIT + DIT) or T_4 (DIT + DIT). Proteolysis of TG releases free T_3 and T_4 into the circulation.

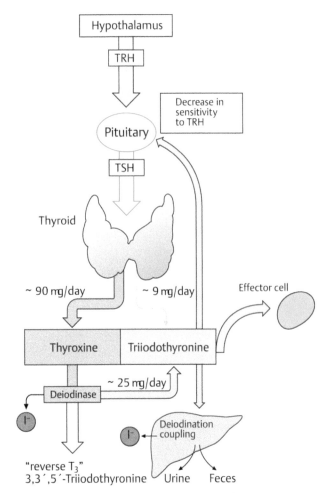

Fig. 16.3 Thyroid hormones: release, effects, and degradation.
Thyrotropin-releasing hormone from the hypothalamus causes thyroid-stimulating hormone (TSH) release from the anterior pituitary. The thyroid secretes the hormones thyroxine (T_4) and triiodothyronine (T_3). T_4 is produced in higher quantities than T_3, but T_3 is the more active form. T_4 is converted to T_3, or the metabolically inactive "reverse T_3," in tissues. T_3 attaches to effector cell receptors, producing its physiological effects. It also causes feedback inhibition of TSH production.

16.3.1 General Properties

Mechanism of Action

Most cells in the body are responsive to thyroid hormones. Within cells, T_4 is converted to T_3, the active form. T_3 binds to its receptor in the cell nucleus to affect gene transcription.

Effects

See ▶ Table 16.6.

Pharmacokinetics

- T_4 has a slower onset, is more extensively bound to plasma proteins, and has a longer duration of action than T_3.
- T_3 is four times more potent than T_4.

Table 16.6 Effects of thyroid hormones

Category	Effects
Development	Essential for CNS development
Growth	↑ protein synthesis ↑ bone formation (with GH and somatomedins) ↑ ossification and fusion of growth plates
Metabolic	↑ intestinal absorption of glucose ↑ gluconeogenesis, glycogenolysis, and glucose oxidation ↑ lipolysis ↑ cholesterol turnover and plasma clearance of cholesterol T_3 potentiates the "hypoglycemic" actions of insulin by increasing glucose uptake into muscle and adipose tissue
BMR	↑ BMR ↑ ATP hydrolysis ↑ O_2 consumption and heat as a consequence of the above
Systemic	Stimulation of adrenergic β-receptors leading to increased heart rate, cardiac output, and ventilation and decreased peripheral vascular resistance. These actions support increased oxygen demand in tissues T_3 facilitates the actions of cortisol, glucagon, and GH

Abbreviations: ATP, adenosine triphosphate; BMR, basal metabolic rate; CNS, central nervous system; GH, growth hormone.

16.3.2 Treatment of Hypothyroidism

Levothyroxine

Levothyroxine, a synthetic form of the thyroxine (T_4), is the drug of choice for replacement therapy.

Uses

- Hypothyroidism, regardless of etiology, including congenital (cretinism).
- Autoimmune thyroiditis (e.g., Hashimoto's thyroiditis).
- Pregnancy and postpartum hypothyroidism.
- Thyroid carcinoma (to suppress TSH).

Toxicity

It causes tachycardia, palpitations, restlessness, tremor, and cardiac arrhythmias.

Clinical Correlation

Hypothyroidism (Myxedema)

Hypothyroidism occurs due to decreased levels of plasma T_3 and T_4. Metabolism is slowed leading to symptoms such as weight gain, constipation, cold intolerance, lethargy, depression, and dementia. Signs of hypothyroidism include bradycardia, dry skin and face, goiter, congestive heart failure, and edema. This condition may be spontaneously acquired, or it may occur after a thyroidectomy, radioiodine treatment, or following drug therapy (e.g., amiodarone and lithium). It is treated by replacement therapy with levothyroxine. More severe, life-threatening hypothyroidism is called myxedema crisis. This can lead to impaired cognition, somnolence (sleepiness), and coma (myxedema coma). Myxedema can be treated with intravenous (IV) levothyroxine or with liothyronine to achieve a more rapid response.

16.3.3 Treatment of Hyperthyroidism and Related Disorders

Propylthiouracil and Methimazole

Mechanism of Action

Propylthiouracil and methimazole inhibit thyroid hormone synthesis by inhibiting the peroxidase enzyme that catalyzes the iodination of tyrosine residues in thyroglobulin and couples iodotyrosines to form T_3 and T_4. Effects are not apparent until the thyroid reserve is depleted.

Pharmacokinetics

- Methimazole is more potent and has a longer duration than propylthiouracil.
- These drugs cross the placenta and are excreted into milk.
- Babies who are exposed to these agents should have thyroid function monitored.

Uses

- To treat hyperthyroidism.

Side Effects

- Rash is common.
- Agranulocytosis (acute low white blood cell count) is rare but serious.

Radioiodine (Sodium Iodide, I^{131})

Mechanism of Action

Radioiodine accumulates in the thyroid gland and destroys parenchymal cells. Clinical improvement may take 2 to 3 months.

Uses

It is the preferred treatment for most patients with hyperthyroidism. Subsequent hypothyroidism occurs in 20 to 80% of patients.

Iodine (Lugol's Solution, Potassium Iodide)

Mechanism of Action

Iodine (supraphysiological dose) inhibits thyroid hormone release, but the effect is not sustained (Wolff–Chaikoff effect); therefore, it only produces a temporary remission of symptoms.

Uses

- Thyrotoxicosis.
- Prior to thyroid surgery (to decrease vascularity of the gland).
- Following radioiodine therapy.

Propranolol, Atenolol, Esmolol, and Metoprolol

The pharmacology of these adrenergic blocking agents was discussed in Chapter 6.

Uses

These agents are used as adjuncts to treat or prevent thyrotoxicosis.

16.4 Parathyroid Hormone and Other Factors Affecting Bone Metabolism

The major hormones involved in bone mineral homeostasis are parathyroid hormone (PTH) and vitamin D (▶ Fig. 16.4). Other endogenous regulators of bone metabolism are calcitonin, glucocorticoids, and estrogens. Numerous exogenous agents are available that affect bone and mineral homeostasis.

Clinical Correlation

Hyperthyroidism (Thyrotoxicosis)

Hyperthyroidism occurs when there are elevated levels of T_3 and T_4 in the blood. Patients may develop hyperthyroidism due to adenomas/carcinomas of the thyroid gland or thyroiditis

(inflammation of the thyroid), or it may be autoimmune in origin. Signs and symptoms are reflective of a hypermetabolic state and include weight loss, increased appetite, frequent stools, tremor, heat intolerance, increased sweating, tachycardia, tremor, ptosis (lid lag), and thyroid enlargement. Severe hyperthyroidism (thyrotoxic storm) is a medical emergency. Treatment depends on the cause.

Foundations

Na⁺–I⁻ Pump

Iodine (from ingested food) is necessary for thyroid hormone synthesis. Because dietary intake inevitably varies, the thyroid gland must sequester iodine so that adequate amounts are always available for thyroid hormone synthesis. It does this via the Na^+–I^- pump on the cell membrane. The pump symports two Na^+ ions into the cytoplasm for every I^- ion. It is driven by the low intracellular $[Na^+]$, via facilitated diffusion, that is maintained by the Na^+–K^+–ATPase pump. TSH is the major physiological stimulator of the iodide pump. High intracellular levels of iodide inhibit the activity of the pump.

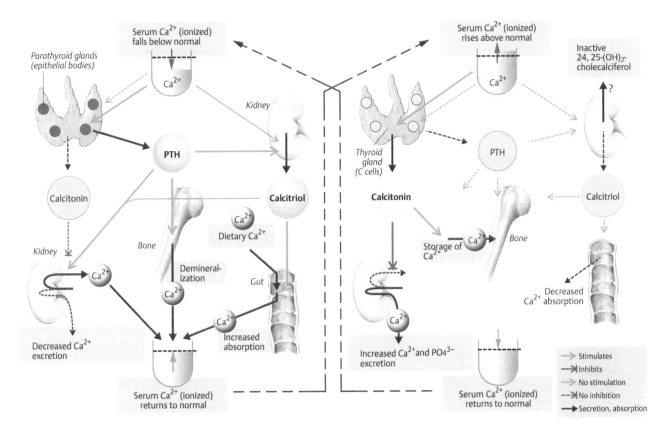

Fig. 16.4 Hormonal regulation of the blood Ca²⁺ concentration.
Ca^{2+} homeostasis is achieved by three main hormones: parathyroid hormone (PTH, from parathyroid gland), calcitonin (from parafollicular cells of the thyroid gland), and calcitriol (mainly produced in the kidney). In low serum Ca^{2+} states, the actions of parathyroid hormone and calcitriol predominate, causing increased Ca^{2+} uptake from the gut and bone and decreased renal excretion. In high serum Ca^{2+} states, the action of calcitonin predominates, causing decreased Ca^{2+} uptake from the gut, increased renal excretion, and storage of excess Ca^{2+} in bone.

Foundations

Wolff–Chaikoff effect

The Wolff–Chaikoff effect results in a reduction in the synthesis and release of thyroid hormones caused by a large amount of iodine. This effect lasts ~ 10 days, after which iodine incorporation into TG and thyroid peroxidase function return to normal. It is widely believed that the resumption of normal functioning is due to downregulation of the iodide pump on the follicular cell membrane. The Wolff–Chaikoff effect is the principle behind the use of iodine for the treatment of hyperthyroidism. Amiodarone may also elicit this side effect, given that it contains iodine.

16.4.1 Parathyroid Hormone

Regulation of Secretion

PTH is released from the parathyroid glands in response to low plasma Ca^{2+} concentrations. High calcium levels suppress PTH secretion.

Effects

See ▶ Table 16.7.

16.4.2 Teriparatide

Mechanism of Action

Teriparatide is a synthetic polypeptide PTH analogue. PTH has both catabolic and anabolic effects on bone, dependent on the duration of exposure. Intermittent administration of teriparatide increases osteoblast activity and bone anabolism.

Pharmacokinetics

Given by daily subcutaneous injection.

Uses

• Osteoporosis in postmenopausal women at high risk of fracture.
• Hypogonadal osteoporosis in men at high risk of fracture.

Table 16.7 Effects of parathyroid hormone (PTH)

Organ/system	Effects
Bone	Mobilization of Ca^{2+} and PO_4^{3-} from bone In the longer term, PTH increases the number of both osteoblasts and osteoclasts and increases the remodeling of bone (▶ Fig. 16.10)[a]
Kidney	↑ Ca^{2+} reabsorption ↑ formation of calcitriol which is the active form of vitamin D
GI tract	↑ absorption of Ca^{2+} (effect mediated via calcitriol)

[a]Daily, intermittent administration of PTH for 1 to 2 hours leads to a net stimulation of bone formation. Continuous exposure to elevated PTH leads to bone resorption.
Abbreviation: GI, gastrointestinal.

16.4.3 Cinacalcet and Etelcalcetide

Mechanism of Action

These agents activate the Ca^{2+}-sensing receptor of the parathyroid gland, which leads to decreased PTH secretion.

Uses

• Hypercalcemia (cinacalcet).
• Primary hyperparathyroidism (cinacalcet).
• Secondary hyperparathyroidism in adults on dialysis with chronic kidney disease.

16.4.4 Vitamin D

The term *vitamin D* refers to cholecalciferol (vitamin D_3) and ergocalciferol (vitamin D_2), which are interchangeable with respect to clinical use. Ergocalciferol is the prescription form of vitamin D and is also used as a food additive. Cholecalciferol is usually used for vitamin D-fortified milk and foods; it is also available in drug combination products. Calcitriol (1α, 25-dihydroxyvitamin D) is the major active metabolite of vitamin D. The metabolism of vitamin D is shown in ▶ Fig. 16.5.

Foundations

Components of Bone

The three major components of bone are osteogenic cells (osteoblasts, osteocytes, and osteoclasts), organic matrix, and mineral. The matrix consists of collagen and proteoglycans and accounts for approximately one-third of bone mass. The mineral component of bone are calcium phosphate crystals deposited as hydroxyapatite (two-thirds of bone mass).

Foundations

Physiological Roles of Calcium

Calcium is vital to normal body functioning, and its levels must be maintained within tight limits. Calcium is the major structural element of bones and teeth, where it is stored in the form of hydroxyapatite crystals $[Ca_{10}(PO_4)_6(OH)_2]$. It is also involved in neural transmission, muscle contraction, vasodilation and vasoconstriction of blood vessels, activation of vitamin K-dependent clotting factors (II, VII, IX, and X), and secretion of hormones (e.g., insulin).

Foundations

Magnesium and Bone Metabolism

Magnesium is the fourth most abundant mineral in the body. About half of the body's magnesium is stored in the hydroxyapatite crystals of bone, and the other half is intracellular. The levels of magnesium in the blood are well regulated and tend to follow those of calcium and phosphate. Like calcium and phosphate, magnesium has a role in bone turnover (but to a much lesser extent). Magnesium deficiency may result from severe

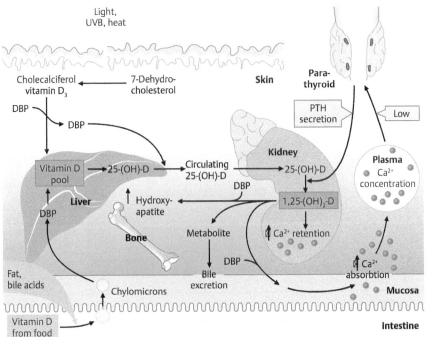

Light, UVB, heat

Cholecalciferol vitamin D₃ ← 7-Dehydro-cholesterol

Skin

Para-thyroid

PTH secretion

Low

DBP

DBP

Vitamin D pool → 25-(OH)-D → Circulating 25-(OH)-D → 25-(OH)-D

Kidney

Plasma Ca²⁺ concentration

Liver

DBP

DBP

↑ Hydroxy-apatite

1,25-(OH)₂-D

Bone

Metabolite

↑ Ca²⁺ retention

DBP

↑ Ca²⁺ absorbtion

Fat, bile acids

Chylomicrons

Bile excretion

Mucosa

Vitamin D from food

Intestine

Fig. 16.5 Vitamin D metabolism.
Ultraviolet light B (UVB) converts 7-dehydrocholesterol to cholecalciferol (vitamin D₃). Ingested vitamin D is fat soluble and is transported to the liver in chylomicrons. All free vitamin D is transported in the blood and liver by a specific vitamin D-binding protein (DBP). The liver converts vitamin D to 25-hydroxycholecalciferol 25-(OH)-D, which is then transported to the kidneys, where it is converted to its active form 1,25-(OH)₂-D, under the influence of parathyroid hormone. The effects of this are increased mineralization of bone, increased calcium and phosphate reabsorption in the kidneys, and increased calcium absorption in the gut. Excess vitamin D is excreted into bile.

IV

diarrhea, alcohol abuse, drugs (e.g., diuretics), and diabetic ketoacidosis. It causes parethesias, seizures, arrhythmias, and tetany (due to accompanying hypocalcemia and hypokalemia). Treatment is by replacement of magnesium.

Clinical Correlation

Chronic Renal Failure and Renal Osteodystrophy

In chronic renal failure, the failing kidneys are unable to perform the necessary 1-α-hydroxylation reactions to produce calcitriol, and they have a reduced capacity to excrete phosphate. This leads to hyperparathyroidism due to hypocalcemia and hyperphosphatemia. Derangement of bone remodeling occurs, which is referred to as renal osteodystrophy. The symptoms of renal osteodystrophy include bone and joint pain, bone deformation, and increased likelihood of bone fractures. Chronic renal failure requires hemodialysis several times per week until renal transplantation can occur. Renal osteodystrophy is treated by calcium and calcitriol, restricting dietary intake of phosphate, and by the administration of medications that bind phosphate, such as calcium carbonate and calcium acetate.

Clinical Correlation

Multiple Endocrine Neoplasia Type I

Multiple endocrine neoplasia type 1 (MEN1) is a rare, inherited disorder that causes multiple tumors (usually benign) in the endocrine glands and duodenum. It affects both genders equally and is usually not detected until adulthood, when tumors start growing. The parathyroid glands are most commonly affected. Tumors in the parathyroid gland cause hyperparathyroidism, which leads to hypercalcemia and its associated symptoms. It also commonly affects the pancreas, causing gastrinomas (from excess gastrin secretion), which, in turn, causes ulcers. These ulcers are more sinister than normal gastric ulcers and are highly prone to perforate. Multiple gastrinomas causing ulcers is referred to as Zollinger–Ellison syndrome. Pancreatic tumors may also cause insulinomas, leading to hypoglycemia; glucagon excess, leading to diabetes; or VIP excess, leading to watery diarrhea. Pituitary tumors may also occur, leading to derangement of its hormones. Patients with MEN1 are more likely to develop cancerous tumors in later life. MEN1 can be detected early by gene testing, and individuals affected have a 50% chance of passing the disease to their children. There is no cure for MEN1, but there are various drugs and surgical options to treat the effects.

Effects

- *Bone:* The effects of vitamin D on bone are a result of its actions that provide the proper balance of Ca²⁺ and PO₄³⁻ to support bone mineralization.
- *Kidney:* Increased reabsorption of Ca²⁺ and PO₄³⁻.
- *GI:* Increased absorption of Ca²⁺.

16.4.5 Cholecalciferol, Ergocalciferol, Calcifediol, and Calcitriol

Uses

- Hypoparathyroidism.
- Hypophosphatemia.
- Prophylaxis of vitamin D deficiency.
- Treatment of rickets.
- Management of hypocalcemia.

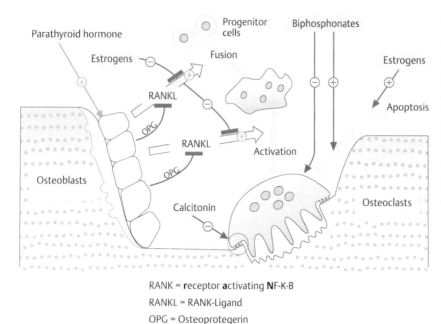

RANK = **r**eceptor **a**ctivating **NF-K-B**

RANKL = RANK-Ligand

OPG = Osteoprotegerin

Bone resorption
Stimulation
Inhibition

Fig. 16.6 Regulation of bone remodeling.
Bone remodeling is complex and is initiated by osteoblasts upon stimulation by parathyroid hormone. Osteoblasts interact directly with osteoclast precursors (that form from progenitor cells) via RANKL (receptor activator of nuclear factor kappa-B ligand). Estrogens (and osteoprotegerin [OPG] secreted by osteoblasts) block RANKL, thus inhibiting the fusion of osteoclast precursors and their activation to osteoclasts. They also promote osteoclast apoptosis. Bisphosphonates inhibit bone resorption by inhibiting osteoclast activity and promoting apoptosis. Calcitonin inhibits bone resorption by transferring active osteoclasts into a resting state.

16.4.6 Calcitonin

Calcitonin is produced by the parafollicular cells (C cells) of the thyroid gland. It is released when there is an elevated level of Ca^{2+} in the blood.

Effects

- *Bone:* Decreases bone resorption by inhibiting osteoclast activity (▶ Fig. 16.6).
- *Kidney:* Decreases reabsorption of Ca^{2+} and PO_4^{3-}, thus increasing their excretion.

16.4.7 Calcitonin (Exogenous)

Pharmacokinetics

Available as a nasal spray or injectable solution.

Uses

- Paget's disease.
- Hypercalcemia.
- Osteoporosis.

16.4.8 Glucocorticoids

Cortisol

Mechanism of Action

Glucocorticoids, such as cortisol, enhance bone loss by decreasing Ca^{2+} absorption, increasing Ca^{2+} excretion, and blocking bone formation.

Uses

- Hypercalcemia of malignancy.
- Vitamin D poisoning.

Side Effects

Prolonged administration leads to osteoporosis.

16.4.9 Estrogens and Selective Estrogen Receptor Modulators (SERMs)

Estrogens: Estradiol, Premarin™, Ethinyl Estradiol, and Mestranol

- Estradiol esters are administered intramuscularly and by a transdermal patch.
- Premarin is a conjugated estrogen that contains estrone and equilin. It is administered orally.
- Ethinyl estradiol and mestranol are synthetic steroid estrogens that are administered orally.

Mechanism of Action

Estrogens decrease osteoclast activity, thus decreasing bone reabsorption. The mechanism by which this occurs is unclear, but it may be that the estrogens cause a decrease in cytokines (small cell-signaling protein molecules) that support osteoclast formation, or they increase the rate of apoptosis of osteoclasts (▶ Fig. 16.6). Estrogens may also decrease other cytokines that decrease osteoblast formation, thus promoting bone formation.

SERM: Raloxifene

See Chapter 17 and ▶ Fig. 17.3 for a further discussion of SERMs.

Uses

Estrogens and SERM agents are used (in the context of bone regulation) to treat postmenopausal osteoporosis. However, estrogens are now only used with caution in patients for whom nonestrogen therapies are not appropriate.

16.5 Bisphosphonates

16.5.1 Alendronate, Etidronate, Ibandronate, Pamidronate, Risedronate, Tiludronate, and Zoledronate

Mechanism of Action

Bisphosphonates are exogenous regulators of bone metabolism. They are analogues of pyrophosphate that accumulate in bone and prevent bone resorption by inhibiting osteoclast activity (▶ Fig. 16.4).

Uses

Prevention and treatment of osteoporosis.

Clinical Correlation

Paget's Disease

Paget's disease is a metabolic bone disease which affects 2 to 3% of the population over the age of 60 years. It consists of increased bone resorption and new bone formation; however, the newly formed bone is disordered, leading to bowing, stress fractures, and arthritis. Additional symptoms may include enlargement of the skull, femur, and clavicle. Nerve compression may occur due to bony overgrowth causing pain, paresthesias, or numbness. Complications include congestive heart failure (due to increased work of the heart) and sarcomas (rarely). Blood biochemistry results show that Ca^{2+} and PO_4^{3-} are usually normal but alkaline phosphatase (ALP) is markedly increased. Because ALP is a by-product of osteoblastic activity, levels of ALP are raised during periods of rapid bone growth (puberty), in bone diseases that cause bone turnover (e.g., Paget's disease and osteomalacia), and during calcium derangement (e.g., hyperparathyroidism). Treatment is with a bisphosphonate and/or calcitonin.

Clinical Correlation

Bisphosphonates and Osteonecrosis of the Jaw

Osteonecrosis is death of bone tissue due to a lack of blood supply. Bisphosphonate usage puts patients at risk of developing osteonecrosis of the jaw that can present following dental extractions. It produces symptoms such as bone pain, swelling, infections, exposed bone, numbness, and loosening of the teeth. This condition usually occurs with IV bisphosphonates, but it can also occur when they are taken orally. Patients who are at risk of developing osteonecrosis should have any sources of infection treated before bisphosphonate therapy is initiated to prevent the condition from developing. However, if osteonecrosis does occur, surgical debridement of necrotic bone and areas of infection is necessary.

16.5.2 Fluoride

Mechanism of Action

Fluoride accumulates in bone and teeth where it slows resorption and promotes calcification.

Uses

- It is added to drinking water to prevent dental caries.
- May have a positive effect in osteoporosis.

16.6 Adrenocortical Hormones

The adrenocortical steroids, or corticosteroids, are steroid hormones produced by the adrenal cortex (▶ Fig. 16.7). They include glucocorticoids, mineralocorticoids, and androgens. The glucocorticoids regulate metabolism and stress responses, and the mineralocorticoids regulate sodium reabsorption. Androgens will be covered in Chapter 17.

16.6.1 Glucocorticoids

Regulation of Secretion

The natural glucocorticoids, cortisol and corticosterone, are synthesized and released in response to ACTH from the anterior pituitary, which is released in response to CRH from the hypothalamus.

Mechanism of Action

Glucocorticoids bind to receptors in the cytosol. These receptors then dissociate from heat shock protein complexes, translocate to the nucleus, and bind to specific sites on DNA within the nucleus, altering gene transcription.

Foundations

The Effect of Corticosteroids on the Respiratory Burst

The respiratory burst is the rapid release of reactive oxygen species (superoxide radical and hydrogen peroxide) from phagocytes (neutrophils and monocytes) when a microbe is encountered and phagocytosed. It is one of the mechanisms by which phagocytes exert their microbicidal effects and is an important immune defense. The reactive oxygen species are generated by the partial reduction of oxygen in the respiratory chain (electron transport chain). They combine with Cl^- to form hypochlorous acid, which dissociates to form hypochlorite ions that kill the microbes. Cortisol (and exogenous corticosteroids) inhibits the respiratory burst and may predispose an individual to infection.

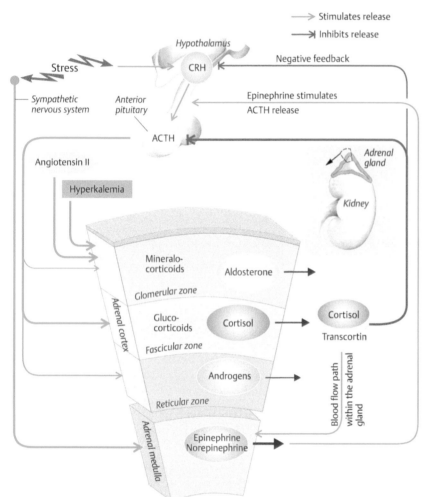

Stimulates release
Inhibits release

Fig. 16.7 Hormonal secretions of the adrenal gland.
Stress causes the release of corticotropin-releasing hormone (CRH) from the hypothalamus, which then stimulates adrenocorticotropic hormone (ACTH) release from the anterior pituitary. ACTH acts on all zones of the adrenal cortex, but it predominantly causes the release of cortisol from the fascicular zone. One of the local actions of cortisol is to stimulate the release of norepinephrine and epinephrine from the adrenal medulla, although the main stimulus for this is sympathetic system activation. Cortisol causes negative feedback inhibition of ACTH (predominantly) and CRH.

At higher concentrations, glucocorticoids are thought to be integrated into the cell membrane, thus altering the physiochemical properties of the cell. The ultimate effect of these changes is that the activation capacity of the cell is reduced (▶ Fig. 16.8).

Effects

▶ Table 16.8 lists the effects of glucocorticoids. These are further illustrated in ▶ Fig. 16.9 and ▶ Fig. 16.10.

16.6.2 Hydrocortisone (Cortisol), Prednisone, Methylprednisolone, Triamcinolone, Dexamethasone, Betamethasone, Beclomethasone, and Fluocinonide

Mechanism of Action

These agents are synthetic glucocorticoids that act like the endogenous hormones.

Pharmacokinetics

These agents are effective orally, parenterally, and topically.
   Note: Beclomethasone and fluocinonide are for local use only.
   ▶ Table 16.9 lists the duration of action of these agents.

Uses

- Endocrine:
  - Adrenocortical insufficiency (Addison's disease).
  - Congenital adrenal hyperplasia (to suppress ACTH release).
- Nonendocrine:
  - Rheumatoid arthritis.
  - Leukemia.
  - Lymphoma.
  - Allergic reactions.
  - Asthma.
  - Inflammatory and autoimmune disorders.
  - Immunosuppression for transplantation.
  - Collagen disorders.
  - Cerebral edema.
  - Bacterial meningitis.

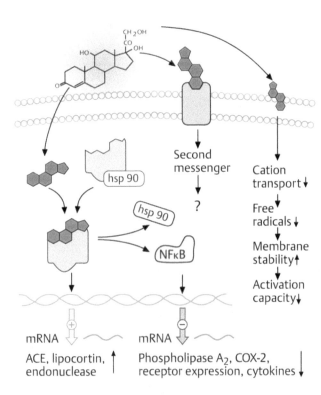

Fig. 16.8 Glucocorticoids: receptors and second messengers.
Glucocorticoids act to alter gene transcription, the effects of which include reduced inflammation. At higher concentrations, they may also act on the cell membrane to reduce the activation capacity of the cell. ACE, angiotensin-converting enzyme; COX-2, cyclooxygenase-2; hsp, heat shock protein; mRNA, messenger RNA.

Table 16.8 Effects of glucocorticoids

Category	Effects
Metabolic	↑ hepatic gluconeogenesis ↑ glycogen synthesis ↑ proteolysis ↑ release of amino acids (key enzymes) for gluconeogenesis ↑ lipolysis, which increases fatty acid and ketone body formation ↓ peripheral glucose utilization
Anti-inflammatory (see also ▶ Fig. 16.10)	↓ transcription of most cytokines and chemokines leads to reduced synthesis of these mediators and decreased activation of leukocytes. ↓ transcription of phospholipase A_2 and cyclooxygenase-2 (COX-2) results in decreased formation of prostaglandins and thromboxanes (see Chapter 32). ↓ expression of adhesion molecules necessary for leukocyte chemotaxis ↑ expression of anti-inflammatory molecules, such as neutral endopeptidase and lipocortins

Side Effects

Large doses of glucocorticoids for 1 week or less do not pose problems, but patients with nonendocrine disorders who receive systemic corticosteroids for longer times develop adverse effects, including inhibition of CRH release from the hypothalamus and ACTH release from the anterior pituitary (▶ Fig. 16.11). Some of the side effects experienced include

- Hyperglycemia.
- Increased susceptibility to infection.
- Weight gain (Cushingoid features).
- Osteoporosis.
- Behavioral and personality changes.
- Myopathy.
- Ocular effects.
- Growth retardation in children.

When possible, glucocorticoids should be administered locally, for example, as an aerosol spray in asthma, to minimize adverse effects, or alternate-day therapy should be used.

Clinical Correlation

Acute Adrenal Crisis (Addisonian Crisis)

Acute adrenal crisis (Addisonian crisis) is due to acute insufficiency of adrenal corticosteroids, mainly cortisol. It usually occurs in people with known Addison's disease who undergo some form of stress, such as surgery, trauma, or infection, but it may also occur on abrupt cessation of long-term steroids. The main sign of acute adrenal crisis is shock (hypotension, tachycardia, or oliguria), but there may also be acute abdominal pain, diarrhea, vomiting, hypoglycemia, fever, weakness, and confusion. It may progress to seizures, coma, and death, if untreated. If there is a high index of suspicion for acute adrenal crisis, treatment should begin before the results of any laboratory tests are known. Treatment involves giving IV fluids, hydrocortisone, antibiotics, and glucose, if necessary. In the longer term, the patient can be switched to oral steroids and the precipitating factor should be treated.

Clinical Correlation

Perioperative Steroid Coverage

Patients who have been on long-term steroids or have stopped steroids recently will have some adrenal suppression. Consequently, the perioperative administration of steroids prior to undergoing the stress of surgery is necessary to prevent adrenal crisis, the major effect of which is shock.

16.6.3 Mineralocorticoids

The major mineralocorticoid produced by the adrenal gland is aldosterone. Aldosterone has a very short half-life and is not used therapeutically.

Regulation of Secretion

Aldosterone secretion is regulated by the renin–angiotensin–aldosterone system (see Chapter 19).

IV

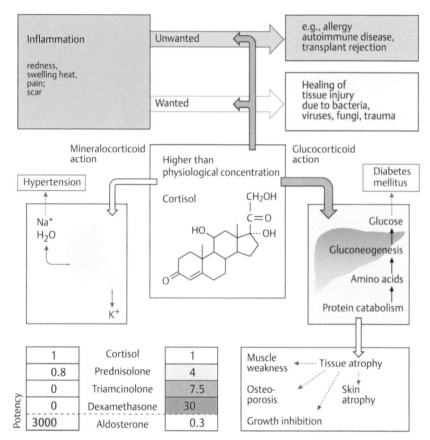

Fig. 16.9 Glucocorticoids: principal and adverse effects.
Therapeutic levels of cortisol suppress the inflammatory response. This is useful in treating conditions such as allergy and autoimmune disease and to prevent transplant rejection, where the inflammatory response is unwanted. However, cortisol also produces a number of adverse effects related to its anti-inflammatory, mineralocorticoid, and glucocorticoid actions. The relative mineralocorticoid potencies (*blue*) and glucocorticoid potencies (*brown*) of some corticosteroids are included.

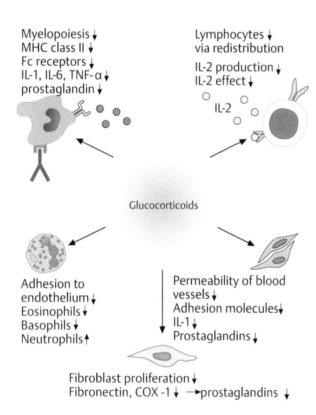

Fig. 16.10 Effects of glucocorticoids on the immune system.
Glucocorticoids act on a wide range of cells, including blood cells, endothelial cells, and fibroblasts, as well as receptor proteins and proinflammatory mediators, to reduce inflammation and its spread. Fc, fragment, crystallizable; IL, interleukin; MHC, major histocompatibility complex; TNF, tumor necrosis factor.

Table 16.9 Duration of action of glucocorticoids

Duration of action	Agent(s)
Short	Hydrocortisone (cortisol)
Intermediate	Prednisone, methylprednisolone, triamcinolone
Long	Dexamethasone, betamethasone

Effects

Mineralocorticoids help maintain normal blood volume by promoting Na^+ reabsorption by the distal tubules. K^+ and H^+ ions are excreted in exchange.

16.6.4 Fludrocortisone

Mechanism of Action

Fludrocortisone is a synthetic corticosteroid that has much greater mineralocorticoid activity than glucocorticoid activity.

Pharmacokinetics

Orally effective.

Uses

Used in salt-losing forms of adrenal insufficiency.

16.6.5 Spironolactone

See Chapter 19 for further discussion of this agent.

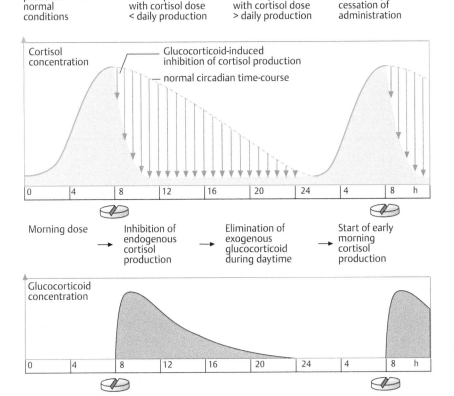

Fig. 16.11 Cortisol release and its modification by glucocorticoids.
Exogenous glucocorticoids cause feedback inhibition of endogenous cortisol production. Depending on the dose, this can cause endogenous cortisol production to decrease or cease completely. If cortisol production is not required by the adrenal cortex, it undergoes atrophy and cannot resume normal cortisol output if exogenous glucocorticoids are abruptly stopped. The dosing regimen of glucocorticoids can minimize adrenocortical atrophy. If they are given when normal cortical secretion is high and feedback inhibition is low (late morning), then the glucocorticoid is eliminated during daytime, and normal cortisol production starts early the following morning.

IV

Mechanism of Action

Spironolactone is an aldosterone receptor antagonist.

Uses

- Primary hyperaldosteronism.
- Cushing syndrome.
- Adrenal adenoma or carcinoma.
- Ectopic ACTH-producing tumors.

16.6.6 Aminoglutethimide

Mechanism of Action

Aminoglutethimide blocks the conversion of cholesterol to pregnenolone, thereby decreasing secretion of all adrenal cortical steroids.

Uses

- Cushing syndrome.
- Adrenal adenoma or carcinoma.
- Ectopic ACTH-producing tumors.

Foundations

Renin–Angiotensin–Aldosterone System

The renin–angiotensin–aldosterone system regulates Na^+ balance, fluid volume, and blood pressure. Renin is released by the kidneys in response to reduced perfusion. Renin then stimulates the production of angiotensin II from angiotensin I in the lungs. Angiotensin II causes vasoconstriction and aldosterone secretion from the adrenal glands. Aldosterone causes Na^+ (and water) reabsorption, thus increasing fluid volume, blood pressure, and renal perfusion.

Foundations

Cholesterol and Steroid Synthesis

Steroid hormones are produced from cholesterol ($C_{27}H_{46}O$). All steroid-producing tissues cleave the side chain of cholesterol between carbons 20 and 22 to form pregnenolone (via cholesterol desmolase). This is the rate-limiting step. In most cases, pregnenolone is then converted to progesterone. In the gonads, progesterone is converted to testosterone via cleavage of the remaining side chain. In many tissues, a 5α-reductase converts testosterone to 5α-dihydrotestosterone (DHT), which is the more active form of the hormone. The ovary also makes testosterone but does not release large quantities of it. Instead, it aromatizes ring A (resulting in the loss of carbon 19) to form 18 carbon steroids (estradiol, estrone). In the adrenal cortex, hydroxylations produce cortisol and aldosterone. Some conversion of pregnenolone to androgens (especially dehydroepiandrosterone [DHEA]) and estrogens may occur.

17 Drugs Used in Reproductive Endocrinology

Summary

The estrogens (estradiol, Premarin, ethinyl estradiol, mestranol, diethylstilbestrol) are used in contraception, in hormone replacement therapy, to correct hormonal imbalances and to treat some cancers. The progestins (progesterone, norethindrone, ethynodiol, norgestrel, medroxyprogesterone) are used in contraception, dysfunctional uterine bleeding, dysmenorrhea, and endometriosis. Estrogen modulators and antagonists include the selective estrogen receptor modulators (tamoxifen, toremifene, ospemifene, raloxifene). Tamoxifen, toremifene, and raloxifene are used to treat breast cancer. Ospemifene is indicated for the treatment of dyspareunia. Clomiphene is used to treat ovulatory dysfunction in women seeking to become pregnant. Fulvestrant is an estrogen receptor antagonist indicated as monotherapy for the treatment of hormone receptor positive metastatic breast cancer. Anastrozole, letrozole, and exemestane block the production of estrogens. Mifepristone is a potent competitive antagonist of progesterone and glucocorticoids that prevents ovulation. The drug terminates pregnancy by blocking the actions of progesterone on the uterus. Misoprostol is administered in combination with mifepristone as an abortifacient. Human chorionic gonadotropin, human menopausal gonadotropin, urofollitropin, and follitropin are used to induce ovulation. Testosterone is used as replacement therapy in hypogonadism. Fluoxymesterone, methyltestosterone, and danazol are used in hypogonadism and endometriosis. Oxymetholone and oxandrolone are anabolic steroids used in the treatment of delayed growth. Antiandrogens (including bicalutamide, enzalutamide, flutamide, nilutamide) are used for treatment of metastatic prostate cancer. The androgen synthesis inhibitor finasteride is used in benign prostatic hyperplasia and male pattern baldness. Abiraterone acetate is used in combination with prednisone to treat prostate cancer. Oxytocin is used to stimulate uterine smooth muscle contraction.

Keywords: estrogen, androgen, progesterone, contraceptives, ovulatory agents

17.1 Introduction to Drugs Used in Reproductive Endocrinology

The estrogens, androgens, and progestins are classes of steroid hormones that play significant roles in male and female reproduction and development. The most well-elucidated activities of all three classes occur by binding of the hormone to nuclear receptors. Ovarian and testicular production of estrogens and androgens are regulated by the anterior pituitary gonadotropins (i.e., luteinizing hormone [LH] and follicle-stimulating hormone [FSH]). LH and FSH are regulated by hypothalamic gonadotropin-releasing hormone (GnRH). Pharmacological therapies that target steroid hormone activity generally act by inhibiting critical enzymes involved in hormone synthesis, exploiting feedback pathways, and functioning as receptor agonists or antagonists. These drugs are used for a variety of conditions ranging from contraception and infertility to breast and prostate cancers.

17.2 Estrogens

The naturally occurring estrogens are the C18 steroids: 17 estradiol, estrone, and estriol, which are secreted by granulosa (follicular) cells within the ovary. 17 estradiol is the major estrogen in premenopausal women, and it maintains reproductive tissues and processes along with progesterone. Estrogens also have important effects on metabolism, for example, on transport proteins, clotting factors, electrolyte balance, and serum lipids. Estrogens are primarily produced by the ovary, placenta, and adipose tissue; however, other tissues synthesize estrogens from androgens for intracrine and paracrine use.

Like other steroids, estrogen binds to receptors in the cytosol and alters DNA transcription. Although the most well-studied effects of estrogens occur through nuclear estrogen receptors (ER), estrogens may also bind with membrane-localized ER, leading to effects on the heart, vasculature, and other systems. These include the classic ERα, ERβ, and the more recently recognized GPR30/G protein-coupled estrogen receptor.

17.2.1 Effects

See ▶ Table 17.1.

Table 17.1 Effects of estrogen

Category	Effects
Ovulation and reproduction	Supports the growth and maturation of ovarian follicles and endometrium (along with progesterone) and stimulates ovulation ↑ the growth and the motility of the smooth muscle of the uterus and increases uterine blood flow ↓ the viscosity of cervical mucus and makes it more alkaline to support the survival of sperm
Puberty	Initiates ductal development in the breasts Controls the female body configuration (e.g., narrow shoulders and broad hips) and the distribution of fat in the breasts and buttocks
Bone	↑ osteoblast activity ↓ apoptosis of osteoblasts ↓ the number and activity of osteoclasts The net result is an increased formation of bone in the presence of estrogen
Brain	Estrogen may have a neuroprotective effect to increase neuronal survival and levels of neuronal growth factors and improve cognition
Cholesterol levels	↓ LDL levels ↑ HDL levels

Abbreviations: HDL, high-density lipoprotein; LDL, low-density lipoprotein.

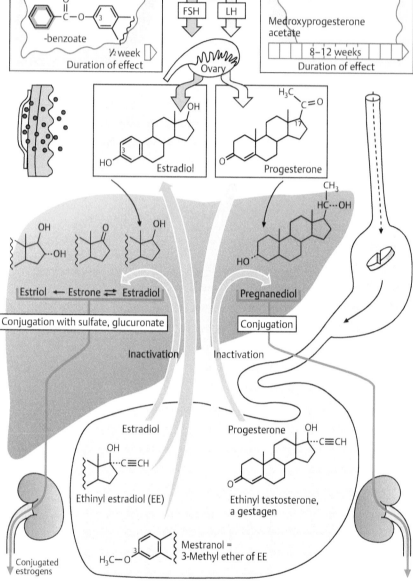

Fig. 17.1 Estradiol, progesterone, and derivatives.
Exogenous estrogen and progesterone mimic the natural hormones at their receptors. Depot preparations are absorbed slowly and thus have a longer duration of action than the natural hormones. Oral preparations undergo a higher degree of first-pass metabolism in the liver. All three estrogen metabolites are water soluble and are excreted by the kidneys. The main metabolite of progesterone is pregnanediol, which is also excreted by the kidneys. FSH, follicle-stimulating hormone; GnRH, gonadotropin-releasing hormone; LH, luteinizing hormone.

17.2.2 Estrogens: Estradiol, Premarin, Ethinyl Estradiol, Mestranol, and Diethylstilbestrol

Several types of estrogen preparations are available with oral, transdermal, topical, or parenteral routes of administration. Oral effectiveness depends on the extent of metabolism in the intestines and the liver.

- Estradiol esters are administered intramuscularly and by a transdermal patch (▶ Fig. 17.1).

- Premarin is a conjugated estrogen that contains estrone and equilin. It is administered orally.
- Ethinyl estradiol and mestranol are synthetic steroid estrogens that are administered orally.

Note: Estrogens are usually administered in cyclic fashion with a progestin (a natural or synthetic steroid hormone that has progesterone-like activity unless the uterus has been removed). The combined use of progestins with estrogen may reduce the risk of endometrial hyperplasia.

Uses

- Contraception.
- To supplement inadequate production in conditions such as constitutional delay of puberty, ovariectomy, menopause, and osteoporosis.
- To correct hormonal imbalance (e.g., dysfunctional uterine bleeding).
- To reverse an abnormal process (e.g., hirsutism or endometriosis; see Chapter 16).
- To treat metastatic breast cancer in select men and postmenopausal women.
- To treat advanced prostate cancer.
- Cross-sex hormone therapy (e.g., transgender feminization).

Note: Estrogens are not indicated for treatment or prevention of cardiovascular or neurodegenerative diseases because of possible untoward side effects including breast cancer, stroke, and adverse coronary events.

Side Effects

- Headache, nausea, and vomiting, breast tenderness, and weight gain due to Na^+ and water retention (usually disappear with continued administration).
- Increased risk of endometrial cancer. This is prevented by the addition of a progestin.
- Reproductive tissue abnormalities and cancers are seen in daughters and sons of women who were prescribed diethylstilbesterol.
- Gallstones (due to increased cholesterol caused by estrogen).

17.3 Progestins

Progesterone is a C21 steroid secreted by the corpus luteum, placenta, and ovarian follicle that supports female reproductive tissues and processes (in conjunction with estrogen). It is also an important intermediate in steroid biosynthesis in tissues that secrete steroid hormones. Like other steroids, progesterone binds to both intracellular receptors that act in the nucleus to regulate gene transcription and less-studied membrane localized progesterone receptors.

17.3.1 Effects

See ▶ Table 17.2.

17.3.2 Progestins: Progesterone, Norethindrone, Ethynodiol, Norgestrel, and Medroxyprogesterone

- Progesterone, the natural hormone, is available in an oily solution for injection (▶ Fig. 17.1).
- Norethindrone, ethynodiol, norgestrel (oral), and medroxyprogesterone (oral, parenteral) are synthetic steroids. Some have slight androgenic activity. Synthetic steroids are the most common progesterone preparations.

Table 17.2 Effects of progesterone

Tissue	Effects
Uterus	During the menstrual cycle, progesterone decreases endometrial proliferation and leads to changes that promote implantation of a fertilized ovum. If implantation does not occur, the decline in progesterone at the end of the cycle is the main signal for the onset of menstruation. Progesterone is essential for the maintenance of pregnancy
Breasts	Stimulates lobular-alveolar development Induces differentiation of ductal tissue that has been stimulated by estrogen
Brain	↑ body temperature and is probably responsible for the rise in basal body temperature at the time of ovulation

Uses

- Contraception.
- Dysfunctional uterine bleeding.
- Dysmenorrhea.
- Endometriosis (see Chapter 16).

Side Effects

- Decreased high-density lipoprotein (androgenic preparations).
- Amenorrhea.
- Weight gain.
- Headache and gastrointestinal (GI) disturbances.

Clinical Correlation

Gallstones

The majority of gallstones (75%) are formed when the amount of cholesterol in bile exceeds the ability of bile salts and phospholipids to emulsify it, causing cholesterol to precipitate out of solution. Gallstones may also be caused by an increased amount of unconjugated bilirubin (often in the form of calcium bilirubinate) in the bile ("pigment stones"). Gallstones may be asymptomatic or they can cause obstruction of a duct causing severe pain, vomiting, and fever. Drugs, such as ursodiol, may be used to dissolve small cholesterol gallstones. Ursodiol decreases secretion of cholesterol into bile by reducing cholesterol absorption and suppressing liver cholesterol synthesis. This alters bile composition and allows reabsorption of cholesterol-containing gallstones. As reabsorption is slow, therapy must continue for at least 9 months. Other treatment includes lithotripsy (shock wave obliteration of gallstones that allow the stone fragments to be excreted) or surgical removal of the gallbladder (cholecystectomy).

Clinical Correlation

Hormone Replacement Therapy

The Women's Health Initiative (WHI) is a long-term study by the National Heart, Lung, and Blood Institute that has focused on the health of postmenopausal women. Prior to this study,

IV

perimenopausal women were routinely prescribed hormone replacement therapy to alleviate the symptoms of menopause. The WHI found that, compared with the placebo group, women taking estrogen plus progestin had slight increases in breast cancer, heart attack, stroke, and thromboembolism in the lungs and legs. The benefits were fewer hip fractures and lower occurrences of colon cancer. Women taking estrogen alone had more strokes, more blood clots in the legs, and fewer hip fractures. Estrogen alone had no effect on breast cancer, heart attacks, or colorectal cancer. The WHI also led to boxed warnings against combined estrogen plus progesterone use for the prevention of both dementia and cardiovascular disease.

17.4 Hormonal Contraception

Estrogen and progesterone are primarily used for hormonal contraception. There are several preparations and modes of administration, which vary in effectiveness. Contraceptive choice largely depends on medical and lifestyle factors.

17.4.1 Combination Oral Contraceptives

A combination of a synthetic estrogen and a progestin is used (e.g., ethinyl estradiol or mestranol combined with norethindrone, ethynodiol, or norgestrel). Monophasic, biphasic, and triphasic preparations are available. In monophasic preparations, each active pill contains the same amount of estrogen and progestin. In biphasic preparations, the estrogen content is the same in each active pill but the level of progestin is increased about halfway through the cycle. In triphasic preparations, the hormone combination changes three times throughout the cycle (approximately every 7 days) (▶ Fig. 17.2).

Mechanism of Action

Combined oral contraceptive agents act by inhibiting ovulation through feedback inhibition of FSH and LH from the anterior pituitary, by thickening cervical mucus, and by inhibition of endometrial proliferation necessary for implantation (▶ Fig. 17.2).

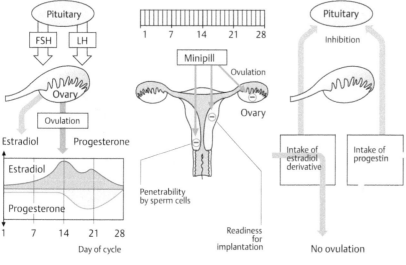

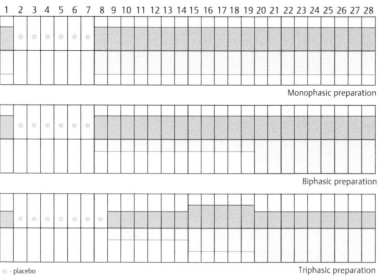

Fig. 17.2 Oral contraceptives.
Oral contraceptives prevent ovulation by feedback inhibition of FSH and LH. The progestin-only minipill primarily acts to increase thick cervical mucus, which is impenetrable to sperm cells. It also inhibits the formation of the endometrial lining, and inconsistently prevents ovulation. Monophasic preparations contain equal amounts of estrogen and progestin. Biphasic preparations have the same estrogen content in each active pill but the level of progestin is increased about halfway through the cycle. Triphasic preparations have three changes to the estrogen and progestin combination throughout the cycle.

Side Effects

Most side effects are related to the estrogen component, but cardiovascular changes may be caused by either component. Adverse reactions other than those associated with estrogen therapy include the following:
- Breakthrough bleeding with low-estrogen preparations.
- Abnormal glucose tolerance.
- Alterations in serum lipids.
- Thromboembolic disease (minimal in low-estrogen preparations).
- Increased risk of myocardial infarction (MI) or stroke, particularly in women 35 years of age or older who smoke.

17.4.2 Progestin-only Oral Contraceptives

Progestin-only "minipills" contain lower doses of progestin than combination oral contraceptives and are taken daily on a continuous regimen.

Mechanism of Action

The contraceptive actions of these agents are due to the formation of impenetrable cervical mucus and prevention of endometrial implantation. Because these preparations do not inhibit ovulation consistently (▶ Fig. 17.2), they are not as effective as combination contraceptives.

Side Effects

Unpredictable bleeding is common.

Note: Oral contraception has a 0.3% failure rate with perfect use and 8% with typical use during the first year.

17.4.3 Emergency Contraception

Hormonal methods of emergency contraception include progestin-only pills, high doses of combined oral contraceptives, and the ovulation-inhibiting selective progesterone receptor modulator ulipristal. A copper bearing intrauterine device (IUD) is also highly effective. The abortifacient drug mifepristone, at lower dosage than used for the termination of pregnancy, is also effective as emergency contraception, but it is not approved for this use in the United States.

Regimen for Emergency Contraception

- The progestin-only pill (i.e., levonorgestrel) should ideally be taken as soon as possible within 72 hours of unprotected intercourse. In a two dose regimen, another pill will be taken 12 hours after the first dose. Treatment is still moderately effective when taken up to 5 days after intercourse. Ulipristal should be taken as soon as possible within 5 days of unprotected intercourse.
- Two combination oral contraceptives immediately plus two more after 12 hours is also effective.

Effectiveness

Emergency contraceptive pills reduce the risk of pregnancy by 88% or more, depending on how soon after intercourse the pills are taken. For instance, progestin-only pills reduce the risk of pregnancy by up to 95% if taken within the first 24 hours after intercourse. Combination pill regimens provide approximately 75% reduction in the risk of pregnancy. The IUD is the most effective form of emergency contraception, with a pregnancy rate of only 0.1%.

Side Effects

Nausea, vomiting, and irregular bleeding are common; however, there is less nausea than seen with a progestin-only regimen.

17.4.4 Transdermal Patch Contraceptives

Progestin, Norelgestromin, and Ethinyl Estradiol

Transdermal patches deliver the progestin, norelgestromin, and ethinyl estradiol daily. The patch is applied to the buttocks, upper outer arm, lower abdomen, or upper torso and left on for 3 weeks, followed by a patch-free week to allow for withdrawal bleeding.

Mechanism of Action

The mechanism of action is the same as that for combination oral contraceptives.

Effectiveness

Generally, transdermal patches are comparable in effectiveness to oral contraceptives; however, women weighing > 90 kg (~ 198 lb) may experience increased contraceptive failure.

Side Effects

Dysmenorrhea and breast tenderness were more frequent with the patch. Otherwise, the side effects are the same as low-dose oral contraceptives.

17.4.5 Subdermal Implant Contraceptives

Etonogestrel

Etonogestrel (a progestin) is available in a 4-cm-long rod for implantation under the skin of the upper arm. This time-release rod is effective for up to 3 years.

Mechanism of Action

As a progestin, this agent thickens the cervical mucus and produces an atrophic endometrium. Ovulation is suppressed in 97% of cycles.

IV

Effectiveness

Effectiveness approaches 100%, but it has not been studied in women weighing more than 130% of their ideal body weight.

Side Effects

The major side effect is irregular menstrual bleeding. Others include headache, vaginitis, weight gain, acne, and breast and abdominal pain.

17.4.6 Intravaginal Ring Contraceptives

Etonogestrel and Ethinyl Estradiol

These agents are contained within a flexible polymer ring with an outer diameter of 54 mm and an inner diameter of 50 mm. It is inserted into the vagina for 3 weeks and then removed to allow bleeding.

Mechanism of Action

The mechanism of action is the same as that for combination oral contraceptives.

Effectiveness

Effectiveness approaches 100%.

Side Effects

Serum levels of hormones are lower, which minimizes side effects. Both women and men have reported feeling the ring during intercourse.

17.4.7 Intrauterine Contraceptive Devices

Levonorgestrel

Levonorgestrel is a progestin.

Mechanism of Action

The mechanism of action is the same as that for progestin-only contraceptives.

Effectiveness

IUDs are very efficacious and provide 5 to 10 years of continuous contraception.

Side Effects

Fewer systemic effects are seen because serum concentrations of hormone are low, but there may still be the following side effects:
- Increased risk of pelvic inflammatory disease related to introduction of bacteria into the genital tract during insertion.
- Increased menstrual blood flow and dysmenorrhea.

17.4.8 Depot Contraceptive Injections

Medroxyprogesterone Acetate

Medroxyprogesterone acetate is a progestin administered by deep intramuscular injection in the gluteal or deltoid muscle or subcutaneously into the abdomen or thigh. It inhibits ovulation for > 3 months.

Mechanism of Action

The mechanism of action is the same as that for progestin-only contraceptives.

Effectiveness

With typical use, 3% of women experience unintended pregnancy.

Side Effects

The side effects are the same as those for oral progestin-only contraceptives.

17.5 Estrogen Modulators and Antagonists

17.5.1 Selective Estrogen Receptor Modulators

Tamoxifen, Toremifene, Ospemifene, and Raloxifene

Mechanism of Action

Tamoxifen and the related compounds toremifene and raloxifene are partial agonists that inhibit the actions of full agonists, such as estradiol, at the estrogen receptor (▶ Fig. 17.3). Tamoxifen is a partial estrogen receptor agonist in endometrial tissue and bone, but an antagonist in breast tissue. Raloxifene is an agonist in bone, but an antagonist in breast and endometrial tissue. Toremifene is an antagonist in breast tissue.

Uses

Tamoxifen, toremifene, and raloxifene are used to treat all stages of breast cancer in both pre- and postmenopausal women, as a palliative treatment for those with advanced disease, and as adjuvant treatment following surgery. Tamoxifen is also approved for the prevention of breast cancer. Ospemifene is indicated for the treatment of painful sexual intercourse (dyspareunia) due to vulvar and vaginal atrophy in menopausal women. Raloxifene may also be used for osteoporosis prevention and treatment.

Side Effects

Hot flashes, nausea, and vomiting are common.

Clinical Correlation

Pelvic Inflammatory Disease

Pelvic inflammatory disease (PID) is an infection of the fallopian tubes (salpingitis) or ovaries, usually due to sexually transmitted bacteria such as chlamydia. Symptoms include pelvic pain, pain during intercourse or urination, irregular menstrual bleeding, heavy vaginal discharge with an unpleasant odor, fever, fatigue, diarrhea, and vomiting. Untreated PID may cause fibrosis and abscesses in the fallopian tubes. This may lead to ectopic pregnancy, infertility, and chronic pelvic pain. Treatment involves the administration of antibiotics and the avoidance of intercourse until both partners are infection free.

Clomiphene

Mechanism of Action

Clomiphene acts by binding estrogen receptors in the hypothalamus and anterior pituitary, thereby preventing the normal feedback inhibition of GnRH and gonadotropin secretion by estrogen (▶ Fig. 17.3). Ovarian stimulation and ovulation result.

Uses

Clomiphene is used to treat ovulatory dysfunction in women seeking to become pregnant.

Side Effects

They include mild menopausal symptoms, ovarian cyst formation, and multiple births.

17.5.2 Antiestrogen

Fulvestrant

Mechanism of Action

Fulvestrant is a competitive estrogen receptor antagonist. It acts by preventing estrogen receptor dimerization, thereby reducing translocation to the nucleus and accelerating estrogen receptor degradation.

Uses

Fulvestrant is indicated as monotherapy for the treatment of hormone receptor positive metastatic breast cancer in post-

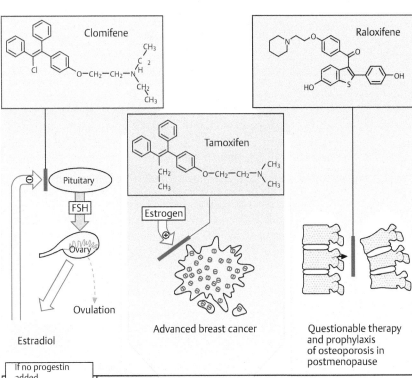

Fig. 17.3 Selective estrogen receptor modulators. Clomiphene is an antagonist at estrogen receptors in the anterior pituitary; because of this, feedback inhibition of gonadotropins by estradiol is suppressed. Raloxifene uses the bone protective effects of estrogen in the prophylaxis and treatment of osteoporosis. Tamoxifen blocks the estrogen stimulus for tumor growth in breast cancer. The relative effects of these agents on cancer and thromboembolism risk, as well as climacteric symptoms (e.g., hot flashes and sweating) and bone mass, are shown.

If no progestin added	Estradiol	Tamoxifen	Raloxifene
Endometrial cancer risk	↑	↑	↓
Breast cancer risk	↑	↓	↓
Thromboembolism	↑	↑	↑
Relief of climacteric complaints	↑	↓	↓
Bone mass	↑	↑	↑

menopausal women following antiestrogen therapy. It is used in combination with palbociclib in women with disease progression following endocrine therapy for human epidermal growth factor receptor 2 (HER2)-negative advanced or metastatic breast cancer.

Side Effects

- Injection-site-related nerve damage and pain.
- GI disturbances such as nausea and vomiting.
- Muscle, bone, and joint pain.
- Headache, fatigue, and anemia.

17.5.3 Estrogen Synthesis Inhibitors

Anastrozole, Letrozole, Exemestane

Mechanism of Action

Aromatase is a key enzyme in the synthesis of estrogens from androgens. In addition to expression in the ovaries and testis, aromatase is expressed in extraglandular sites such as the brain, bone, and breast adipose tissue. Aromatase inhibitors bind to and inhibit the aromatase enzyme, thereby blocking the production of estrogens and reducing estrogen-dependent tumor growth.

Uses

- First-line therapy for hormone-receptor-positive or unknown hormone receptor status locally advanced or metastatic breast cancer.
- Adjuvant treatment of early stage hormone-receptor-positive cancer in postmenopausal women.
- Breast cancer prevention in high-risk postmenopausal women.
- Off-label uses include infertility treatment in anovulatory women with polycystic ovary syndrome, recurrent ovarian cancer, and treatment for endometrial or uterine cancers.

Side Effects

- Loss of bone density and increased risk of osteoporosis and osteonecrosis.
- Arthralgia and myalgia.
- Hot flashes, vaginal dryness, nightsweats, and other menopausal symptoms.

17.6 Progesterone Antagonists

17.6.1 Mifepristone

Mechanism of Action

Mifepristone (RU-486) is a potent competitive antagonist of progesterone and glucocorticoids. When administered in the follicular phase of the menstrual cycle, the drug prevents ovulation by inhibiting the effects of progesterone on the pituitary or hypothalamus. When given later, the drug terminates pregnancy by blocking the actions of progesterone on the uterus (▶ Fig. 17.4).

Uses

RU-486 is used for the medical termination of pregnancy. However, some countries use RU-486 as an emergency contraceptive. It is also used to control hyperglycemia secondary to hypercortisolism in certain patients with Cushing syndrome. Misoprostol is administered in combination with RU-486 as abortifacient.

Side Effects

GI disturbances and pelvic or abdominal pain may occur. Vaginal bleeding requiring medical intervention occurs in up to 5% of patients.

17.7 Ovulatory Agents

17.7.1 Selective Estrogen Receptor Modulator

Clomiphene

See section 17.5.1 above for a discussion of this agent.

17.7.2 Gonadotropins

Human Chorionic Gonadotropin, Human Menopausal Gonadotropin, Urofollitropin, and Follitropin

Mechanisms of Action

- Human chorionic gonadotropin (hCG), which is isolated from the urine of pregnant women, mimics the actions of LH.

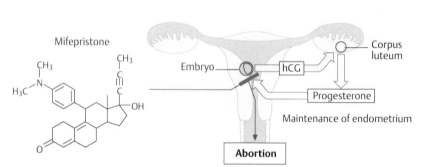

Fig. 17.4 Progesterone receptor antagonist. Implantation of the embryo causes the secretion of human chorionic gonadotropin (hCG) which acts on the corpus luteum to secrete progesterone. Progesterone is responsible for maintaining the endometrial lining. Mifepristone is an antagonist of progesterone at its receptors. This agent causes abortion of the embryo due to shedding of the endometrial lining.

- Human menopausal gonadotropin (hMG), or menotropin, which is isolated from the urine of postmenopausal women, contains equal amounts of FSH and LH, as well as other urinary proteins.
- Urofollitropin is highly purified FSH.
- Follitropin is recombinant FSH (rFSH).

Uses

- To induce ovulation.
- To cause the testicle to move to the scrotum in cases of cryptorchidism (undescended testicle), and hypogonadotropic hypogonadism in men (absent or decreased function of the testes) to encourage maturation of Leydig cells.

Side effects

- Multiple births.
- Ovarian enlargement with possible pain and ascites (excess fluid in the peritoneal cavity).

This is known as ovarian hyperstimulation syndrome (see Chapter 16).

17.7.3 Prolactin-inhibiting Hormone Agonists

Cabergoline and Bromocriptine Uses

Used for infertility (male and female) secondary to hyperprolactinemic states. See Chapter 16 for a further discussion of these agents.

17.8 Androgens, Anabolic Steroids, and Antiandrogens

The hormone testosterone is produced by the testis, adrenal glands, and ovaries (in small amounts). It has androgenic effects that are important in the development and maintenance of male sex characteristics and anabolic effects to increase muscle size and strength. Testosterone is converted to 5-dihydrotestosterone (DHT), which is the more active form, in cells that contain the 5α-reductase enzyme (skin, prostate, seminal vesicles, and epididymis). Like other steroids, testosterone and 5-DHT bind to intracellular receptors that alter gene transcription.

17.8.1 Effects

See ▶ Table 17.3.

Table 17.3 Effects of testosterone

Androgenic effects	Stimulates the growth of the penis, testes, and scrotum
	Induces pubic, axillary, and facial hair
	Thickens the vocal cords and growth of the larynx, producing a lower-pitched voice
	↑ libido
	↑ activity of sebaceous glands
Anabolic effects	↑ muscle growth and bone mass
	↑ production of red blood cells

17.8.2 Synthetic Testosterone Esters

Synthetic agents vary in the ratio of anabolic to androgenic effects. Unaltered testosterone is not suitable for oral or parenteral administration because of its rapid absorption and hepatic metabolism.

Testosterone Cypionate and Testosterone Enanthate

Pharmacokinetics

These agents are given intramuscularly in oily solutions.

Uses

Replacement therapy in hypogonadism (primary, secondary, or tertiary).

17.8.3 Synthetic Androgens

Fluoxymesterone, Methyltestosterone, and Danazol

These agents contain 17α-alkyl substitutions to retard hepatic degradation.

Pharmacokinetics

Orally effective.

Uses

- Replacement therapy in hypogonadism (primary, secondary, or tertiary).
- Endometriosis (Chapter 16), fibrocystic breast disease, and hereditary angioneurotic edema (danazol).

Side Effects

The substituted androgens produce liver dysfunction.

17.8.4 Anabolic Steroids

Oxymetholone and Oxandrolone

These agents also have 17α-alkyl substitutions. They are weak androgens designed to provide anabolic activity. It is impossible to completely separate androgenic and anabolic effects.

Uses

Anabolic steroids are used in the treatment of constitutional delay of growth.

Side Effects

- Androgenic effects: acne, facial hair, and deepening of the voice are the earliest effects, followed by priapism (a persistent, usually painful, erection of the penis) and prostatic hyperplasia.
- Gynecomastia.

- Cholestatic hepatitis (with 17α-alkylated compounds).
- Atherogenic changes in blood lipids (when taken in large doses, e.g., by athletes).
- Na$^+$ retention and edema.
- Benign and malignant tumors of the liver (rare).

17.8.5 Antiandrogens

Bicalutamide, Enzalutamide, Flutamide, Nilutamide

Mechanisms of Action

These nonsteroidal drugs block androgenic effects by binding androgen receptors, thereby preventing androgens from binding and activating the receptor.

Uses

Treatment of metastatic prostate cancer. Flutamide and bicalutamide are indicated for use in combination with an LH-releasing hormone agonist. Nilutamide is used in combination with surgical castration. Enzalutamide is approved as monotherapy in patients previously treated with docetaxel.

Side Effects

Gynecomastia, hot flushes, GI disturbances, breast tenderness, and abnormal liver function test results are associated with all of these agents. Nilutamide is associated with visual disturbances and alcohol intolerance. Enzalutamide may additionally cause seizures and asthenia.

17.8.6 Androgen Synthesis Inhibitors

Finasteride and Abiraterone Acetate

Mechanism of Action

Finasteride blocks the conversion of testosterone to DHT by inhibiting the enzyme 5α-reductase (▶ Fig. 17.5). Abiraterone acetate selectively inhibits 17α-hydroxylase/C17,20-lyase, an enzyme responsible for catalyzing two steps in androgen biosynthesis. Abiraterone acetate will therefore reduce both adrenal and testicular androgen production, whereas finasteride will not directly reduce adrenal androgen or testosterone production.

Uses

Finasteride is used in benign prostatic hyperplasia and male pattern baldness in men. Abiraterone acetate is used in combination with prednisone to treat metastatic, castration-resistant prostate cancer.

Side Effects

Both agents may cause edema, swelling, change of weight, sexual dysfunction, and impotence. Abiraterone acetate may also cause hypertension, hypokalemia, and abnormal liver function test results.

17.9 Drugs Acting on the Uterus

17.9.1 Oxytocin

Oxytocin is a posterior pituitary hormone that can now be synthetically produced for pharmacological use. The uterus is more sensitive to vasopressin than oxytocin except in the third trimester of pregnancy. During the third trimester, uterine oxytocin receptors increase in number, with sensitivity to oxytocin being maximal at term (vasopressin sensitivity decreases in parallel).

Effects

- Stimulates uterine smooth muscle contraction to facilitate parturition (birth).
- Causes myoepithelial cells of the mammary gland to contract and stimulates milk "letdown."
- Oxytocin-containing parvocellular neurons of the hypothalamus send axonal projections throughout the brain to regulate memory and maternal behaviors.

Pharmacokinetics

- Oxytocin is ineffective orally (destroyed by stomach enzymes) and is usually given intravenously or intramuscularly.
- Uterine contractions occur within seconds after intravenous injection and last ~ 20 minutes.

Uses

Oxytocin is used for the induction of labor and control of postpartum hemorrhage.

Side Effects

- Transient fall in blood pressure when injected intravenously.
- Na$^+$ and water retention.

Note: Do not use oxytocin in patients with uterine abnormalities.

17.9.2 Ergot Alkaloids

Ergot (*Claviceps purpurea*) is a fungus that grows on rye. Extracts of ergot contain a variety of pharmacologically active substances (histamine, tyramine, etc.). Ergot alkaloids per se are derivatives of lysergic acid. Ergot alkaloids have varied actions as agonists or antagonists on tryptaminergic, dopaminergic, and adrenergic receptors.

See Chapter 32 for a discussion of ergot alkaloids in relation to migraine.

Ergonovine

Mechanism of Action

Ergonovine is the most potent ergot compound for oxytocic effect with a relatively selective action on the uterus. It is also a partial α-adrenergic receptor agonist.

Pharmacokinetics

Rapid absorption after oral administration provides prompt onset of action.

Effects

Ergonovine can cause forceful, prolonged, or sustained contractions.

Uses

- Prevention and treatment of postpartum hemorrhage (after delivery of the placenta).
- Hastens involution of the uterus (the process where the uterus returns to its normal prepregnant size and state after childbirth).

Note: Ergonovine is not approved for use in the United States.

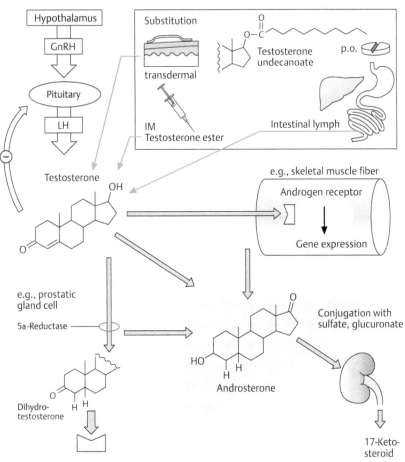

Fig. 17.5 Testosterone.
Natural testosterone (or its synthetic derivatives) is reduced in target cells to dihydrotestosterone (DHT) by 5α-reductase. DHT has a higher affinity than testosterone for androgen receptors. The liver rapidly metabolizes testosterone to androsterone, which undergoes renal elimination. 5α-reductase inhibitors inhibit the production of DHT and the androgenic activity in tissues where this is active (e.g., the prostate). They have little or no effect on testosterone-dependent tissues (e.g., skeletal muscle). Androgen receptor antagonists inhibit all androgen effects.

IV

Methylergonovine

Methylergonovine is a semisynthetic derivative with similar properties as ergonovine.

Anatomy and Innervation of the Uterus

The uterus is composed of a thick layer of smooth muscle with a central cavity that is lined by glandular epithelium. This cavity is continuous laterally with the fallopian tubes and inferiorly with the lumen of the vagina. The uterus is completely under autonomic control. It is innervated by the inferior hypogastric plexus (sympathetic) and the pelvic splanchnic nerves (parasympathetic from S2 to S4). Afferent signals from the uterus travel with the sympathetic efferents to T10-T12 and L1 spinal cord segments.

18 Insulin, Hypoglycemic, and Antihypoglycemic Drugs

Summary

Diabetes mellitus is characterized by hyperglycemia and may be insulin-dependent (type 1) or noninsulin-dependent (type 2). Rapid-acting insulin (insulin lispro, insulin aspart, and insulin glulisine) is typically injected prior to meals to reduce postprandial blood glucose elevations. Technosphere is normal insulin for pulmonary delivery. Regular insulin is identical to human insulin. Neutral protamine Hagedorn (NPH) insulin is produced by combining insulin with protamine. Long-acting insulins include insulin detemir, insulin glargine, and insulin degludec. Pramlintide is used as an adjunct for patients who take insulin with meals. Oral hypoglycemic agents are used in the treatment of type 2 diabetes. Metformin is widely used as first-line therapy. Sulfonylureas (chlorpropamide, tolazamide, tolbutamide, glimepiride, glipizide, and glyburide) are insulin secretagogues. Acarbose and miglitol are competitive reversible inhibitors of intestinal α-glucosidase that cause delayed absorption of carbohydrates, thereby blunting postprandial hyperglycemia. Pioglitazone and rosiglitazone increase insulin sensitivity in tissues. Nateglinide, and repaglinide block ATP-sensitive K+ channels in pancreatic beta cells and increase insulin release. Glucagon-like peptide 1 (GLP-1) receptor agonists (exenatide, liraglutide, albiglutide, dulaglutide, and lixisenatide) lower blood glucose by mimicking the actions of GLP-1. Sitagliptin, alogliptin, linagliptin, and saxagliptin are dipeptidyl peptidase 4 inhibitors that enhance the action of GLP-1. Sodium–glucose cotransporter 2 inhibitors (canagliflozin, dapagliflozin, and empagliflozin) increase the urinary excretion of glucose, thereby lowering plasma glucose concentration. In patients with diabetes who are taking insulin, hypoglycemia may occur from insufficient caloric intake or sudden, excessive physical exertion, or an excess of injected insulin. Primary therapy is to raise the glucose level in the blood with glucagon.

Keywords: diabetes, insulin, glucose, hyperglycemia, hypoglycemia, antidiabetic agents

18.1 Diabetes Mellitus

Diabetes mellitus is a group of chronic metabolic disorders characterized by hyperglycemia that result from inadequate insulin-related activity. Insulin-dependent diabetes mellitus (IDDM; type 1) is caused by destruction of the insulin-producing beta cells of the pancreas by antibodies (autoimmune disease). Noninsulin-dependent diabetes mellitus (NIDDM; type 2) occurs due to insufficient production of insulin or insulin resistance. The effects of insulin deficiency are shown in ▶ Fig. 18.1, and ▶ Table 18.1 lists the signs, symptoms, and complications of diabetes mellitus.

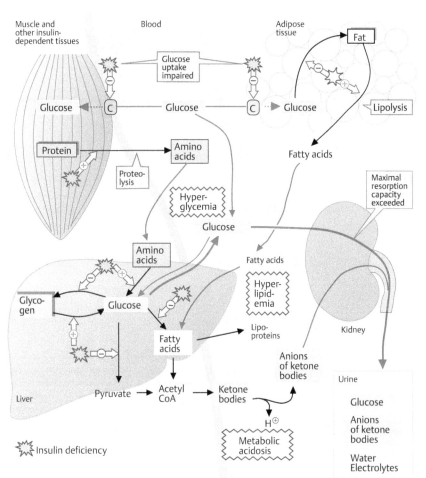

Fig. 18.1 Effects of insulin deficiency.
Insulin deficiency causes hyperglycemia. In muscle, glucose uptake is impaired and protein catabolism is increased. In addition, the uptake of glucose into fat is reduced, glucose conversion to fat is inhibited, and lipolysis is stimulated. The amino acids produced are transported in the blood to the liver, where they are converted to ketone bodies and lipoproteins. Gluconeogenesis is stimulated in the liver, leading to more glucose being transported to the blood than is taken up by the liver. Glucose conversion to glycogen is also inhibited. In the kidneys, glucose is secreted when their capacity to reabsorb glucose is exceeded, along with ketones, water, and electrolytes. CoA, coenzyme A. C, Solute carrier, insulin-stimulated glucose transporter type 4 (GLUT-4).

IV

Table 18.1 Signs, symptoms, and complications of diabetes mellitus

Signs	Symptoms	Complications
Hyperglycemia Glycosuria Poor wound healing Predilection to infection	Thirst (polydipsia) Increased frequency of urination (polyuria) Dehydration Fatigue Nausea and vomiting	Microvascular disease: • Retinopathy (can cause blindness) • Nephropathy • Neuropathy Accelerated atherosclerosis causing strokes, coronary heart disease, and hypertension Gangrene

18.2 Insulin

18.2.1 Synthesis

Insulin is produced by the beta cells of the pancreatic islets. Pre-proinsulin is processed to proinsulin which is cleaved to form three peptide chains. Insulin, consisting of the A (21 amino acids) and B (30 amino acids) chains connected by disulfide bonds, is secreted from the beta cells along with the C peptide. The beta cells also secrete amylin, a 37-amino acid peptide.

18.2.2 Mechanism of Action

The insulin receptor is a tyrosine kinase receptor that dimerizes upon binding insulin, leading to receptor autophosphorylation and the activation of intracellular signaling molecules. The activated receptor initiates a complex cascade that mediates the effects of insulin (▶ Fig. 18.2). Examples include stimulation of the translocation of glucose transporters and increased glycogen synthesis which lowers elevated blood glucose levels. It also stimulates protein synthesis and lipogenesis.

Clinical Correlation

Diagnosis of Diabetes Mellitus

The diagnosis of diabetes mellitus is made by the evaluation of symptoms and the blood tests listed below. If type 1 diabetes is diagnosed, the patient will also be screened for autoantibodies that are commonly associated with type 1 diabetes.

1. *Glycated hemoglobin (A1C) test:* This test measures the percentage of blood sugar attached to hemoglobin and indicates the patient's average blood sugar levels over the past 2 to 3 months. An A1C ≥ 6.5% on two separate tests is diagnostic of diabetes. A1C values between 5.7 and 6.4% indicate prediabetes, and a value below 5.7% is considered normal.
2. *Random blood sugar level:* A random blood test is taken and blood sugar measured. A value of > 200 mg/dL (11.1 mmol/L) is suggestive of diabetes, especially if the patient has associated symptoms.
3. *Fasting blood sugar test:* The patient fasts overnight and a blood sample is taken in the morning. A value of ≥ 126 mg/dL (≥ 7 mmol/L) on two separate occasions allows for a diagnosis of diabetes. A value ranging between 100 and 125 mg/

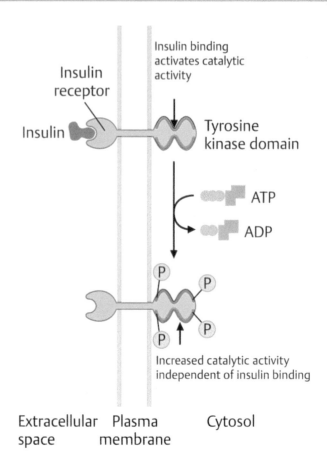

Fig. 18.2 Signal transduction: insulin.
The insulin receptor is a glycoprotein consisting of two alpha chains, located on the outside of the cell, and two beta chains that are membrane bound and reach into the cytosol. Insulin binds to the exterior alpha chains, which phosphorylates part of the internal beta chains. This activates tyrosine kinase, which then phosphorylates tyrosine groups of a peptide (insulin receptor substrate), which in turn triggers further phosphorylation and dephosphorylation reactions, leading to the physiological effects of insulin. ADP, adenosine diphosphate; ATP, adenosine triphosphate.

dL (5.6 to 6.9 mmol/L) is indicative of prediabetes, and values below 100 mg/dL are considered normal.
4. *Oral glucose tolerance test:* (see call-out box below).

Clinical Correlation

Oral Glucose Tolerance Test

Glucose tolerance is used to test for type 2 diabetes and gestational diabetes. It involves giving the patient a known oral dose of glucose, following an 8- to 12-hour fasting period, then measuring plasma glucose levels at intervals thereafter to determine how quickly plasma glucose levels fall and homeostasis is regained. When testing for type 2 diabetes, measurements of plasma glucose taken after 2 hours should be < 140 mg/dL (7.8 mmol/L). Glucose levels of 140 to 199 mg/dL (7.8 to 11 mmol/L) indicate impaired glucose tolerance (prediabetes), and levels of 200 mg/dL (11.1 mmol/L) or higher suggest a diagnosis of diabetes. An additional test or evaluation of symptoms may be used to confirm the diagnosis of type 2 diabetes. To diagnose gestational diabetes, the oral glucose tolerance test will last for 3 hours with different cut off limits.

Clinical Correlation

Diabetic Ketoacidosis

Diabetic ketoacidosis (DKA) is a life-threatening complication of diabetes. It mostly occurs in type 1 diabetes but may occur in type 2 diabetes also. In DKA, there is a shortage of insulin, so the body cannot process enough glucose and increases the metabolism of fatty acids. The increased acetyl coenzyme A (CoA) from fatty acid oxidation leads to ketone body (acetoacetic acid, β hydroxybutyric acid, and acetone) production. The overabundance of ketones lowers the blood pH. Dehydration occurs, followed by metabolic acidosis and coma. Signs may include hyperventilation and the breath smelling of ketones ("fruity" smell). DKA usually occurs in known diabetics and can be triggered by illness or inadequate/inappropriate insulin therapy. Treatment involves giving insulin, K^+, and fluid replacement.

Foundations

Ketone Formation

Ketones provide an alternative source of energy during periods of low glucose after glycogen stores have been consumed. They are formed by the beta oxidation of acetyl CoA which is derived from fatty acids in liver mitochondrial cells. Beta oxidation also yields the reduced form of nicotinamide adenine dinucleotide (NADH) and the hydroquinone form of flavin adenine dinucleotide ($FADH_2$), which then undergoes oxidative phosphorylation, producing adenosine triphosphate (ATP). Acetyl CoA from fatty acid catabolism would normally enter the citric acid cycle, producing energy (via the oxidative phosphorylation of NADH and $FADH_2$). However, in periods of low glucose, oxaloacetate (a citric acid cycle intermediate) is used for gluconeogenesis; thus acetyl CoA is diverted for ketone formation. There are three ketones: acetoacetic acid, β-hydroxybutyric acid, and acetone. Acetone is a result of the spontaneous decarboxylation of acetoacetic acid and is produced in the least quantity of all the ketones. Furthermore, acetone cannot be converted back to acetyl CoA, so it is excreted in urine and exhaled (giving the breath a characteristic "fruity" smell in ketotic states).

18.2.3 Effects of Insulin

- Increased transport of glucose into fat and muscle, and increased muscle and hepatic glycogen synthesis.
- Increased K^+ uptake into cells.
- Decreased lipolysis and increased triglyceride synthesis.
- Decreased protein catabolism, increased amino acid transport, and ribosomal protein synthesis.

- Decreased hepatic glucose production (gluconeogenesis).
- Decreased glucagon secretion.

Note: The overall effect of insulin is to control hyperglycemia and keto acid formation.

Clinical Correlation

Gestational Diabetes

Gestational diabetes occurs during pregnancy and resembles type 2 diabetes. It is thought to occur in ~2 to 5% of all pregnancies and may improve or disappear after delivery of the baby. Gestational diabetes can be dangerous for both mother and baby. The baby may have macrosomia (high birth weight), congenital cardiac and central nervous system anomalies, and skeletal muscle malformations. They may also have respiratory distress syndrome after birth due to decreased production of surfactant, a substance that causes maturation of the lungs.

Foundations

Insulin and K^+ Balance

K^+ is an important ion in the body, with 98% being intracellular. The ratio of intracellular to extracellular K^+ determines cell membrane potential. Immediate K^+ balance is controlled by intracellular and extracellular K^+ exchange driven by the $Na^+–K^+$–ATPase pump. This is controlled by insulin and p_2 receptors. Long-term K^+ balance is controlled by renal excretion. In hyperkalemic (high K^+) states, glucose and insulin are used to drive K^+ into cells by increasing the activity of the $Na^+–K^+$–ATPase pump.

18.2.4 Insulin Preparations

Insulin is used to lower elevated blood glucose levels in type 1 diabetes mellitus, as well as in some cases of type 2 diabetes mellitus. Insulin preparations have been developed to delay absorption of insulin and prolong its action, but they act in the same way as regular insulin and have the same side effects. ▶ Table 18.2 provides a summary of the pharmacokinetic properties of different insulin preparations, and ▶ Fig. 18.3 describes two different approaches to insulin replacement. To approximate physiological insulin release, insulin preparations may be combined such that intermediate or long-acting insulins are used to provide basal coverage while rapid or short-acting insulins are utilized for postprandial glucose control. All insulin preparations are administered by injection or infusion with the exception of inhaled insulin.

Rapid-acting Insulins: Insulin Lispro, Insulin Aspart, and Insulin Glulisine

Rapid-acting insulin is typically taken prior to meals to reduce postprandial blood glucose elevations.
- Insulin lispro differs from human insulin by inversion of the B-chain amino acids proline and lysine at positions 28 and 29, respectively.

Table 18.2 Pharmacokinetic properties of insulin preparations

Type	Preparations	Onset	Peak[b]	Duration
Rapid-acting insulin	Insulin lispro	0.25–0.5 h	0.5–2.5 h	≤5 h
	Insulin aspart	~0.2–0.3 h	1–3 h	3–7 h
	Insulin glulisine	0.2–0.5 h	1.6–2.8 h	3–4 h
	Technosphere[a]	~0.2 h	~0.5–0.9 h	1.5–4.5 h
Short-acting insulin	Regular insulin	0.5–1 h	2–4 h	6–8 h
Intermediate-acting insulin	Insulin NPH	1–2 h	4–12 h	10–20 h
Long-acting insulin	Insulin detemir	3–4 h	3 to 9 h	6–23 h
	Insulin glargine	4–6 h	None	~24 h
	Insulin degludec	~1 h	None	24–>42 h

Abbreviation: NPH, neutral protamine Hagedorn.
[a]All preparations are administered by subcutaneous injection except for Technosphere, which is inhaled.
[b]Peak effect.
Reference numbers are estimates and may vary by source.

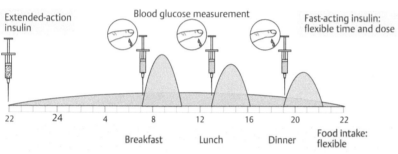

1. Intensified insulin therapy

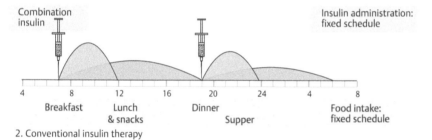

2. Conventional insulin therapy

Fig. 18.3 Methods of insulin replacement.
In intensified insulin therapy, long-acting insulin is administered late in the evening to generate a basal level. A fast-acting insulin is then injected before meals, the dose being dependent on blood glucose concentration measurement and the meal-dependent demand. This approach allows the patient flexibility in meal times and insulin injection. In conventional insulin therapy, a fixed-dosage schedule is maintained. Insulin (a combination of regular insulin and insulin suspension) is injected in the morning and evening, and carbohydrate ingestion is synchronized with this.

- Insulin aspart differs from human insulin by replacement of the proline at position 28 (B chain) by aspartic acid.
- Insulin glulisine is formulated by substituting an asparagine for lysine at position 3 and glutamic acid for lysine at position 29 of the B chain.

Inhaled (Rapid-acting) Insulin: Technosphere

Technosphere is normal insulin that is adsorbed onto carrier particles for pulmonary delivery. It is administered by inhalation at the beginning of a meal. Technosphere is contraindicated in patients with lung diseases, such as asthma or COPD, due to the potential for acute bronchospasm. Pulmonary lung function may also decline over time.

Short-acting (Regular) Insulin: Regular Novolin R, Regular Humulin R

Regular insulin, produced by recombinant DNA techniques, is identical to human insulin. It has a delayed absorption into the bloodstream which necessitates that subcutaneous administration occurs approximately 30 minutes before mealtime.

Intermediate-acting Insulin: Neutral Protamine Hagedorn Insulin

Neutral protamine Hagedorn (NPH) insulin is produced by combining insulin with the positively charged polypeptide protamine. Following subcutaneous administration, proteolytic enzymes must degrade the protamine to release the insulin. This results in a delayed onset of action as compared to regular insulin. The variability of NPH absorption is high, and its use is declining due to the availability of more predictable long-acting insulin preparations.

Long-acting Insulin: Insulin Detemir, Insulin Glargine, and Insulin Degludec

Similar to NPH insulin, long-acting insulins exploit delayed absorption techniques to extend activity. Long-acting insulins may also bind to albumin, additionally extending the active time period.

- Insulin detemir is produced by covalently binding myristic acid to lysine 29 and omitting lysine 30 on the B chain.
- Insulin glargine is produced by replacing the asparagine residue at position 21 of the A chain with glycine and adding two arginine residues to the C terminus of the B chain.
- Insulin degludec has a deletion of threonine at the B-30 position with a C16 fatty acid side chain attached at position B-29 via a glutamic acid spacer.

18.2.5 Side Effects of Insulin Therapy

Hypoglycemia is the most common adverse effect in patients with well-controlled diabetes. This may be caused by any of the following factors:

- Wrong dose.
- Exercise inappropriate for the dose of insulin (exercise increases glucose uptake by insulin-independent mechanisms).
- Not eating at a regular time or eating insufficient amounts.
- Drugs enhancing insulin-induced hypoglycemia include anabolic steroids, captopril, ethyl alcohol, and salicylates.
- Beta-adrenergic-blocking drugs that may mask symptoms of hypoglycemia and delay the onset of treatment. These drugs also impair counter-regulatory responses.
- Allergic reactions and localized atrophy are less common with newer, single-component insulin preparations.

Hypoglycemia should be treated with oral glucose (tablets or gel) to relieve the symptoms. Patients and their families may be instructed for the use of a glucagon emergency kit for treating severe hypoglycemic reactions.

18.3 Amylin Analogue: Pramlintide

18.3.1 Mechanism of Action

Pramlintide is a synthetic analogue of amylin, a neuroendocrine hormone synthesized by pancreatic beta cells. Amylin delays gastric emptying and reduces digestive secretion. In addition, amylin reduces the postprandial secretion of plasma glucagon. This improves postprandial glucose control. It may also increase satiety, leading to decreased caloric intake and weight loss. Pramlintide, which mimics the effect of amylin, is used as an adjunct for patients with type 1 or type 2 diabetes who take insulin with meals. Pramlintide alone does not reduce blood glucose. It is given by subcutaneous injection with every meal to reduce postprandial hyperglycemia. To reduce the risk of hypoglycemia, it is recommended that prandial insulin is reduced by 50% at the initiation of pramlintide treatment and subsequently adjusted based on glycemic control and tolerability.

18.3.2 Uses

Type 1 or type 2 diabetes mellitus.

18.3.3 Side Effects

- Hypoglycemia.
- Mild nausea that decreases over time.

18.4 Oral Hypoglycemic Drugs

18.4.1 Uses

Oral hypoglycemic agents are used in the treatment of type 2 diabetes mellitus, although diet and exercise are the primary treatments for this condition. These agents are ineffective in type 1 diabetes mellitus.

18.4.2 Sulfonylurea Derivatives

Chlorpropamide, Tolazamide, Tolbutamide, Glimepiride, Glipizide, Glyburide

Sulfonylureas are insulin secretagogues that induce the release of insulin regardless of the presence of glucose. They are classified by relative potency, with first-generation sulfonylureas having a lower potency as compared with second-generation sulfonylureas.

- First-generation agents: Chlorpropamide, tolazamide, and tolbutamide.
- Second-generation agents: Glimepiride, glipizide, glyburide.

Mechanism of Action

These agents block ATP-sensitive K^+ channels on the surface of pancreatic beta cells. This causes membrane depolarization and increased insulin secretion (▶ Fig. 18.4).

Side Effects

- Hypoglycemia.
- Chlorpropamide may cause water retention because of augmentation of antidiuretic hormone action.

18.4.3 Biguanides

Metformin

Metformin is widely used as first-line therapy for type 2 diabetics. It reduces hepatic glucose production, increases insulin sensitivity, and stimulates glucose uptake and glycolysis in peripheral tissue. Metformin also has a low risk of hypoglycemia and does not induce weight gain, which is beneficial for overweight diabetic patients. Potentially fatal lactic acidosis is associated with metformin overdose. The elimination of metformin primarily occurs by renal tubular secretion and glomerular filtration; therefore, the risk of lactic acidosis increases with drug accumulation in cases of renal insufficiency.

Mechanism of Action

- The exact mechanism of metformin action is unclear. Reduction of hepatic glucose production may occur through

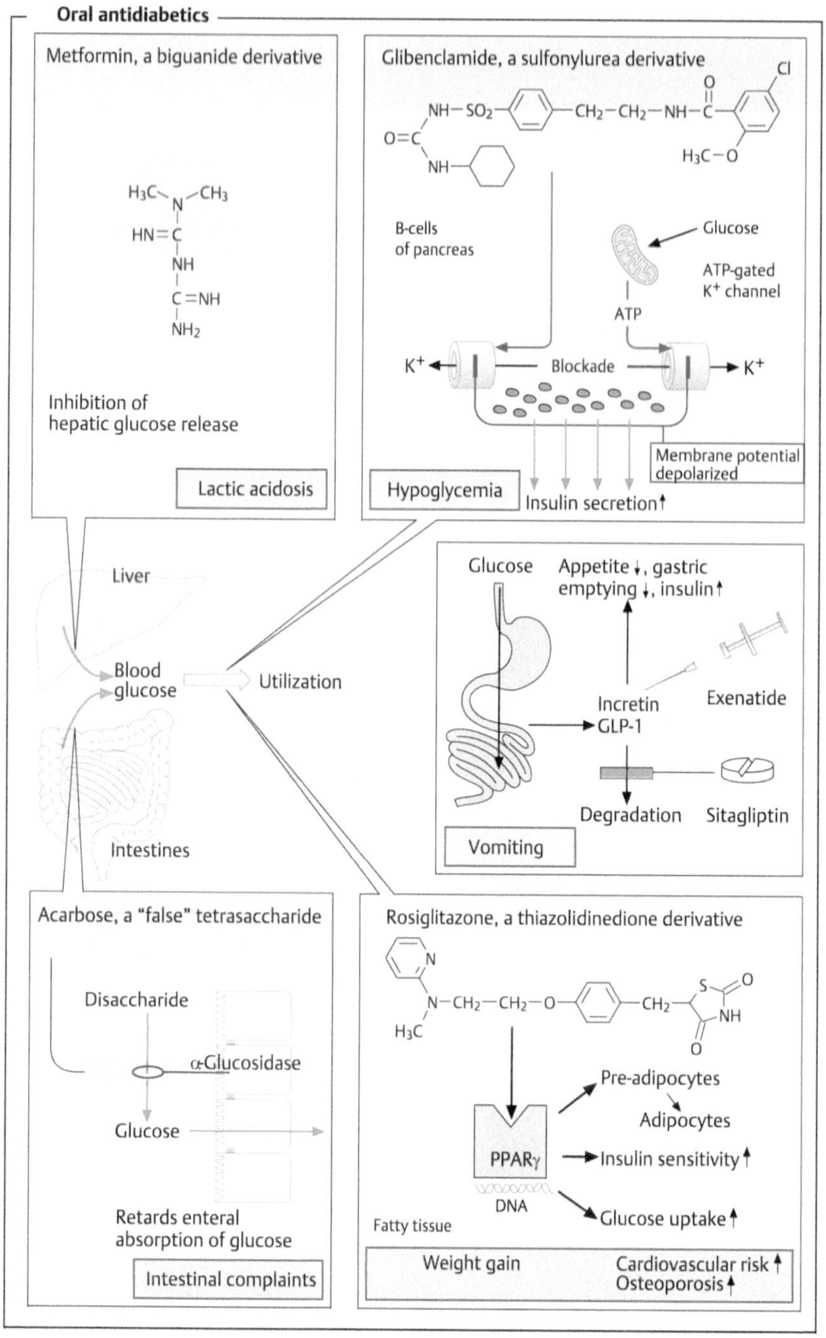

Fig. 18.4 Oral antidiabetics.
Blood glucose concentration depends on the inflow of glucose (mainly from the liver and intestines) and the outflow from the blood into tissues and then cells where it is utilized. Metformin and acarbose both inhibit glucose inflow into the blood, and sulfonylureas and thiazolidinedione derivatives positively affect the outflow of glucose into tissues by stimulating insulin secretion and increasing insulin sensitivity, respectively. Exenatide acts on the glucagon-like peptide 1 (GLP-1) receptor to stimulate glucose-dependent insulin release and inhibit glucagon secretion. Sitagliptin is a dipeptidyl peptidase 4 (DPP-4) inhibitor that inhibits the degradation of GLP-1 by DPP-4, the enzyme that metabolizes GLP-1 in the intestine. PPAR, peroxisome proliferator-activated receptor.

inhibition of the mitochondrial respiratory-chain class 1, inducing a reduction in cellular energy status and activation of AMP-dependent kinase (AMPK). Activated AMPK is also involved in metformin-enhanced insulin sensitivity. Decreases hepatic gluconeogenesis and absorption of glucose from the gastrointestinal (GI) tract.
• Increases insulin sensitivity of skeletal muscle and adipose tissue.

Note: Metformin does not increase the release of pancreatic insulin; therefore, the risk of hypoglycemia is less than that seen for the sulfonylurea agents.

Side Effects

GI disturbances, including diarrhea.

18.4.4 Alpha-Glucosidase Inhibitors

Acarbose and Miglitol

Mechanism of Action

These agents are competitive reversible inhibitors of intestinal α-glucosidase, which normally hydrolyzes oligosaccharides, trisaccharides, and disaccharides to glucose and other monosaccharides.

They cause delayed absorption of carbohydrates, thereby blunting postprandial hyperglycemia (▶ Fig. 18.2).

Pharmacokinetics

These agents are not absorbed systemically.

Side Effects

High incidence of GI pain, discomfort, flatulence, and diarrhea.

18.4.5 Thiazolidinediones

Pioglitazone and Rosiglitazone

Mechanism of Action

These agents increase insulin sensitivity in tissues, for example, muscle, adipose tissue, and the liver (▶ Fig. 18.2).

Side Effects

- Edema.
- Weight gain.

18.4.6 Meglitinides

Nateglinide and Repaglinide

Mechanism of Action

Meglitinides block ATP-sensitive K^+ channels in pancreatic beta cells, leading to membrane depolarization and increased insulin release.

18.4.7 Glucagon-like Peptide 1 Receptor Agonists

Exenatide, Liraglutide, Albiglutide, Dulaglutide, and Lixisenatide

Mechanism of Action

Glucagon-like peptide 1 (GLP-1) is a hormone secreted from intestinal L cells in response to nutrient ingestion. It acts on the GLP-1 receptor to stimulate glucose-dependent insulin release and inhibit glucagon secretion. It potentiates the first- and second-phase insulin responses, slows gastric emptying, and reduces food intake. Postprandial GLP-1 secretion is reduced in type 2 diabetes. GLP-1 receptor agonists lower blood glucose by mimicking the actions of GLP-1.

Uses

Exenatide is used to improve glycemic control in patients with type 2 diabetes.

Side Effects

- Hypoglycemia, primarily when combined with insulin enhancing agents.
- Nausea.
- Pancreatitis.

18.4.8 Dipeptidyl Peptidase 4 Inhibitors

Sitagliptin, Alogliptin, Linagliptin, and Saxagliptin

Mechanism of Action

Dipeptidyl peptidase 4 (DPP-4) is the enzyme that rapidly metabolizes endogenously released GLP-1 in the intestine, terminating its effects. DPP-4 inhibitors inhibit the degradation of GLP-1 by DPP-4, thereby enhancing the action of GLP-1. This results in increased insulin release and decreased glucagon levels. They do not slow gastric emptying.

Uses

Management of type 2 diabetes as monotherapy or in combination with metformin and thiazolidinediones.

18.4.9 Sodium–Glucose Cotransporter 2 Inhibitors

Canagliflozin, Dapagliflozin, Empagliflozin, and Ertugliflozin

Mechanism of Action

Sodium–glucose cotransporter 2 (SGLT2) in the proximal renal tubules is involved in the reabsorption of filtered glucose. Inhibition of SGLT2 results in an increase in urinary excretion of glucose, thereby lowering plasma glucose concentration. The efficacy of SGLT2 inhibitors is reduced with declining renal function.

Side Effects

- Yeast and urinary tract infections.
- Hyperkalemia and hyponatremia.

18.5 Antihypoglycemic Drugs

In patients with diabetes who are taking insulin, hypoglycemia may occur from insufficient caloric intake or sudden, excessive physical exertion, or an excess of injected insulin. Primary therapy is to raise the glucose level in the blood.

18.5.1 Glucagon

Glucagon is a polypeptide produced by the alpha cells of the pancreas. It acts by increasing the catabolism of hepatic glycogen, and it also stimulates gluconeogenesis. This leads to increased release of glucose from the liver into the blood. Other effects of glucagon include ionotropic and chronotropic effects on the heart, as well as relaxation of intestinal smooth muscle. Cardiac effects, such as increased blood pressure and pulse, are transient due to glucagon's short half-life. Glucagon is available as an emergency kit that contains freeze-dried glucagon as a powder and a 1 mL syringe of glycerin. The glycerin is mixed with the glucagon powder prior to injection and may be given intravenously, intramuscularly, or subcutaneously.

IV

Mechanism of Action

Glucagon binds to G protein-coupled receptors, mainly in the liver. Signal transduction occurs by means of increased cyclic adenosine monophosphate (cAMP), leading to stimulation of gluconeogenesis and glycogenolysis in the liver and an increase in blood glucose.

Uses

- Hypoglycemic emergency.
- Diagnosis of endocrine disorders.

Side Effects

Nausea and vomiting.

Unit IV Review Questions

1. Which of the following is contraindicated in patients with COPD?
   A. Technosphere.
   B. Pramlintide.
   C. Pioglitazone.
   D. Metformin.
   E. Acarbose.

2. A couple visits the physician after unsuccessfully attempting to conceive a child for a year. Examination and analysis do not reveal ovulatory dysfunction related to pituitary or ovarian failure. Which of the following drugs could be used to enhance LH and FSH secretion and stimulate ovulation?
   A. Clomiphene.
   B. Danazol.
   C. Medroxyprogesterone acetate.
   D. Metformin.
   E. Betamethasone.

3. A 31-year-old man with acromegaly was found to have a large pituitary tumor secreting growth hormone. Surgical removal of the tumor was partially successful, but the patient still requires additional pharmacotherapy. Which of the following drugs would be the best choice to treat the patient?
   A. Lanreotide.
   B. Mecasermin.
   C. Somatropin.
   D. Growth hormone.
   E. Glucagon.

4. A patient is brought to the emergency room with tachycardia, muscle weakness, nervousness, fever, vomiting, extreme sweating, and delirium. Laboratory tests show an elevated serum free tetraiodothyronine, or thyroxine (T_4), and a decreased thyroid-stimulating hormone (TSH) level. To rapidly prevent the synthesis of thyroid hormones, methimazole is given. What is the prescribed action of this drug?
   A. To inhibit tyrosine hydroxylase, thereby decreasing norepinephrine formation.
   B. To inhibit thyroid peroxidase, thereby decreasing the formation of thyroxine (T_4) and triiodothyronine (T_3).
   C. To inhibit Ca^{2+} uptake by the endoplasmic reticulum.
   D. To increase the secretion of thyroxine.
   E. To inhibit growth of parenchymal cells.

5. One hour later, the patient in question 4 is given stable iodine as a saturated solution of potassium iodide. What is the purpose of giving high iodide concentrations?
   A. To inhibit thyroid hormone release.
   B. To replenish depleted iodine stores.
   C. To overcome the thyroid effects of methimazole.
   D. To prevent cardiac side effects of methimazole.
   E. To replace salts lost by sweating.

6. Iodides cannot be used long term to control thyrotoxicosis (hyperthyroidism) because the inhibitory actions of iodide decrease within several weeks. Which of the following treatments can be used to produce a long-term decrease in thyroid hormone levels?
   A. Levothyroxine.
   B. Fluorouracil.
   C. Parathyroid hormone.
   D. Calcitriol.
   E. Radioactive iodine (^{131}I).

7. A 62-year-old postmenopausal Caucasian woman experienced menopause in her early 50 s and has been under hormone replacement therapy with a conjugated estrogen preparation since that time. She is not on any other medications. She has become concerned about the dangers associated with long-term hormone replacement therapy. If the goal of therapy is primarily for prevention of osteoporosis, which of the following therapies might be an appropriate substitute?
   A. Estrogen only.
   B. Progestin only.
   C. A second-generation sulfonylurea.
   D. Ergonovine.
   E. A bisphosphonate.

8. The effectiveness of glucocorticoids for nonadrenal disorders such as allergic reactions is related to the glucocorticoids' ability to
   A. Suppress inflammatory and immune responses.
   B. Reduce receptor sensitivity to stress associated cytokines.
   C. Increase glucose utilization and subsequent response to insulin.
   D. None of the above.
   E. All of the above.

9. A 25-year-old man reports becoming exhausted easily and having intestinal pains. The patient also reports being irritable, vomiting for many days, and having a sore throat. Examination shows purple spots on his rib cage and legs. His skin appears tanned even in un-exposed areas. The patient has also lost weight. The morning cortisol level after intravenous cosyntropin is unchanged. What would be the primary drug therapy for this patient?
   A. Corticorelin.
   B. Aminoglutethimide.
   C. Levothyroxine.
   D. Hydrocortisone.
   E. Mifepristone.

10. Although the patient in question 9 reports feeling much better after primary drug therapy, he still feels dizzy when standing. Serum Na + is low, and urinary Na + is increased. This patient may benefit from the addition of which of the following drugs?
    A. Cortisol (p.o.).
    B. Spironolactone.
    C. Dexamethasone.
    D. Fludrocortisone.
    E. Mifepristone.

11. Which one of the following is an adverse effect of high-dose estrogen therapy?
    A. Acne.
    B. Lymphopenia.

C. Weight loss.

D. Thromboembolism.

12. Which of the following is an androgen synthesis inhibitor that blocks the activity of CYP17, the enzyme that catalyzes the biosynthesis of androgens from pregnane precursors?

A. Prednisone.

B. Abiraterone.

C. Mifepristone.

D. Hydrocortisone.

E. Spironolactone.

13. A known diabetic patient is brought to the emergency room in a deep coma. There is an obvious need for immediate treatment, but the instrument used to determine plasma glucose concentration is not working, and the laboratory cannot supply the result in less than 1 hour. The best emergency procedure is the prompt administration of which of the following?

A. Crystalline (regular) insulin.

B. Neutral protamine Hagedorn (NPH) insulin.

C. A second-generation sulfonylurea.

D. Oral glucose.

E. Intravenous glucose.

14. There are several therapeutic options available for postmenopausal women with hormone-receptor-positive cancer. Which of the following is a major difference between tamoxifen and anastrozole?

A. Anastrozole inhibits the conversion of estrogens to androgens, while tamoxifen is a competitive inhibitor of the estrogen receptor.

B. Anastrozole is a 5α-reductase inhibitor, while tamoxifen is a competitive inhibitor of the estrogen receptor.

C. Anastrozole inhibits the conversion of androgens to estrogens and tamoxifen is a selective estrogen receptor modulator.

D. Anastrozole is a selective progesterone receptor modulator and tamoxifen is a selective estrogen receptor modulator.

15. Pamela J. is a 33-year-old woman in her 43rd week of gestation. Her physician would like to induce labor. Which of the following agents may be used to facilitate this process?

A. Tamoxifen.

B. Oxytocin.

C. Leuprolide.

D. Prolactin.

E. Serotonin.

16. A patient on chlorpromazine, a dopamine receptor antagonist used for the treatment of schizophrenia, complains of breast enlargement. This would be related to

A. Increased estrogen secretion from the ovaries due to increased aromatase activity.

B. Increased progesterone levels resulting from 17alpha-hydroxylase deficiency.

C. Increased prolactin secretion from the anterior pituitary gland.

D. Decreased pregnenolone levels resulting from 17alpha-hydroxylase deficiency.

17. A1C testing provides the practitioner with an indication of the patients' average blood glycemia for the past

A. 2-3 months.

B. 6 months.

C. 12 months.

D. 3 years.

E. 3 days.

18. Which of the following therapies will benefit a patient with pediatric short stature and growth hormone deficiency?

A. Somatropin.

B. Somatostatin.

C. Octreotide.

D. Bromocriptine.

E. Technosphere.

19. George B. is a 95-year-old type 2 diabetic with a history of cigar smoking. He was admitted to the hospital with signs of mental confusion and severe dehydration after a case of pneumonia. Lab tests report a blood glucose concentration of 622 mg/dL and a serum osmolality of 335 mmol/L. What is George likely suffering from?

A. Hyperglycemic hyperosmolar syndrome.

B. Diabetic nephropathy (kidney damage) leading to dehydration and neuroglycopenia.

C. Diabetic ketoacidosis.

D. Severe hypoglycemia.

20. Which of the following is a selective progesterone receptor modulator used for emergency contraception?

A. Clomiphene.

B. Faslodex.

C. Raloxifene.

D. Ulipristal acetate.

E. Estradiol.

21. Thomas J., a 72-year-old man with poorly controlled diabetes, was determined to have an insufficient increase in insulin secretion in response to sulfonylurea therapy. The mechanism by which sulfonylureas induce insulin secretion is

A. Increasing the activity of incretins.

B. Sensitizing pancreatic beta cells to glucagon.

C. Blocking ATP-sensitive K^+ channels on the surface of pancreatic beta cells.

D. Activating ATP-sensitive K^+ channels on the surface of pancreatic beta cells.

22. Arthur H. is a 33-year-old man who recently switched to a different medication for his T2DM. On a check-up, it was noted that although his blood hyperglycemia decreased, there was an increase in his urinary glucose. Which of the following drugs would be responsible for this effect?

A. Nateglinide.

B. Empagliflozin.

C. Liraglutide.

D. Pioglitazone.

E. Metformin.

23. A synthetic form of tetraiodothyronine (T_4) is

A. Propylthiouracil.

B. Levothyroxine.

C. Iodide.

D. Liotrix.

E. Radioactive iodine(^{131}I).

24. An antiprogestin that is effective in terminating pregnancy within the first 9 weeks of gestation is
A. Mifepristone.
B. Diethylstilbestrol.
C. Clomiphene.
D. Mestranol.
E. Norethindrone.

25. In the treatment of infertility, clomiphene
A. Directly stimulates the ovaries.
B. Acts as an antiprogestin.
C. Acts at progestin receptors.
D. Acts by binding to estrogen receptors.

26. Continuous administration of high doses of leuprolide
A. Increases the release of both luteinizing hormone (LH) and follicle-stimulating hormone (FSH).
B. Increases the release of FSH and not LH.
C. Restores normal ovulation in a patient with hypothalamic disease.
D. Desensitizes gonadotropin-releasing hormone (GnRH) receptors and leads to decreased release of FSH and LH.
E. Should be considered for a patient with hypogonadotropic hypogonadism.

27. Which of the following is effective in treating type 1 (insulin-dependent) diabetes mellitus?
A. Insulin.
B. Tolbutamide.
C. Glyburide.
D. Metformin.

28. Which of the following is classified as an intermediate-acting insulin preparation?
A. Neutral protamine Hagedorn (NPH) insulin.
B. Insulin lispro.
C. Metformin.
D. Glyburide.

29. In the treatment of infertility, gonadotropins
A. Directly stimulate the ovaries.
B. Act as antiprogestins.
C. Block the actions of follicle-stimulating hormone (FSH).
D. Increase the release of luteinizing hormone (LH) and FSH from the adenohypophysis.
E. Are effective when administered orally.

30. Which of the following will provide the most rapid onset of action to treat myxedema coma?
A. Thyroglobulin.
B. Thyroid extract.
C. Liothyronine (T$_3$).
D. Levothyroxine (T$_4$).

31. A dopamine receptor agonist that is sometimes used to treat hyperprolactinemia is
A. Chlorpromazine.
B. Phenytoin.
C. Diazepam.
D. Lithium carbonate.
E. Bromocriptine.

32. Which one of the following is caused by methyltestosterone but not by testosterone cypionate?
A. Facial hair.
B. Acne.
C. Deepening voice.
D. Jaundice.
E. Increased muscle strength.

33. Long-term therapy with the corticosteroids can predispose patients to which one of the following conditions?
A. Acute adrenal insufficiency.
B. Lymphocytic leukemia.
C. Insulin-dependent diabetes.
D. Dermatological conditions.
E. Increased susceptibility to infection.

34. The most common adverse effect of acarbose is
A. Hypoglycemia.
B. Hepatotoxicity.
C. Lactic acidosis.
D. Weight gain.
E. Flatulence.

35. A 51-year-old African American woman complains of constipation. The patient's last bowel movement was 1 week ago, and she has not had any bowel movements since, despite taking multiple laxatives. She also admits to feeling depressed. Laboratory tests show the level of serum free tetraiodothyronine (T$_4$) is low, and thyroid-stimulating hormone (TSH) is elevated. What would be an appropriate drug therapy for the primary disease?
A. Levothyroxine.
B. Propylthiouracil.
C. Psyllium laxative.
D. Selective serotonin reuptake inhibitor (SSRI).
E. Radioactive iodine (^{131}I).

36. A 62-year-old postmenopausal Caucasian woman experienced menopause in her early 50 s and has been under hormone replacement therapy with a conjugated estrogen preparation since that time. She is not on any other medications. What are the long-term risks of continuing hormone replacement therapy?
A. Stroke and thromboembolism.
B. Hot flashes and flushing.
C. Hirsutism and lower voice.
D. Hypercalcemia and kidney stones.
E. Nausea and vomiting.

37. A 28-year-old woman and her husband have been trying unsuccessfully to conceive for the past 2 years. Both are healthy with no significant medical history. Neither of them takes any medications. They have coitus about three times a week. Her menstrual periods have been irregular, with the length varying. She is diagnosed with anovulation and a course of clomiphene therapy is prescribed. Why is clomiphene appropriate for infertility treatment?
A. It increases the secretion of follicle-stimulating hormone (FSH) and luteinizing hormone (LH).
B. Inhibits proteolysis of zona pellucida glycoproteins.
C. It increases the chance that a fertilized ovum will be implanted.

D. It increases libido in ovulating women.

E. It inhibits androgen production by the adrenals.

38. Following an episode of orchitis that was treated with antibiotics, a 32-year-old man is experiencing a decreased libido and an inability to maintain a penile erection. The patient has lost weight, and gynecomastia is noted. Morning testosterone is 150 ng/dL (270–1070 ng/dL), and luteinizing hormone (LH) is 12 mIU/L (normal = 2–12 mIU/L). Which one of the following drugs is the best choice for long-term treatment of hypogonadism in men?

    A. Methyltestosterone.

    B. Testosterone cypionate.

    C. Fluoxymesterone.

    D. Danazol.

    E. Norethindrone.

39. A 51-year-old man who has had type 1 diabetes since he was a teenager is being treated with insulin and complains of his increasing weight. He walks regularly for exercise. The patient monitors his blood glucose four to six times per day and treats low blood glucose with food. His most recent A1C (glycated hemoglobin) reading was 6.8. He is 71 inches (5 ft 11 in, 180 cm) tall and weighs 215 lb (97.5 kg), giving him a body mass index of 30 kg/m². To achieve better control of his blood glucose levels and decrease hypoglycemia and weight gain, the patient was given a drug that is a synthetic analogue of a neuroendocrine hormone synthesized by pancreatic β cells. At the same time, his insulin dosage was reduced. What is the naturally occurring hormone that this drug mimics?

    A. Insulin.

    B. Vasopressin.

    C. Amylin.

    D. Glucagon.

    E. Oxytocin.

Unit IV Answers and Explanations

1. A. Technosphere is administered by inhalation. It is contraindicated in people with chronic pulmonary diseases such as asthma or COPD.

B, C, D, E. Pramlintide, metformin, pioglitazone, and acarbose are also used to treat diabetes, but are not administered in a fashion that may impact respiratory function.

2. A. Clomiphene blocks estrogen receptors in the pituitary, thereby decreasing negative feedback and enhancing gonadotropin release.

B. Danazol is androgenic and will suppress gonadotropin release.

C. Medroxyprogesterone acetate is a contraceptive.

D. Metformin is used to treat diabetes.

E. Betamethasone is a corticosteroid.

3. A. Lanreotide is an analogue of somatostatin and will reduce growth hormone secretion.

B, C, D. Mecasermin (B) is an analogue of IGF-1, and would stimulate growth rather than inhibit it. Somatropin (C) is identical to growth hormone (D), and both would have the effect of enhancing growth and worsening the patients' condition.

E. Glucagon is not indicated for acromegaly.

4. B. The symptoms indicate hyperthyroidism, which is confirmed by the laboratory results. Thus, a drug is needed that will decrease thyroid hormone levels. Methimazole inhibits thyroid peroxidase, decreasing the formation of thyroxine (T_4) and triiodothyronine (T_3), and thus is an effective treatment for hyperthyroidism.

A, C-E. None of the other choices describe the mechanism of action of methimazole.

5. A. Iodine (supraphysiological dose) inhibits thyroid hormone release.

B-E. None of the other choices describe the rationale for giving iodine.

6. E. Radioactive iodine accumulates in the thyroid gland and destroys parenchymal cells thereby producing a long-term decrease in thyroid hormone levels.

A. Levothyroxine is the synthetic sodium salt of T_4, or thyroxine and is the drug of choice for replacement therapy of thyroid hormone in hypothyroidism.

B. Fluorouracil is a pyrimidine analogue used in treating cancer.

C. Parathyroid hormone is a hormone released from the parathyroid gland and is involved in calcium homeostasis.

D. Calcitriol ($1\alpha,25$-[OH]$_2$D$_3$) is the active form of vitamin D.

7. E. Biphosphonates are analogues of pyrophosphate that accumulate in bone and prevent bone resorption in osteoporosis by inhibiting osteoclast activity.

A. Because the goal is to stop taking estrogens, choice A is not valid.

B. Progestin does not have beneficial effects on bone.

C. Second-generation sulfonylureas are used to treat type 2 (noninsulin-dependent) diabetes mellitus.

D. Ergonovine is an ergot alkaloid used to prevent and treat postpartum hemorrhage and to hasten involution of the uterus.

8. A. Glucocorticoids suppress immune and inflammatory responses. Allergic reactions are caused by the immune response. None of the other choices describe the reasons for glucocorticoid effectiveness in allergic reactions.

9. D. These are signs and symptoms of primary adrenal insufficiency (Addison disease). The lack of cortisol response to intravenous administration of cosyntropin, an adrenocorticotropic hormone (ACTH) agonist, is confirmatory. Treatment is to replace the lack of cortisol with hydrocortisone, a synthetic glucocorticoid, given orally once or twice per day.

A. Corticorelin, or ovine corticotropin-releasing hormone, is used to differentiate pituitary ACTH-dependent Cushing disease from ectopic ACTH-secreting tumors (Cushing syndrome).

B. Aminoglutethimide suppresses the adrenal cortex by inhibiting enzymatic conversion of cholesterol to pregnenolone and inhibiting synthesis of adrenal steroids.

C. Levothyroxine is used for replacement therapy in hypothyroidism.

E. Mifepristone is a competitive antagonist of progesterone.

10. D. The symptoms indicate that the patient also has a deficiency of the mineralocorticoid aldosterone. Fludrocortisone is a synthetic mineralocorticoid used to treat aldosterone deficiency.

A. Cortisol is the natural glucocorticoid hormone and is not effective orally.

B. Spironolactone is an aldosterone antagonist that would worsen the patient's symptoms.

C. Dexamethasone is a synthetic glucocorticoid that would be unhelpful in treating the mineralocorticoid aspect of the disease.

E. Mifepristone is a competitive antagonist of progesterone.

11. D. Of the side effects listed, thromboembolism is the one most likely to be seen with estrogen therapy.

A and B. Acne is often seen in anabolic steroid usage (androgen effects) or progesterone therapy.

B. Lymphopenia is not seen with estrogen therapy.

C. Estrogen therapy may cause weight gain, not loss.

12. B. Abiraterone blocks the activity of CYP17. CYP17 catalyzes key reactions involved in the production of sex steroids, the conversion of pregnenolone to 17α-hydroxypregnenolone and progesterone to 17α-hydroxyprogesterone, as well as the conversion of 17α-hydroxypregnenolone to DHEA (Δ^5 pathway) and 17α-hydroxyprogesterone to androstenedione (Δ^4 pathway). Reducing the formation of these precursor androgens results in a decrease in all androgen production.

A, D. Prednisone and hydrocortisone are corticosteroids.

C. Mifepristone acts at the progesterone receptor and, at higher doses, the glucocorticoid receptor. It is also used as an abortifacient.

E. Spironolactone is a mineralocorticoid receptor antagonist.

13. E. This is a hypoglycemic emergency, and the patient is unable to take oral glucose (D). A bolus of dextrose (glucose) should be given, followed by continuous infusion of a dextrose-containing solution.

A-C. Insulin and the sulfonylureas are antihyperglycemics and would worsen the patient's condition.

14. B. Anastrozole is an aromatase inhibitor; it blocks CYP19 which is essential in the conversion of androgens to estrogens. Tamoxifen is a selective estrogen receptor modulator. The former reduces synthesis of estrogens, whereas the latter reduces the ability of estrogen to bind to the estrogen receptor. None of the other choices describe the difference between these two drugs.

15. B. Oxytocin is used for the induction or stimulation of labor.

A. Tamoxifen is a SERM used for breast cancer.

C. Leuprolide is an agonist of the GnRH receptor, used in conditions that require modulation of gonadotropin signaling such as central precocious puberty and endometriosis.

D. Prolactin is involved in lactation.

E. Serotonin is a neurotransmitter with many effects in areas such as the CNS and the gut, but is not used for inducing labor.

16. C. Dopamine is an inhibitor of prolactin secretion. Therefore, dopamine antagonists may cause disinhibition of prolactin secretion leading to hyperprolactinemia and subsequent effects on the breast.

A, B, D. Chlorpromazine does not increase aromatase activity, or decrease CYP17 activity, at any known significant levels.

17. A. The lifetime of the average red blood cell is approximately 3 months. The fraction of glycated hemoglobin is proportionate to glucose concentration experienced over that time. The other answers do not reflect this.

18. A. Somatropin is growth hormone and may be used to treat growth hormone deficiency.

B, C, D. Somatostatin, Octreotide, and Bromocriptine are used to treat excess growth hormone.

E. Technosphere is inhaled insulin.

19. A. The diagnosis of hyperglycemic hyperosmolar syndrome includes a plasma glucose of over 600 mg/dL, a calculated serum osmolality higher than 320 mmol/L, dehydration, declining mental status and possible seizures.

B, C, D. None of these matches the patient's presentation. Neuroglycopenia typically results from hypoglycemia, and ketoacidosis was not described in the patient's presentation. The patient has hyperglycemia, not hypoglycemia.

20. D. Ulipristal acetate is the only drug listed that matches the description.

A, C. Raloxifene and clomiphene are selective estrogen receptor modulators.

B. Faslodex is an estrogen receptor antagonist.

E. Estradiol binds to the estrogen receptor and is not a selective progesterone receptor modulator.

21. C. Blocking ATP-sensitive K^+ channels on the surface of pancreatic beta cells results in depolarization, increased intracellular calcium, and subsequent release of insulin.

A, B, D. None of these represents the mechanism of action of sulfonylureas.

22. B. Empagliflozin is a SGLT2 inhibitor. It acts by reducing the reabsorption of filtered glucose in the renal tubular lumen, thereby increasing the amount of glucose excreted in the urine.

A. Nateglinide stimulates insulin release and improves glucose uptake.

C. Liraglutide is an incretin mimetic.

D. Pioglitazone improves the target cell response to insulin, thereby enhancing glucose uptake.

E. Metformin reduces hepatic glucose output and improves insulin sensitivity.

23. B. Levothyroxine is the synthetic sodium salt of T_4, or thyroxine.

24. A. Mifepristone is a potent competitive antagonist of progesterone that terminates pregnancy by blocking the actions of progesterone on the uterus.

B. Diethylstilbestrol is a nonsteroidal synthetic estrogen used to treat postmenopausal osteoporosis.

C. Clomiphene is an antiestrogen used to stimulate ovulation.

D. Mestranol is a synthetic estrogen used in combination oral contraceptives.

E. Norethindrone is a synthetic progesterone used in combination oral contraceptives and for the treatment of dysfunctional uterine bleeding, dysmenorrhea, and endometriosis.

25. D. Clomiphene binds competitively to estrogen receptors, decreasing the sites available to endogenous estrogen. This decreases the normal feedback inhibition of endogenous estrogen to hypothalamic and pituitary estrogen receptors and results in increased secretion of gonadotropin-releasing hormone (GnRH), luteinizing hormone (LH), and follicle-stimulating hormone (FSH).

IV

26. D. Leuprolide is a GnRH analogue agonist. By activating the GnRH receptor, leuprolide initially stimulates the release of LH and FSH. Continuous exposure of the receptors to leuprolide, however, leads to their desensitization and a decreased release of FSH and LH.

C, E. Leuprolide does not restore normal ovulation in a patient with hypothalamic disease nor should it be considered for a patient with hypogonadotropic hypogonadism.

27. A. Type 1 diabetes mellitus is caused by autoimmune destruction of the insulin-producing β cells of the pancreas. Therefore, replacement of insulin is the most effective treatment.

B–D. Tolbutamide, glyburide, and metformin are oral hypoglycemic agents that are effective only in type 2 (noninsulin-dependent) diabetes mellitus.

28. A. NPH insulin is an intermediate-acting insulin.

B. Insulin lispro is a rapid-acting insulin.

C. Metformin is an oral hypoglycemic agent for type 2 (non-insulin-dependent) diabetes mellitus.

D. Glyburide is a second-generation sulfonylurea derivative that increases insulin secretion by blocking ATP-sensitive K^+ channels on the surface of pancreatic β cells.

29. A. The gonadotropins contain FSH and LH; FSH stimulates the development and maturation of the ovarian follicle. LH causes ovulation and stimulates the development of the corpus luteum.

B. Gonadotropins are not antiprogestins.

C. Gonadotropins contain FSH and therefore enhance, not block, its actions.

D. The gonadotropins contain FSH and LH; they do not increase their release.

E. Gonadotropins are not effective orally because they are metabolized in the gut.

30. C. Myxedema is another name for hypothyroidism, a condition in which the thyroid does not produce enough thyroid hormones (T_3 and T_4). In severe cases, the patient may go into a coma and a rapidly acting therapy is required. Liothyronine is the synthetic sodium salt of triiodothyronine (T_3) and acts more rapidly than T_4.

A. Thyroglobulin is a protein found in the thyroid that plays a critical role in thyroid hormone synthesis.

B. Thyroid extract, or desiccated thyroid, contains a mix of T_3 and T_4 and was used to treat hypothyroidism prior to the development of synthetic T_3 and T_4.

D. Levothyroxine has a slower onset and a longer duration of action.

31. E. Bromocriptine and cabergoline are dopamine analogue agonists at the D^2 dopamine receptor. Activation of D^2 receptors inhibits prolactin release.

A. Chlorpromazine is a D^2 antagonist antipsychotic agent.

B–D. Phenytoin is an anticonvulsant, diazepam is a benzodiazepine, and lithium is an antimanic drug.

32. D. Methyltestosterone is a 17α-alkylated form of testosterone. It acts like testosterone to increase facial hair, cause acne, deepen the voice, and increase muscle strength. Unlike testosterone, it also may produce liver dysfunction leading to jaundice.

33. E. Glucocorticoids suppress inflammatory responses, including neutrophil actions, eicosanoid release, and late-phase allergic reactions, which can increase susceptibility to infection.

A-D. Corticosteroids do not predispose patients to the other choices.

34. E. Acarbose is an α-glucosidase inhibitor that delays absorption of carbohydrates, thus blunting the postprandial increase in blood glucose. Gastrointestinal (GI) disturbances, e.g., flatulence, are common with this drug.

A-D. The drug is not absorbed from the GI tract and does not produce any of the other listed symptoms.

35. A. The symptoms indicate hypothyroidism, which is confirmed by the laboratory results. Levothyroxine is the synthetic sodium salt of T_4, or thyroxine and is the drug of choice for replacement therapy.

B. Propylthiouracil inhibits the synthesis of thyroid hormones and is used in hyperthyroidism.

C. Psyllium is a bulk-forming laxative effective for constipation, but this patient has already tried laxatives to no avail.

D. SSRIs are effective for depression, but the patient's other symptoms indicate that the depression is secondary to hypothyroidism, so the primary cause should be treated.

E. Radioactive iodine accumulates in the thyroid gland and destroys parenchymal cells; it is used to treat hyperthyroidism.

36. A. Long-term therapy with estrogens increases the risk of stroke and thromboembolism.

B–E. Estrogen replacement therapy is not associated with the other choices.

37. A. Clomiphene is an antiestrogen with weak estrogenic activity. It binds to estrogen receptors and prevents the normal feedback inhibition by estrogen of gonadotropin-releasing hormone (GnRH) secretion. GnRH in turn stimulates the secretion of LH and FSH which stimulate ovulation.

38. B. Of the drugs listed, testosterone is the best choice for treatment of hypergonadism.

A, C, D. Methyltestosterone, fluoxymesterone, and danazol contain 17α-alkyl substitutions to retard hepatic degradation. Although these drugs are orally effective, they have a less favorable side effect profile compared with testosterone.

F. Norethindrone is a synthetic progesterone.

39. C. The drug the patient was given was pramlintide, a synthetic analogue of amylin. Amylin is a neuroendocrine hormone synthesized by pancreatic β cells. Pramlintide improves postprandial glucose control and may also increase satiety, leading to decreased caloric intake and weight loss. It is given by subcutaneous injection with every meal to reduce postprandial hyperglycemia and requires a reduction in the dose of insulin.

A. Insulin is a hormone produced by β cells, but the patient is already taking insulin.

B. Vasopressin, also known as arginine vasopressin or antidiuretic hormone (ADH), is a peptide hormone that controls the reabsorption of water and other molecules in the kidney.

D. Glucagon is a natural hormone synthesized and secreted by the α cells of the pancreas. It is used in emergency situations to treat hypoglycemia.

E. Oxytocin is a pituitary hormone synthesized in the hypothalamus and released into the blood from the posterior lobe (neurohypophysis) of the pituitary gland. It is involved in birth and breastfeeding.

Unit V

Drugs Acting on the Renal and Cardiovascular Systems

By June Yun

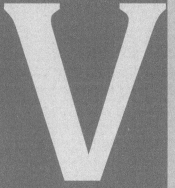

19 Renal Pharmacology

Summary

There are two major types of drugs that affect the kidney—diuretics and antidiuretics. Diuretics are drugs that promote the excretion of urine. Antidiuretics decrease urine production. Antidiuretic drugs and inhibitors are used in cases of insufficient or excess antidiuretic hormone (ADH). Diuretics are the main class of drug used in renal pharmacology to decrease edema, treat heart failure, and as antihypertensives. Mannitol is an osmotic diuretic used to reduce cerebrospinal or intraocular pressure in acute renal failure or to dilute toxins in urine. Acetazolamide is a carbonic anhydrase inhibitor used in the treatment of glaucoma, acute mountain sickness, and metabolic alkalosis. Furosemide, bumetanide, and ethacrynic acid are loop (high-ceiling) diuretics for edema due to congestive heart failure, acute oliguria, hypertension, and acute hypercalcemia. Thiazide diuretics (hydrochlorothiazide, chlorothiazide, and chlorthalidone) are the standard of therapy in mild to moderate hypertension. Spironolactone and eplerenone are potassium-sparing diuretics used to treat primary aldosteronism, heart failure, resistant hypertension, hyperuricemia, hypokalemia, or glucose intolerance. Triamterene and amiloride are used to treat hypertension when given along with the thiazides to prevent K^+ depletion. Vasopressin (8-arginine vasopressin), also known as ADH, is a peptide hormone. Desmopressin (1-deamino-8-D-arginine vasopressin) is a synthetic arginine analogue of vasopressin used to treat diabetes insipidus of pituitary origin, primary nocturnal enuresis (bedwetting) in children and adults, and as an adjunct in hemophilia therapy (vasopressin increases circulating levels of blood clotting factor VIII). The vasopressin antagonists conivaptan, tolvaptan, and demeclocycline are used to treat hyponatremia.

Keywords: diuretic, antidiuretic, kidney, thiazide, loop diuretic, carbonic anhydrase, potassium sparing

19.1 Introduction

There are two major types of drugs that affect the kidney—diuretics and antidiuretics. Diuretics are drugs that promote the excretion of urine. Antidiuretics decrease urine production. Antidiuretic drugs are used in cases of insufficient or excess antidiuretic hormone (ADH). Diuretics are widely used as one of the primary therapies for hypertension and for heart failure. They are also used to increase urine production in a variety of situations.

19.2 Overview of Renal Physiology

The major functions of the kidneys are to eliminate metabolic waste and foreign substances from the body; control the excretion of water and electrolytes (salts) to maintain fluid volume, osmolality, and acid–base balance; to produce renin and other hormones that regulate erythropoiesis and Ca^{2+} metabolism; and aid in the metabolism of glucose (▶ Fig. 19.1).

19.2.1 Renal Transport Systems

The functional unit of the kidney is the nephron. Each section of the nephron and its effects on water and electrolyte excretion are explained in ▶ Table 19.1 and illustrated in ▶ Fig. 19.2.

19.2.2 Renin–Angiotensin–Aldosterone Relationship

Renin

Renin is an enzyme released by juxtaglomerular cells in the kidney. The enzyme cleaves the serum protein angiotensinogen

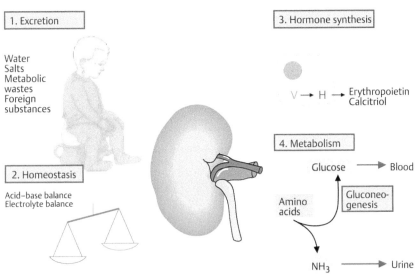

Fig. 19.1 Functions of the kidney.
The kidneys play an important role in excretion, homeostasis, hormone synthesis, and metabolism. H, hormone; V, prohormone.

Table 19.1 Water and electrolyte movement at different sections of the nephron

Section of the nephron	Effects
Proximal convoluted tubule	Approximately 60 to 70% of the filtered Na^+ and K^+ ions are removed isotonically from the proximal tubule. After passing the length of the proximal tubule, the volume of the filtrate is reduced by 30 to 40% without altering Na^+ or K^+ ion concentrations. Actively transported species include Na^+, K^+, and HCO_3^-. If Na^+ and K^+ ion reabsorption is inhibited at this site, the transport mechanisms in the remaining nephron (loop of Henle and distal convoluted tubule) can fully compensate, and the final urine composition is not altered. HCO_3^- reabsorption and urine pH are primarily controlled in the proximal tubule
Ascending loop of Henle	Approximately 15 to 20% of the total filtered Na^+ and Cl^- load are reabsorbed at this site by Na^+–K^+–$2Cl^-$ cotransporter
Distal convoluted tubule	Approximately 8 to 10% of the Na^+ and K^+ load is reabsorbed in the distal convoluted tubule. Active transport mechanisms are present in the distal convoluted tubule for Na^+, K^+, and Cl^-. Cotransport or exchange transport mechanisms exist in the distal convoluted tubule for both Na^+–H^+ exchange and Na^+–K^+ exchange
Collecting tubule and duct	Na^+–K^+ exchange and, to some extent, Na^+–H^+ ion exchange are controlled by aldosterone and urine Na^+ concentrations. When the Na^+ concentrations increase in the distal tubule, Na^+ ions are absorbed in exchange for K^+ ion and H^+ ion excretion. Increased aldosterone thus increases Na^+ ion retention in the plasma and urinary K^+ excretion. There is a resultant decrease in urine pH (H^+ ion excretion in the urine)

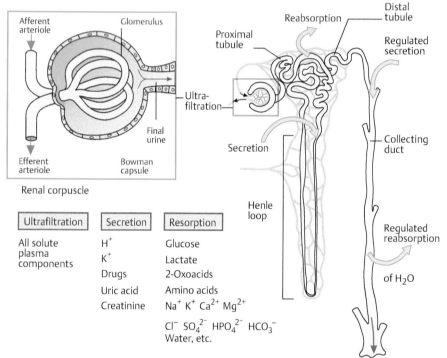

Fig. 19.2 Urine formation.
Urine is formed by the ultrafiltration, secretion, and reabsorption of substances at different parts of the nephron. The relative quantities are regulated by the kidneys to maintain homeostasis.

into the decapeptide angiotensin I (▶ Fig. 19.3). Angiotensin I is then further acted upon by angiotensin-converting enzyme (ACE) in the lung to produce the octapeptide angiotensin II. Angiotensin II acts directly as a vasoconstrictor and also stimulates aldosterone release from the adrenal cortex. The renin–angiotensin mechanism for aldosterone release is dependent upon the actions of both renin and ACE for the activation of angiotensinogen. Increased quantities of renin are released by the kidneys into the systemic circulation under conditions of

- Low plasma (Na^+).
- Low arterial blood pressure.
- Increased sympathetic nervous system stimulation.

Foundations

Ultrafiltration and Starling Forces

Ultrafiltration of plasma occurs as plasma moves from glomerular capillaries into Bowman's capsule under the influence of Starling forces. Glomerular filtration is the same mechanism as systemic capillary filtration, that is, the balance between hydrostatic and oncotic forces across the glomerular membrane determines the direction of fluid movement. Glomerular capillary hydrostatic pressure is the main driving force for ultrafiltration across the glomerular membrane. This is opposed by the hydrostatic pressure in Bowman's capsule and glomerular capillary oncotic pressure.

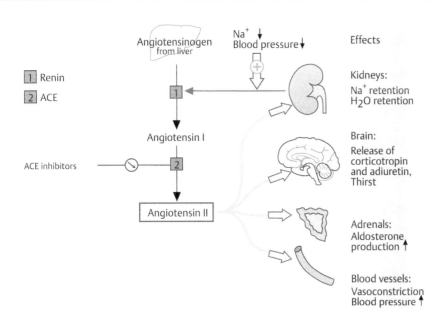

Fig. 19.3 Renin–angiotensin system.
The kidneys produce renin in response to low blood pressure or low plasma Na^+ concentration. Renin acts on angiotensinogen in plasma to form angiotensin I. Angiotensin I is converted to angiotensin II in the lungs by the action of angiotensin-converting enzyme (ACE). Angiotensin II acts as a hormone and a neurotransmitter on different organs to produce changes that help restore blood pressure and Na^+ homeostasis.

Foundations

Glomerular Versus Systemic Capillaries

The glomerular capillaries are much more permeable than average systemic capillaries, due to both increased permeability and surface area. Approximately 180 L/day of fluid are filtered across glomerular capillaries, while only 4 L/day of fluid would have been filtered if these were systemic capillaries. The ultrafiltration coefficient (Kf = membrane permeability × surface area) for glomerular capillaries is about 40 to 50 times greater than for systemic capillaries.

Foundations

Vasa Recta

The vasa recta of the kidneys are capillaries derived from efferent arterioles of juxtamedullary nephrons and are the blood supply of the medulla. These vessels are U-shaped, composed of thin, fenestrated epithelial cells, and run parallel with the loops of Henle. Blood flow through them is very slow and they are permeable to water and solutes. These properties allow the efficient exchange of water and solutes with the surrounding interstitial fluid, which is fundamental to maintaining the osmotic gradient in the medulla that is ultimately responsible for the production of concentrated urine. The vasa recta eventually drain into the renal vein. Due to the slow blood flow, the vasa recta are potential sites for thrombosis in hypercoagulable states.

Aldosterone

The mineralocorticoid aldosterone is secreted from the adrenal cortex and plays an important role in the control of renal Na^+ excretion and extracellular electrolyte balance. Secretion of aldosterone is controlled primarily by circulating levels of angiotensin II. In the nephrons, aldosterone acts in the distal tubule, connecting tubule, and collecting ducts to regulate ion channels that lead to increased Na^+ and water retention, and increased K^+ and H^+ secretion. The net results of the actions of aldosterone are as follows:

- Na^+ ion retention.
- Increased extracellular fluid volume.
- Increased K^+ and H^+ excretion.
- Mild metabolic alkalosis.

19.3 Diuretics

Diuretics are the main class of drug used in renal pharmacology. They increase the production of urine by acting in the kidney to alter salt and water excretion. The major indications for use of diuretics are to decrease edema, treat heart failure, and as antihypertensives.

Most diuretics increase urine flow by altering the reabsorption of Na^+ ions, and, along with them, Cl^- and water, at different sites in the nephron (▶ Fig. 19.4). Osmotic diuretics, however, increase urine flow directly. The capacity to increase urine flow make diuretics effective in treating conditions such as hypertension and heart failure (HF).

Clinical Correlation

Mannitol in Head Injury Management

Mannitol is widely used to reduce intracranial pressure (ICP), which can result from traumatic brain injury. In this setting, mannitol is preferentially administered as an intravenous (IV) bolus. Two mechanisms are thought to contribute to mannitol's beneficial effects. First, volume expansion reduces blood viscosity, and increasing cerebral blood flow induces an autoregulatory vasoconstriction of cerebral vessels, reducing cerebral blood volume. Second, mannitol creates an osmotic gradient that draws water out of brain tissue and into the intravascular space, thus decreasing edema (and ICP).

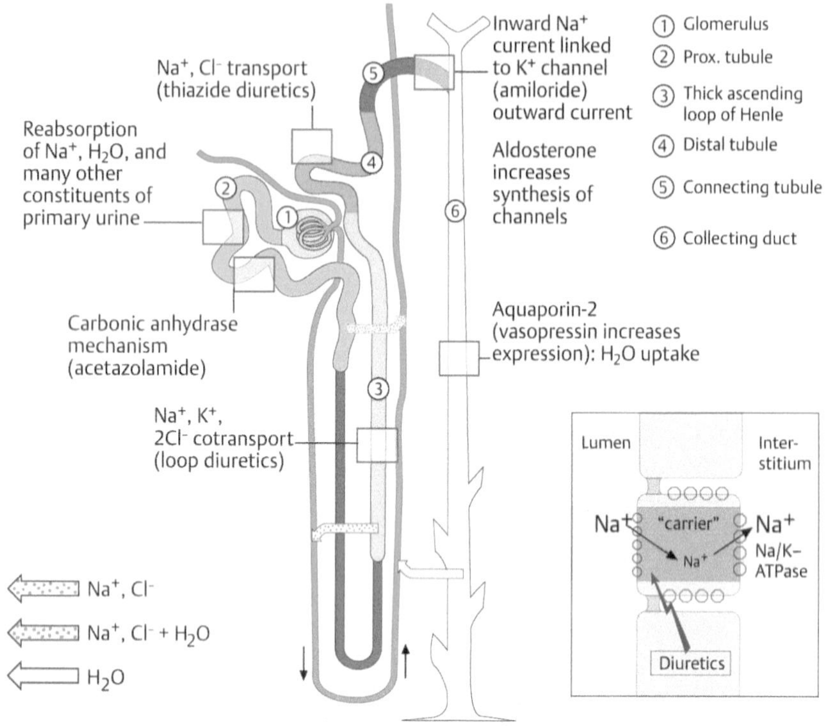

Fig. 19.4 Renal actions of diuretics.
Na^+ ions are normally transported into cells from the lumen of the tubules by carrier molecules. They are then secreted into the interstitium by the Na^+–K^+–ATPase pump. Diuretics act at different parts of the nephron to inhibit Na^+ reabsorption. The higher Na^+ load in urine increases its osmolarity, which causes water to be drawn into it and excreted.

Labels in figure:

- Na$^+$, Cl$^-$ transport (thiazide diuretics)
- Reabsorption of Na$^+$, H$_2$O, and many other constituents of primary urine
- Carbonic anhydrase mechanism (acetazolamide)
- Na$^+$, K$^+$, 2Cl$^-$ cotransport (loop diuretics)
- Inward Na$^+$ current linked to K$^+$ channel (amiloride) outward current
- Aldosterone increases synthesis of channels
- Aquaporin-2 (vasopressin increases expression): H$_2$O uptake

① Glomerulus
② Prox. tubule
③ Thick ascending loop of Henle
④ Distal tubule
⑤ Connecting tubule
⑥ Collecting duct

Na$^+$, Cl$^-$
Na$^+$, Cl$^-$ + H$_2$O
H$_2$O

Lumen — Interstitium
Na$^+$ — "carrier" — Na$^+$ — Na/K–ATPase
Na$^+$
Diuretics

Clinical Correlation

Osmotic Diuresis with Diabetes

Glucose is normally freely filtered at the glomerulus and is completely reabsorbed in the proximal tubule of the kidneys. In diabetes, however, high plasma glucose levels exceed the maximum tubular transport capacity (Tm), as transporter proteins become saturated. Glucose remains in the tubule and exerts an osmotic pressure that prevents water reabsorption along the nephron. More water in the filtrate disrupts the Na$^+$ concentration gradients needed for Na + reabsorption leading to more Na$^+$ being excreted. These factors explain polyuria (excessive urination), polydipsia (excessive thirst), and dehydration that are common presenting symptoms in diabetes.

Clinical Correlation

Diabetic Nephropathy

Diabetes mellitus is a leading cause of chronic renal failure. The main pathogenic feature is glomerular disease with thickening of the glomerular basement membrane and glomerulosclerosis. This leads to alterations in glomerular filtrations and causes proteinuria to develop; eventually the glomerular filtration rate is irreversibly reduced. Clinically, signs and symptoms include those seen with diabetes and its associated disorders, such as retinopathy, neuropathy, hypertension, peripheral vascular disease, coronary artery disease, nonhealing ulcers, as well as frothy urine, proteinuria, and edema (if nephrotic syndrome develops [see call-out box]). Patients show albuminuria (> 30 mg/day), reduced glomerular filtration rate, and elevated arterial blood pressure. Treatment involves meticulous glycemic control and ACE inhibitors to slow progression to chronic renal failure. Ultimately dialysis or renal transplantation may be needed.

19.3.1 Osmotic Diuretics

Mannitol

Mechanism of Action

Osmotic diuretics are freely filtered at the glomerulus but not reabsorbed. Mannitol is the prototypical drug in this class.

Osmotic diuretics remain in the lumen and exert an opposing osmotic force that prevents water from being reabsorbed in the proximal tubule and the descending limb of the Loop of Henle (LOH). Sodium continues to be reabsorbed but this declines as more water is retained in the lumen and the sodium gradient becomes disrupted. Thus, although both sodium and water are lost, a greater proportion of water is lost than sodium. Sodium will also be reabsorbed in distal nephron sites. Dilution of the luminal fluid also disrupts the reabsorption of most other electrolytes (e.g., K$^+$, Ca^{2+}, Mg^{2+}). Mannitol is unable to freely cross cell membranes. Therefore, mannitol in the extracellular space draws water from cells, leading to extracellular volume expansion. Renal blood flow is increased, resulting in wash out of the corticomedullary osmotic gradient, and inhibition of urine concentration (▸ Fig. 19.5).

Pharmacokinetics

Mannitol is available for IV administration.

Uses

- Acute reduction of cerebrospinal or intraocular pressure.
- Oliguric acute renal failure.
- To dilute toxins in urine.

Contraindications

- Anuria.
- Severe pulmonary edema or congestion.
- Active intracranial bleeding.

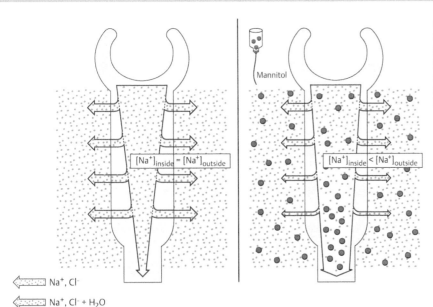

Fig. 19.5 Sodium chloride (NaCl) reabsorption in the proximal tubule and the effect of mannitol. Mannitol increases the osmolality of the glomerular filtrate. In the proximal tubule this causes reduced reabsorption of water relative to Na$^+$. Overall this causes increased urine flow with little increase in Na$^+$ excretion.

Na$^+$, Cl$^-$

Na$^+$, Cl$^-$ + H$_2$O

[Na$^+$]$_{inside}$ = [Na$^+$]$_{outside}$

[Na$^+$]$_{inside}$ < [Na$^+$]$_{outside}$

Mannitol

Side Effects

Increase in extracellular fluid volume (ECF) can lead to pulmonary edema and complicate HF. The increased ECF can dilute plasma and cause symptoms of hyponatremia, whereas greater loss of water over sodium can lead to hypernatremia.

19.3.2 Carbonic Anhydrase Inhibitors

Torsemide, Acetazolamide, Brinzolamide, Dorzolamide, Methazolamide

Mechanism of Action

Carbonic anhydrase (CA) inhibitors inhibit both cytoplasmic and luminal CA in the proximal convoluted tubule to reduce the reabsorption of HCO$_3^-$ ions from the glomerular filtrate (▶ Fig. 19.6). This also leads to sodium and water loss in urine.

By inhibiting CA, HCO$_3^-$, and H$^+$ concentrations in tubular lumen increase. Disruption of H$^+$ concentration reduces Na$^+$–H$^+$ antiporter activity reducing Na$^+$ (and water) reabsorption. However, the overall diuretic effect is modest since the sodium can be reabsorbed in more distal nephron segments. The loss of bicarbonate can cause metabolic acidosis, which further limits their use as diuretics. Because of these reasons, CA inhibitors are not used for their diuretic properties.

Uses

- Treatment of glaucoma (inhibits aqueous humor formation to reduce ocular pressure).
- Prophylaxis and treatment of acute mountain sickness.
- Metabolic alkalosis.
- Epilepsy.

Side Effects

These include drowsiness and paresthesias (sensations of numbness or tingling of the skin), metabolic acidosis, potential hypersensitivity (these are sulfonamide drugs), and formation of kidney stones.

Contraindications

- Liver cirrhosis.

19.3.3 Loop (High-Ceiling) Diuretics

Furosemide, Bumetanide, and Ethacrynic Acid

Mechanism of Action

The loop diuretics bind to the Cl$^-$ binding site of the Na$^+$–K$^+$–2Cl$^-$ cotransporter (NKCC2) in the thick ascending limb of LOH to inhibit the reabsorption of Na$^+$, K$^+$, and Cl$^-$ (▶ Fig. 19.6). Reabsorption of Mg^{2+} and Ca^{2+} is also reduced, by disrupting the lumen-positive transepithelial potential that drives paracellular reabsorption of these cations. Increased delivery of Na$^+$ to the distal tubule and cortical collecting duct results in increased Na$^+$ reabsorption here, which is coupled to increased K$^+$ and H$^+$ secretion (▶ Fig. 19.6). This can lead to hypokalemic metabolic alkalosis. Inhibition of NKCC2 also disrupts the generation of a hyperosmotic gradient in the renal interstitium, preventing formation of a concentrated urine. The loop diuretics are actively secreted into the proximal convoluted tubule from plasma and are the most effective natriuretic and diuretic agents available. They can inhibit the reabsorption of up to 25% of the filtered sodium.

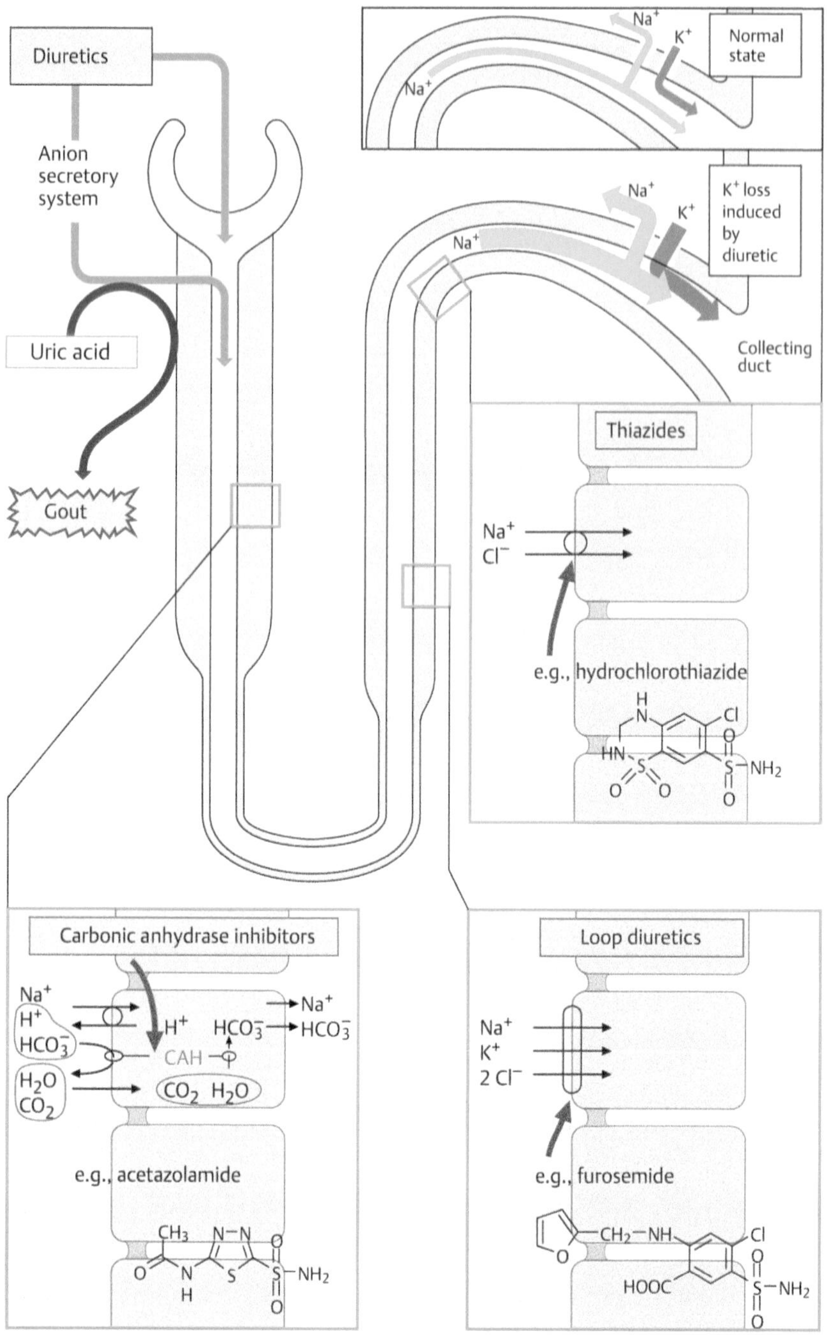

Fig. 19.6 Action of thiazides, loop diuretics, and carbonic anhydrase inhibitors.
Thiazide diuretics inhibit the Na^+–Cl^- cotransporter on the luminal membrane of tubular cells. This leads to reduced reabsorption of NaCl and water. Loop diuretics produce a strong diuresis by inhibiting the Na^+–K^+–$2Cl^-$ cotransporter in the thick ascending loop of Henle. Carbonic anhydrase (CA) inhibitors inhibit the production and absorption of bicarbonate in tubular cells. This causes less Na^+ reabsorption because fewer H^+ ions are available for the Na^+–H^+ antiporter.

Foundations

Metabolic Acidosis

Metabolic acidosis occurs when there is excess production of H^+ in the body causing blood pH to fall. One of the situations in which this occurs is diabetic ketoacidosis (DKA), when acidic ketone bodies (acetoacetic acid, β hydroxybutyric acid, and acetone) are produced from the breakdown of fat. Bicarbonate ions (HCO_3^-) buffer some of the excess H^+ ions by binding to them, producing carbonic acid, which then dissociates to form carbon dioxide (CO_2) and water. Centrally, the fall in blood pH stimulates the respiratory center in the medulla to initiate hyperventilation. This hyperventilation (known as Kussmaul respiration) "blows off" CO_2, thus lowering partial pressure of CO_2 (pCO_2), causing blood pH to rise. Renal compensation involves virtually complete reabsorption of HCO_3^-, which replenishes that used to buffer the excess acid. There is also increase in excretion of titratable acid and NH_4^+.

V

Clinical Correlation

Kidney Stones

Kidney stones in the renal pelvis and ureters will increase hydrostatic pressure in the Bowman's capsule and therefore greatly reduce the glomerular filtration rate. Uric acid kidney stones may sometimes be dissolved by alkalinizing the urine with potassium citrate. Kidney stones that are less than 0.5 inch in diameter can be fragmented by applying focused ultrasound waves (lithotripsy).

Pharmacokinetics

These agents have a rapid onset of action (within 10–20 minutes following IV administration).

Uses

- Edema due to heart failure (HF), pulmonary edema, cirrhosis.
- Acute oliguria (by maintaining urine formation).
- Hypertension (less effective than thiazides, used in glomerular filtration rate < 30 mL/minute).
- Acute hypercalcemia.

Side Effects

Loop diuretics are more potent than thiazides and thus have more potential for side effects, which may include:
- Dehydration.
- Electrolyte disturbances: hypokalemia, hypocalcemia, hypomagnesemia.
- Ototoxicity (greater risk with ethacrynic acid).
- Metabolic alkalosis (loss of Cl^-, but not HCO_3^-).
- Hyperuricemia (interferes with secretion of uric acid in the proximal convoluted tubules and may precipitate gouty arthritis [see Chapter 33 for a discussion of gout]).
- Allergic reactions as these drugs (except ethacrynic acid) are related to the antibacterial sulfonamides.
- Increased renin production.

19.3.4 Thiazide Diuretics

Hydrochlorothiazide, Chlorothiazide, Chlorthalidone, Indapamide, and Meolazine

Note: Chlorthalidone, indapamide, and meolazine are not chemically thiazides, but have the same mechanism of action.

Mechanism of Action

The thiazide diuretics are actively secreted into the proximal convoluted tubule and inhibit Na^+ reabsorption in the distal convoluted tubule by inhibiting the Na^+–Cl^- cotransporter (NCC) (▶ Fig. 19.6). Reducing intracellular Na^+ increases basolateral Na^+–Ca^{2+} exchange (via NCX), resulting in greater Ca^{2+} reabsorption. The thiazide diuretics are weak inhibitors of CA, but diuresis is not dependent upon an inhibition of CA. Incomplete inhibition of CA does produce a small increase in urine pH. All thiazide diuretics share a common mechanism of action and common side effects. They differ from each other in potency and duration of action.

Pharmacokinetics

Orally effective.

Uses

- Thiazide diuretics are the standard of therapy in mild to moderate hypertension. They are frequently given along with other antihypertensive medications and can potentiate the action of other antihypertensive drugs. Thiazides are more effective in lowering blood pressure than loop diuretics in patients without edema.
- Nephrogenic diabetes insipidus (paradoxical antidiuretic effect [see call-out box]).

Side Effects

- Renal failure due to a decreased glomerular filtration rate.
- Hyperuricemia, which may precipitate gouty arthritis.
- Hypokalemic alkalosis (due to K^+ loss). This is rarely a problem in normal patients, but it may be problematic in patients with cardiac arrhythmias, especially if they are on digitalis or have severe liver disease.
- Hyperglycemia (decreased glucose tolerance).
- Hypercholesterolemia and hypertriglyceridemia (mild effect).

Clinical Correlation

Pulmonary Edema

Pulmonary edema is fluid accumulation in the lungs. Its acute formation constitutes a medical emergency. It is usually caused by left ventricular failure, which renders the heart unable to adequately drain fluid from the lung. Left ventricular failure may be caused by such conditions as myocardial infarction and hypertension. Other causes of pulmonary edema are direct injury to the lung parenchyma, pneumonia, toxins, and high altitude. Signs and symptoms include difficulty in breathing, coughing up blood (hemoptysis), anxiety, sweating, pale skin, and pink, frothy sputum. Treatment involves sitting the patient up, oxygen therapy, administering a loop diuretic, nitrate administration, and treating the underlying cause.

Clinical Correlation

Acute Renal Failure

Acute renal failure produces a sharp rise in urea, creatinine, K^+ (hyperkalemia) and Na^+ (hypernatremia) usually with oliguria (low urine output) or anuria (no urine output). There may also be vomiting, confusion, bruising, or GI bleeding. A metabolic acidosis (usually with a normal anion gap) will occur due to the failure to excrete H^+ as titratable acid and NH_4^+. Acute renal failure may occur due to disease of the kidneys themselves, which may be vascular, septic, neoplastic, due to drugs, or due to pregnancy. Extra renal causes include burns, sepsis, trauma, heart failure, and obstruction. Treatment should be aimed at the underlying cause but hyperkalemia may require urgent correction to avoid cardiac complications (see call-out box). Loop diuretics are given for oliguria/anuria.

Clinical Correlation

Nephrotic Syndrome

Nephrotic syndrome results in severe proteinuria (loss of proteins into the urine), hypoalbuminemia, and edema due to the decrease in capillary oncotic pressure. Causes of nephrotic syndrome include glomerulonephritis (inflammation of the glomerulus), diabetes, neoplasia, and drugs. Signs include peripheral edema, ascites, and swelling of the eyelids. Venous thrombosis and emboli may occur due to excretion of certain clotting factors and antithrombin III in the urine. Treatment involves addressing the underlying cause plus the administration of a loop diuretic with a K^+-sparing agent, plasma protein replacement (without salt), and anticoagulation (if necessary).

Clinical Correlation

Hyperkalemia

Hyperkalemia (elevated potassium levels) usually occurs due to metabolic acidosis when K^+ is taken up by tubular cells in exchange for H^+ secretion via the H^+–K^+–ATPase antiporter. Hyperkalemia may also be caused by renal failure, severe tissue damage (e.g., rhabdomyolysis), massive blood transfusions, Addison's disease, and potassium-sparing diuretics. Symptoms include palpitations, malaise, and muscle weakness. Severe hyperkalemia (> 6.5 mmol/L) is a medical emergency as it can cause ventricular fibrillation and sudden death. Electrocardiography findings in hyperkalemia include small P waves, widened QRS complexes, and peaked T waves. Treatment is aimed at the underlying cause. In an emergency, calcium gluconate is given IV to reduce myocardial excitability; insulin and 50% glucose are given IV to shift K^+ into cells (via activity of Na^+–K^+–ATPase); and bicarbonate is given to correct acidosis. Hemodialysis may also be necessary to increase K^+ elimination.

19.3.5 Potassium-sparing Diuretics

Spironolactone, Eplerenone

Mechanism of Action

Spironolactone and eplerenone act as competitive antagonists of aldosterone at the cytosolic mineralocorticoid receptor in epithelial cells of the late distal convoluted tubule and collecting duct to reduce reabsorption of Na^+, Cl^-, and water.

Aldosterone normally increases the synthesis and number of ENaC Na^+ channels and Na^+–K^+–ATPases expressed in cell membranes. Inhibiting aldosterone leads to a reduction in the number of membrane-localized channels and transporters, thereby reducing reabsorption of Na^+, Cl^-, and water. As K^+ secretion is coupled to Na^+ reabsorption at these sites, K^+ is retained.

Uses

- Primary aldosteronism (overproduction of aldosterone).
- Heart failure.
- Resistant hypertension: spironolactone is adjunctive therapy for hypertension that remains uncontrolled despite a three-drug regimen.

- May be useful in patients with hyperuricemia, hypokalemia, or glucose intolerance.

Side Effects

- Hyperkalemia (high blood K^+).
- Diarrhea, nausea, and vomiting.
- Headaches, confusion, and somnolence.
- Gynecomastia (with spironolactone).

Triamterene and Amiloride

Mechanism of Action

These drugs directly interfere with Na^+ transport in the distal convoluted tubule by directly inhibiting epithelial sodium channels (▶ Fig. 19.7). Although the drugs do not act on the renin–angiotensin axis, the net effect on urinary composition is similar.

Uses

Triamterene and amiloride are used to treat hypertension. They are weak diuretics and have little hypotensive action when given alone. However, they are useful when given along with the thiazides to prevent K^+ depletion.

Side Effects

- Hyperkalemia.

Note: Do not use potassium-sparing diuretics and potassium supplements together.

19.3.6 Over-the-Counter Drugs as Diuretics

Most over-the-counter drugs promoted as diuretic agents contain caffeine (100 mg) and/or ammonium chloride (~ 500 mg). The drugs have, at best, only a mild diuretic action. Caffeine mildly inhibits Na^+ reabsorption in renal tubules, and ammonium chloride metabolism results in urea formation and excretion of a Cl^- ion. Na^+ passively follows the increased Cl^- load, resulting in mild diuresis.

19.4 Antidiuretic Drugs

19.4.1 Vasopressin

Vasopressin (8-arginine vasopressin), also known as ADH, is a peptide hormone composed of nine amino acids. It is synthesized in the hypothalamus and transported to its site of release in the posterior pituitary (see also Chapter 16). The main stimuli for vasopressin release are hyperosmolality of the blood and volume depletion. Two types of vasopressin receptors are known:

- V_1 receptors stimulate contraction of vascular smooth muscles (▶ Fig. 19.8).
- V_2 receptors stimulate water reabsorption in the renal tubule through a cyclic adenosine monophosphate (cAMP)-dependent mechanism.

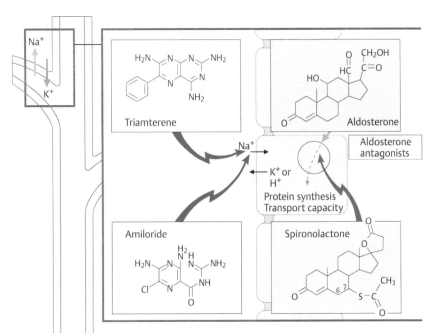

Fig. 19.7 Potassium-sparing diuretics.
These drugs inhibit Na^+ reabsorption and K^+ secretion in the tubules and proximal part of the collecting duct. This produces a mild diuresis without depleting potassium. Aldosterone increases the synthesis of Na^+ channel proteins and Na^+–K^+–ATPases, which promotes the reabsorption of Na^+, Cl^-, and water. Spironolactone is an antagonist at the aldosterone receptor and inhibits the normal action of aldosterone.

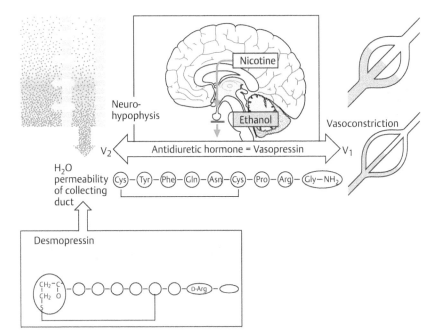

Fig. 19.8 Vasopressin (antidiuretic hormone [ADH] and derivatives).
Vasopressin acts on V_2 receptors to promote the reabsorption of water. This occurs due to an increased expression of aquaporins, which increases the permeability of collecting duct epithelium to water. Vasopressin also acts on V_1 receptors on vascular smooth muscle, producing vasoconstriction. Desmopressin is an analogue of vasopressin that produces a varying amount of antidiuretic and vasoconstrictive effects. Nicotine increases and ethanol decreases vasopressin secretion.

Vasopressin is found in other areas of the brain and may promote learning and improve long-term memory.

Clinical Correlation

Treatment of Nephrogenic Diabetes Insipidus

In nephrogenic diabetes insipidus, the kidneys are unresponsive to vasopressin, and thiazide diuretics cause a paradoxical reduction in polyuria. The mechanism for this effect is uncertain, but is presumed to be due to an increase in proximal tubular sodium and water reabsorption due to hypovolemia. Thiazides inhibit NaCl reabsorption in the early segments of the distal tubule but have little effect in the thick ascending limb, which

is involved in concentrating the urine. In the ascending limb, water is reabsorbed along with Na^+.

Clinical Correlation

Syndrome of Inappropriate Secretion of Antidiuretic Hormone

Syndrome of inappropriate ADH secretion (SIADH) occurs when excessive amounts of ADH are secreted from the posterior pituitary gland. This leads to hyponatremia (low plasma Na^+) and fluid overload. Causes include head injury, meningitis, infections (e.g., brain abscess), pneumonia, and cancer. Treatment involves addressing the cause and using demeclocycline or lithium carbonate for symptomatic control.

19.4.2 Desmopressin

Desmopressin (1-deamino-8-D-arginine vasopressin) is a synthetic arginine analogue of vasopressin with the highest ratio of antidiuretic:vasopressor activities and the longest duration of action.

Uses

- Diabetes insipidus of pituitary origin (neurogenic diabetes insipidus).
- Primary nocturnal enuresis (bedwetting) in children and adults.
- Adjunct in hemophilia therapy (vasopressin increases circulating levels of blood clotting factor VIII).

Side Effects

- Vasoconstriction (may be dangerous in patients with angina).
- Contraction and cramps of smooth muscles.
- Water intoxication.

19.5 Vasopressin Antagonists

High levels of circulating plasma arginine vasopressin (AVP), also known as ADH, are characteristic of a SIADH. This leads to decreased water diuresis, an increase in body water, and a relative decrease in sodium (hyponatremia). There are many varied causes of SIADH, including CNS disorders (stroke, infection, trauma), drugs, surgery, and tumors, or it may be idiopathic.

Conivaptan, tolvaptan, and demeclocycline are used to treat hyponatremia.

19.5.1 Conivaptan, Tolvaptan, and Demeclocycline

Mechanism of Action

Conivaptan and tolvaptan are vasopressin receptor antagonists. Demeclocycline blocks the renal action of vasopressin, but does not directly antagonize the receptor.

Uses and Precautions

Conivaptan is for intravenous use in a hospital setting. Tolvaptan is given orally but should be initiated and reinitiated in patients only in a hospital where serum sodium can be monitored closely.

Too-rapid correction of hyponatremia with either of these drugs can cause osmotic demyelination of nerves resulting in serious side effects.

Oral demeclocycline may be used for chronic treatment.

20 Antihypertensive Drugs

Summary

Hypertension is a major risk factor for cardiovascular disease and necessitates pharmacological treatment when lifestyle changes alone fail to reach blood pressure goals. A number of different drug classes are used in the treatment of hypertension. The drug classes that are recommended for initial therapy include thiazide diuretics, calcium channel blockers (amlodipine, felodipine, isradipine, nifedipine, nicardipine, nisoldipine, verapamil, and diltiazem), angiotensin-converting enzyme (ACE) inhibitors (captopril, enalapril, benazepril, fosinopril, moexipril, perindopril, quinapril, ramipril, and trandolapril), and angiotensin receptor blockers (ARBs) (losartan, valsartan, and candesartan). Beta blockers (propranolol, nadolol, pindolol, timolol, atenolol, betaxolol, metoprolol, carvedilol, labetalol, and nebivolol) may be considered after an acute myocardial infarction or in patients with atrial fibrillation for rate control. Other drug classes are less often used as initial therapy but are considered in the presence of compelling indications. These include alpha1-adrenergic receptor-blocking agents (prazosin, terazosin, and doxazosin) and the alpha2-adrenergic receptor agonist clonidine. In resistant cases, the direct vasodilator hydralazine may be used. Hydralazine administered parenterally, minoxidil, diazoxide, and sodium nitroprusside are used in acute hypertensive emergencies. While monotherapy is advantageous for increasing compliance and limiting adverse effects, most patients will require combination therapy from classes with different mechanisms of action in order to achieve blood pressure goals.

Keywords: hypertension, blood pressure control, antihypertensive, adrenergic, angiotensin, calcium channel blocker, vasodilator

20.1 Hypertension

Hypertension is a major risk factor for cerebrovascular disease, heart failure, renal insufficiency, and myocardial infarction (see ▶ Fig. 20.1 for the causes and mechanism of hypertension). It is often asymptomatic until organ damage reaches a critical point, so frequent monitoring is vital. Antihypertensive therapy initially consists of lifestyle changes, such as weight reduction, smoking cessation, reduction of salt, saturated fat, and excessive alcohol intake, and increased exercise before drug therapy is initiated.

Generally, pharmacological intervention is initiated when lifestyle changes alone do not reduce blood pressure to target goals. Typically, an adult with sustained systolic pressure ≥ 140 mm Hg and/or a diastolic pressure ≥ 90 mm Hg will warrant drug therapy.

20.1.1 Drug Management of Hypertension

A number of drug classes are used in treatment of hypertension. Monotherapy is desirable due to increased compliance and fewer side effects; however, most patients on antihypertensive therapy will require two or more drugs with different mechanisms of action. Combination therapy with drugs from different classes may have additive effects on lowering blood pressure and also offset compensatory mechanisms that may arise. The choice of drug(s) depends on various factors, including comorbid conditions. Guidelines recommend the use of diuretics, angiotensin antagonists, or calcium channel blockers (CCBs) as initial monotherapy or combinations thereof in the treatment of uncomplicated hypertension. However, other drug classes are sometimes used depending on comorbidities. The following drugs are used either as the sole agent or in combination with other agents:

1. Diuretics (mainly thiazides).
2. Angiotensin antagonists: angiotensin-converting enzyme (ACE) inhibitors, angiotensin II receptor antagonists, and renin inhibitors.
3. CCBs (long acting).
4. β-blockers and mixed antagonists.
5. α_1-adrenergic receptor blocking agents.
6. α_2-adrenergic receptor agonists and neuronal blockers.
7. Direct vasodilators.

20.2 Diuretics

These drugs are discussed in detail in Chapter 19. The precise mechanism by which diuretics reduce blood pressure is poorly understood; however, antihypertensive effects during the early stage of treatment have been related to a decrease in circulating blood volume and decreased cardiac output. However, these parameters return to nearly normal values after a few weeks of therapy. Their action may, in part, be related to a depletion or redistribution of Na^+ or a direct arteriolar dilation.

20.3 Angiotensin Antagonists

20.3.1 Angiotensin-converting Enzyme Inhibitors

Captopril, Enalapril, Benazepril, Fosinopril, Moexipril, Perindopril, Quinapril, Ramipril, and Trandolapril

Mechanism of Action

These agents competitively inhibit ACE by acting as a false substrate to reduce the conversion of angiotensin I (a decapeptide) to angiotensin II (an octapeptide). Reducing angiotensin II formation results in several effects that contribute to reduction in blood pressure. First, vasodilation is elicited by preventing direct vasoconstrictive effects of angiotensin II on blood vessels. Also, because angiotensin II is a stimulator of aldosterone secretion in the adrenal cortex, ACE inhibition prevents aldosterone release, which will reduce sodium and water retention (▶ Fig. 20.2). ACE inhibitors also prevent the degradation of

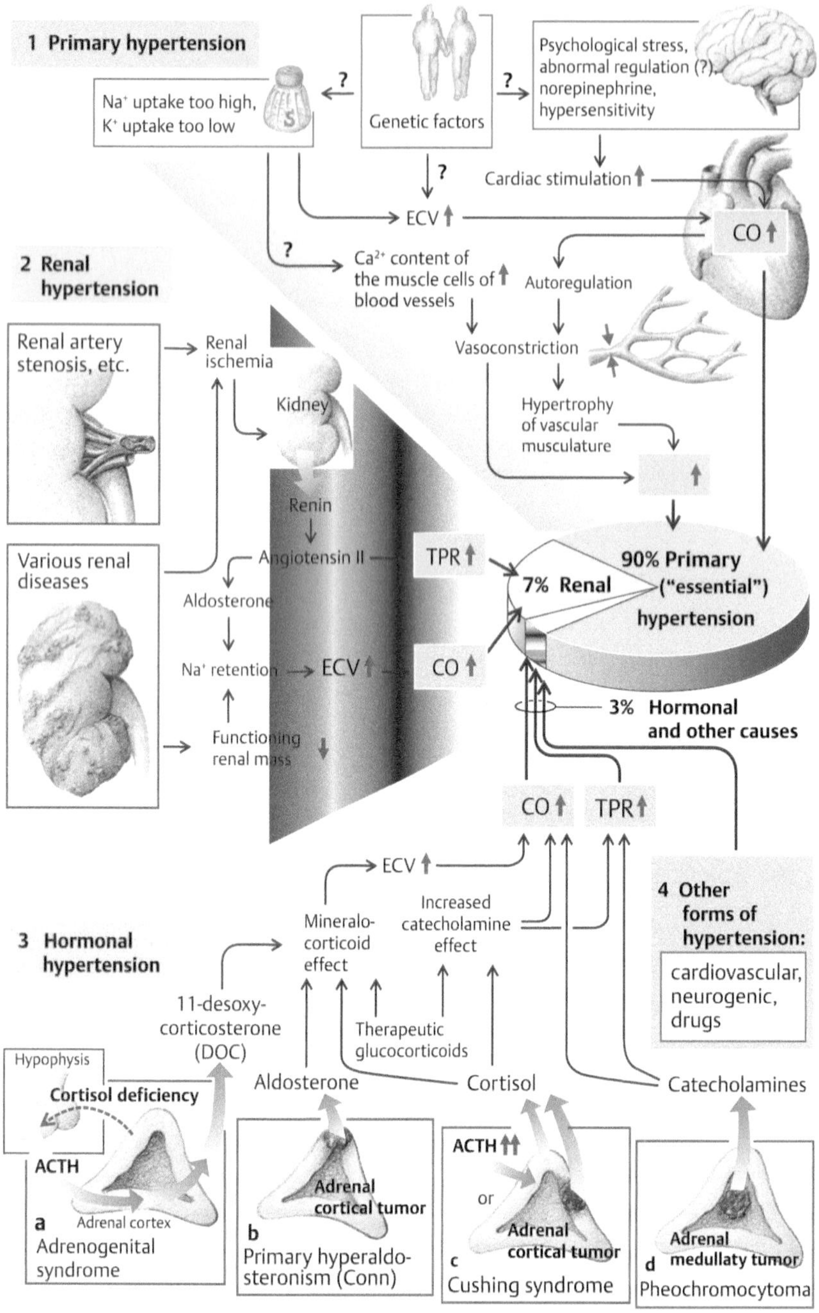

Fig. 20.1 Causes and mechanism of hypertension.
This illustration shows the mechanisms by which cardiac output (CO) and/or total peripheral resistance (TPR) are increased in primary and secondary hypertension (renal hypertension, hormonal hypertension, and other forms of hypertension). ACTH, adrenocorticotropic hormone; ECV, extracellular volume.

bradykinin (ACE is also called kininase II). Bradykinin is a vasodilator, and increasing its amount may contribute to the effects of ACE inhibitors.

ACE inhibitors are particularly beneficial in diabetic patients as they reduce proteinuria and can protect against diabetic nephropathy. These drugs may be considered as an initial agent to treat hypertension in diabetes. Diabetics are also sometimes treated with ACE inhibitors for their renoprotective effects in the absence of hypertension. Of note, ACE inhibitors are less effective in African American patients as monotherapy. Greater reductions in blood pressure can be achieved when combined with a thiazide diuretic or calcium channel blocker in these patients.

Clinical Correlation

Causes of Hypertension

Primary or essential hypertension has no identifiable cause and accounts for about 90% of all cases. The other 10% of hypertension cases have an identifiable cause. These causes may include diseases such as renal artery stenosis, chronic kidney disease, diabetes mellitus, Cushing syndrome, Conn syndrome, pheochromocytoma, hyperparathyroidism, coarctation of the aorta, and preeclampsia. Hypertension can also occur due to medications such as oral contraceptives or nonsteroidal anti-inflammatory agents. Pain can also be a cause of hypertension.

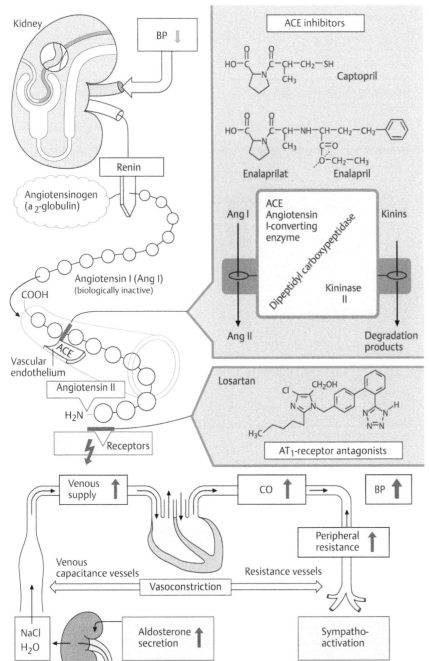

Fig. 20.2 Renin–angiotensin–aldosterone system and inhibitors.
Angiotensin-converting enzyme (ACE) inhibitors inhibit the ACE in the luminal side of vascular epithelium that is primarily responsible for the conversion of angiotensin I to angiotensin II. ACE, or kininase II, also contributes to the inactivation of kinins (e.g., bradykinin). The net result is a reduction in blood pressure and in the work of the heart. Angiotensin receptor antagonists produce effects similar to ACE inhibitors, but they do not affect kinin degradation. BP, blood pressure; CO, cardiac output.

Clinical Correlation

End Organ Damage in Hypertension

Examples of end organ damage that may result from chronic hypertension include left ventricular hypertrophy, renal failure, peripheral vascular disease, stroke, transient ischemic attacks, myocardial infarction, congestive heart failure, and cerebral encephalopathy.

Clinical Correlation

Baroreceptor Reflex

The baroreceptor reflex allows the body to compensate rapidly for changes in arterial pressure. It is mediated by receptors sensitive to mechanical stretch that are located in the carotid sinuses and in the walls of the aortic arch. A decreased arterial pressure reduces the amount of stretch of the arterial wall, which is sensed by the baroreceptors. The carotid sinus baroreceptors respond by decreasing the rate of action potential firing in the carotid sinus nerve, a branch of the glossopharyngeal nerve. The baroreceptors in the aortic arch, which is innervated by branches of the vagus nerve, act in a similar manner. Impulses from baroreceptors are then relayed to the vasomotor center in the medulla oblongata which increases sympathetic outflow, resulting in increased heart rate, contractility, and stroke volume. Venoconstriction increases which reduces venous compliance, resulting in an increase in venous return to the heart. According to the Frank–Starling mechanism, increased venous return increases filling pressures (preload) such that cardiac output is increased. Increased vasoconstriction of arterioles also occurs.

Pharmacokinetics

- Orally effective.
- Enalapril is more potent and longer acting than captopril. It is a prodrug that is hydrolyzed in the body to enalaprilat, an active metabolite.

Uses

- Heart failure.
- Hypertension (normal and high renin).
- Hypertension in diabetes (first choice along with angiotensin receptor blockers [ARBs]).
- Prevention of diabetic nephropathy.

Side Effects

- Persistent dry cough (due to bradykinin in lungs).
- Angioedema (due to increased bradykinin).
- Hyperkalemia (Avoid concurrent potassium supplements or potassium-sparing diuretics).
- Increased renin (due to reduction of angiotensin II-mediated inhibition of renin release [negative feedback]).
- First-dose hypotension (can be greater in the setting of volume depletion, that is, when combined with a diuretic).
- Taste disturbances.

Contraindications

- Pregnancy. ACE inhibitors can cause fetal abnormalities and potential death. Discontinue immediately upon pregnancy confirmation.
- Bilateral renal artery stenosis. In this condition, glomerular filtration rate (GFR) is maintained by angiotensin II-mediated vasoconstriction of efferent arteriole. ACE inhibitors can reduce GFR to cause acute renal failure.

20.3.2 Angiotensin II Receptor Antagonists

Losartan, Valsartan, Candesartan, Eprosartan, Irbesartan, Telmisartan, and Olmesartan

Mechanism of Action

These agents are competitive inhibitors of angiotensin II at the AT_1-type angiotensin receptor (▶ Fig. 20.2). Also called ARBs.

Uses and Side Effects

They are similar to ACE inhibitors, but they do not produce a cough or significant angioedema as these adverse effects are due to bradykinin accumulation resulting from ACE (kininase) inhibition. Similar to ACE inhibitors, ARBs are beneficial in diabetic patients.

20.3.3 Direct Renin Inhibitors

Aliskiren

Mechanism of Action

Aliskiren binds to renin and produces a dose-dependent reduction in plasma renin activity. Inhibiting renin reduces angiotensin I (inhibits formation from angiotensinogen), angiotensin II, and aldosterone, with a concomitant reduction in blood pressure.

Uses and Side Effects

Direct renin inhibitors are effective orally and used in treatment of hypertension. Side effect profile is similar to ACE inhibitors. Of note, aliskiren combined with ACE inhibitors or ARBs is contraindicated in diabetes or renal failure due to increased incidence of renal impairment, hyperkalemia, and hypotension.

Note: Drugs that act directly on the renin–angiotensin system, including ACE inhibitors, angiotensin II receptor antagonists, and direct renin inhibitors, can cause injury and death to the developing fetus and their use in pregnancy should be avoided.

20.4 Calcium Channel Blockers

CCBs, also termed *calcium antagonists* and *calcium entry blockers*, are pharmacological agents capable of reducing Ca^{2+} entry through the cell membrane via voltage-dependent, L-type calcium channels (slow, long-lasting inward current).

20.4.1 Amlodipine, Felodipine, Isradipine, Nifedipine, Nicardipine, Nisoldipine, Verapamil, Diltiazem

- *Dihydropyridine CCBs*: amlodipine, felodipine, isradipine, nifedipine, nicardipine, and nisoldipine.
- *Nondihydropyridine CCBs*: verapamil and diltiazem.

Mechanism of Action

Two major types of Ca^{2+} channels exist in cardiac and vascular smooth muscle, the T type and the L type. The L-type channel is targeted by CCBs. CCBs are referred to as either dihydropyridines or nondihydropyridines based on their tissue selectivity (▶ Fig. 20.3).
- The dihydropyridines (amlodipine, nifedipine, and nicardipine) inhibit Ca^{2+} entry and smooth muscle contractility with a relative absence of direct effects on the myocardium. The drugs can also prevent or reverse biliary–esophageal spasm.
- The nondihydropyridines are more cardioselective. Diltiazem and verapamil have relatively greater effects on myocardial

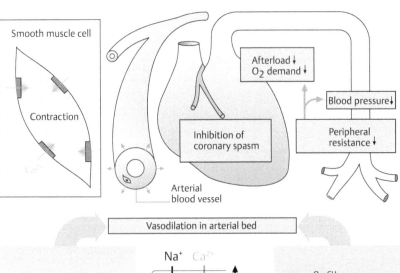

Fig. 20.3 Vasodilators: calcium antagonists.
Calcium channel blockers inhibit Ca²⁺ entry into cells. In smooth muscle cells, this produces arterial vasodilation, decreased blood pressure, and reduced coronary artery spasm. In heart muscle cells, these agents inhibit cardiac functions, causing decreased heart rate, atrioventricular (AV) conduction, and contractility. Nifedipine acts predominantly on smooth muscle cells to produce vasodilation and has almost no effect on cardiac function at therapeutic doses. Verapamil acts on both smooth muscle and heart muscle cells.

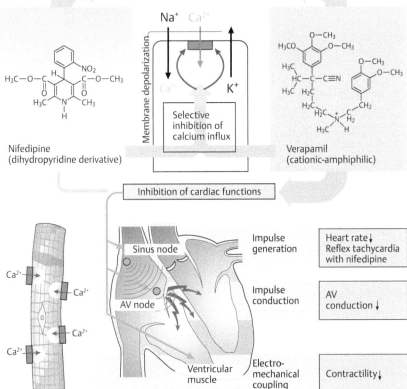

Ca²⁺ channels than those in vascular smooth muscle. They significantly reduce heart rate, contractility, and conduction velocity in the heart, reducing myocardial oxygen demand. All CCBs prevent coronary vasospasm and increase myocardial oxygen supply.

Uses

- Hypertension (all agents).
- Angina pectoris, both classical and variant types (all agents).
- Supraventricular tachycardia (diltiazem and verapamil only).

Side Effects

- Cardioselective verapamil and diltiazem can cause bradycardia, reduce inotropy (force of contraction), impair electrical conduction, and cause atrioventricular nodal block. These agents should be avoided in combination with beta-blockers due to potential additive effects on depressed inotropy and electrical conduction.
- Dihydropyridines can cause excess hypotension, headache, and pedal edema, resulting from profound vasodilation and fluid retention. Reflex tachycardia due to profound vasodilation can occur with some dihydropyridines, but not with others, mostly longer-acting CCBs, for example, amlodipine. The nondihydropyridine agents act more directly on the heart (with relatively less vasodilator activity) so reflex tachycardia is limited.

▶ Table 20.1 summarizes the electrophysiological and hemodynamic effects of these agents.

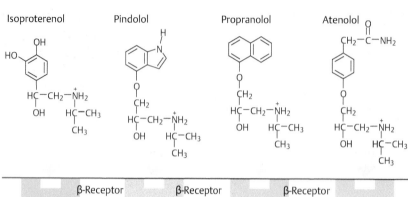

Isoproterenol   Pindolol   Propranolol   Atenolol

Fig. 20.4 Effects of some β sympatholytics and their presystemic elimination. Isoproterenol, a synthetic catecholamine, is an agonist at both β_1 and β_2 receptors. Pindolol, a partial agonist at β receptors, is classed as a β sympatholytic, as it prevents full agonists from achieving their maximal effect. Propranolol blocks Na^+ channel function and so has a "membrane-stabilizing" effect. Atenolol possesses a higher affinity for β_1 receptors than β_2 receptors and is said to be cardioselective.

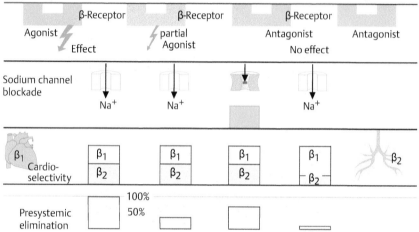

Table 20.1 Summary of electrophysiological and hemodynamic effects of calcium channel blocker agents

	Electrophysiology				Hemodynamics			
	Sinus node conduction	AV node conduction						
Agent(s)	Direct effect	Indirect effect	Direct effect	Indirect effect	Contractility	Preload	Afterload	Oxygen consumption
Amlodipine Nifedipine Nicardipine	None	Increased	None	Increased	No change	No change	Decreased	Reduced
Diltiazem Verapamil	Decreased	Increased	Decreased	Increased	Decreased	No change	Decreased	Reduced

Abbreviation: AV, atrioventricular.

20.5 Sympatholytic Drugs

These are also discussed in Chapter 6.

20.5.1 Beta Adrenergic Receptor Blocking Agents

Propranolol, Nadolol, Pindolol, Timolol, Atenolol, Betaxolol, Metoprolol

Mechanisms of Action

- Propranolol (▶ Fig. 20.4), nadolol, pindolol, and timolol are all nonselective β_1 and β_2 blockers.
- Atenolol, betaxolol, bisoprolol, and metoprolol are more "cardiac" selective β_1 blockers.

All beta blockers are effective as antihypertensives. Their effects on lowering blood pressure are the result of a reduction in cardiac output. Long-term effectiveness may also include the reduction in renin release or other central nervous system (CNS) effects to reduce sympathetic activity. They are not recommended as a first-line choice in uncomplicated hypertension due to increased risk of cardiovascular events; however, they may be used in treatment of hypertension in patients who may benefit from beta blocker therapy due to other indications such as angina, migraines, myocardial infarction, arrhythmias, or certain cases of heart failure.

Effects

- Reduce myocardial oxygen consumption by decreasing resting heart rate and myocardial contractility.
- Delay atrioventricular (AV) conduction.
- Decrease renin release.

Uses

- Hypertension.
- Effort-induced angina.

- Myocardial infarction.
- As antiarrhythmics.
- Systolic heart failure.
- Open-angle glaucoma (timolol) (see Chapter 6).

Side Effects

There are generally mild side effects, except in patients with accompanying disease, but may include the following:
- Bradycardia.
- Reduced tolerance to exercise.
- AV nodal block.
- Bronchoconstriction.
- Use caution in diabetes (masking of hypoglycemia symptoms).

Foundations

Excitation–Contraction Coupling in Cardiac Muscle

Depolarization of the cardiac muscle cell membrane triggers an action potential which passes through the T-tubules. During phase 2 (plateau) of the action potential, there is increased Ca^{2+} conductance causing inward Ca^{2+} flow. This inward Ca^{2+} flow initiates the release of Ca^{2+} from the sarcoplasmic reticulum (Ca^{2+}-induced Ca^{2+} release). The result of this is an increase in intracellular $[Ca^{2+}]$. Ca^{2+} binds to troponin-C and tropomyosin moves out of its blocking position allowing actin and myosin to form cross-bridges. The thick and thin filaments of actin and myosin slide past each other resulting in cardiac muscle cell contraction. The contraction ends when intracellular $[Ca^{2+}]$ is removed by the reuptake of Ca^{2+} into the sarcoplasmic reticulum via the sarco/endoplasmic reticulum Ca^{2+}–ATPase (SERCA) or extracellular transport of Ca^{2+} by the Na^+–Ca^{2+} exchanger (NCX).

Note: The force of contraction of cardiac muscle cells is proportional to the amount of Ca^{2+} release, which varies depending on conditions.

Contraindications

- Asthma/obstructive airways disease due to bronchoconstriction (β_2 effect). Cardioselective agents can be used in asthmatics if a beta blocker is necessary, but require caution.
- Sinus bradycardia.
- Heart block.

Beta Blockers with Additional Effects: Carvedilol, Labetalol, Nebivolol

Mechanism of Action

Carvedilol and labetalol are mixed antagonists and block both α_1- and β-adrenergic receptors, therefore having the combined actions and side effects of both. Nebivolol has nitric oxide vasodilating effects in addition to beta blocking properties, which contribute to lowering blood pressure.

Uses

- Similar to other beta blockers.
- Labetalol used in hypertension in pregnancy.

20.5.2 Alpha₁ Adrenergic Receptor-blocking Agents: Prazosin, Terazosin, and Doxazosin

Mechanism of Action

These agents act selectively on the postsynaptic α_1 receptor of vascular smooth muscle, causing vasodilation and lowering total peripheral resistance.

Uses

- Hypertension.
- Benign prostatic hyperplasia.

Side Effects

Orthostatic (postural) hypotension and reflex tachycardia are frequent, especially after the first dose.

20.5.3 Alpha₂ Adrenergic Receptor Agonists (Central Sympatholytics)

Alpha-Methyldopa

Mechanism of Action

Methyldopa is metabolized to α-methylnorepinephrine (α-MNE) which acts as an agonist of central α_2 receptors to inhibit sympathetic outflow. Also, by inhibiting presynaptic α_2 autoreceptors there is inhibition of norepinephrine release from peripheral nerves. There is also a reduction in renin secretion.

Uses

- Hypertension (the antihypertensive effect occurs via CNS reduction of sympathetic outflow.).
- Hypertension in pregnancy.

Side Effects

- Drowsiness.
- Depression.
- Dry mouth.

Clonidine

Mechanism of Action

Clonidine causes stimulation of CNS α_2 adrenergic receptors, which in turn causes inhibition of sympathetic tone (see ▶ Fig. 6.7). Effects are long lasting and are antagonized by yohimbine (*Pausinystalia yohimbe*), an alkaloid with stimulant and aphrodisiac properties.

Pharmacokinetics

Clonidine is very lipophilic; therefore, it can be administered orally or through a transdermal patch.

V

Uses

- Hypertension.
- Migraine.
- Menopausal flushing.

Side Effects

- Xerostomia (dry mouth).
- Sedation.
- Fluid retention (use with a diuretic).

Note: Withdrawal may precipitate hypertensive crisis, which may be treated with labetalol (a β blocker).

20.5.4 Adrenergic Neuron Blockers Reserpine

Mechanism of Action

Reserpine is an irreversible inhibitor of vesicular monoamine transporter on storage vesicles of peripheral nerve terminals. This prevents the uptake of dopamine and norepinephrine (and serotonin) into vesicles and depletes norepinephrine stores in the peripheral nerve terminals and in the brain (see ▸ Fig. 6.10).

Uses

- Hypertension (rarely used).

Side Effects

These are largely due to unopposed parasympathetic effects and include the following:
- Bradycardia.
- Nasal stuffiness.
- Diarrhea, increased motility, and aggravation of peptic ulcers.
- Depression (contraindicated in history of depression).
- Excessive sedation, extrapyramidal symptoms, and impotence.

Guanethidine

Mechanism of Action

Guanethidine has complex effects on the adrenergic neuron. It prevents norepinephrine release during nerve stimulation by blocking transmission of the action potential into the terminal nerve ending, as well as by causing the depletion of peripheral stores of norepinephrine and blocking its reuptake. It does not cross the blood–brain barrier; therefore, there are no CNS effects (see ▸ Fig. 6.10).

Pharmacokinetics

- Slow onset (2–3 days) with long duration of action (effects persist for about 1 week after the drug is stopped.)

Uses

- Hypertension.

Side Effects

Same as for reserpine.

20.5.5 Ganglionic Blocking Agent Trimethaphan

Mechanism of Action

The hypotensive action of trimethaphan is primarily due to reduced vasomotor tone, decreased venous return, and lowered cardiac output.

Pharmacokinetics

- Given by a slow intravenous (IV) infusion.

Uses

- Occasionally used for hypertensive crisis or in surgery to reduce blood pressure.

Side Effects

Potential side effects limit the usage of trimethaphan and may include the following:
- Precipitous falls in blood pressure.
- Histamine release from mast cells and basophils that may lead to asthma.
- Urinary retention, constipation, and dry mouth.

20.6 Direct Vasodilators

Agents that cause vasodilation will reduce blood pressure, but this stimulates counterregulatory responses that are designed to maintain blood pressure (▸ Fig. 20.5). Additional drugs (e.g., ACE inhibitors, diuretics, and β blockers) are given to inhibit these responses.

20.6.1 Arterial Vasodilators

Arterial vasodilators all cause K^+ channel activation, leading to hyperpolarization and vascular smooth muscle relaxation.

Hydralazine

Mechanism of Action

Hydralazine directly relaxes vascular smooth muscle and decreases peripheral resistance through an unknown mechanism thought to involve activation of K^+ channels. It also causes reflex cardiac stimulation (increased cardiac output and tachycardia), which can be blocked with propranolol. Increased fluid retention can be inhibited with a diuretic.

Pharmacokinetics

- Well absorbed after oral administration and generally well tolerated.

Uses

- Resistant hypertension.
- Hypertension in pregnancy.
- Especially useful in acute hypertensive crisis (administered parenterally).

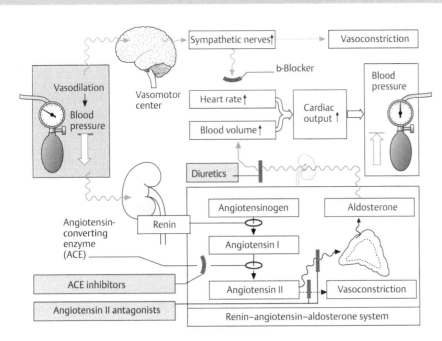

Fig. 20.5 Counterregulatory responses in hypotension due to vasodilators.
Vasodilation causes a decrease in blood pressure. To counteract this, the body activates the sympathetic nervous system and the renin–angiotensin system. However, because these homeostatic mechanisms are undesired when using vasodilator drugs in hypertension, heart failure, and angina, additional drugs are given to block them.

Side Effects

- Headache.
- Palpitations.
- Gastrointestinal disturbances.
- The most serious toxicity is a lupus-like syndrome occurring with long-term therapy. This side effect limits its chronic use and is reversible if the drug is stopped.

Minoxidil

Mechanism of Action

The mechanism of action is the opening of K⁺ channels. Minoxidil is longer acting than hydralazine. Reflex cardiac stimulation and fluid retention occur and coadministration of a beta blocker and diuretic is usually necessary.

Uses

- Severe and uncontrollable hypertension.

Side Effects

- Salt and water retention.
- Hypertrichosis (excessive growth of hair).

Diazoxide

Diazoxide is a nondiuretic congener of the thiazide diuretic drugs.

Mechanism of Action

Diazoxide is a K⁺ channel activator that has direct effects on the arterioles to lower blood pressure.

Uses

- Acute hypertensive emergencies (given IV).

Side Effects

- Hyperglycemia (inhibits insulin release from the beta cells of the pancreas).
- Hyperuricemia.
- Pancreatic necrosis.

20.6.2 Arterial and Venous Vasodilators

Sodium Nitroprusside

Mechanism of Action

This agent spontaneously releases nitric oxide that acts on vascular smooth muscle to result in both veno- and arteriodilation.

Uses

- Acute hypertensive emergencies.

Note: Nitroprusside is not considered suitable for chronic management of hypertension.

Side Effects

Nitroprusside can precipitate marked hypotension when administered as an IV dosage. It is also light sensitive, and accumulation of its metabolite, thiocyanate, can lead to symptoms such as tinnitus, weakness, seizures, and psychosis. As nitroprusside breaks down in the body, cyanide is produced. Cyanide toxicity can occur, resulting in metabolic acidosis, respiratory arrest, coma, or death.

Table 20.2 Summary of mechanisms of antihypertensive agents

Antihypertensive agent(s)	Parameter of BP affected	Mechanism
Diuretics	TPR	Initial decrease in CO, followed by sustained decrease in TPR (exact mechanism unclear)
ACE inhibitors	TPR	Indirect vasodilation by decreasing angiotensin II levels
Angiotensin II receptor antagonists	TPR	Indirect vasodilation by blocking angiotensin II receptor
Calcium channel blockers	TPR	Decrease influx of Ca^{2+} into vascular smooth muscle
β blockers	CO, TPR	Decrease heart rate and force of contraction by sympathetic inhibition Decrease renin production, leading to decreased circulating angiotensin II
α_2 adrenergic receptor agonists	TPR	Stimulate presynaptic α_2 adrenergic receptors in brainstem to decrease sympathetic activity
α_1 adrenergic receptor-blocking agents	TPR	Block α_1-receptor-mediated contraction of vascular smooth muscle
Adrenergic neuron blockers, ganglionic blockers	TPR	Depletes NE or prevents NE release
Direct vasodilators	TPR	Direct vasodilation of vascular smooth muscle

Abbreviations: ACE, angiotensin-converting enzyme; BP, blood pressure; CO, cardiac output; NE, norepinephrine; TPR, total peripheral resistance.

▶ Table 20.2 lists the antihypertensive agents and provides an at-a-glance reference to the parameters of blood pressure that they reduce and the mechanisms by which they do it.

21 Drugs Used in the Treatment of Heart Failure

Summary

Pharmacological management of heart failure is aimed at reducing symptoms and increasing survival. Inotropic agents and vasodilators are used to improve ejection fraction and cardiac function while diuretics are primarily used to relieve symptoms. Loop (furosemide) and thiazide (hydrochlorothiazide) diuretics are first-line agents in heart failure therapy. Beta blockers (bisoprolol, carvedilol, metoprolol), angiotensin-converting enzyme inhibitors (captopril, enalapril, benazepril, fosinopril, moexipril, perindopril, quinapril, ramipril, and trandolapril), angiotensin receptor blockers (ARBs; losartan, valsartan, candesartan), aldosterone antagonists (spironolactone, eplerenone), and hydralazine plus nitrate have been shown to reduce symptoms and improve mortality. Other drugs that may be used in heart failure include phosphodiesterase inhibitors (milrinone and inamrinone), ivabradine (selectively inhibits the pacemaker current to reduce heart rate without affecting myocardial contractility), and sacubitril, a neprilysin inhibitor available in combination with valsartan (an ARB). Dobutamine is used for short-term support in severe heart failure. Digoxin also has benefit in reducing hospitalizations.

Keywords: heart failure, congestive, inotropy, diuretic, ACE inhibitor

21.1 Heart Failure

Heart failure is a pathophysiological state in which cardiac output is inadequate to meet the demands of the body tissues. The basic cardiac dysfunction of decreased cardiac output, combined with activation of compensatory mechanisms, produces the commonly recognized spectrum of clinical symptoms and signs, including tachycardia, dyspnea (shortness of breath), decreased exercise tolerance, edema, and cardiomegaly. Peripheral or pulmonary edema (i.e., congestion) is also commonly seen. Heart failure with reduced ejection fraction ($\leq 40\%$) is characterized as systolic heart failure which occurs due to impaired heart pumping. Heart failure with preserved ejection fraction is called diastolic heart failure, and it occurs due to a defect in filling or cardiac relaxation. Drug treatment is not curative, but involves attempts to reduce symptoms, improve cardiac function, and reduce mortality.

21.2 Drug Management of Heart Failure

The following drug classes are utilized in the management of heart failure:

1. Diuretics.
2. Angiotensin-converting enzyme (ACE) inhibitors.
3. Angiotensin receptor blockers (ARBs).
4. β blockers.
5. Positive inotropic agents.
6. Direct vasodilators.
7. Other drugs.

These drugs either directly stimulate the mechanical action of the heart or have effects on the compensatory mechanisms that are activated in heart failure. In heart failure, the reduced cardiac output leads to activation of the sympathetic nervous system and the renin–angiotensin–aldosterone system in order to maintain cardiac output. Both systems, however, can cause increases in preload and afterload which can be detrimental to the heart. Many of the drugs used improve cardiac function by decreasing preload and afterload (▶ Fig. 21.1). The positive inotropic agents act directly on the heart to increase contractility.

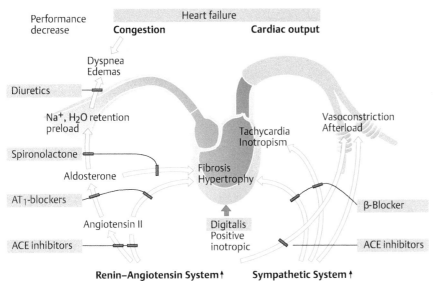

Fig. 21.1 Heart failure (HF).
In HF, the heart is failing as a pump; cardiac output is therefore insufficient to meet the metabolic demand for oxygen in the body. HF also causes fluid congestion in the lungs and venous circulation. Compensatory mechanisms, such as the activation of the sympathetic system and the renin–angiotensin system, are designed to increase cardiac output on a short-term basis but eventually place further strain on the heart if the heart failure is chronic. Drug therapy in chronic HF aims to inhibit these unhelpful compensatory mechanisms. ACE, angiotensin-converting enzyme.

The mechanism of the beneficial effect of the β blockers in heart failure is not well understood but these drugs can reduce cardiac remodeling and inhibit excess sympathetic signals that contribute to worsening heart failure. A mortality benefit has been seen with β blockers, ACE inhibitors/ARBs, mineralocorticoid receptor antagonists, and hydralazine/nitrate combination. The diuretics and digoxin are used for symptom relief.

Clinical Correlation

Etiology of Heart Failure

Heart failure can occur due to several etiologic factors such as intrinsic disease of the heart muscle (e.g., cardiomyopathy, ischemia, and infarction); chronic elevated preload (e.g., fluid overload and mitral regurgitation); chronic elevated afterload (e.g., aortic stenosis and hypertension); disorder of cardiac filling (e.g., cardiac tamponade); and when there is an inadequate heart rate, for example, following myocardial infarction (MI), β blocker therapy, or negatively inotropic drug therapy (e.g., antiarrhythmic drug).

Foundations

Jugular Venous Pressure

The internal jugular vein passes medial to the clavicular head of the sternocleidomastoid muscle up behind the angle of the mandible. It is a reliable indicator of right atrial pressure. It is not normally visible or palpable but may become distended in right ventricular failure.

Foundations

Preload

Up to a point, the heart pumps more when it is filled more during diastole. This is referred as Starling's law of the heart or the Frank–Starling mechanism. The amount of filling is called preload. It is a reflection of forces in the vasculature acting to fill the ventricle. The amount of preload can be expressed in several ways, such as end diastolic volume, end diastolic pressure, or stretch (sarcomere length). It will be low in cases of hypovolemia or low systemic venous tone and high in cases of fluid retention, many cases of heart failure, or excessive venous sympathetic stimulation. If the right ventricle is impaired, but not the left, right ventricular preload will tend to be high, while left ventricular preload will tend to be low.

Foundations

Contractility

Contractility expresses the ability of the heart to contract at a given preload. Greater contractility manifests as greater systolic pressure or greater systolic ejection. At the cellular level, contractility reflects the amount of Ca^{2+} released from the sarcoplasmic reticulum with each heartbeat (positive inotropy). The supply of Ca^{2+} in the sarcoplasmic reticulum is increased by anything that stimulates more Ca^{2+} to enter the cell through Ca^{2+} channels, or that stimulates the Ca^{2+}–ATPase (SERCA) pump to take up Ca^{2+} from the cytosolic space. Both effects increase the amount of Ca^{2+} stored in the sarcoplasmic reticulum between beats. Positive inotropic effectors include agents that increase heart rate and force of contractions (increase cytosolic Ca^{2+}), including β adrenergic agonists and cardiac glycosides (e.g., digitalis) that reduce efflux of Ca^{2+} via Na^+–Ca^{2+} antiport. Negative inotropic effectors include β adrenergic antagonists.

Foundations

Afterload

Afterload is the pressure against which the ventricle works to eject blood during systole. At rest it is primarily a function of total peripheral resistance, that is, it requires greater systolic pressure to eject blood in the face of high peripheral resistance. Afterload also depends on output of the heart, because pressure in the peripheral circulation is a function of the amount of blood ejected. For example, during exercise peripheral resistance is low, which by itself would decrease afterload, but afterload is actually somewhat elevated because the heart is ejecting so much blood that mean arterial pressure is increased.

21.3 Diuretics

21.3.1 Loop and Thiazide

Diuretics are first-line agents in heart failure therapy. They are used to resolve the signs and symptoms of volume overload, which are pulmonary and/or peripheral edema (▶ Fig. 21.2). Once this goal has been achieved, diuretics are used to maintain a euvolemic state. The diuretics used for heart failure are the loop diuretics (e.g., furosemide) or the thiazides (e.g., hydrochlorothiazide). The loop diuretics are used most often because they are highly effective and work quickly; thiazides are less potent when used on their own. The pharmacology of diuretics is discussed in detail in Chapter 19.

21.3.2 Spironolactone and Eplerenone

Spironolactone and eplerenone are potassium-sparing diuretics that act as antagonists of aldosterone at the mineralocorticoid receptor. The addition of these drugs to standard chronic heart failure treatment regimen reduces morbidity and mortality. These drugs help preserve serum potassium to reduce the risk of arrhythmias; secondly, these drugs inhibit aldosterone-mediated cardiac hypertrophy and fibrosis in heart failure.

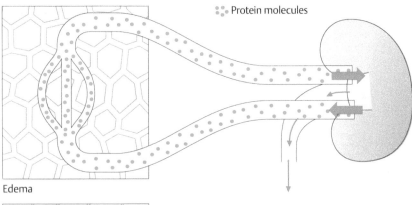

Edema

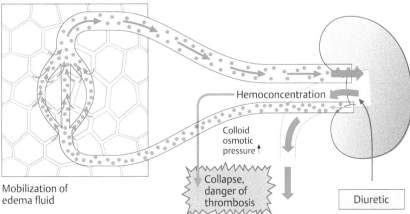

Mobilization of edema fluid

Hemoconcentration

Colloid osmotic pressure ↑

Collapse, danger of thrombosis

Diuretic

Protein molecules

Fig. 21.2 Mechanism of edema fluid mobilization by diuretics.
Edema is caused by the accumulation of fluid mostly in the interstitial space. Diuretics counteract this by increasing the renal excretion of Na⁺ and water. This causes a reduction in plasma volume and the concentration of plasma proteins, which increases plasma colloid osmotic pressure and attracts water from the interstitium into the plasma.

21.4 Angiotensin-converting Enzyme Inhibitors and Angiotensin Receptor Blockers

21.4.1 Angiotensin-converting Enzyme inhibitors

ACE inhibitors are discussed in Chapter 20. Specific points in relation to heart failure are as follows:
- ACE inhibitors are considered as first-line drugs for heart failure therapy and have been shown to reduce mortality.
- These agents acutely decrease systemic vascular resistance, venous tone, and mean blood pressure while producing a sustained increase in cardiac output.
- There is symptomatic improvement and reduced mortality in patients with heart failure.
- Exercise tolerance in patients with refractory heart failure is improved, and both salt and water retention are reduced.

21.4.2 Angiotensin Receptor Blockers

ARBs may be used in patients who are intolerant of ACE inhibitors. Similar to ACE inhibitors, these drugs can improve survival in heart failure. Use of combined therapy with ARBs and ACE inhibitors is generally not recommended due to increased risk of side effects. These drugs are discussed in Chapter 20.

21.5 Beta Blockers

21.5.1 Bisoprolol, Carvedilol, Metoprolol

Although administration of a β blocker to improve cardiac function is seemingly paradoxical, several clinical trials have demonstrated that bisoprolol, carvedilol, and metoprolol have beneficial effects to improve cardiac function, decrease symptoms, and improve survival rates in chronic heart failure. Trials with other β blockers have not been shown to be as effective. Bisoprolol and metoprolol are selective for the β_1 receptor (cardiac). Carvedilol blocks β_1, β_2, and α_1 receptors. The mechanism of the beneficial effect of β blockers likely involves the inhibition of sympathetic nervous system activity to inhibit pathologic changes of the myocardium that occur in heart failure. Heart rate, renin release, and cardiac fibrosis are reduced with β blocker therapy. β blockers are not used in cases of acute decompensated heart failure. β blockers are discussed in Chapters 6 and 20.

21.6 Positive Inotropic Agents

21.6.1 Digoxin

Digoxin, also known as digitalis, is a cardiac glycoside that was previously one of the mainstays in the treatment of heart failure. Its use is now reserved for when symptoms are not fully treated by standard therapy with diuretics and ACE inhibitors. It can decrease symptoms and lower the rate of hospitalization for heart failure, but it does not decrease mortality.

Uses

- Chronic heart failure.
- Atrial fibrillation.

Mechanism of Action

The therapeutic and toxic effects of digoxin are attributable to inhibition of the Na^+–K^+–ATPase pump (sodium pump, the digitalis receptor) located on the sarcolemma of the myocardial cells. Normally, this Na^+–K^+–ATPase pumps sodium ions out of, and potassium ions into, the cell. When the pump is inhibited, Na^+ accumulates intracellularly. Secondarily, the decreased Na^+ concentration gradient affects Na^+–Ca^{2+} exchange, causing Ca^{2+} to accumulate inside the cell. Consequently, more Ca^{2+} is available in the sarcoplasm and for storage in the sarcoplasmic reticulum. This results in greater amounts of Ca^{2+} being available for release and interaction with the contractile proteins during the excitation–contraction coupling process. At therapeutic doses of digoxin, there is an increase in contractile force. Toxicity to digitalis also relates to inhibition of the Na^+–K^+–ATPase pump. Inhibition of the Na^+–K^+–ATPase pump affects the K^+ gradient; this may lead to a significant reduction of intracellular K^+, predisposing the heart toward arrhythmias. Likewise, Ca^{2+} overload may contribute to serious arrhythmias. Digoxin also stimulates indirectly an increase in parasympathetic activity while decreasing sympathetic tone. Although the exact manner in which digoxin does this is unknown, these effects involve modulation of baroreceptor sensitivity, regulation of plasma neurohormone levels, central actions of digoxin, and secondary compensation due to increased cardiac output.

Pharmacokinetics

- Digoxin can be given orally or intravenously (IV).

Effects

- The fundamental action of digoxin is to increase the force and velocity of cardiac contraction, resulting in a marked increase in cardiac output of the failing heart. The decrease in end-diastolic volume and pressure leads to a decrease in heart size, decreased venous pressure, and decreased edema.
- Another important action of digitalis is to slow the heart rate (negative chronotropic action). The magnitude of slowing is dependent upon preexisting vagal or sympathetic tone. Both direct and indirect actions, mediated by the vagus nerve, contribute to the decrease in heart rate, decreasing the O_2 demand of the myocardium. The decreased sympathetic tone also increases renal blood flow and leads to diuresis and decreased edema.

Side Effects

Digoxin has a low therapeutic index, so toxicities are common and can be dangerous. They may include the following:

- *Cardiac arrhythmias:* as therapeutic concentrations are exceeded, the automaticity of secondary latent, ectopic pacemaker cells is increased. Premature ventricular contractions, ventricular tachycardia, and ventricular fibrillation are serious arrhythmias that occur in digitalis-toxic patients.
- Due to stimulation of vagal tone, sinus bradycardia or atrioventricular (AV) conduction block may also occur.
- Digoxin also shows characteristic changes on electrocardiograph: increased PR, decreased QT, inverted T wave.
- Gastrointestinal effects are common and are among the earliest signs of toxicity. Anorexia, nausea, vomiting, and abdominal pain occur.
- Fatigue, headache, and drowsiness are also early signs of toxicity. More serious signs are disorientation, delirium, visual disturbances (photophobia, halos, and yellow vision), and, rarely, hallucinations or convulsions.

Treatment of Toxicity

Discontinue the drug, correct K^+ deficiency, and use digoxin antibodies (Fab fragments).

Drug Interactions

- Digitalis toxicity can be exacerbated by K^+ depletion with diuretics. Hypokalemia can increase digoxin binding to Na^+–K^+–ATPase to enhance digoxin effects (and toxicity).
- Amiodarone, quinidine, verapamil can reduce renal excretion of digoxin, which can cause toxicity.
- Arrhythmias are enhanced by interaction with sympathomimetic agents.

21.7 Phosphodiesterase Inhibitors

21.7.1 Milrinone and Inamrinone

Mechanism of Action

Milrinone and inamrinone inhibit phosphodiesterase type 3, leading to increased cyclic adenosine monophosphate (cAMP) in cardiac and vascular smooth muscle cells. In cardiac muscle, this causes an increase in intracellular Ca^{2+} levels while cAMP in smooth muscle inhibits myosin light-chain kinase to promote relaxation. These agents have positive inotropic effects and vasodilator activity.

Uses

These agents are used infrequently. They are only given parenterally for short-term management of patients with heart failure that is refractory to digoxin, diuretics, and vasodilators. They are unacceptable for long-term use.

Side Effects

These include possible arrhythmias, fever, nausea, vomiting, hypersensitivity reactions, hepatotoxicity, and thrombocytopenia. Milrinone is better tolerated.

21.8 Beta Adrenergic Receptor Agonists

21.8.1 Dobutamine

Mechanism of Action

Dobutamine is a synthetic catecholamine that stimulates α_1 and β_1 receptors in both heart and blood vessels but selectively stimulates the cardiac β_1 receptors to produce its inotropic action.

Pharmacokinetics

Dobutamine must be given by IV infusion.

Uses

Dobutamine is used for short-term support in severe heart failure but is not used long-term, as it may cause arrhythmias and increase O_2 consumption.

21.9 Vasodilators

21.9.1 Direct Smooth Muscle Relaxants

Hydralazine, Isosorbide Dinitrate, Nitroprusside, and Nitroglycerin

See ▶ Fig. 21.3 for an overview of the venous and arterial vasodilation of these agents.

Uses

The addition of the vasodilators hydralazine and isosorbide dinitrate added to an ACE inhibitor β blocker, and mineralocorticoid receptor antagonist reduces mortality in patients, especially African Americans with more severe, class III and IV, heart failure.

Specific points in relation to heart failure

• Hydralazine is primarily an arteriolar vasodilator and may be beneficial in reducing afterload in congestive heart failure.

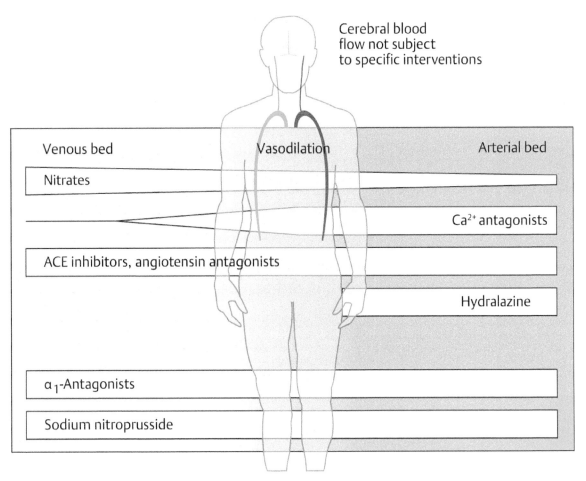

Fig. 21.3 Vasodilators.
Venous tone regulates the volume of blood returned to the heart and thus affects stroke volume and cardiac output. Arterial tone determines peripheral resistance. Vasodilator drugs may act preferentially on venous tone (nitrates) or on arterial tone (Ca^{2+} antagonists and hydralazine). They may also affect the tone of both (ACE inhibitors, α_1-antagonists, and sodium nitroprusside).

V

Tolerance may develop to this drug. It may worsen fluid retention.

- Isosorbide dinitrate is an orally active agent similar in action to nitroglycerin and nitroprusside. It is combined with hydralazine in the treatment of heart failure.
- Nitroprusside is a potent relaxant for both veins and arteries. Its use is limited to short-term IV therapy. Its short half-life allows for titration and makes it beneficial in acute or severe refractory heart failure.
- Nitroglycerin is used for short-term IV treatment of severe heart failure. It dilates large capacitance veins and reduces preload. Development of tolerance limits its therapeutic usefulness. See Chapter 22 for a more detailed discussion of nitroglycerin.

21.10 Ivabradine

21.10.1 Mechanism of Action

Ivabradine selectively inhibits the pacemaker I_f (funny) current to reduce heart rate without effects on myocardial contractility. It is used to treat chronic heart failure with reduced ejection fraction, and it has been shown to reduce hospitalizations. Ivabradine is used in addition to, or instead of, beta blockers.

21.10.2 Side effects

- Bradycardia.
- Visual disturbances.
- Contraindicated in sick sinus syndrome, AV block.

21.11 Neprilysin Inhibitors

21.11.1 Sacubitril

Mechanism of Action

Neprilysin is an endopeptidase enzyme that degrades vasoactive peptides including natriuretic peptides and bradykinin.

Inhibitors of neprilysin increase levels of these peptides showing benefit in heart failure, including reduction in vasoconstriction and reduced fibrosis, and other effects.

Use

Sacubitril is available in combination with valsartan (ARB) in treating chronic heart failure. This combination may replace ACE inhibitors or ARBs in a specific subset of patients and appears to be effective in reducing morbidity and mortality in clinical trials. Avoid in history of angioedema.

Foundations

Stages of Heart Failure

In order to determine the best course of therapy for heart failure, physicians often assess the stage of heart failure according to the New York Heart Association (NYHA) functional classification system. This system relates symptoms to everyday activities and the patient's quality of life. In class I (mild) heart failure, there is no limitation of physical activity; ordinary physical activity does not cause undue fatigue, palpitations, or dyspnea (shortness of breath). In class II (mild) heart failure, there is slight limitation of physical activity. The patient is comfortable at rest, but ordinary physical activity results in fatigue, palpitations, or dyspnea. In class III (moderate) heart failure, there is marked limitation of physical activity. The patient is comfortable at rest, but less than ordinary activity causes fatigue, palpitations, or dyspnea. In class IV (severe) heart failure, the patient is unable to carry out any physical activity without discomfort. There are symptoms of cardiac insufficiency at rest. If any physical activity is undertaken, discomfort is increased.

22 Antianginal Drugs

Summary

Angina is characterized by sudden chest pain that is caused by an imbalance between oxygen supply and demand. The drugs used to treat angina work to reduce oxygen demand or to increase oxygen supply. The vasodilators (nitroglycerin, isosorbide dinitrate, isosorbide mononitrate, and amyl nitrite) and calcium channel blockers are used in treating and preventing chronic stable and variant angina. Nitrates are used in the termination of acute pain. The beta blockers are only used in preventing episodes of pain in chronic stable angina. These drugs are not used in variant angina due to unopposed alpha adrenergic effects which can aggravate vasospasm. Unstable angina is an acute coronary syndrome treated with antiplatelets and thrombolytics.

Keywords: angina, ischemia, anti-anginals, nitroglycerin

22.1 Angina

Angina or angina pectoris is characterized by sudden, temporary, substernal chest pain that often radiates to the shoulders, neck, or jaw. The anginal pain may consist of a feeling of tightness or pressure in the chest. It results from an imbalance of the supply of oxygenated blood to cardiac muscle and the oxygen demand of the tissue (▶ Fig. 22.1). The primary goal in the treatment of angina is to restore the balance between oxygen supply and oxygen demand.

- Classic, typical, stable, or exertional angina is induced by exercise or stress and is caused by atherosclerosis of the coronary arteries (▶ Fig. 22.2). Stenosis in the coronaries can result in reduced blood flow during periods of exertion, resulting in myocardial ischemia, caused by increased myocardial oxygen demand.
- Variant angina (Prinzmetal's angina) is angina caused by coronary vasospasm, reducing myocardial oxygen supply. This type of angina occurs predominantly at rest.
- Unstable angina is due to the rupture of an atherosclerotic plaque, and resultant platelet aggregation and thrombus formation. Unstable angina causes ischemia but does not cause death of cardiomyocytes, and it requires immediate treatment due to potential for myocardial infarction (MI).

22.2 Drug Management of Angina

Foundations

Coronary Blood Flow

The major right and left coronary arteries that serve the heart tissue are the first vessels to branch off the aorta. These arteries, when healthy, maintain coronary blood flow at levels appropriate to the needs of the heart muscle. When flow through a coronary artery is reduced to the point that the myocardium it supplies becomes hypoxic, angina pectoris develops. Some individuals have angina only on exertion; others have more severe restriction of blood flow and have anginal pain at rest. If the decrease in myocardial blood flow is severe and prolonged, irreversible changes occur in the muscle, and the result is a myocardial infarction (MI). Partially occluded coronary arteries can be constricted further by vasospasm, producing MI, or, most commonly, rupture of an atherosclerotic plaque triggers the formation of a coronary-occluding clot at the site of the plaque and leads to ischemia and MI.

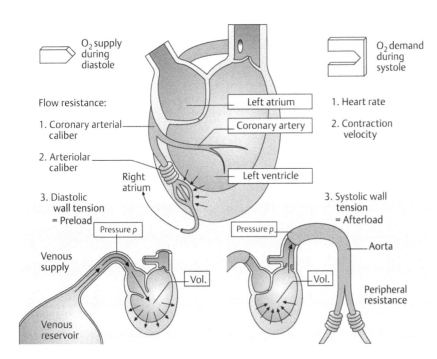

Fig. 22.1 Oxygen supply to, and demand of, the myocardium.

Oxygen supply to the myocardium occurs during diastole and is determined by the caliber of the coronary arteries and arterioles, as well as by preload. Oxygen demand occurs during systole and is determined by heart rate, contraction velocity, and afterload. Angina occurs when there is myocardial hypoxia due to inadequate myocardial blood flow (i.e., when oxygen demand exceeds supply). Therapy for angina, therefore, aims to restore balance, whether by increasing oxygen supply or decreasing oxygen demand.

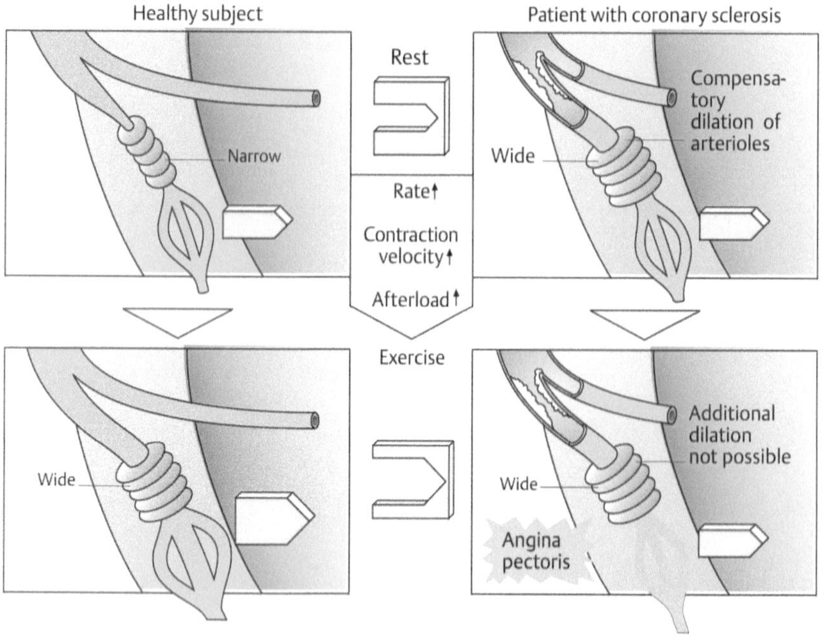

Fig. 22.2 Pathogenesis of classic angina in coronary sclerosis.

In a healthy person, the caliber of coronary arterioles determines myocardial oxygen supply and is adjusted automatically during exercise to meet the increased demand by increasing heart rate, contraction velocity, and afterload. In a patient with atherosclerosis of the coronary arteries, there is a dilation of arterioles at rest to compensate for the flow resistance caused by the atheroma, and myocardial oxygen supply is maintained. However, during exercise, further dilation cannot occur, leading to myocardial ischemia and pain.

Clinical Correlation

Coronary Artery Bypass Graft

Coronary artery bypass graft (CABG) is a surgical procedure performed to bypass atherosclerotic narrowings of the coronary arteries that are the cause of anginal pain. These narrowings can eventually occlude if untreated, leading to myocardial infarction (MI). There are two main coronary arteries, left and right, and these have several branches. A CABG is denoted as single, double, triple, and so on, depending on the number of arteries that are to be bypassed. The internal thoracic artery that supplies the anterior chest wall and breasts is usually harvested to use as the bypass artery.

Foundations

Cardiac Muscle Metabolism

Cardiac muscle requires an abundant supply of oxygen-rich blood, because it depends almost exclusively on aerobic metabolism to supply the adenosine triphosphate (ATP) for its contractions. Other tissues can vary their extraction of oxygen from blood and can survive on anaerobic metabolism. Cardiac tissue has a very high fractional extraction of oxygen and can only increase its uptake of oxygen by increasing coronary blood flow. At rest the heart uses oxidation of fatty acids for its ATP; only small quantities of glucose are utilized. When cardiac workload is increased, cardiac muscle removes lactic acid from coronary blood and oxidizes it directly.

Foundations

Myocardial Infarction

Myocardial infarction (MI) is death of heart muscle. It is caused by complete occlusion of one or more coronary arteries by thrombosis. The pain of an MI is similar to that of angina but it is more severe and of longer duration. It is also accompanied by nausea, vomiting, diaphoresis (sweating), and dyspnea (shortness of breath). Patients also describe a feeling "as if they are going to die." Common complications of MI include arrhythmias, heart failure, hypertension, and emboli formation. Electrocardiography analysis shows ST elevation, T wave inversion, and Q waves in the leads that "look at" the infarction. Cardiac enzymes are also measured and used as a basis for diagnosis of MI. Immediate treatment of an MI involves the use of thrombolytic drugs such as tissue plasminogen activator (tpa, given as soon as possible after infarction) and aspirin, as well as morphine and nitrates. Longer-term treatment involves the use of β blockers and angiotensin-converting enzyme inhibitors. Surgical treatment is the same as for angina.

Clinical Correlation

Cardiac Enzymes

Several enzymes are released when cardiac muscle cells are damaged such as troponin I, creatine kinase, myoglobin, and lactate dehydrogenase. Increased blood levels of troponin I and troponin T reflect cardiac muscle damage and are routinely measured to help diagnose MI.

22.3 Vasodilators

22.3.1 Organic Nitrates: Nitroglycerin, Isosorbide Dinitrate, Isosorbide Mononitrate, and Amyl Nitrite

Mechanism of Action

Organic nitrates act like the endogenous compound nitric oxide. They activate guanylate cyclase to increase cyclic guanosine monophosphate in smooth muscle. This leads to relaxation of vascular smooth muscle and both arterial and venous dilation (▶ Fig. 22.3). By reducing preload and afterload, myocardial oxygen consumption is reduced. In the presence of a fixed stenosis, coronary blood flow is not altered. The decrease in mean blood pressure produces reflex activation of the sympathetic nervous system. Increases in heart rate and contractility partially reverse the decrease in oxygen consumption produced by arterial and venous vasodilation and can be blocked by β adrenergic receptor antagonists. In patients with variant angina, the organic nitrates can prevent or reverse coronary artery spasm. Organic nitrates are effective for the treatment of classic and variant angina.

Pharmacokinetics

- Isosorbide dinitrate and mononitrate are effective orally.
- Amyl nitrite is administered by inhalation.
- Nitroglycerin and isosorbide dinitrate given sublingually are rapidly absorbed through the oral mucosa. Their therapeutic effects are observed within 2 to 4 minutes but last for only 1 to 2 hours.
- Nitrates are well absorbed through skin from ointments and sustained-release patches. The therapeutic effects of the

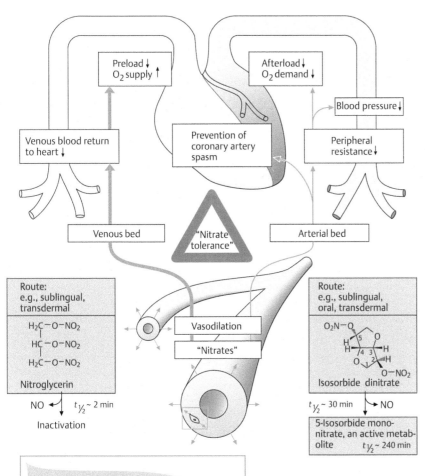

Fig. 22.3 Vasodilators: nitrates.
Nitrates cause vasodilation by acting like endogenous nitric oxide (NO), causing activation of guanylate cyclase and increased cyclic guanosine monophosphate (cGMP) levels in vascular smooth muscle cells. This vasodilation reduces cardiac work by reducing preload and afterload. Nitroglycerin and isosorbide dinitrate are both highly membrane permeable. GTP, guanosine triphosphate; SH, sulfhydryl.

ointment persist for 4 to 8 hours, and the sustained-release preparation can maintain stable blood levels of nitroglycerin for 24 hours. Usefulness is limited by rapid tolerance.

- Nitroglycerin may be given as an intravenous infusion in the treatment of MI.
- Amyl nitrite is volatile and is administered by inhalation.

Side Effects

- Headache (subsides with repeated use).
- Orthostatic (postural) hypotension.

Tolerance

The uninterrupted use of organic nitrates results in tolerance, with subsequent doses of nitrates producing little hemodynamic response. The use of dermal nitrates should not extend for more than 12 to 16 hours of any 24-hour period and must include a nitrate-free interval between doses.

22.4 Beta Blockers

Beta blockers are discussed in Chapter 20.

22.4.1 Specific Points in Relation to Angina

- The β adrenergic receptor antagonists are useful for the prophylaxis of effort-induced angina but are not effective for the acute termination of effort-induced angina or for the treatment of coronary artery spasm.
- When used in combination with organic nitrates, β blockers antagonize the reflex increase in sympathetic nervous system activity observed with the organic nitrates.
- Contraindicated in variant angina due to unopposed alpha adrenergic receptor effects that may aggravate angina.

▶ Table 22.1 compares the effects of nitrates and β blockers on the heart.

22.5 Calcium Channel Blockers

Calcium channel blockers are discussed in Chapter 20.

22.5.1 Specific Points in Relation to Angina

- In angina, calcium channel blockers act to increase coronary blood flow by dilating coronary vessels and decreasing myocardial oxygen demand by blocking Ca^{2+} channels on cardiac myocytes.

22.6 Ranolazine

22.6.1 Mechanism of Action

The main mechanism of ranolazine is to inhibit the late inward sodium current in cardiac myocytes. This current is enhanced in ischemia (and other pathological conditions), and it leads to an intracellular calcium overload. Inhibiting this current leads to reduced intracellular calcium. The major effect is a reduction in diastolic calcium levels, which improves myocardial relaxation and reduces myocardial oxygen demand. Coronary blood flow is also improved. Ranolazine is used to treat chronic stable angina as first-line therapy in those patients who are intolerant to other drugs, or used as an adjunctive agent when angina persists despite standard therapy.

22.6.2 Pharmacokinetics

- Ranolazine is effective orally.
- Hepatically metabolized.

22.6.3 Side Effects

- Risk of prolonged QT interval at higher doses.
- Contraindicated in hepatic cirrhosis.

▶ Table 22.2 provides a summary of the mechanisms by which antianginal drugs act.

Table 22.1 Summary of effects of nitrates and β blockers

Class of drug	Heart rate	Contractility	Preload	Afterload	Oxygen consumption
Nitrates	Small increase	Small increase	Large decrease	Small decrease	Moderate decrease
β blockers	Large decrease	Large decrease	Small increase	Small increase	Moderate decrease

Note: The hemodynamic actions of the nitrates complement those of the β blockers and are the basis for their concomitant use in the therapy of effort-induced angina.

Table 22.2 Summary of mechanisms of antianginal drugs

Drug class	Parameter affected	Mechanism
Nitrates	↓ preload and afterload ↓ myocardial O_2 consumption ↓ coronary artery spasm ↑ blood flow to ischemic areas of the heart	Activates guanylate cyclase to ↑ cGMP
β blockers	↓ heart rate and contractility ↓ myocardial O_2 consumption	Blocks sympathetic activation
Calcium channel blockers	↑ coronary blood flow ↓ myocardial O_2 consumption	Blocks L-type Ca^{2+} channels to dilate blood vessels and decrease contractility of cardiac muscle
Ranolazine	↑ myocardial relaxation ↓ myocardial O_2 consumption	Inhibits late inward sodium current in cardiac myocytes

Abbreviation: cGMP, cyclic guanosine monophosphate.

23 Antiarrhythmic Drugs

Summary

The antiarrhythmic drugs act to reduce abnormal impulse generation or abnormal conduction in order to suppress and prevent arrhythmias. Consideration of the proarrhythmic propensity and other adverse effects of these agents should be undertaken before use. The four major classes of antiarrhythmic drugs are: Na^+ channel blockers (Class I), beta blockers (Class II), K^+ channel blockers (Class III), and Ca^{2+} channel blockers (Class IV). In supraventricular arrhythmias (atrial fibrillation and flutter), pharmacological therapy is usually used to control the ventricular rate. The most often used drugs are the beta blockers and the calcium channel blockers (verapamil and diltiazem). Amiodarone can be considered if these drugs are ineffective. Class IA (quinidine, procainamide, and disopyramide), class IC (flecainide and propafenone), and class III (amiodarone, dronedarone, sotalol, ibutilide, and dofetilide) agents may be considered to maintain suppression of arrhythmias but are less used due to serious side effect risks. Typically, pharmacological therapy is adjunctive to implantable devices in treatment of ventricular arrhythmias. Class IA, IB (lidocaine, mexiletine, tocainide, and phenytoin), IC, II, III, and IV agents are available for use in treatment; however, due to the potential for serious adverse effects, the most commonly recommended drugs are beta blockers or amiodarone for suppression of ventricular arrhythmia. Lidocaine may be considered for patients who are refractory to amiodarone or beta blockers. Digoxin may be used in atrial fibrillation or atrioventricular (AV) node reentrant arrhythmias. Intravenous (IV) adenosine may be used for acute termination of AV node reentry. Atropine may be useful in bradycardia.

Keywords: arrhythmia, action potential, electrocardiogram, atrial arrhythmia, ventricular arrythmia

23.1 Electrophysiology of the Heart

23.1.1 Conduction System of the Heart

The sinoatrial (SA) node is the primary pacemaker of the heart, since it is able to spontaneously generate action potentials (inherent automaticity). These action potentials are conducted rapidly through the right atrial myocardium to the atrioventricular (AV) node, which delays the impulse before conducting it to the ventricles via the bundle of His and Purkinje fibers. This provides an orderly contraction sequence from apex to base for efficient ejection of blood from the ventricles (▶ Fig. 23.1).

- The SA node spontaneously generates action potentials at a rate of ~ 80 to 100 beats per minute.
- The AV node also has inherent automaticity but at a slower rate than the SA node. If the SA node fails, the AV node will take over the pacemaker activity of the heart.
- The delay of the cardiac impulse at the AV node gives the contracting atria adequate time to empty their contents into the ventricles before ventricular contraction is initiated.

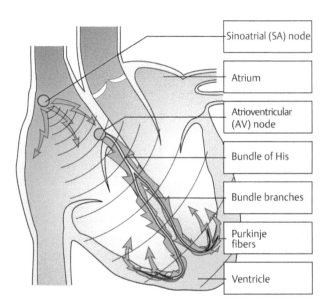

Fig. 23.1 Cardiac conduction system.
An impulse-initiating cardiac contraction begins in the sinoatrial (SA) node. It travels through the atrial myocardium to the atrioventricular (AV) node. From the AV node, the impulse spreads to the ventricular myocardium via the bundle of His and Purkinje fibers. Contraction of the ventricular myocardium occurs from the inside to the outside and from the apex to the base of the heart.

Note: The typical resting heart rate is 65 to 75 beats per minute. This is due to vagal slowing of the heart below the intrinsic rate set by the SA node.

23.1.2 Cardiac Action Potentials

The ionic conductances that are a feature of action potential phases at the SA node, cardiac muscle, and branches of the conduction system are discussed in this section.

Action Potential Phases at the Sinoatrial Node

Refer to the action potential waveforms of slow response tissue (nodal cells) in ▶ Fig. 23.2.

Phase 0

- This slow upstroke of the action potential shows membrane depolarization (it becomes less negative).
- It results from an increase in Ca^{2+} conductance, causing inward Ca^{2+} flow.

Phases 1 and 2

- These phases do not occur at the SA node.

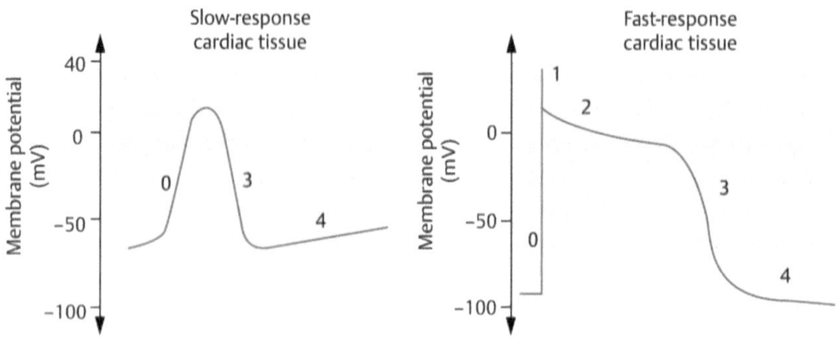

Fig. 23.2 Membrane potential changes in cardiac muscle fibers.
Slow-response tissue includes the sinoatrial (SA) node and atrioventricular (AV) node. Fast-response tissue includes the atrial and ventricular myocardium, the bundle of His, and Purkinje fibers. Slow- and fast-response tissues have distinct electrochemical properties. This causes them to react differently to antiarrhythmic drugs.

Phase 3

- This is the repolarization phase.
- It results from an increase in K⁺ conductance, which causes outward K⁺ flow and repolarization of the membrane toward the K⁺ equilibrium potential (the resting potential).

Phase 4

- The SA node does not have a stable resting membrane potential. During phase 4, it slowly depolarizes (which is responsible for its inherent automaticity).
- It results from an increase in Na⁺ conductance, causing inward Na⁺ flow and a decrease in K⁺ conductance.

Note: The events at the AV node are similar to those at the SA node but slower. As a result, the AV node normally does not generate its own action potentials. This is because action potentials are conducted to the AV node more frequently than its own slow inherent rate of action potential generation.

Action Potential Phases at the Atrial and Ventricular Myocardium, Bundle of His, and Purkinje Fibers

Refer to the action potential waveforms of fast response (non-pacemaker) tissue in ▶ Fig. 23.2.

Phase 0

- This rapid upstroke of the action potential shows membrane depolarization (it becomes less negative).
- It results from an increase in Na⁺ conductance, causing rapid inward Na⁺ flow.
- This inward Na⁺ flow stops after a few milliseconds due to inactivation of Na⁺ channels.
- The maximum rate of voltage change during phase 0 (dV/dt) determines the conduction velocity.

Phase 1

- This is an early slight membrane repolarization (membrane becomes more negative).
- It results from rapid outward K⁺ flow (due to a favorable electrochemical gradient) and a decrease in Na⁺ conductance.

Phase 2

- This is the plateau phase.

- In this phase, there is increased Ca²⁺ inward flow through L-type Ca²⁺ channels which approximately balances outward K⁺ flow.
- Ca²⁺ entry during phase 2 is necessary for cardiac muscle contraction.

Phase 3

- This is the repolarization phase.
- It results from a decrease in Ca²⁺ conductance and an increase in K⁺ conductance. The net effect of this is that there is a rapid outward K⁺ flow which repolarizes the membrane toward the K⁺ equilibrium potential (the resting potential).

Phase 4

- This is the resting membrane potential.
- It is determined by high K⁺ conductance and its value is therefore close to the K⁺ equilibrium potential (−96 mV). At this potential, K⁺ outflow and K⁺ inflow are equal.

23.1.3 Measuring the Electrical Activity of the Heart: The Electrocardiogram

Recording an Electrocardiogram

The electrocardiogram (ECG) is an overall representation of the electrical activity in the heart (▶ Fig. 23.3). It is measured by recording voltages through surface electrodes that "look" at the heart from different positions. A wave of depolarization moving toward a lead causes an upward deflection of the ECG. Analysis of the results of an ECG allows clinicians to diagnose a variety of cardiac disorders, including arrhythmias, ischemia, and the location of myocardial infarction (MI).

Interpretation of ECG Waves, Segments, and Intervals

Waves

- The P wave corresponds to atrial depolarization.
- The QRS complex corresponds to ventricular depolarization that occurs from apex to base.
- The T wave corresponds to ventricular repolarization that occurs from base to apex.

Note: Repolarization of the atria is masked by the QRS complex.

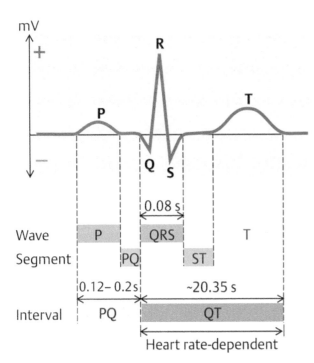

Fig. 23.3 Electrocardiogram (ECG) curve.
The ECG depicts electrical activity in the heart. The P wave corresponds to atrial depolarization. The QRS complex represents ventricular depolarization, and the T wave represents ventricular repolarization.

Foundations

Excitation–Contraction Coupling in the Heart

Contraction of cardiac muscle occurs when the excitation produced by an action potential is transmitted to cardiac myofibrils. Depolarization of the cardiac muscle cell membrane triggers an action potential that passes through T tubules. During phase 2 (plateau) of the action potential, there is increased Ca^{2+} conductance, causing inward Ca^{2+} flow. This inward Ca^{2+} flow initiates the release of Ca^{2+} from the sarcoplasmic reticulum (Ca^{2+}-induced Ca^{2+} release) which increases intracellular $[Ca^{2+}]$. Ca^{2+} binds to troponin C, and tropomyosin moves out of its blocking position, allowing actin and myosin to form cross-bridges. The thick and thin filaments of actin and myosin slide past each other, resulting in cardiac muscle cell contraction. The contraction ends when Ca^{2+} ATPase facilitates the reuptake of Ca^{2+} into the sarcoplasmic reticulum, reducing the intracellular $[Ca^{2+}]$. The force of contraction of cardiac muscle cells is proportional to the amount of Ca^{2+} release, which varies depending on conditions.

Foundations

Cardiac Axis

The cardiac axis is the mean direction of electrical current flow through the ventricles during depolarization. It is calculated by analysis of the QRS complexes in the ECG leads. Many factors can alter the cardiac axis, including abnormal cardiac anatomy or position, MI, ischemia, pulmonary embolism, cardiomyopathy, and conduction abnormalities.

Clinical Correlation

Cardioversion

Cardioversion is a procedure in which an electrical shock is delivered to the heart via paddles or electrodes to convert an arrhythmia to a normal rhythm. It does this by causing all of the cardiac muscle cells to contract simultaneously. This brief interruption to the arrhythmia gives the SA nodes an opportunity to regain control over the pacing of the heart.

Clinical Correlation

Valsalva Maneuver

The Valsalva maneuver involves forceful expiration against a closed glottis, resulting in increased intrathoracic pressure that causes a reduction in venous return, a reduction in cardiac output due to decreased preload (via the Starling mechanism), reduced heart rate, and a fluctuation in aortic pressures (increased initially, then decreased). The Valsalva maneuver can be used to arrest episodes of supraventricular tachycardia and as a diagnostic aid to clinicians for some cardiac diseases (e.g., hypertrophic cardiomyopathy) that are worsened by the Valsalva. It is also used by swimmers and people on aircraft to normalize ear pressures. A similar effect to the Valsalva maneuver is seen in people straining during a bowel movement. This is particularly dangerous for patients with pulmonary embolism.

Segments

- The PQ segment is an isoelectric period between the P wave and the QRS complex. During this time, the wave of depolarization is traveling through the AV node into the bundle of His.
- The ST segment corresponds to the plateau phase of the cardiac action potential when all ventricular fibers are simultaneously depolarized.

Intervals

- The PQ (or PR) interval corresponds to the conduction of the action potential through the AV node.
- The QT interval corresponds to ventricular depolarization and repolarization.

23.2 Arrhythmias

▶ Table 23.1 provides a classification of arrhythmias.

An *arrhythmia* is a disorder of the heart rate or rhythm. Arrhythmias arise due to abnormal impulse generation (automaticity, triggered activity) or abnormal conduction (reentry). Dysfunction in automaticity of pacemaker cells can cause slowed (sinus bradycardia, heart rate < 60 beats per minute) or increased (sinus tachycardia, heart rate > 100 beats per minute) heart rate. Increased impulse generation in abnormal pacemaker sites within the atria or ventricles, known as *ectopic foci*, can also result in abnormal rhythms. Under normal circumstances, ectopic pacemaker activity is overridden by the pace set by the SA node; however, in cardiac disease states, they can cause tachycardia or bradycardia depending on their site and

Table 23.1 A classification of arrhythmias

Arrhythmia	Rhythm	Comment
Atrial flutter	The atrial rhythm is very rapid but regular (300–400 beats/min)	One of every two (2:1 block) or three (3:1 block) atrial beats is conducted to the ventricle through the AV node. The ventricular heart rate (133–200 beats/min) is regular but too rapid to allow optimal ventricular filling during diastole
Atrial fibrillation	The atrial rhythm is rapid (400–600 beats/min) and irregular. The ventricular rhythm is also rapid and irregular (100–150 beats/min)	No distinct P waves seen on ECG
Ventricular premature beats		These beats originate in the ventricles. They usually do not reduce cardiac output. Many patients with frequent premature ventricular beats may be bothered by palpitations
Ventricular tachycardia	Rapid rhythm (200–400 beats/min) originating in the ventricles	Ventricular tachycardia can be self-terminating or sustained (lasting > 30 s). Patients with ventricular tachycardia and heart disease have a high probability of developing ventricular fibrillation. Ventricular tachycardia leading to ventricular fibrillation is the leading cause of death in the United States
Ventricular fibrillation	Rapid rhythm (> 400 beats/min) originating in the ventricles	Ventricular fibrillation is invariably fatal unless electrical defibrillation is performed

Abbreviations: AV, atrioventricular; ECG, electrocardiogram.

the disease involved. Abnormal conduction through the AV node can lead to bradycardia, and arrhythmias may also occur due to abnormal (reentry) conduction. This results when action potentials travel in a circuit within the heart rather than in one direction causing persistent excitation. Multiple reentry circuits within a chamber of the heart can lead to incoordination of cardiac muscle contraction known as *fibrillation*.

23.3 Antiarrhythmic Drugs

▶ Table 23.2 outlines the classification of antiarrhythmic agents on the basis of ion channel or receptor that they block and the effects they have on the action potential. However, these drugs often target multiple proteins in order to impart their effects. The grouping of the agents represents the Vaughan Williams classification of antiarrhythmics, which is based on mechanism of action and effects on the action potential. Although limited, this classification system is widely used.

23.3.1 Class I Antiarrhythmic Drugs: Sodium Channel Blockers (Local Anesthetics)

All class I antiarrhythmic agents inhibit sodium channels by binding to them in the open or inactivated states. These drugs show use dependence, that is, they have greater effects at faster heart rates than normal ones. Subclassification of agents is based on effects on the action potential by acting on other ion currents and the degree of sodium channel inhibition. By inhibiting sodium channels involved in phase 0 depolarization of myocardium action potentials (fast response), class I antiarrhythmics slow conduction in atrial and ventricular tissue reducing the amplitude of the action potential and the slope of phase 0. These agents are categorized into three groups based on the magnitude of sodium channel inhibition and other effects. The effects of class I agents on channel opening, ionic conductances, and cardiac excitability are depicted in ▶ Fig. 23.4.

Table 23.2 Classification of antiarrhythmic agents

Drug class	Mechanism of action	Effect on action potential
Class IA	Moderate Na^+ channel blockers	Slow phase 0, increase the action potential duration, and slow conduction
Class IB	Weak Na^+ channel blockers	Shorten phase 3, slightly decrease in action potential duration, and slow conduction
Class IC	Strong Na^+ channel blockers	Markedly slow phase 0, no effect on action potential duration, and slow conduction
Class II	β blockers	Slow phase 4, automaticity, and conduction
Class III	K^+ channel blockers	Prolong phase 3, increase action potential duration, and slow conduction
Class IV	Ca^{2+} channel blockers (verapamil and diltiazem only)	Slow phase 0 to decrease automaticity, decrease amplitude and duration of phase 2

Class IA Agents: Quinidine, Procainamide, and Disopyramide

Mechanism of Action

Class IA agents moderately inhibit sodium channels with preferential binding in the open state. They also block potassium channels. This slows the rate of repolarization in nodal and nonnodal cells, increasing the effective refractory period and prolonging the action potential duration and QT interval. Reduced ventricular conduction can increase QRS interval. Class IA drugs have anticholinergic (vagolytic) actions to varying degrees, possibly by inhibiting acetylcholine-mediated activation of potassium channels or inhibiting acetylcholine release. Procainamide has the least amount of vagolytic activity. By inhibiting cholinergic activity, these drugs can improve AV nodal conduction; however, because they also directly depress AV nodal conduction, there is a variable net effect on AV nodal conduction.

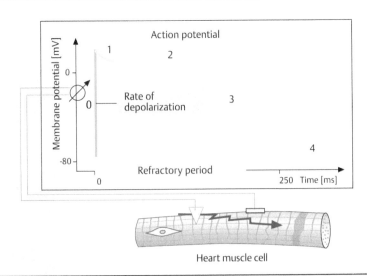

Fig. 23.4 **Effects of antiarrhythmic drugs of the Na⁺ channel blocking type.** Antiarrhythmics of the Na⁺ channel blocking type inhibit Na⁺ channel opening. This can result in a decreased rate of depolarization (phase 0), suppression of action potential (AP) generation, or an increase in the refractory period (phases 1–3).

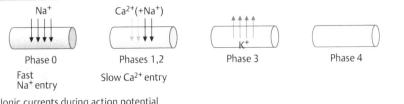

Ionic currents during action potential

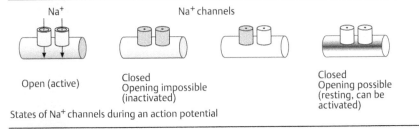

States of Na⁺ channels during an action potential

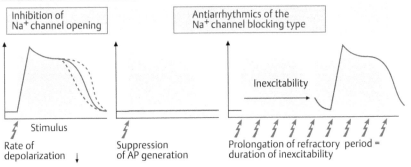

Uses

- Atrial fibrillation.
- Atrial flutter.
- Ventricular tachycardia.
- Ventricular fibrillation.

Note: These drugs should not be used alone for the treatment of atrial flutter or atrial fibrillation because the ventricular heart rate may dramatically increase through a combination of the anticholinergic effect which enhances AV nodal conduction and an increase in impulses passing though the AV node. This can cause a reduction in cardiac output. All three drugs depress myocardial contractility and can worsen existing heart failure.

Side Effects

- May cause life-threatening arrhythmias (ventricular tachycardia or ventricular fibrillation). One life-threatening ventricular arrhythmia produced by both class IA and class III agents is torsades de pointes. The procainamide metabolite *N*-acetylprocainamide (NAPA) has class III (potassium channel blocking) activity, which can further contribute to inducing arrhythmias.
- Heart failure due to negative inotropic effects.
- Anticholinergic: dry eyes, dry mouth, and urinary retention (disopyramide > quinidine > procainamide).
- Skin rash, muscle weakness, and arthralgia (joint pain).
- Cinchonism (quinidine only [quinidine is the d-isomer of quinine]): tinnitus (ringing in the ears), blurred vision, delirium, gastrointestinal upset (with or without cinchonism).

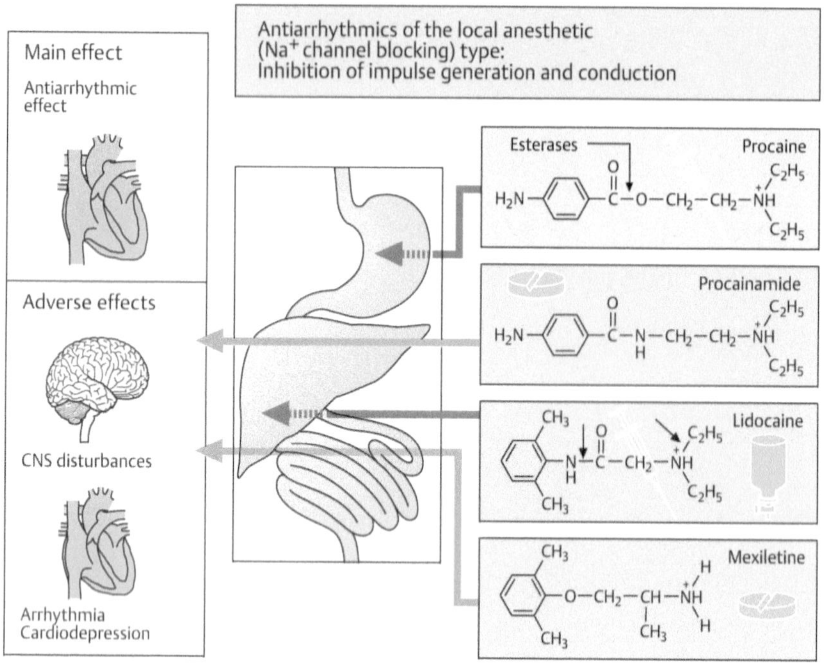

Fig. 23.5 Antiarrhythmic drugs of the Na⁺ channel blocking type.
Procaine and lidocaine are rapidly degraded in the body by cleavage (at the points indicated by *arrows* in the chemical structure box). These drugs must be given intravenously or by intravenous infusion. The orally administered drugs procainamide and mexiletine are not subject to such rapid degradation and are thus more likely to cause adverse effects. CNS, central nervous system.

• Acute lupus erythematosus (procainamide only): chronic administration increases antinuclear antibody levels.

Clinical Correlation

Torsades de pointes

Torsades de pointes is a rare form of ventricular tachycardia accompanied by distinctive ECG changes. It translates as "twisting of the points," which refers to the twisting of QRS complexes around the baseline electrical axis of the heart by at least 180 degrees. The QT interval is also prolonged. This arrhythmia can degenerate to ventricular fibrillation causing sudden death if untreated. Causes include therapy with class IA and III antiarrhythmic agents (which inhibit K⁺ channels), hypomagnesemia (low plasma Mg^{2+}), and hypokalemia (low plasma K⁺).

Class IB Agents: Lidocaine, Mexiletine, Tocainide, and Phenytoin

Mechanism of Action

Class IB agents bind to sodium channels in both open and inactivated states, and may have greater effects in ischemic myocardium where membrane depolarization increases the propensity for sodium channels to be open or inactivated. Slow conduction and prolonged QRS interval occur at fast heart rates. Unlike class IA agents, these drugs do not inhibit potassium channels. These agents typically shorten the action potential duration, which is attributed to inhibition of late sodium channels in phase 2. Class IB drugs have little effect on AV nodal conduction or myocardial contractility.

Pharmacokinetics

• Lidocaine is rapidly metabolized in the liver. It has a short plasma half-life and is used as an IV infusion only in a hospital setting (▶ Fig. 23.5).
• Mexiletine and tocainide are analogues of lidocaine and are used orally for long-term therapy.

Uses

• In ventricular arrhythmias as an alternative to amiodarone (class III antiarrhythmic agent). These drugs are not effective in atrial arrhythmias.
• Phenytoin is an antiepileptic agent that is also classified as a class IB antiarrhythmic. It is used sometimes when other drugs have failed.

Side Effects

• Central nervous system: act as local anesthetics in the brain.
• Sedation at low doses.
• Muscle twitching and vertigo with moderate dosages.
• Convulsions at higher doses.

Class IC Agents: Flecainide and Propafenone

Mechanism of Action

Class IC agents have prominent sodium channel blocking effects resulting in slow conduction and prolonged QRS interval at slow, moderate, and fast heart rates. These agents slow conduction in all cardiac tissues (including the AV node) and also depress cardiac contractility. They have no effect on the duration of the action potential.

Uses

- Paroxysmal atrial flutter.
- Paroxysmal atrial fibrillation.
- Life-threatening ventricular arrhythmias.

Side Effects

- Heart failure (due to negative inotropic effects of all class IC drugs).
- Worsening of cardiac arrhythmias. Use is limited by proar-rhythmic properties.
- Worsening of conduction abnormalities.
- Avoid in post-MI cases. These drugs may increase mortality when administered to patients post MI.
- Headache.

23.3.2 Class II Antiarrhythmic Drugs: Beta Blocking Agents

Beta Adrenergic Receptor Antagonists: Propranolol, Metoprolol, Esmolol and Others

Mechanism of Action

Class II β adrenergic receptor antagonists are used to treat arrhythmias by inhibiting sympathetic effects on cardiac tissue. These drugs slow phase 4 depolarization, thus slowing automaticity and AV nodal conduction, and decreasing heart rate and contractility.

Uses

Class II agents are used to depress AV nodal conduction with atrial flutter-fibrillation and prevent ventricular fibrillation following MI. Esmolol has a short duration of action so it is often used to prevent acute arrhythmias, that is, during or after surgery.

23.3.3 Class III Antiarrhythmic Drugs: Potassium Channel Blockers

Amiodarone, Dronedarone, Sotalol, Ibutilide, Dofetilide

Mechanism of Action

The class III antiarrhythmic drugs prolong action potential duration, QT interval, and effective refractory period mostly by inhibiting potassium channels. Most of the drugs in this class impart this effect at slower heart rates (reverse use dependence).

Amiodarone is the most commonly used drug in this class. In addition to blocking potassium channels, it also blocks sodium and calcium channels, and has beta blocking activity.

Pharmacokinetics

- The half-life of amiodarone is ~ 30 days. There is a prolonged time to achieve efficacy with oral administration, and effects are prolonged after drug withdrawal.

Uses

Treatment of atrial and ventricular arrhythmias.

Note: Due to the high incidence of serious side effects, the class III drugs are restricted for life-threatening arrhythmias.

Side Effects

- Torsades de pointes: amiodarone is not as prone to inducing arrhythmias as others in this class.
- Sinus bradycardia.
- Amiodarone: corneal opacities, photosensitivity that produces a gray-blue skin rash, thyroid dysfunction (drug contains iodine atoms), peripheral neuropathy, and life-threatening pulmonary toxicity (pulmonary fibrosis and interstitial pneumonitis) that may not remit with drug withdrawal.
- Sotalol: all adverse effects seen with β blockers and torsades de pointes.

23.3.4 Class IV Antiarrhythmic Agents: Calcium Channel Blockers

Nondihydropyridines: Verapamil and Diltiazem

Mechanism of Action

Class IV drugs inhibit calcium entry through L-type calcium channels in the myocardium and depress AV nodal transmission.

Note: Nifedipine and nicardipine, although excellent vasodilators and antianginal drugs, are poor inhibitors of AV nodal transmission and are ineffective as antiarrhythmic drugs.

Uses

- Treatment of atrial flutter-fibrillation.
- Acute termination of AV nodal reentry.

Side Effects

- Sinus arrest or complete AV nodal blockade, especially in the presence of β adrenergic receptor blockade (verapamil).

23.3.5 Miscellaneous Antiarrhythmic Agents

Adenosine

Mechanism of Action

Adenosine binds to adenosine receptors in the heart, resulting in increased potassium conductance and reduced calcium current. Conduction velocity is decreased, especially at the AV node.

Pharmacokinetics

Adenosine is administered as an IV bolus and has a plasma half-life of a few seconds (it is taken up by red blood cells). A repeat bolus can be given again within minutes if the first dose is ineffective.

Uses

Acute termination of AV node reentry.

Side Effects

- Transient dyspnea.
- Flushing.

Digoxin

Mechanism of Action

The mechanisms of action, effects, and side effects of digoxin are discussed in detail in Chapter 21. The action to enhance vagal effects on the atrium and AV node contribute to its usefulness as an antiarrhythmic.

Uses

- Atrial fibrillation.
- AV node reentrant arrhythmias.

Atropine

Mechanism of Action

The mechanisms of action, effects, and side effects of atropine are discussed in detail in Chapter 5. Atropine is a muscarinic cholinergic receptor antagonist. Thus, it blocks effects of the vagus nerve on the heart.

Pharmacokinetics

Given IV.

Use

Bradyarrhythmias.

Clinical Correlation

Nondrug Therapies for Arrhythmias

Surgical interventions have an important role in addition to or in place of drug therapy for arrhythmias. Catheter ablation of the source or conduction path of the arrhythmia by application of radiofrequency current applied through a large-tip electrode on a steerable catheter may be useful for supraventricular tachycardias, atrial arrhythmias, atrial fibrillation, and ventricular tachycardia. In patients with SA node dysfunction or AV nodal block, or if heart block persists following an ablative procedure, implantation of a permanent pacemaker may be indicated. In ventricular fibrillation or ventricular tachycardia, implantation of a cardioverter-defibrillator is superior to drug therapy in certain patient populations.

24 Drugs Acting on the Blood

Summary

Drugs that act on blood are used in the prevention and treatment of blood clotting disorders and cytopenias. Anticoagulants, antiplatelets, and thrombolytics are the mainstay in therapy for prevention and treatment of stroke, thromboembolism, and acute coronary syndrome. Aspirin and dipyridamole are two antiplatelet drugs. Clopidogrel, prasugrel, and ticlopidine are irreversible antagonists of the purinergic P2Y12 receptors on platelets. Ticagrelor and cangrelor are reversible inhibitor or P2Y12 receptors. Abciximab, eptifibatide, and tirofiban are glycoprotein IIb/IIIa receptor antagonists. The anticoagulants include heparin and the low-molecular-weight heparins enoxaparin and dalteparin. Direct thrombin inhibitors include bivalirudin, lepirudin, and argatroban. Direct factor Xa inhibitors include rivaroxaban, apixaban, and edoxaban. Warfarin is an anticoagulant that antagonizes the hepatic synthesis of the vitamin K-dependent clotting factors. Thrombolytic drugs include streptokinase, urokinase, alteplase, reteplase, and tenecteplase. Aminocaproic acid and tranexamic acid inhibit plasmin and plasminogen activator. They can be used to prevent bleeding. Desmopressin and pentoxifylline also decrease bleeding. Iron deficiency anemia is treated with ferrous sulfate or iron dextran. Megaloblastic anemia is treated with leucovorin or vitamin B_{12}. Filgrastim and sargramostim are recombinant granulocyte colony stimulating factors (CSFs) and granulocyte-macrophage CSFs, respectively, used to stimulate bone marrow cell reconstitution after transplantation or cancer chemotherapy. Epoetin alfa is recombinant erythropoietin used to increase the number of red blood cells. Interleukin 11 is used to speed platelet recovery in patients undergoing chemotherapy with nonmyeloid malignancies.

Keywords: hemostasis, coagulation, anticoagulants, anemia, iron, heparin, warfarin, bone marrow growth factors

24.1 Introduction

Traumatic injury to blood vessels results in a series of events aimed at achieving hemostasis (cessation of bleeding), including vasoconstriction, platelet aggregation, and the deposition of fibrin (▶ Fig. 24.1).

24.2 Hemostasis

An intact, undamaged endothelium normally produces substances to prevent blood from clotting. These include inhibitors of platelet aggregation, such as nitric oxide (NO) and prostacyclin, and thrombomodulin and heparans, which inhibit clotting. The process of hemostasis begins upon damage to the endothelium.

Foundations

Role of Endothelial Cells in Preventing Thrombus Formation

Endothelial cells produce NO and prostacyclin that inhibit platelets from adhering to undamaged, healthy endothelium. Diseases that impair endothelial function (e.g., elevated blood glucose, chronic hypertension, and smoking) increase the tendency for platelets to adhere to endothelium and so predispose an individual to thrombosis.

When there is physical damage to endothelium, platelets adhere to exposed subendothelial collagen fibers directly via glycoprotein 1a receptors on the platelet surface. This interaction is also bridged by von Willebrand factor (vWF) in the vascular endothelium interacting with glycoprotein 1b receptors on the surface of platelets. This adhesion activates platelets, which release a number of factors that aid hemostasis: vasoconstrictors serotonin, thromboxane A_2, and mediators that increase platelet activation

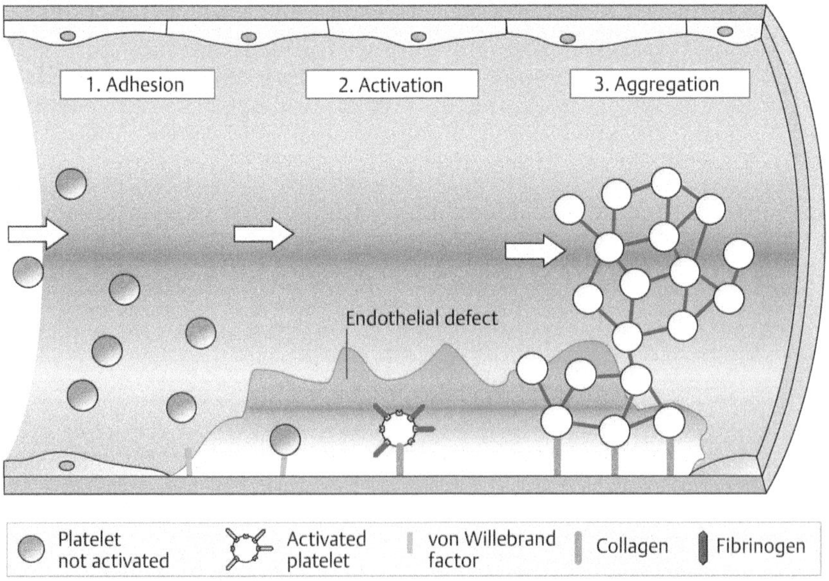

Fig. 24.1 Platelet-mediated hemostasis.
Vascular injury and endothelial defects in vessel walls expose collagen and extracellular matrix. Platelet interaction with exposed subendothelial collagen and von Willebrand factor in vascular endothelium cause fast-flowing platelets to slow down at the site of an endothelial defect. This activates platelets and causes them to change shape and gain an affinity for fibrinogen. The platelets then become linked to each other via fibrinogen bridges, causing thrombus formation.

1. Adhesion   2. Activation   3. Aggregation

Endothelial defect

Platelet not activated | Activated platelet | von Willebrand factor | Collagen | Fibrinogen

such as vWF, adenosine diphosphate (ADP), platelet-activating factor (PAF), and thrombin. Of note, ADP binds to puringeric receptors (P2Y1 and P2Y12) on platelet surfaces that increase mobilization of intracellular calcium and inhibit cyclic adenosine monophosphate (cAMP); both effects are involved in promoting platelet aggregation. Once activated, platelets change shape and glycoprotein IIb/IIIa receptors change their conformation which promotes the affinity of platelets for fibrinogen. Fibrinogen, by binding to IIb/IIIa receptors on two platelets, can act to increase platelet adhesion and further platelet aggregation.

Endothelial injury also stimulates the coagulation (clotting) cascade via the release of tissue factors and by mediators released by activated platelets. This results in the formation of thrombin (Factor IIa) which then catalyzes the hydrolysis of fibrinogen to fibrin. Fibrin forms a meshwork within the platelet plug (aggregated platelets). Overall, a platelet–fibrin clot is produced that achieves hemostasis (▶ Fig. 24.1 and ▶ Fig. 24.2).

24.2.1 Thrombosis and Embolism

Thrombosis is the formation of an unwanted blood clot in a blood vessel or within the heart. It is an inappropriate response of the hemostatic process to alterations in the circulatory system, lesions in vascular walls, or other stimuli (▶ Fig. 24.2).

Embolism occurs when thrombi are dislodged and are carried by the circulation to small vessels, where they may cause occlusions and tissue ischemia.

Thrombosis is treated by pharmacological agents designed to inhibit platelet function, inhibit fibrin deposition, or enhance fibrinolysis.

24.3 Antiplatelet Drugs

When platelets are stimulated to aggregate, arachidonic acid is liberated from platelet phospholipids and may be metabolized

to thromboxane A_2 by the sequential actions of cyclooxygenase-1 (COX-1) and thromboxane synthetase. As this occurs, platelet levels of cAMP decrease, and ADP is released. Both ADP and thromboxane A_2 are potent stimuli for platelet aggregation.

24.3.1 Aspirin

Aspirin is discussed in more detail in Chapter 33.

Mechanism of Action

Aspirin acetylates platelet COX-1 and irreversibly inhibits the enzyme (▶ Fig. 24.3). This reduces the formation of thromboxane A_2. Because platelets cannot generate new COX-1, the effects of aspirin last for the duration of the platelet lifespan, about 8 to 10 days.

Pharmacokinetics

Aspirin is usually given at a dose of 50 to 100 mg daily for its antithrombotic effects.

Uses

- Prophylaxis or treatment of stroke or myocardial infarction (MI).
- Also used after vascular surgery, such as percutaneous coronary intervention, carotid endarterectomy, or coronary artery bypass surgery to prevent thrombosis.

Side Effects

The major side effects of aspirin are gastrointestinal (GI) distress and bleeding.

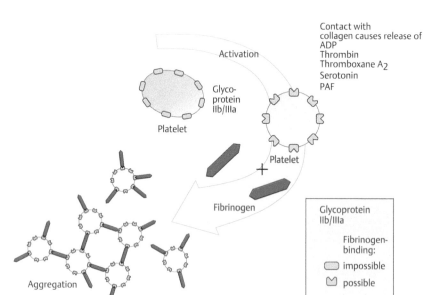

Contact with collagen causes release of
ADP
Thrombin
Thromboxane A_2
Serotonin
PAF

Activation

Glycoprotein IIb/IIIa

Platelet

Platelet

Fibrinogen

Aggregation

Glycoprotein IIb/IIIa

Fibrinogen-binding:
⬭ impossible
⬒ possible

Fig. 24.2 Aggregation of platelets by glycoprotein IIb/IIIa and fibrinogen.
Glycoprotein IIb/IIIa in the platelet membrane change their conformation when platelets are activated by adhesion to the site of vascular injury. This causes the platelets to gain an affinity for fibrinogen. Activated platelets release other substances, for example, ADP and thromboxane A_2, which can activate other platelets. ADP, adenosine diphosphate; PAF, platelet-activating factor.

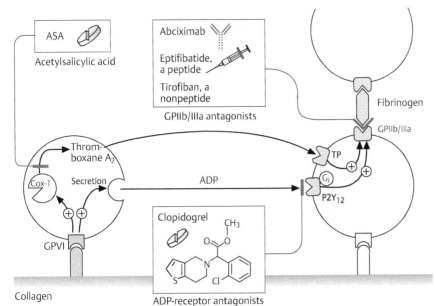

Fig. 24.3 Inhibitors of platelet aggregation.
Platelets attach to collagen via glycoprotein VI (GPVI) on platelet membranes. This activates them and causes them to secrete adenosine diphosphate (ADP) and serotonin, as well as increasing production of thromboxane A_2 to be produced from arachidonic acid via cyclooxygenase-1 (COX-1). Glycoprotein IIb/IIIa (GPIIb/GPIIIa) activation also leads to platelet aggregation. Acetylsalicylic acid (ASA) inhibits COX-1, which prevents thromboxane formation. Clopidogrel is an ADP receptor antagonist at the P2Y12 receptor. Other agents (e.g., abciximab) block the binding of fibrinogen to GPIIb/GPIIIa. TP, thromboxane prostanoid receptor.

Clinical Correlation

Stroke

Stroke is death of brain tissue due to either cerebral ischemia or intercerebral hemorrhage. Ischemic strokes are usually caused by thromboembolism but may rarely be caused by severe hypotension or vasculitis. Hemorrhagic strokes are usually due to rupture of an aneurysm. There are many risk factors for stroke including hypertension, diabetes, heart disease, peripheral vascular disease, atrial fibrillation, drugs (e.g., contraceptive steroids), and excess alcohol intake. Symptoms occur shortly after the cerebral event and relate to the area of brain affected. They may include difficulty speaking, understanding language, or walking; vision problems; contralateral paralysis or numbness; and headache. Treatment for ischemic stroke includes aspirin and tissue plasminogen activator (t-PA) anticoagulation. Hemorrhagic strokes require surgical removal of the clot and clipping or coiling of the aneurysm.

24.3.2 Dipyridamole

Mechanism of Action

Dipyridamole inhibits platelet aggregation by increasing cAMP levels in platelets. This is accomplished in two ways. By acting as a phosphodiesterase inhibitor, dipyridamole prevents cAMP catabolism, which increases cellular levels of cAMP. A second mechanism of dipyridamole is to inhibit the uptake of extracellular adenosine into red blood cells (RBCs) and inhibit its metabolism. Adenosine can act on platelets via adenosine receptors, which stimulate adenylyl cyclase to increase cAMP levels. This mechanism is also important in dipyridamole's effects as a vasodilator. Dipyridamole also decreases the adhesion of platelets to artificial surfaces.

Uses

This agent is used in combination with coumarins to prevent clot formation after heart valve replacement. In combination with aspirin, dipyridamole is used to prevent stroke.

Side Effects

Produces vasodilation that may lead to flushing, headache, dizziness, and hypotension.

24.3.3 P2Y12 Purinergic Receptor Blockers

The purinergic receptor P2Y12 that binds the platelet activator ADP to impart platelet activation is a target for antiplatelet therapy. Two classes are currently in use clinically—irreversible and reversible blockers of the P2Y12 receptor.

Clopidogrel, Prasugrel, and Ticlopidine

Mechanism of Action

Clopidogrel, prasugrel, and ticlopidine are irreversible antagonists of the purinergic P2Y12 ADP receptors on the platelets. The effects of these drugs last for the life of the platelet (▶ Fig. 24.3). Ticlopidine is rarely used due to a worse adverse effect profile.

Pharmacokinetics

Clopidogrel requires metabolism to its active form by CYP2C19. Other drugs that interfere with CYP2C19 activity can interfere with clopidogrel's effects. Genetic poor metabolizers of CYP2C19 may require monitoring or use of a different agent (i.e., prasugrel).

All agents are prodrugs, with ticlopidine having the longest time to onset and prasugrel having the shortest.

Uses

- Used in patients undergoing coronary stent placement to prevent thrombosis and restenosis.
- Used for patients who have experienced or are at risk for cerebrovascular or cardiovascular thrombotic events (i.e., stroke or MI) and is recommended for patients who cannot take aspirin, or in combination with aspirin.

Side Effects

These drugs are generally well tolerated. Prasugrel has greater risk of bleeding than clopidogrel and is contraindicated in patients with history of cerebrovascular events. Ticlopidine may produce agranulocytosis (acute low white blood cell count) and patients must be monitored for evidence of neutropenia. Thrombocytopenia and thrombotic thrombocytopenic purpura (tTP) have also been associated with ticlopidine.

Ticagrelor and Cangrelor

Ticagrelor and cangrelor are reversible inhibitors of P2Y12 ADP receptors. They are not prodrugs so they have a faster onset of action than the irreversible antagonists. Ticagrelor is available for oral administration and cangrelor is available for intravenous (IV) administration.

24.3.4 Glycoprotein IIb/IIIa Receptor Antagonists

Abciximab, Eptifibatide, and Tirofiban

Abciximab is a monoclonal antibody, eptifibatide is a cyclic peptide, and tirofiban is a small molecule.

Mechanism of Action

This class of drugs prevents platelet aggregation by competing with fibrinogen and vWF for occupancy of platelet receptors (▶ Fig. 24.2 and ▶ Fig. 24.3).

Pharmacokinetics

These agents are given IV for acute treatment or prophylaxis.

Uses

- Stent placement and coronary angioplasty (abciximab).
- Prevention of thrombosis in acute coronary syndrome (eptifibatide and tirofiban).

Side Effects

- Bleeding at arterial sites.
- Acute thrombocytopenia (low platelet count) may occur with abciximab.

24.4 Anticoagulants

24.4.1 Heparin

Heparin is an endogenous sulfated mucopolysaccharide found in mast cells bound to histamine. The drug is commercially prepared from pork stomach and beef lung.

Clinical Correlation

Heparin Therapy in Pregnancy

Heparins are used in the treatment of thromboembolic disease in pregnancy because they do not cross the placenta. Low-molecular-weight heparins are preferred because they have a lower risk of heparin-induced thrombocytopenia and osteoporosis.

Mechanism of Action

Heparin combines with, and catalytically activates, a plasma cofactor named antithrombin III. Binding of heparin is through a pentasaccharide sequence that is present on heparin. This complex neutralizes several activated clotting factors, particularly factors IIa (thrombin) and Xa (▶ Fig. 24.4 and ▶ Fig. 24.5). Heparin is active to a lesser extent against activated forms of factors VIII, IX, XI, and XII. It has no therapeutic effects other than the inhibition of clotting. Heparin causes the release of lipoprotein lipase from tissues which hydrolyzes plasma triglycerides and has a "clearing" effect on turbid plasma.

Clinical Correlation

Heparin-Associated Osteoporosis

The exact mechanism of heparin-associated osteoporosis is unknown. It is thought that it may be due to the following: overactivation of osteoclasts by parathyroid hormone (PTH), reduced activity of osteoblasts, and/or increased bone resorption due to disruption of vitamin D metabolism and collagen activation. The fact that heparin has an affinity for Ca^{2+}, leading to reduced Ca^{2+} in the blood and activation of PTH, may support the first two theories.

Pharmacokinetics

- Heparin can be given IV or subcutaneously.
- Dosage is adjusted according to coagulation time (activated partial thromboplastin time [PTT]) in therapy of acute thrombotic episodes. Unfractionated heparin therapy requires regular monitoring (e.g., aPTT).
- For prophylaxis, low doses of heparin are given that cause little change in clotting time.

Uses

- Percutaneous coronary intervention.
- Treatment and prevention of venous thromboembolism.

Side Effects

- Hemorrhage.
- Heparin-induced thrombocytopenia: This may be mild and transient, or severe if antiplatelet antibodies are formed.
- Osteoporosis: This occurs when long-term heparin therapy is necessary.
- Allergy: This probably develops to animal proteins in the solution.

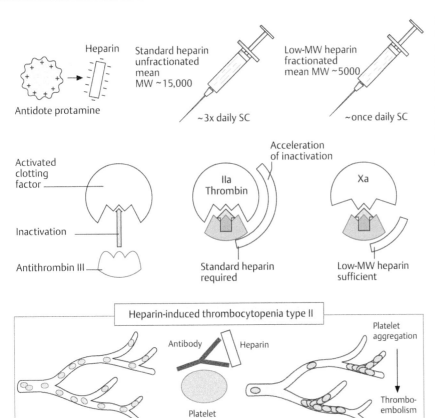

Fig. 24.4 Heparins: origin, structure, and mechanism of action.
Antithrombin III (ATIII) is a glycoprotein that can inactivate clotting factors. Heparin inhibits clotting by increasing the activity of ATIII. Different chain lengths of heparin are required to inactivate different clotting factors. The inactivation of thrombin (factor IIa) requires that heparin contact it and ATIII simultaneously; to inactivate factor Xa, contact between heparin and ATIII is sufficient. A serious complication of heparin usage is thrombocytopenia. This occurs when antibodies attach to heparin and platelet factor 4 complexes on platelets, causing platelet aggregation. This can lead to thromboembolism or hemorrhage. MW, molecular weight; SC, subcutaneously.

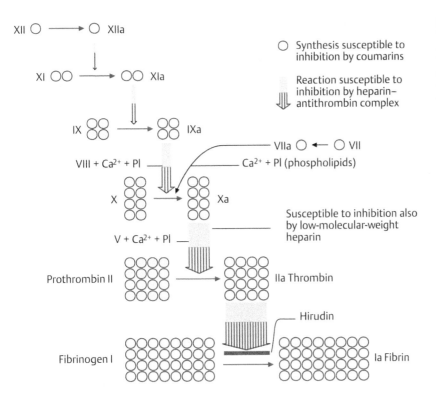

Fig. 24.5 Inhibition of clotting cascade in vivo.
The clotting cascade requires the synthesis and activation of many clotting factors, so it can be inhibited at various steps. Coumarin anticoagulants decrease the synthesis of factors II, VII, IX, and X in the liver. Heparin and antithrombin III neutralize the protease activity of activated factors.

241

Clinical Correlation

Heparin-Induced Hyperkalemia

Inhibition of aldosterone by heparin (including low-molecular-weight heparin) can result in hyperkalemia (high plasma K^+), especially with prolonged treatment. Patients with diabetes mellitus, chronic renal failure, acidosis, or raised plasma K^+, and those taking potassium-sparing diuretics are particularly at risk of hyperkalemia and should have their potassium levels monitored.

Clinical Correlation

Thrombocytopenia

Thrombocytopenia is the term for a low platelet count. Causes include decreased production of platelets (e.g., due to leukemia or aplastic anemia), increased breakdown of platelets (e.g., due to autoimmune disease, viruses, drugs such as heparin and sulfa-containing antibiotics), tTP, idiopathic thrombocytopenic purpura (ITP), and hypersplenism. Symptoms include nosebleeds, bruising, prolonged bleeding from cuts, and bleeding gums. Treatment may not be required for mild thrombocytopenia. Otherwise, treatment is aimed at the underlying cause.

Heparin treatment can cause thrombocytopenia (heparin-induced thrombocytopenia [HIT]). Type I HIT is transient, mild low platelet count that appears 1 to 2 days after heparin initiation but normalizes after continued administration. Type II HIT is more serious and is antibody mediated. It takes more time to develop, usually about 4 to 10 days after heparin exposure. Antibodies develop against platelet factor 4 (PF4) and heparin complexes, which increases platelet activation and can cause potentially fatal thrombosis and thrombocytopenia. Discontinuation of heparin is necessary in such cases. HIT is most associated with unfractionated heparin.

Clinical Correlation

Percutaneous Coronary Intervention

Percutaneous means "through the skin," so it refers to procedures in which access to organs or tissues is achieved via needle puncture of the skin. Percutaneous coronary interventions include balloon angioplasty, implantation of stents, and rotational or laser atherectomy to clear atherosclerotic vessels.

Clinical Correlation

Deep Vein Thrombosis

Deep vein thrombosis (DVT) is a blood clot (thrombosis) that most commonly occurs in the deep veins of the lower leg. It is precipitated by factors that cause abnormal blood clotting or venous circulation. Risk factors for developing DVT include immobility (e.g., sitting or lying for prolonged periods of time), surgery, obesity, pregnancy, malignancy, and estrogen-containing drugs. DVT is often asymptomatic, but it can present with swollen, hot, painful calves with distended veins. There may also be increased resistance and pain on dorsiflexion of the foot (Homan's sign). DVT is diagnosed by venograph or Doppler ultrasound and is treated by heparin, then warfarin anticoagulation. Deep vein thrombi may break off and cause a pulmonary embolism.

Antidote

Protamine sulfate is an antidote for heparin and forms a 1:1 complex with the anticoagulant.

24.4.2 Enoxaparin and Dalteparin

Mechanism of Action

These agents are low-molecular-weight heparins that also bind to antithrombin III, but the complex is less effective than the heparin-activated complex against thrombin. As a result, low-molecular-weight heparins exert an antithrombotic effect (primarily attributed to inhibition of clotting factor Xa) but have little effect on bleeding time. The effects are more predictable and thus may require less monitoring than unfractionated heparin.

Pharmacokinetics

Enoxaparin and dalteparin are given by subcutaneous injection.

Uses

- Thromboembolism prevention and treatment.
- Unstable angina.
- Non-ST elevation myocardial infarction (NSTEMI).
- Acute MI with ST elevation.
- Percutaneous cardiac intervention.

Note: These agents cannot be used interchangeably (unit for unit) with heparin or other low-molecular-weight heparin preparations.

Side Effects

May produce mild thrombocytopenia; thus, periodic platelet counts should be carried out.

Contraindications

Patients with major bleeding.

Fondaparinux is a synthetic drug made up of the pentasaccharide sequence of heparin that binds to antithrombin III. It has activity against factor Xa, but is unable to inhibit thrombin. It is given by subcutaneous injection and is used to prevent venous thromboembolism. It has a longer half-life than heparin, which may or may not be advantageous depending on setting. It does not have a neutralizing antidote.

24.4.3 Direct Thrombin Inhibitors

Bivalirudin, Lepirudin, and Argatroban

Clinical Correlation

Warfarin and International Normalized Ratio

Dosages of warfarin depend on the measurement of prothrombin time (PT), reported as International Normalized Ratio (INR). This is usually measured daily in the early days of treatment and then at appropriate intervals thereafter. A normal INR is 1, and the target INR in oral anticoagulant therapy is different depending on the condition for which anticoagulation is required. For example, for treatment of DVT, an INR of 2.5 may suffice, whereas for patients with a prosthetic heart valve, a target INR of 3.5 may be more appropriate.

Mechanism of Action

These agents inhibit clot-bound and circulating thrombin.

Pharmacokinetics

Given IV.

Uses

- Bivalirudin can be used instead of heparin in patients undergoing coronary angioplasty.
- Lepirudin and argatroban are indicated for use in patients with heparin-induced thrombocytopenia.

Side Effects

The main side effect of these agents is bleeding.

Dabigatran

Mechanism of Action

Dabigatran etexilate is an orally active direct thrombin inhibitor that binds to both circulating and clot-bound thrombin to prevent clot formation.

Use

- It is used to prevent stroke in patients with nonvalvular atrial fibrillation.

- It is contraindicated in renal failure as it is primarily eliminated by the kidneys.

Antidote

Idarucizumab is a monoclonal antibody that binds free and thrombin-bound dabigatran and its metabolites to reverse the anticoagulant effects of dabigatran.

24.4.4 Direct Factor Xa Inhibitors

Rivaroxaban, Apixaban, and Edoxaban

These drugs are orally effective inhibitors of factor Xa by binding to factor Xa and preventing the cleavage of prothrombin to thrombin.

Recombinant human factor Xa, andexanet alfa, is available as an antidote to reverse the effects of these agents.

Use

Used to treat venous thromboembolism and prevent stroke in patients with nonvalvular atrial fibrillation.

24.4.5 Warfarin

Mechanism of Action

Warfarin is a coumarin oral anticoagulant drug that antagonizes the hepatic synthesis of the vitamin K-dependent clotting factors II (prothrombin), VII, IX, and X (▶ Fig. 24.5 and ▶ Fig. 24.6).

Pharmacokinetics

- Well absorbed after oral administration.
- Highly bound to plasma proteins (99% bound).
- Metabolized in liver prior to excretion.
- Onset of action in 2 to 3 days, during which time preexisting levels of clotting factors are diminished.
- Highly variable effects are seen from patient to patient; dosage is adjusted on the basis of the PT (a standard clotting test). Patients on warfarin therapy require regular monitoring for dosage adjustments (e.g., INR).

Uses

- Long-term anticoagulant therapy.
- Acute venous thromboembolism.
- Atrial fibrillation (to reduce the risk of thromboembolic stroke).

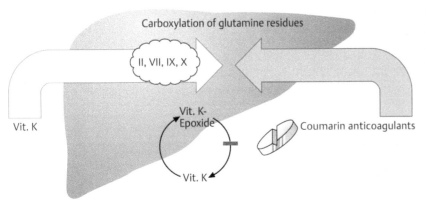

Fig. 24.6 Vitamin K antagonists of the coumarin type and vitamin K.
Vitamin K promotes the carboxylation of glutamine residues on factors II, VII, IX, and X in the liver. Carboxyl groups are required for Ca^{2+}-mediated binding of factors to phospholipids. Coumarin anticoagulants (e.g., warfarin) act as "false" vitamin K molecules and prevent the regeneration of active vitamin K from vitamin K epoxide.

Side Effects

- Hemorrhage.
- Skin necrosis.
- Teratogenesis, especially during the first trimester. This may be explained by the fact that other vitamin K-dependent functions are affected by warfarin administration. Contraindicated in pregnancy.
- Liver and kidney toxicity are seen only with indanedione derivatives which limits the usefulness of this chemical class of anticoagulants.
- Drug interactions occur between the oral anticoagulants and many other drugs (▶ Fig. 24.7).

Antidote

Phytonadione (vitamin K_1) is a warfarin antagonist that is used to neutralize warfarin's effects.

Therapeutics

Clotting Tests

There are four tests used to gauge hemostatic activity:
1. Quick test: plasma is made incoagulable with a Ca^{2+} chelating agent (citrate, oxalate, or ethylenediaminetetraacetic acid). Excessive amounts of Ca^{2+} and tissue thrombokinase are then added. Clotting time is compared with normal values (70–125%).
2. PTT: kephalin, kaolin, and Ca^{2+} are added to citrated plasma, and clotting time is measured (normal clotting time: 25–38 seconds).
3. PT: thrombin is added to citrated plasma (normal clotting time: 18–22 seconds).
4. Bleeding time: bleeding time is measured (e.g., prick in earlobe).

Note: Platelet counts are also extremely important in monitoring hemostatic activity.

Therapeutics

Pulmonary Embolism

Pulmonary embolism is an obstruction in the pulmonary arterial system, usually caused by blood clots from the periphery, particularly the deep veins of the legs, which are transported to the lung. Symptoms include dyspnea (shortness of breath), chest pain exacerbated by taking a deep breath or coughing, cough +/– hemoptysis. Pulmonary embolism decreases the area available for diffusion of gases (increases dead space) and so a ventilation/perfusion (V/Q) scan will show a mismatch. In severe cases pulmonary embolism can cause death due to hypoxia and cor pulmonale (right heart failure due to chronic pulmonary hypertension). Treatment involves the use of the anticoagulants heparin and warfarin or thrombolytics, for example, streptokinase (not normally required). Surgical clot removal may be necessary for large pulmonary emboli.

Therapeutics

Myocardial Infarction and Fibrinolysis

Thrombolytic drugs, such as streptokinase, have been shown to reduce mortality in patients having an acute MI. These drugs need to be given within 12 hours of symptom onset but ideally within 1 hour. They should be used with caution if there is a risk of bleeding and are absolutely contraindicated if the patient has had a recent hemorrhage, trauma, or surgery, or has a known bleeding disorder.

24.5 Thrombolytic Drugs

24.5.1 Mechanism of Action

These agents promote the dissolution of thrombi by stimulating the conversion of endogenous plasminogen to plasmin (fibrinolysis). Plasmin limits the growth of a clot and dissolves the

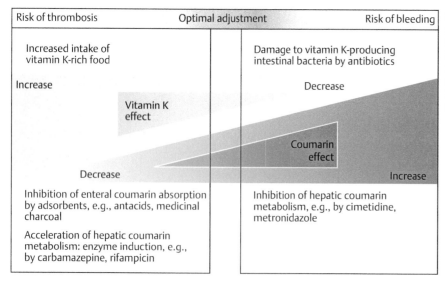

Risk of thrombosis	Optimal adjustment	Risk of bleeding
Increased intake of vitamin K-rich food		Damage to vitamin K-producing intestinal bacteria by antibiotics
Increase	Vitamin K effect	Decrease
Decrease	Coumarin effect	Increase
Inhibition of enteral coumarin absorption by adsorbents, e.g., antacids, medicinal charcoal		Inhibition of hepatic coumarin metabolism, e.g., by cimetidine, metronidazole
Acceleration of hepatic coumarin metabolism: enzyme induction, e.g., by carbamazepine, rifampicin		

Fig. 24.7 Possible interactions of vitamin K antagonists and vitamin K.
Dosages of coumarin anticoagulants must be balanced to protect against thrombosis while minimizing the risk of bleeding. Extrinsic factors, such as pharmacological interactions, may threaten this vitamin K–coumarin balance, so dosage adjustment is necessary.

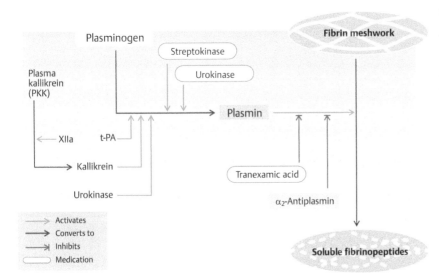

Fig. 24.8 Fibrinolysis.
Fibrinolysis occurs when plasminogen is activated to plasmin under the influence of factors such as kallikrein (a peptidase), urokinase, and tissue plasminogen activator (t-PA). Plasmin then acts on the fibrin meshwork to dissolve the clot into fibrinopeptides. Streptokinase and urokinase act as thrombolytic drugs by activating plasminogen. Some anticoagulant drugs (e.g., tranexamic acid), as well as endogenous substances (α_2-antiplasmin), act by inhibiting plasma-mediated fibrinolysis.

fibrin meshwork as the endothelial injury heals (▶ Fig. 24.8). Bleeding is the primary adverse effect of these drugs. Patients may also require anticoagulant therapy to prevent reocclusion of blood vessels.

24.5.2 Uses

These agents are used to degrade existing thrombi in cases of MI, stroke, or pulmonary embolism.

24.5.3 Streptokinase

Streptokinase is produced from cultures of β-hemolytic streptococci and is therefore antigenic but readily available. Streptokinase is a protein that binds to plasminogen both free and in clots to form a complex that converts plasminogen to plasmin.

Side Effects

Allergic and febrile reactions are the most common nonhemorrhagic side effects.

24.5.4 Urokinase

Urokinase is obtained from human urine or kidney tissue culture and directly converts plasminogen to plasmin.

24.5.5 Tissue Plasminogen Activators: Alteplase, Reteplase, and Tenecteplase

Mechanism of Action

- t-PA is a human protein that specifically cleaves plasminogen, thus leading to the formation of plasmin. The activity of t-PA is accelerated in the presence of fibrin. Thus, it preferentially activates plasminogen bound to fibrin, which provides "clot-specific" thrombolytic activity. It has less bleeding risk associated with it than streptokinase.
- Alteplase is human t-PA produced by recombinant DNA methods.
- Reteplase and tenecteplase are bioengineered recombinant mutant forms of t-PA.

Pharmacokinetics

- Alteplase has a short plasma half-life (4–5 minutes) and requires a constant infusion to maintain a therapeutic level.
- The modifications of reteplase result in less fibrin binding, a longer half-life, and greater thrombolytic potency than t-PA. Tenecteplase also has a longer plasma half-life, but it has enhanced fibrin specificity.

Therapeutics

Hemophilia A and B

Hemophilia A is an autosomal recessive deficiency of factor VIII causing impairment of blood clotting. Symptoms depend on the severity of the factor VIII deficiency and include extensive nosebleeds, bruising, prolonged bleeding from cuts, bleeding gums, hemarthroses (bleeding into joints), muscle hematomas, and blood in the urine or stool. Hemarthroses may lead to arthritis and hematomas may cause nerve damage. Treatment involves the use of desmopressin and concentrated factor VIII replacement. Nonsteroidal anti-inflammatory drugs (NSAIDs) and intramuscular injections should be avoided in these patients.

Hemophilia B (Christmas disease) is caused by a deficiency of factor IX. Clinically, it behaves the same as hemophilia A.

Therapeutics

Von Willebrand Disease

Von Willebrand disease is an autosomal dominant deficiency of a protein called vWF and factor VIII that is carried along with this. This causes reduced platelet adherence producing symptoms such as nosebleeds, bruising, prolonged bleeding from cuts, and bleeding gums. However, unlike hemophilia, hemarthroses and muscle hematomas are rare in this. Treatment is by concentrated vWF and factor VIII replacement, desmopressin, or antifibrinolytic drugs.

24.6 Drugs Used in the Treatment of Bleeding

24.6.1 Aminocaproic Acid and Tranexamic Acid

Mechanism of Action

These agents inhibit plasmin and plasminogen activator (▸ Fig. 24.8).

Uses

They can be used to prevent bleeding in hemophiliacs undergoing dental extractions, as well as in hemorrhage secondary to aplastic anemia, hepatic cirrhosis, or nephrotic disease.

24.6.2 Desmopressin (Antidiuretic Hormone)

Desmopressin is also discussed in Chapter 19.

Mechanism of Action

Desmopressin stimulates the release of clotting factor VIII from the vascular endothelium.

Uses

Desmopressin is used preoperatively in hemophilic patients with low circulating levels of this factor.

24.6.3 Pentoxifylline

Mechanism of Action

Pentoxifylline is a dimethylxanthine derivative that decreases blood viscosity and increases erythrocyte flexibility.

Uses

Pentoxifylline is indicated for muscle pain during exercise associated with occlusive arterial diseases of the limbs (intermittent claudication).

24.7 Anemia and Antianemia Drugs (Hematinics)

24.7.1 Iron Deficiency Anemia

Iron deficiency anemia is a condition in which there is insufficient hemoglobin in RBCs due to a lack of iron (which is an essential component of heme). Approximately two-thirds of the iron content of the body (women: 2 g, men: 5 g) is bound to hemoglobin.

Iron deficiency anemia is usually caused by blood loss from menses in premenopausal women, but it can also be due to inadequate dietary intake of iron, GI bleeding (e.g., from peptic ulcers, long-term use of NSAIDs, or certain GI cancers), GI conditions that decrease the absorption of iron (e.g., Crohn disease), or pregnancy (where the need for iron is increased due to the increase in maternal blood volume and for fetal hemoglobin synthesis).

Therapeutics

Blood Smear in Anemia

Iron deficiency anemia is referred to as a microcytic, hypochromic anemia because when a blood smear is viewed through a microscope, the RBCs appear smaller and paler than usual. Megaloblastic anemia is characterized by immature (megaloblastic) RBCs that are macrocytic and hyperchromic. Flow cytometry is used in laboratories to measure RBC count; hemoglobin concentration; mean corpuscular volume, which reports the size of the RBC; and RBC distribution width, which measure the deviation of the volume of RBCs. These can then be used to calculate the patient's hematocrit (percentage of the blood that is composed of RBCs); mean corpuscular hemoglobin, which is the mean hemoglobin content of each RBC; and mean corpuscular hemoglobin concentration, which is the mean hemoglobin content of a given volume of RBCs. All of these measurements are used clinically to distinguish the different causes and the severity of anemia.

24.8 Drugs Used to Treat Iron Deficiency Anemia

24.8.1 Ferrous Sulfate

Pharmacokinetics

- See ▸ Fig. 24.9 for absorption of iron and other pharmacokinetic factors.
- Ferrous sulfate is given orally, three or four times daily, preferably on an empty stomach to increase iron absorption.

Uses

Drug of choice for iron deficiency anemia.

Side Effects

GI symptoms, resulting from the direct toxic effect of iron. This may cause patient noncompliance and is the most common cause of therapeutic failure. This problem can usually be resolved by an adjustment in dosage.

Therapeutics

Hematocrit

The hematocrit is the percentage of blood volume that is composed of RBCs. It is normally ~ 48% for men and ~ 38% for women. The hematocrit is elevated in polycythemia (a disorder in which the bone marrow produces excessive RBCs), and in diseases which cause hypoxia (e.g., chronic obstructive pulmonary disease) as the body attempts to compensate by producing more RBCs. It can also be elevated in dehydration. The hematocrit is lowered in hemorrhage and iron deficiency anemia.

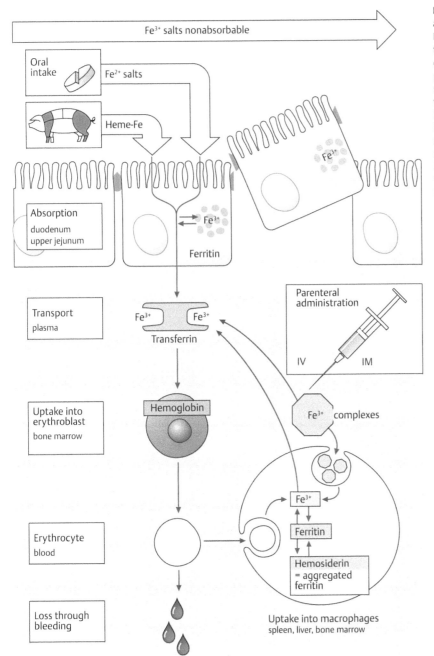

Fe³⁺ salts nonabsorbable

Oral intake — Fe²⁺ salts

Heme-Fe

Fe³⁺

Absorption
duodenum
upper jejunum

Fe³⁺

Ferritin

Transport
plasma

Fe³⁺   Fe³⁺

Transferrin

Parenteral administration

IV   IM

Uptake into erythroblast
bone marrow

Hemoglobin

Fe³⁺ complexes

Erythrocyte
blood

Fe³⁺

Ferritin

Hemosiderin
= aggregated
ferritin

Loss through bleeding

Uptake into macrophages
spleen, liver, bone marrow

Fig. 24.9 Iron: possible routes of administration and fate in the organism.
Ferrous iron (Fe²⁺) and heme are well absorbed in the small bowel, where they are oxidized and deposited as ferritin or transported in the plasma protein transferrin to erythroblasts for hemoglobin synthesis. Macrophages degrade erythrocytes, which liberate iron from hemoglobin. This iron can be stored as ferritin or recycled for erythropoiesis in bone marrow via transferrin. Iron is usually given orally for therapeutic replacement. When this is not possible, parenteral iron is given in the form of Fe³⁺ (ferric) complexes. This prevents free iron toxicity, as Fe³⁺ can bind to transferrin or be stored in macrophages.

24.8.2 Iron Dextran

Pharmacokinetics

- Iron dextran may be given by intramuscular or IV (preferred) injection.
- Parenterally administered iron is associated with several adverse effects and is indicated only when the need for iron cannot be met by oral administration (e.g., malabsorption).
- Dosages must be carefully calculated so that the body's storage capacity is not exceeded ("iron overload").
- Rare risk of potentially fatal anaphylaxis.
- Other forms of parenteral iron include ferric gluconate and iron sucrose.

Antidote

Deferoxamine mesylate is a specific chelating agent for iron. It may be administered orally or parenterally for treatment of acute iron poisoning or iron overload.

Therapeutics

Signs and Symptoms of Anemia

Anemia may be asymptomatic or there may be any of the following signs and symptoms: fatigue, pallor (seen most readily by inspection of the conjunctiva or mucous membranes), dizziness, particularly upon standing (postural hypotension), headache, dyspnea (shortness of breath), coldness of the hands and feet, palpitations, and glossitis (swelling and soreness of the tongue). In severe cases, anemia can cause chest pain (angina due to hypoxia of cardiac muscle) and heart failure (as the heart has to work harder to oxygenate tissues). Iron deficiency anemia also commonly causes brittle nails, cracks at the corner of the mouth, and predilection to infection. Pernicious anemia causes neurologic symptoms, such as numbness, tingling, weakness, and impairment of coordination and memory.

24.8.3 Megaloblastic Anemia

Megaloblastic anemia is a condition caused by inhibition of DNA synthesis in RBC production. It is caused by a lack of vitamin B_{12} and/or folic acid.

Folic acid is widely available in the diet and deficiency due to dietary insufficiency alone is uncommon in the United States. Alcohol and some drugs (e.g., anticonvulsants) are folate antagonists and may exacerbate megaloblastic anemia caused by folate deficiency. Folic acid is necessary for the biosynthesis of thymidylate and subsequent formation of DNA. Orally administered folic acid is usually adequate for all folate deficiency conditions.

The daily requirement for vitamin B_{12} is extremely low (2–5 µg), and because this vitamin is found in many foods of animal origin, a deficiency due to dietary insufficiency is rare. However, the absorption of vitamin B_{12} from the GI tract requires the presence of intrinsic factor, a protein secreted in the stomach. The absence of intrinsic factor, as in pernicious anemia, results in inadequate vitamin B_{12} absorption.

Therapeutics

Hemochromatosis

Hemochromatosis is a condition in which there is failure of regulation of iron absorption in the bowel. This leads to excessive iron in the body, which then gets deposited in organs, such as the liver, heart, pancreas, and pituitary. Signs include fatigue, arthralgia (joint pain), changes in skin pigmentation, liver disease, cardiomyopathy, and diabetes. Management is by venesection until the patient is iron deficient.

24.8.4 Drugs Used to Treat Megaloblastic Anemia

Leucovorin (Folinic Acid)

Mechanism of Action

Folinic acid is a folic acid derivative with vitamin activity equal to folic acid. It does not require reduction by dihydrofolate reductase to be converted to tetrahydrofolate.

Uses

- Injected to "rescue" normal cells after high-dose methotrexate treatment in cancer chemotherapy.
- Can also be given as a folate supplement if oral therapy is not feasible.

Therapeutics

Erythrocyte Sedimentation Rate

The erythrocyte sedimentation rate (ESR) is a nonspecific test that is a marker for conditions associated with acute and chronic inflammation. It does not provide a conclusive diagnosis but rather prompts the clinician to do further investigations. It measures the rate of sedimentation of RBCs in anticoagulated blood over 1 hour. If certain proteins cover red cells, these will stick together and will fall faster. The ESR rises with age and anemia.

Therapeutics

Folic Acid and Prevention of Neural Tube Defects

Folic acid supplement taken before and during pregnancy can reduce the occurrence of neural tube defects, such as spina bifida. Dosages of folic acid are different depending on the couple's risk factors for neural tube defects.

Vitamin B_{12}

Mechanism of Action

Vitamin B_{12} is required for the normal metabolism of folic acid, and a vitamin B_{12} deficiency will cause a pernicious anemia (a type of megaloblastic anemia) because of diminished folate-dependent DNA synthesis. However, neurologic symptoms observed in pernicious anemia apparently develop from defective biosynthesis of myelin, which does not involve folic acid.

Pharmacokinetics

See ▶ Fig. 24.10 for the metabolism of vitamin B_{12} and folate.
- Parenteral vitamin B_{12} is used for treatment of pernicious anemia.
- Oral vitamin B_{12} preparations with intrinsic factor derived from animals give erratic and unreliable results.

Uses

- Pernicious anemia.
- Dietary deficiency.

Vitamin B_{12} Absorption

Vitamin B_{12} absorption from the GI tract involves several steps: B_{12} is released from dietary proteins by gastric acid. It then binds to R protein (transcobalamin 1, haptocorrin) which is secreted in saliva. In the duodenum, trypsin digests the R protein, liberating B_{12} which then forms a complex with intrinsic factor (IF), a glycoprotein secreted by gastric parietal cells. This B_{12}–IF complex is resistant to the effects of trypsin and travels to the terminal ileum where it binds to specific receptors and is absorbed via receptor-mediated endocytosis.

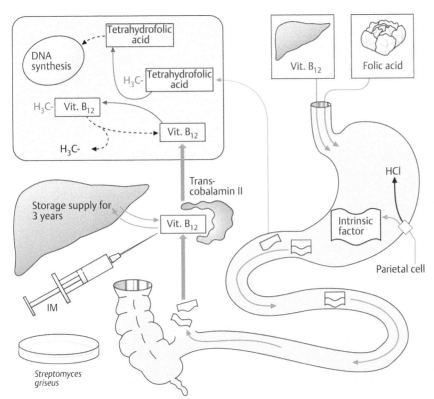

Fig. 24.10 Vitamin B$_{12}$ and folate metabolism.
Vitamin B$_{12}$ is absorbed in the small intestine but requires intrinsic factor, produced by parietal cells in the stomach. It is transported in the blood by transcobalamin II to the liver for storage or to erythropoietic cells to facilitate the conversion of methyltetrahydrofolic acid to tetrahydrofolic acid (THF), which is important in DNA synthesis. Therapeutically, vitamin B$_{12}$ is given parenterally. Folic acid is also absorbed in the small intestine and is taken up into erythropoietic cells. Therapeutically, it can be administered orally.

24.9 Hematopoietic Growth Factors

Hematopoietic growth factors are the agents used to increase the number of specific cell types in distinct cytopenias that occur often after cancer chemotherapy.

24.9.1 Filgrastim and Sargramostim

Granulocyte (G) and granulocyte-macrophage (GM) colony stimulating factors (CSF) are naturally occurring peptide growth factors that increase the production of granulocytes, especially neutrophils. Filgrastim and sargramostim are recombinant G-CSF and GM-CSF, respectively.

Uses

- Stimulation of bone marrow growth (myeloid cell reconstitution) after transplantation or cancer chemotherapy.
- Neutropenia.
- Mobilization of stem cells.

24.9.2 Epoetin Alfa

It is a recombinant erythropoietin used to increase the number of RBCs.

Uses

- Anemia due to renal failure, bone marrow disease, or cancer chemotherapy, or in patients with acquired immunodeficiency syndrome (AIDS) receiving AZT (zidovudine, formerly called azidothymidine).

24.9.3 Interleukin 11 (Oprelvekin)

Mechanism of Action

Interleukin 11 stimulates the formation of platelet progenitor cells.

Uses

It is used to speed up platelet recovery in patients undergoing chemotherapy with nonmyeloid malignancies.

Erythropoietin

Erythropoietin (epoetin alpha) is a renal hormone that regulates the production of RBCs in the bone marrow. Patients with chronic renal failure develop anemia secondary to inadequate levels of erythropoietin. Human recombinant erythropoietin has been shown to be effective in treatment of anemia associated with uremia. There are no direct adverse effects of replacement therapy, although ~ 25% of patients experience hypertension during treatment, and there is a risk of thrombotic events. Many patients may require supplemental iron during treatment with erythropoietin due to the increased production of RBCs.

25 Antihyperlipidemic Drugs

Summary

Regulation of lipid levels is effective in primary and secondary prevention of cardiovascular events. In approaching lipid disorders, lifestyle and dietary modifications are employed prior to initiating drug therapy. The most effective and most frequently used agents to reduce low-density lipoprotein (LDL) cholesterol are the 3-hydroxy-3-methylglutaryl-coenzyme A reductase-inhibiting statins (atorvastatin, fluvastatin, lovastatin, pravastatin, rosuvastatin, simvastatin, and pitavastatin). These drugs inhibit the rate-limiting step in cholesterol biosynthesis. Bile acid sequestrants (cholestyramine, colestipol, and colesevelam) bind bile acids in the gut, leading to increased hepatic synthesis of bile acids, which reduces cholesterol levels. Ezetimibe inhibits cholesterol absorption in the small intestine by binding to the Niemann–Pick C1–like protein 1, which is required for intestinal cholesterol uptake. Nicotinic acid (niacin) shows beneficial effects on overall lipid profile, as it increases high-density lipoprotein while decreasing LDL and triglycerides. Fibrates, such as gemfibrozil, fenofibrate, clofibrate, ciprofibrate, and bezafibrate, are usually used to treat increased triglyceride and LDL levels. Alirocumab and evolocumab inhibit the enzyme proprotein convertase subtilisin/kexin type 9 (PCSK9). Lomitapide and mipomersen are apolipoprotein B inhibitors indicated as adjuncts to other lipid-lowering treatments in patients with homozygous familial hypercholesterolemia. Combination therapy with different classes of hypolipidemic drugs can be highly effective in obtaining desired lipid levels. However, care must be taken to ensure that adverse effects are minimized.

Keywords: cholesterol, triglyceride, lipid, LDL, HDL, statin

25.1 Lipoproteins

Lipids, such as triglycerides and cholesterol, are nonpolar compounds that are insoluble in water. Most dietary fats are triglycerides, which are composed of glycerol and three fatty acids. They are stored by the body and provide an energy source when required. Cholesterol is also ingested in smaller amounts. It is an essential component of cell membranes. In order to be transported in the blood, lipids are formed into particles called lipoproteins. Lipoproteins are made up of lipids (cholesterol, triglycerides, phospholipids) and proteins called apolipoproteins (or apoproteins) which provide structural stability to lipoproteins and can act as ligands for interactions with cellular lipoprotein receptors. Hydrophobic lipids such as cholesteryl esters and triglycerides situated in the core are surrounded by a phospholipid layer which contains apolipoproteins and unesterified cholesterol. The different types of lipoproteins contain different relative quantities of triglycerides and cholesterol as well as different types of apolipoproteins in the phospholipid layer. Lipoproteins are designated as chylomicrons (lowest density due to high fat vs. protein content), very-low-density lipoproteins (VLDLs), low-density lipoproteins (LDLs), or high-density lipoproteins (HDLs, high density due to high protein vs. fat content). Lipoprotein metabolism is illustrated in ▶ Fig. 25.1.

25.1.1 Dyslipidemias and Related Diseases

Dyslipidemia is a general term used to describe high levels of LDL cholesterol (LDL-C) or triglycerides, or low levels of HDL cholesterol (HDL-C). Dyslipidemias are major contributors to atherosclerosis and atherosclerosis-related conditions, such as coronary heart disease (CHD), ischemic cerebrovascular disease, and peripheral vascular disease. Genetic disorders and lifestyle may contribute to the dyslipidemias. Therapy for dyslipidemias is based on the blood levels of LDL-C, HDL-C, and triglycerides (found mainly in VLDL cholesterol).

Notes

Lipoprotein Levels

The optimal level for LDL-C is < 100 mg/dL. It is considered high when it is ≥ 160 mg/dL. HDL-C should ideally be > 40 mg/dL. HDL-C > 60 mg/dL is considered to be protective against heart disease. Total cholesterol should be < 200 mg/dL. It is considered high if it is > 240 mg/dL.

25.1.2 Antihyperlipidemic Therapy

Initial therapy is to institute lifestyle changes, including reduction of dietary intake of cholesterol and saturated fats and increased intake of soluble fiber and omega-3 fatty acids. In addition, weight management and increased physical activity should be initiated. If these are insufficient to lower LDL-C to the desired level, drug therapy is indicated.

The National Cholesterol Education Program serves as the basis for guidelines for initiation of drug therapy in dyslipidemias based on the blood levels of the lipoproteins. The presence of other major risk factors, such as cigarette smoking, hypertension, low HDL-C (< 40 mg/dL), family history of premature CHD, and age, determine the level to which cholesterol should be lowered.

Foundations

Role of Genetics in Hyperlipidemic Diseases

Genetic defects in the production of chylomicrons, lipoprotein lipase, the synthesis of LDL receptors, and overproduction of the lipids/lipoproteins can be familial causes for hyperlipidemic diseases.

25.2 Antihyperlipidemic Drugs

Antihyperlipidemic drugs are used to treat primary hyperlipidemias or hyperlipoproteinemias. Lipid-lowering treatment is also recommended to prevent cardiovascular events in conditions that can secondarily elevate plasma levels of cholesterol or triglycerides, for example, type 2 diabetes and metabolic syndrome. Diabetics usually have high triglycerides, moderate elevations of total cholesterol and LDL-C, and low HDL-C.

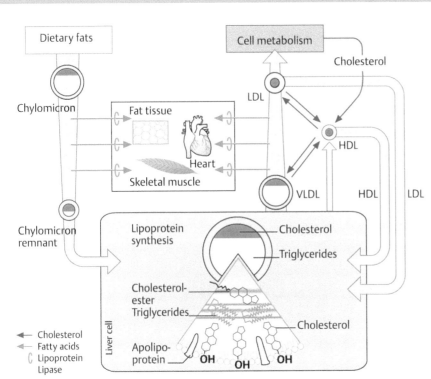

Fig. 25.1 Lipoprotein metabolism.
Enterocytes release absorbed dietary lipids in the form of triglyceride-rich chylomicrons. These are acted upon by lipoprotein lipases in endothelial cells and other sites to produce fatty acids which are stored in tissues. Chylomicron remnants, enriched for dietary cholesterol, are transported to liver cells. VLDLs synthesized in the liver supply tissues with fatty acids. As the triglyceride content in VLDLs decreases, VLDL remnants become cholesterol-rich low-density lipoproteins (LDLs). LDLs supply cells with cholesterol, or are taken up by the liver. High-density lipoprotein (HDL) functions in reverse-cholesterol transport. HDL precursors synthesized in liver and intestine collect cholesterol from peripheral tissues to form mature HDL particles, which delivers cholesterol to the liver. HDLs also transfer cholesterol to VLDL and LDL. In hepatocytes, cholesterol is either secreted in bile or used to synthesize bile acids or very low density lipoproteins (VLDLs).

25.2.1 Statins

The statins (3-hydroxy-3-methylglutaryl [HMG]-coenzyme A [CoA] reductase inhibitors) have become the most widely prescribed drugs for lowering plasma cholesterol levels.

Clinical Correlation

Metabolic Syndrome

Metabolic syndrome is a combination of medical disorders that increases the risk of developing atherosclerotic disease, for example, coronary heart disease, peripheral vascular disease, and stroke. It also increases the risk of developing type 2 diabetes. Its etiology is unknown, but weight gain, advancing age, lifestyle factors, and genetics are all known to be involved. Signs of metabolic syndrome include fasting hyperglycemia, hypertension, abdominal obesity, high levels of triglycerides, and low levels of HDL-C. Treatment primarily involves weight management and increasing exercise, then drug management for hypertension, diabetes, and to correct lipid levels as appropriate.

Atorvastatin, Fluvastatin, Lovastatin, Pravastatin, Rosuvastatin, Simvastatin, and Pitavastatin

Mechanism of Action

The major mechanism of these agents is to competitively inhibit HMG-CoA reductase, the rate-limiting enzyme in cholesterol synthesis (▶ Fig. 25.2). This causes reductions in LDL-C by reducing hepatic cholesterol synthesis. Reductions in cholesterol also lead to increased expression of LDL receptors on hepatocytes which contribute to statin effect by increasing removal of LDL from the blood (▶ Fig. 25.3). VLDL and remnants also contain apolipoprotein E (apoE), which is the ligand for LDL receptors; thus, by increasing LDL receptors, statins also increase clearance of VLDL which can reduce blood triglyceride levels. Those individuals with two dysfunctional alleles of the LDL receptor show limited responses to statin therapy (e.g., homozygous familial hypercholesterolemia). Statins can also cause small increases in HDL.

Other effects of statins that likely contribute to their therapeutic effects include anti-inflammatory, plaque-stabilizing, and reduced platelet-aggregating effects.

Effects

- Lowers LDL (variable depending on statin; up to 50% at higher doses).
- Lowers triglyceride levels.
- Increases HDL levels.

Uses

- First-line treatment for hypercholesterolemia.
- Used prophylactically to prevent adverse vascular events in patients with diabetes mellitus or cardiovascular disease.

Side Effects

A major adverse effect is myopathy or rhabdomyolysis, either when administered alone or in combination with fibrates.

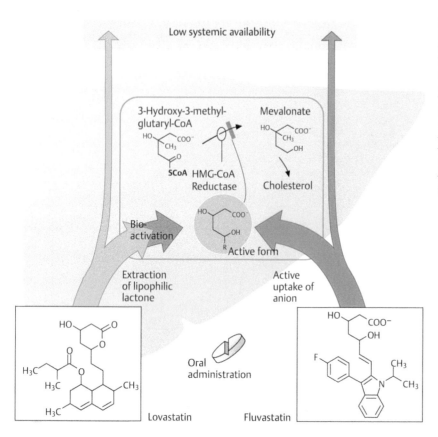

Fig. 25.2 Accumulation and effect of 3-hydroxy-3-methylglutaryl-coenzyme A (HMG-CoA) reductase inhibitors in the liver.
The HMG-CoA reductase inhibitors mimic the normal enzyme substrate, which renders it unavailable for cholesterol synthesis in the liver. These drugs accumulate in the liver, as they have a high rate of presystemic elimination. This accumulation is advantageous because it concentrates the actions of these drugs where they are needed. The liver maintains its requirement for cholesterol by the uptake of low-density lipoproteins (LDL) from the blood, thus lowering plasma cholesterol levels.

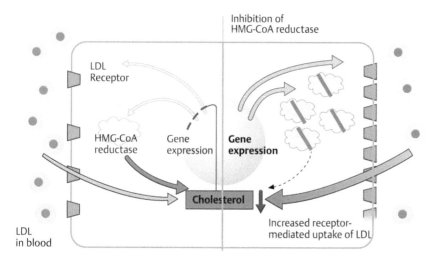

Fig. 25.3 Regulation by cellular cholesterol concentration of 3-hydroxy-3-methylglutaryl-coenzyme A (HMG-CoA) reductase and LDL receptors.
In the presence of HMG-CoA reductase inhibitors, hepatocytes increase the production of low-density lipoprotein (LDL)-receptor proteins. This allows LDL uptake from the blood to increase.

Drugs that are metabolized by CYP3A4 can reduce statin metabolism to increase possible myopathy. Statins can alter liver enzymes and should be used cautiously or avoided in the setting of liver disease.

Drug Interactions

The HMG-CoA reductase inhibitors increase warfarin levels so prothrombin times (expressed as International Normalized Ratio [INR]; see Chapter 24) should be monitored. Drugs that increase the levels of statins through pharmacokinetic interference (e.g., erythromycin, fibrates) can increase toxicity.

Clinical Correlation

Rhabdomyolysis

Rhabdomyolysis is the rapid breakdown of skeletal muscle due to injury to muscle tissue. The muscle breakdown product, myoglobin, is harmful to the kidney and can precipitate acute kidney failure. Signs and symptoms include pain, tenderness, and swelling of the affected muscle, as well as nausea, vomiting, confusion, arrhythmias, coma, anuria, and later disseminated intravascular coagulation (DIC). This is a rare complication of treatment with statins and fibrates.

25.2.2 Bile Acid Sequestrants

Cholestyramine, Colestipol, and Colesevelam

Mechanism of Action

These agents are insoluble resins that are not absorbed by the body, but bind bile acids in the gut, resulting in elimination and depletion of the bile acid pool. This interrupts enterohepatic circulation of bile acids, leading to increased hepatic synthesis of bile acids, which reduces cholesterol levels. This can also cause an increase in triglyceride levels, which may be clinically relevant in those patients who are already hypertriglyceridemic. This effect is typically transient in those with normal triglycerides. ▸ Fig. 25.4 illustrates the effect of cholesterol-lowering drugs like cholestyramine on cholesterol metabolism in the liver.

Pharmacokinetics

Given orally, these drugs bind with bile acids in the intestine and produce an insoluble complex that is excreted in the feces.

Effects

- Decrease LDL levels.
- May increase triglycerides, or they may remain unchanged (contraindicated in hypertriglyceridemia).
- Increase HDL levels.

Uses

These agents can be used alone to treat increased LDL; however, they are not as efficacious as statins. They are most often used as secondary agents if statin therapy alone is not optimal.

Side Effects

- Bloating, nausea, constipation.
- Steatorrhea (the presence of excess fat in feces), and these may prevent absorption of fat-soluble vitamins (A, D, E, K).

Note: Compliance may be a problem due to the unpleasant taste of the drug.

Drug Interactions

These agents may interfere with the absorption of other drugs given concurrently (e.g., warfarin, levothyroxine, digoxin, and others); therefore, all drugs should be taken ~1 to 2 hours before or several hours after taking bile acid sequestrants.

25.2.3 Ezetimibe

Mechanism of Action

Ezetimibe inhibits cholesterol absorption in the small intestine by binding to the Niemann–Pick C1–like protein 1, which is required for intestinal cholesterol uptake.

Effects

It lowers LDL-C levels by up to 20%.

Uses

It is used primarily as adjunctive therapy with statins. Ezetimibe can elicit a compensatory increase in cholesterol biosynthesis; therefore, the combination therapy with statins to inhibit cholesterol biosynthesis can lower LDL-C by 50% or more.

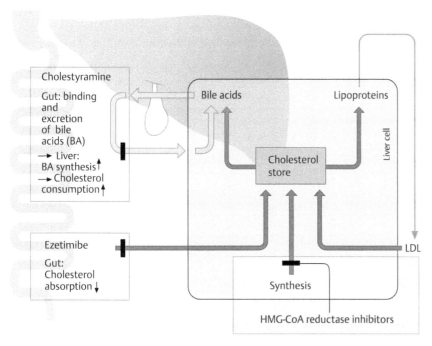

Fig. 25.4 Cholesterol metabolism in liver cell and cholesterol-lowering drugs.
Cholesterol-lowering drugs may act in the gut to reduce the absorption of dietary cholesterol, they may inhibit cholesterol synthesis in the liver, or they may act to increase the consumption of cholesterol.

Side Effects

It may increase the hepatotoxicity and myopathy of statins.

25.2.4 Nicotinic Acid (Niacin)

Niacin

Niacin has multiple favorable effects on lipoproteins. It reduces LDL-C and triglycerides along with increasing HDL-C.

Mechanisms of Action

- Inhibition of hepatocyte diacylglycerol acyltransferase-2, a key enzyme for triacylglycerol synthesis, decreasing secretion of VLDL and LDL-C.
- Enhancing of lipoprotein lipase activity, which increases the clearance of chylomicrons and VLDL.
- Decreased hepatic catabolism of apolipoprotein A-I increases the half-life and concentrations of HDL-C.
- Niacin also reduces vascular inflammatory genes involved in atherosclerosis.

Effects

- Decreases levels of LDL and triglycerides.
- Increases HDL levels (most effective agent).

Uses

Niacin is used to treat hypertriglyceridemias and hypercholesterolemia. It is especially useful in patients with both hypertriglyceridemia and low HDL-C levels.

Note: Nicotinamide is not effective in lowering lipids, although it acts interchangeably with nicotinic acid as a vitamin.

Side Effects

- Cutaneous flushing, burning, and itching are common, as is GI irritation, nausea, and vomiting. The niacin flush results from the stimulation of prostaglandins D_2 and E_2 from subcutaneous Langerhans cells by a G protein-coupled niacin receptor. Flushing can be minimized by taking a daily aspirin.
- Activation of peptic ulcers, abnormal elevation of liver enzyme levels, hyperglycemia, and hyperuricemia occur infrequently.

Contraindications

- Chronic liver disease.
- Gout (see Chapter 33).
- Pregnancy (potential for birth defects).
- May be inappropriate for use in peptic ulcer disease, hyperuricemia, and diabetes.

25.2.5 Fibrates

Gemfibrozil, Fenofibrate, Clofibrate, Ciprofibrate, and Bezafibrate

Mechanism of Action

These drugs lower VLDLs and plasma triglycerides by binding to peroxisome proliferator-activated receptors alpha (PPARalpha) to regulate gene transcription leading to stimulation of lipoprotein lipase. They also lower cholesterol by inhibiting its synthesis and enhancing excretion in the bile.

Effects

- Decreases LDL and triglyceride levels.
- Increases HDL levels.

Uses

For treatment of hypertriglyceridemia and hypercholesterolemia.

Side Effects

Side effects include GI disturbances (nausea, diarrhea, and cramps), muscle weakness, and rash. Long-term use may increase the incidence of thromboembolism, angina, arrhythmias, or gallstones (see call out box in Chapter 17).

Contraindications

- Pregnancy.
- Impaired renal or hepatic function.

Drug Interactions

These agents displace acidic drugs (e.g., warfarin and phenytoin) from plasma proteins; thus a reduced dose of anticoagulant (or other drug) is required.

25.2.6 PCSK9 Inhibitors

Alirocumab and Evolocumab

Mechanism of Action

These drugs are monoclonal antibodies that bind to and inhibit the enzyme proprotein convertase subtilisin/kexin type 9 (PCSK9). PCSK9, much of it produced in liver, binds to LDL receptors to increase their degradation, resulting in reduced LDL clearance. These agents are administered by subcutaneous injection and most often used in combination with statins in familial hypercholesterolemia or other conditions that require greater LDL lowering effects than can be achieved with other means.

Side Effects

Hypersensitivity, neurocognitive events (e.g., amnesia, confusion).

25.3 Drug Combinations

The following drugs are apolipoprotein B inhibitors indicated as adjuncts to other lipid-lowering treatments in patients with homozygous familial hypercholesterolemia.

25.3.1 Lomitapide

Lomitapide inhibits microsomal triglyceride transfer protein (MTP). Normally, MTP is required for proper formation of apolipoprotein B (apoB) and apoB-containing lipoproteins.

Therefore, inhibiting MTP leads to reduced synthesis of chylomicrons, VLDL, and LDL. Lomitapide is administered orally.

25.3.2 Mipomersen

Mipomersen is an antisense oligonucleotide that binds to and inhibits the messenger RNA of apoB-100, thus reducing synthesis of VLDL and LDL. Mipomersen is administered by subcutaneous injection.

Use and Adverse Effects

With both lomitapide and mipomersen, there is a serious risk of liver toxicity. Both drugs are available through a risk evaluation and mitigation strategy (REMS) program and are used to treat patients with homozygous familial hypercholesterolemia.

V

Unit V Review Questions

1. A patient with edema is being treated with a drug that inhibits the absorption of bicarbonate ions from the glomerular filtrate. The effectiveness of this drug for long-term therapy is limited by drug-induced acidosis, which appears within the first weeks of therapy. With which of the following drugs is the patient being treated?
   A. Metolazone.
   B. Ethacrynic acid.
   C. Amiloride.
   D. Acetazolamide.
   E. Spironolactone.

2. Which of the following produces an acute increase in the urinary excretion of 20 to 30% of the filtered load of calcium and is therefore useful in treating symptomatic hypercalcemia, provided the plasma volume is maintained?
   A. Furosemide.
   B. Chlorthalidone.
   C. Hydrochlorothiazide.
   D. Desmopressin.
   E. Mannitol.

3. A patient admitted to the hospital for severe heart failure was treated with an IV diuretic as part of therapeutic regimen. Shortly after a bolus dose of the drug, he complained of muffled hearing. Which of the following was he most likely administered?
   A. Triamterene.
   B. Hydrochlorothiazide.
   C. Furosemide.
   D. Spironolactone.
   E. Mannitol.

4. A 49-year-old man with high blood pressure tried to lower his blood pressure through diet and exercise. After 1 year, his blood pressure is slightly decreased, but it remains at 150/100 mm Hg. In the past year, he has been to your office once with a red, tender, and swollen first metatarsophalangeal joint at the base of the big toe. Which of the following drugs would have to be prescribed with caution in this patient?
   A. Nifedipine.
   B. Labetalol.
   C. Prazosin.
   D. Chlorothiazide.
   E. Spironolactone.

5. A 72-year-old man is being treated for HF with a thiazide diuretic, an angiotensin-converting enzyme (ACE) inhibitor, and a β adrenergic receptor blocking agent. During a routine examination, serum electrolyte values were found to be the following: $Na^+ = 135$ mEq/L, $Cl^- = 105$ mEq/L, $K^+ = 2.8$ mEq/L, $HCO_3^- = 24$ mEq/L. The electrolyte values could be balanced by which of the following drugs?
   A. Acetazolamide.
   B. Amiloride.
   C. Furosemide.
   D. Hydrochlorothiazide.
   E. Aldosterone.

6. Which of the following is useful in the treatment of diabetes insipidus of pituitary origin?
   A. Triamterene.
   B. Amiloride.
   C. Ethacrynic acid.
   D. Desmopressin.
   E. Furosemide.

7. Which of the following is useful in the treatment of nephrogenic diabetes insipidus?
   A. Triamterene.
   B. Hydrochlorothiazide.
   C. Furosemide.
   D. Desmopressin.
   E. Mannitol.

8. A 70-year-old Caucasian woman is brought to the emergency room with heart palpitations and an erratic, irregular pulse. She is admitted to the hospital and diagnosed with hypertension complicated by paroxysmal atrial fibrillation. She had been taking a blood pressure medication but ran out of pills 1 week before the incident. Which of the following antihypertensive agents was she most likely taking?
   A. Propranolol.
   B. Enalapril.
   C. Hydrochlorothiazide.
   D. Losartan.
   E. Clonidine.

9. Which of the following antihypertensive drugs is contraindicated in patients with asthma?
   A. Reserpine.
   B. Hydrochlorothiazide.
   C. Nifedipine.
   D. Verapamil.
   E. Propranolol.

10. Which of the following antihypertensive drugs is less effective as monotherapy for African American patients?
   A. Clonidine.
   B. Enalapril.
   C. Labetalol.
   D. Nifedipine.
   E. Prazosin.

11. A 62-year-old woman is being treated for hypertension with captopril and hydrochlorothiazide. She has had a cough for the last 6 months that started 2 months after she began antihypertensive therapy. Her blood pressure is well controlled. Chest radiograph (X-ray) and spirometry are normal. The cough is most likely a result of which of the following?
   A. Pneumonia.
   B. The common cold.
   C. Poorly controlled blood pressure.
   D. A side effect of hydrochlorothiazide.
   E. A side effect of captopril.

12. Given that the patient in question 11 has shown a favorable response to decreasing the function of angiotensin II, you decide to replace the drug with a drug that blocks the

binding of angiotensin II to the angiotensin type I (AT^1) receptor. Which of the following drugs is prescribed?
A. Clonidine.
B. Enalapril.
C. Labetalol.
D. Nifedipine.
E. Losartan.

13. A 48-year-old African American man has had a blood pressure of 160/90 mm Hg, 170/95 mm Hg, and 165/95 mm Hg on three monthly visits. The patient's hypertension is treated with nifedipine. How does this drug reduce hypertension?
A. By blocking α_2 adrenergic receptors.
B. By inhibiting ACE.
C. By blocking β adrenergic receptors.
D. By blocking L-type calcium channels.
E. By inhibiting sodium reabsorption in the loop of Henle.

14. Abrupt cessation of antihypertensive therapy may cause a serious rebound hypertension with which of the following drugs?
A. Prazosin.
B. Clonidine.
C. Guanethidine.
D. Enalapril.
E. Reserpine.

15. A 68-year-old man with asthma, long-standing hypertension, and diabetes mellitus who is receiving digoxin, hydrochlorothiazide, and 35 units of neutral protamine Hagedorn (NPH) insulin gradually develops HF. Why would the addition of captopril to the patient's medication be potentially harmful?
A. It results in hypokalemia.
B. It blocks the subjective warning signs of hypoglycemia.
C. It aggravates the patient's asthmatic condition.
D. It may cause severe hypotension.
E. It activates the cytochrome P-450 enzymes that metabolize digoxin.

16. A 58-year-old man is being treated for heart failure with a diuretic, an ACE inhibitor, and a β adrenergic receptor blocking agent. He continues to experience dyspnea on exertion. The patient may benefit from the addition of a drug that inhibits which of the following proteins on the membrane of cardiac myocytes?
A. α_2 adrenergic receptors.
B. Glucose transporter 1 (GLUT1).
C. Na$^+$–K$^+$–ATPase.
D. L-type Ca^{2+} channels.
E. Delayed rectifier K$^+$ channels.

17. Digoxin is a cardiac glycoside used for the treatment of heart failure. The drug has a low therapeutic index, in part because it may affect the intracellular K$^+$ concentration of cardiac myocytes. What would be the expected effect of digoxin on intracellular K$^+$ levels?
A. It would lead to membrane hyperpolarization.
B. It would lead to membrane depolarization.
C. It would lead to no change in membrane potential.
D. It would decrease automaticity.
E. It would decrease contractility.

18. An elderly man comes to the emergency room with an acute myocardial infarction. He is in cardiogenic shock in which the cardiac output is very low, and there is a reflex vasoconstriction. Which of the following drugs would be most appropriate to administer?
A. Dobutamine.
B. Isoproterenol.
C. Bethanechol.
D. Propranolol.
E. Phenylephrine.

19. Relief of pulmonary congestion after administration of nitroglycerin to a patient in HF is primarily due to
A. Arteriolar dilation.
B. Inotropic stimulation.
C. Increased cardiac output.
D. Increased venous capacitance.

20. A 62-year-old patient is experiencing chest pain on exertion. Effort-induced angina is diagnosed, and treatment is begun. Nitroglycerin and isosorbide dinitrate are given sublingually and are rapidly absorbed through the oral mucosa. Once in the bloodstream, they increase the level of which signaling molecule in smooth muscle?
A. Inositol triphosphate.
B. Phospholipase Cß.
C. RAF kinase.
D. Cyclic guanosine monophosphate (cGMP).
E. Cyclooxygenase-3 (COX-3).

21. The patient in question 20 is prescribed another drug to take daily to prevent the effort-induced angina attacks. This drug is most likely which of the following?
A. Diltiazem.
B. Nitroglycerin.
C. Metoprolol.
D. Isosorbide dinitrate.
E. Verapamil.

22. Organic nitrates may relieve angina by which of the following mechanisms?
A. Reduction of the heart rate.
B. Reduction of myocardial contractility.
C. Increase in the left ventricular residual volume.
D. Reduction of ventricular wall stress.
E. Increase in venous pressure.

23. A common property of all class I antiarrhythmic drugs is
A. Reduction of sodium influx.
B. Prolongation of the effective refractory period.
C. Hyperpolarization of the membrane.
D. Atropine-like effect.

24. A 58-year-old female patient with recurrent ventricular tachycardia requires treatment with an antiarrhythmic drug. She has a previously been diagnosed with systemic lupus erythematosus (SLE). Which of the following drugs would be contraindicated in this patient?
A. Flecainide.
B. Procainamide.
C. Quinidine.
D. Amiodarone.
E. Verapamil.

25. A 69-year-old man is taking mexiletine for prevention of ventricular arrhythmia. He has experienced some ataxia, paresthesias, and tremor 2 to 3 hours after taking the medicine. These effects result from mexiletine acting as which of the following?
    A. Calcium channel blocker.
    B. β blocker to decrease blood flow.
    C. Local anesthetic to affect neuronal conduction.
    D. Alcohol dehydrogenase inhibitor.
    E. Benzodiazepine receptor agonist.

26. Following an acute myocardial infarction, a patient is given an antiarrhythmic drug that has beneficial effects that include prevention of supraventricular and ventricular arrhythmias. Which of the following drugs was the patient given?
    A. Phenylephrine.
    B. Isoproterenol.
    C. Norepinephrine.
    D. Nitroglycerin.
    E. Propranolol.

27. A hospitalized patient is receiving heparin for prevention of deep vein thrombosis. One of the drugs the patient received during the procedure was eptifibatide. What is the action of this drug?
    A. To block the synthesis of factor II in liver.
    B. To inhibit platelet aggregation by reversibly binding to the platelet receptor glycoprotein IIb/IIIa.
    C. To inhibit the release of adenosine diphosphate (ADP) by increasing cyclic adenosine monophosphate (cAMP) levels.
    D. To acetylate platelet cyclooxygenase.
    E. To inhibit ADP-induced platelet fibrinogen binding.

This case is for questions 28–30.

A 44-year-old man has swelling and pain in his right leg, ankle, and foot. At first he thought he had a cramp, but then he noticed his calf had become red and warm. The swelling has not decreased after 3 days. He has chest pain but no shortness of breath. Blood pressure is 145/85 mm Hg, heart rate is 105 beats per minute, and respiration is 30 breaths per minute. Auscultation reveals a loud pulmonary heart sound. Arterial partial pressure of oxygen (pO_2) is slightly decreased. Pulmonary embolism is suspected, and the patient is admitted to the hospital. Heparin therapy is initiated. Two days later, the patient's activated partial thromboplastin time (aPTT) is found to be excessively prolonged.

28. Which of the following drugs could be used to restore the patient's aPTT to within an acceptable range?
    A. Protamine sulfate.
    B. Warfarin.
    C. Vitamin K.
    D. Enoxaparin.
    E. Bivalirudin.

29. In addition to monitoring aPTT, what other parameter should be monitored for patients receiving heparin?
    A. Platelet count.
    B. Bone density.
    C. Vitamin K levels.
    D. Cytokine levels.
    E. Vitamin C levels.

30. A transition from heparin to warfarin anticoagulant therapy is initiated while the patient is in the hospital. After discharge of the patient from the hospital, warfarin anticoagulant therapy is continued. Following discharge, the patient decides to institute lifestyle changes, including diet and exercise. His dietary plan is to dramatically decrease his intake of meat to try to become a vegetarian. How would an increased consumption of green leafy vegetables (which contain vitamin K) be expected to alter the patient's International Normalized Ratio (INR)?
    A. It would be increased.
    B. It would be decreased.
    C. It would be unchanged.
    D. It would be doubled.
    E. It would be halved.

31. Which of the following decreases cholesterol synthesis by inhibition of HMG-CoA reductase?
    A. Lovastatin.
    B. Cholestyramine.
    C. Nicotinic acid.
    D. Clofibrate.

32. A 56-year-old man has a total cholesterol of 245 mg/dL, LDL = 160 mg/dL, HDL = 60 mg/dL, and triglycerides = 107 mg/dL. He is 69 inches (5 ft 9 in, 175 cm) tall and weighs 160 lb (72.5 kg). His father had a heart attack at age 45, and his older brother has had coronary angioplasty. He was started on the initial recommended dose of lovastatin 6 months ago. The National Cholesterol Education Program goal for this patient is to reduce his LDL cholesterol to < 130 mg/dL. Which of the following would be most optimal for further lowering the patient's cholesterol?
    A. Increase the dose of lovastatin.
    B. Add a bile acid sequestrant.
    C. Add niacin.
    D. Add clofibrate.
    E. Lose more weight.

33. The main side effect of which of the following drugs is flushing of the skin?
    A. Lovastatin.
    B. Cholestyramine.
    C. Nicotinic acid.
    D. Probucol.

34. A 58-year-old Caucasian female patient has a total cholesterol of 299 mg/dL, LDL = 240, HDL = 30, and triglycerides = 928 mg/dL. She is 62 inches (5 ft 2 in, 157 cm) tall and weighs 220 lb (~ 100 kg). Which of the following drugs would be most effective for this patient?
    A. Nonselective β blocker.
    B. $β_1$ selective adrenergic receptor blocker.
    C. Ezetimibe.
    D. Gemfibrozil.
    E. Verapamil.

35. Which of the following requires the presence of aldosterone to be an effective diuretic?
    A. Triamterene.
    B. Hydrochlorothiazide.
    C. Furosemide.

D. Spironolactone.
E. Mannitol.

36. The drug-induced acidosis that appears within the first week of therapy terminates the diuretic action of which of the following drugs?
A. Chlorothiazide.
B. Ethacrynic acid.
C. Amiloride.
D. Acetazolamide.
E. Spironolactone.

37. Which of the following diuretics is most likely to cause hyperkalemia?
A. Acetazolamide.
B. Chlorothiazide.
C. Ethacrynic acid.
D. Triamterene.
E. Furosemide.

38. Which of the following may cause bradycardia, bronchoconstriction, and heart failure?
A. Propranolol.
B. Captopril.
C. Hydralazine.
D. Diazoxide.
E. Hydrochlorothiazide.

39. The antihypertensive effect of which of the following drugs results from a direct action on vascular smooth muscle?
A. Hydralazine.
B. Methyldopa.
C. Losartan.
D. Guanethidine.
E. Enalapril.

40. Which of the following drugs is used for hypertensive emergencies?
A. Propranolol.
B. Captopril.
C. Clonidine.
D. Diazoxide.
E. Hydrochlorothiazide.

41. Prazosin decreases blood pressure by
A. Acting centrally to decrease peripheral sympathetic nerve activity.
B. Decreasing cardiac output.
C. Directly acting on myofibrils of vascular smooth muscle.
D. Inhibiting the release of renin from the kidney.
E. Preventing the vasoconstrictor effects of neuronally released norepinephrine on vascular smooth muscle.

42. Which of the following inhibits activated and inactivated voltage-gated Na^+ channels to decrease the sodium conductance in cardiac cells?
A. Acetazolamide.
B. Lidocaine.
C. Hydrochlorothiazide.
D. Digoxin.
E. Furosemide.

43. Which of the following drugs will decrease resting heart rate and reduce the maximal heart rate response during exercise?
A. Isoproterenol.
B. Nitroglycerin.
C. Atropine.
D. Metoprolol.
E. Nifedipine.

44. Toxicity is enhanced by hypokalemia for which of the following?
A. Digoxin.
B. Sodium nitroprusside.
C. Diltiazem.
D. Nifedipine.
E. Triamterene.

45. Drugs that affect which of the following are potentially teratogenic?
A. β-Adrenergic receptors.
B. Calcium channels.
C. Potassium excretion.
D. Renin-angiotensin system.
E. Antithrombin III.

46. Which of the following drugs directly inhibits renin activity?
A. Aliskiren.
B. Captopril.
C. Candesartan.
D. Angiotensinogen.
E. Aldosterone.

47. Which of the following is not effective for most forms of supraventricular arrhythmias?
A. Digitalis.
B. Procainamide.
C. Verapamil.
D. Propranolol.
E. Lidocaine.

48. A synthetic catecholamine that increases myocardial contractility and renal blood flow but whose usefulness for long-term treatment of heart failure is limited by its short half-life, lack of effect after oral administration, and side effects is
A. Digoxin.
B. Dobutamine.
C. Prazosin.
D. Captopril.
E. Lidocaine.

49. Nitroglycerin decreases congestive symptoms of heart failure primarily by decreasing which of the following parameters?
A. Preload.
B. Afterload.
C. Myocardial contractility.
D. Ventricular automaticity.

50. What is the preferred initial drug therapy for a white asthmatic man with moderate hypertension and angina pectoris?
    A. An orally active diuretic.
    B. A calcium channel blocker.
    C. A β-adrenergic receptor blocker.
    D. An angiotensin-converting enzyme (ACE) inhibitor.
    E. An α1 -adrenergic receptor blocking agent.

51. An orally active class IB antiarrhythmic that has minimal effects on cardiac contractility is
    A. Procainamide.
    B. Propranolol.
    C. Mexiletine.
    D. Flecainide.
    E. Verapamil.

52. A sodium channel blocker that has predominant action on phase 0 depolarization and conduction but not much effect on the duration of the action potential is
    A. Procainamide.
    B. Propranolol.
    C. Mexiletine.
    D. Flecainide.
    E. Verapamil.

53. Use of propranolol for relief of angina pectoris may safely be used in patients who have
    A. A blood pressure of 190/mm Hg.
    B. A first- or second-degree atrioventricular (AV) block.
    C. Dyspnea, wheezing, and eosinophilia in the sputum.
    D. Signs of heart failure with a normal sinus rhythm.
    E. Diabetes mellitus.

54. Which of the following acts by binding bile acid salts, which leads to their increased fecal elimination?
    A. Lovastatin.
    B. Cholestyramine.
    C. Nicotinic acid (niacin).
    D. Clofibrate.

55. Patients using which of the following drugs must be advised to contact their physician immediately if they experience muscle pain, tenderness, or weakness?
    A. Lovastatin.
    B. Cholestyramine.
    C. Nicotinic acid.
    D. Probucol.

56. An increased incidence of cholelithiasis (gallstones) is seen with
    A. Cholestyramine.
    B. Clofibrate.
    C. Nicotinic acid.
    D. Probucol.

57. The effects of which of the following can be counteracted by protamine sulfate?
    A. Heparin.
    B. Warfarin.
    C. Tissue plasminogen activator (t-PA).
    D. Streptokinase.
    E. Bivalirudin.

58. Which of the following is not effective when taken orally?
    A. Aspirin.
    B. Warfarin.
    C. Aliskiren.
    D. Heparin.
    E. Lovastatin.

59. Which of the following binds to specific sites on fibrin?
    A. Heparin.
    B. Warfarin.
    C. Tissue plasminogen activator (t-PA).
    D. Streptokinase.
    E. Bivalirudin.

60. The anticoagulant action of warfarin is due to
    A. Direct binding to prothrombin, resulting in inhibition of prothrombin activity.
    B. Increased breakdown of fibrin.
    C. Inhibition of thromboplastin activity.
    D. Inhibition of the synthesis of prothrombin.
    E. Reduction of heparin content in mast cells.

61. The mechanism of the antiplatelet activity of aspirin is
    A. Activation of cyclooxygenase.
    B. Reversible inhibition of phosphodiesterase.
    C. Covalent (irreversible) inhibition of cyclooxygenase.
    D. Irreversible inhibition of phosphodiesterase.
    E. Reduction of heparin content in mast cells.

62. An antiplatelet drug for patients who have experienced thrombotic stroke or stroke precursors and who cannot take aspirin is
    A. Deferoxamine.
    B. Desmopressin.
    C. Ferrous sulfate.
    D. Erythropoietin.
    E. Ticlopidine.

63. A 76-year-old woman with existing cardiomyopathy has severe dyspnea and labored breathing. Her legs are swollen. Auscultation reveals rales at the base of the lungs bilaterally. Which of the following diuretics would be the best choice for immediate treatment of this patient?
    A. Furosemide.
    B. Mannitol.
    C. Acetazolamide.
    D. Chlorothiazide.
    E. Spironolactone.

64. A patient with a head injury is exhibiting signs of increased intracranial pressure. Which of the following drugs would be the best choice for immediate treatment of this patient?
    A. Labetalol.
    B. Mannitol.
    C. Acetazolamide.
    D. Chlorothiazide.
    E. Spironolactone.

65. A 48-year-old African American man has had a blood pressure of 160/mm Hg, 170/mm Hg, and 165/mm Hg on three monthly visits. The patient's hypertension is treated with nifedipine. How does this drug reduce hypertension?

A. By blocking α2-adrenergic receptors.
B. By inhibiting angiotensin-converting enzyme.
C. By blocking β-adrenergic receptors.
D. By blocking L-type calcium channels.
E. By inhibiting sodium reabsorption in the loop of Henle.

66. A 58-year-old African American woman is being treated for heart failure with a diuretic, an angiotensin-converting enzyme (ACE) inhibitor, and a β-adrenergic receptor blocking agent. She continues to experience dyspnea on exertion. She is more likely than a Caucasian patient to benefit from the addition of which of the following drugs?

A. A direct vasodilator.
B. A positive inotropic agent.
C. An angiotensin receptor antagonist.
D. A calcium channel blocker.
E. An oral antihyperglycemic.

67. A patient is diagnosed as having stable angina. He also has overt congestive heart failure, chronic obstructive pulmonary disease, and insulin-dependent diabetes mellitus. Which agent would be the drug of choice to initiate the treatment of the angina?

A. Nonselective β-blocker.
B. B1 selective adrenergic blocker.
C. Diltiazem.
D. Isosorbide dinitrate.
E. Verapamil.

68. A 62-year-old patient is experiencing chest pain on exertion. Effort-induced angina is diagnosed, and treatment is begun. The patient is given one drug to take daily to prevent the effort-induced angina attacks and a second drug to take if an acute attack occurs. The second drug is most likely which of the following?

A. Diltiazem.
B. Nitroglycerin.
C. Metoprolol.
D. Propranolol.
E. Verapamil.

69. A patient is being treated with verapamil to prevent the recurrence of atrial flutter. Which of the following changes would you expect to observe in the patient's electrocardiogram (EKG)?

A. Q-T prolongation.
B. Increased P-R interval.
C. Inverted T wave.
D. Increased R wave amplitude.
E. Appearance of a prominent Q wave.

70. A 54-year-old male patient has a total cholesterol of mg/dL, low-density lipoprotein (LDL) = mg/dL, high-density lipoprotein (HDL) = mg/dL, and triglycerides = mg/dL. He quit smoking years ago. One year ago, his values were total cholesterol of mg/dL, LDL = mg/dL, HDL = mg/dL, and triglycerides = mg/dL. At that time, he instituted dietary changes and began walking at least minutes per day. He is inches (5 ft 9 in, cm) tall and weighs lb (kg). His father has a history of atherosclerosis, and his mother has suffered cerebrovascular strokes. What laboratory test must be conducted prior to prescribing a 3-hydroxy-3-methylglutaryl (HMG)–coenzyme A (CoA) reductase inhibitor to this patient?

A. Complete blood count.
B. Serum glucose level.
C. Serum creatine kinase level.
D. Serum alanine aminotransferase level.
E. Serum apolipoprotein E level.

V

Unit V Answers and Explanations

1. D. Acetazolamide is a carbonic anhydrase inhibitor that acts in the proximal convoluted tubule to reduce the absorption of bicarbonate ions from the glomerular filtrate. The effectiveness of its diuretic action decreases as plasma bicarbonate is depleted. This causes a metabolic acidosis.

A. Metolazone is a thiazide–like diuretic.

B. Ethacrynic acid is a loop diuretic that inhibits the Na^+–K^+–$2Cl^-$ cotransporter in the thick ascending loop of Henle.

C. Amiloride is a potassium-sparing diuretic used that directly interferes with sodium transport in the distal convoluted tubule.

E. Spironolactone is a competitive antagonist to aldosterone and so inhibits the synthesis of Na^+ channel proteins and Na^+–K^+–ATPases which promotes the reabsorption of Na^+, Cl^-, and water.

2. A. Furosemide and the loop (or high-ceiling) diuretics increase calcium ion excretion into the urine and are therefore useful in treating symptomatic hypercalcemia.

B, C. Thiazide diuretics, such as chlorthalidone and hydrochlorothiazide, decrease calcium excretion.

D. Desmopressin is the synthetic replacement for antidiuretic hormone (ADH), the hormone that reduces urine production.

E. Mannitol is an osmotic diuretic that increases the solute load (solutes cannot be absorbed but bind to water), causing increased urine production.

3. C. Loop diuretics, such as furosemide, can cause ototoxicity, especially when given at higher doses. These symptoms include tinnitus or hearing loss, which are usually reversed upon drug discontinuation but can be permanent in some cases.

4. D. The foot inflammation in a male patient of this age indicates a gout attack. Thiazide diuretics, such as chlorothiazide, produce hyperuricemia (elevated blood uric acid level), which may precipitate further attacks.

5. B. The patient has hypokalemia (normal range 3.5–5.0 mEq/L). Amiloride is a potassium-sparing diuretic that is useful when given along with a thiazide to prevent potassium depletion.

A. Acetazolamide is a carbonic anhydrase inhibitor that will increase the excretion of bicarbonate.

C. Furosemide is a loop diuretic that may worsen the hypokalemia.

D. The patient is already taking hydrochlorothiazide, a thiazide diuretic.

E. Aldosterone is an endogenous mineralocorticoid hormone that increases sodium reabsorption and potassium excretion.

6. D. Diabetes insipidus of pituitary origin is the most common type of diabetes insipidus and is caused by a deficiency of arginine vasopressin (AVP). Desmopressin (1-deamino-8-D-arginine vasopressin) is a synthetic analogue of AVP used as replacement therapy for AVP.

A, B. Triamterene and amiloride are potassium-sparing diuretics used in combination with a thiazide diuretic to treat hypertension.

C, E. Ethacrynic acid and furosemide are loop diuretics used to treat chronic heart failure, pulmonary edema due to left ventricular failure, hypertension, acute oliguria, and hypercalcemia.

7. B. Nephrogenic diabetes insipidus is caused by a defect in the tubules of the kidney, leading to an improper response to ADH and overproduction of dilute urine. Thiazide diuretics, such as hydrochlorothiazide, exert a paradoxical effect to decrease the urine output of patients with nephrogenic diabetes insipidus.

A. Triamterene is a potassium-sparing diuretic used in combination with a thiazide diuretic to treat hypertension.

C. Furosemide is a loop diuretic used to treat chronic heart failure, pulmonary edema due to left ventricular failure, hypertension, acute oliguria, and hypercalcemia.

D. Desmopressin is the synthetic replacement for ADH, the hormone that reduces urine production.

E. Mannitol is an osmotic diuretic that increases the solute load (solutes cannot be absorbed but bind to water), causing increased urine production.

8. A. The patient's symptoms suggest that the antihypertensive drug she was taking may also have been preventing the atrial fibrillation.

Propranolol, a nonselective β blocker, has both antihypertensive and antiarrhythmic effects.

B. Enalapril is an ACE inhibitor that has antihypertensive but no antiarrhythmic effects.

C. Hydrochlorothiazide is a thiazide diuretic that has antihypertensive but no antiarrhythmic effects.

D. Losartan is an angiotensin II receptor antagonist that has antihypertensive but no antiarrhythmic effects.

E. Clonidine is an α_2 adrenergic receptor agonist that has antihypertensive but no antiarrhythmic effects.

9. E. The nonselective β adrenergic receptor blocking agents, such as propranolol, may worsen asthma by blocking the bronchodilation produced via β_2 adrenergic receptor activation.

A. Reserpine is an adrenergic neuron blocker that reduces blood pressure by depleting norepinephrine stores and by preventing its reuptake and storage. It will have no effect on asthma.

B. Hydrochlorothiazide is a thiazide diuretic. It will have no effect on asthma.

C, D. Nifedipine and verapamil are calcium-channel blockers. Nifedipine acts on vascular smooth muscle causing vasodilation and so reducing blood pressure. Verapamil also causes vasodilation of vascular smooth muscle but it also acts on cardiac muscle cells to reduce heart rate, force of contraction, and velocity of contraction. It is therefore also useful in the treatment of angina and some arrhythmias. Both nifedipine and verapamil have no effect on asthma.

10. B. ACE inhibitors, such as enalapril, are less effective in African American patients than in other patient groups unless combined with a thiazide diuretic.

A, C–E. The other drugs listed are not associated with this reduced effectiveness.

11. E. The test results are negative for other causes for her cough, and cough is a common side effect of ACE inhibitors, such as captopril.

12. E. Losartan blocks the binding of angiotensin II to the angiotensin I–type angiotensin receptor. Its side effects are similar to those of captopril, but it does not produce a cough.

A–D. The other drugs do not affect the angiotensin system directly.

13. D. Nifedipine is a dihydropyridine calcium channel antagonist that acts by blocking L-type (long-lasting) calcium channels. This causes vasodilation of vascular smooth muscle and a reduction in blood pressure.

14. B. Clonidine stimulates α_2 adrenergic receptors in the medulla, which in turn decreases sympathetic tone and blood pressure. Persistent activation of α_2 adrenergic receptors leads to their downregulation. Upon cessation of clonidine, this decrease in α_2 adrenergic receptor function leads to a rebound in blood pressure that may last a day or two until the normal level of α_2 adrenergic receptors is restored.

A. Prazosin is an α_1 adrenergic receptor antagonist that reduces blood pressure by vasodilation of vascular smooth muscle. Orthostatic hypotension is common after the first dose.

C. Guanethidine is an adrenergic neuron blocker that reduces blood pressure by preventing norepinephrine release, depleting norepinephrine stores, and blocking its reuptake.

D. Enalapril is an ACE inhibitor that reduces blood pressure by preventing the vasoconstrictive effects of angiotensin II on vascular smooth muscle.

E. Reserpine is an adrenergic neuron blocker that reduces blood pressure by depleting norepinephrine stores and by preventing its reuptake and storage.

15. D. Hypotension is a side effect of captopril, an ACE inhibitor. This effect is amplified when it is combined with hydrochlorothiazide and is more frequently observed in patients with heart failure.

A–C, E. The other results are not normally associated with captopril.

16. C. Because the patient is already being treated with a diuretic, an ACE inhibitor, and a β blocker, a logical next choice would be digoxin. Both the therapeutic and toxic effects of digoxin are attributable to inhibition of Na$^+$–K$^+$–ATPase (the digitalis receptor) located on the outside of the myocardial cell membrane.

A, B, D, E. The other choices are not valid mechanisms for drugs that treat heart failure.

17. B. As an inhibitor of Na$^+$– K$^+$–ATPase, which pumps Na$^+$ out of the cell and K$^+$ into the cell, digoxin would be expected to decrease the level of intracellular K$^+$. According to the Nernst equation, membrane potential is proportional to the level of K inside the cell/K outside the cell. Decreasing the K inside the cell will decrease membrane potential (i.e., depolarize the cell).

A, C–E. The other effects listed are not typical of digoxin.

18. A. Dobutamine is used for short-term support in severe heart failure. It acts by stimulating cardiac β_1 receptors to increase cardiac contractility. It is not used long term, as it may cause arrhythmias and increase oxygen consumption.

B. Isoproterenol is a nonselective β adrenergic receptor agonist that increases heart rate and contractility. It is more likely than dobutamine to cause arrhythmias and increase oxygen consumption. It is used to improve cardiac output in patients with heart block.

C. Bethanechol is a cholinergic muscarinic receptor agonist that would decrease, not improve, cardiac function.

D. Propranolol is a nonselective β adrenergic receptor blocker and would have a negative inotropic effect.

E. Phenylephrine is an α adrenoceptor agonist that would produce vasoconstriction, but reflex vasoconstriction is already present.

19. D. In HF, the main therapeutic actions of nitroglycerin are due to dilation of large capacitance veins.

A. Nitroglycerin will cause some arteriolar dilation but this is not its primary effect.

B, C. Nitroglycerin does not increase cardiac contractility (inotropism) or increase cardiac output.

20. D. Organic nitrates are converted to nitric oxide, which activates guanylate cyclase, increases intracellular cGMP concentrations, and causes vasodilation of venous and arterial blood vessels.

21. C. Metoprolol is a β adrenergic receptor antagonist. It is useful for the prophylaxis of effort-induced angina but is not effective for the acute termination of effort-induced angina or for the treatment of coronary artery spasm.

A, E. The calcium channel blockers diltiazem and verapamil are more appropriate for variant or unstable angina due to coronary vasospasm.

B, D. Nitroglycerin and isosorbide dinitrate are indicated for acute relief of an angina pectoris attack. They are given sublingually and rapidly absorbed through the oral mucosa. Therapeutic effects are observed within 2 to 4 minutes but last for only 1 to 2 hours.

22. D. Organic nitrates act like the endogenous compound nitric oxide. They activate guanylate cyclase to increase the level of cyclic guanosine monophosphate (cGMP) in smooth muscle. This leads to relaxation of vascular smooth muscle and both arterial and venous dilation. This results in a decrease in ventricular preload and a reduction of ventricular wall stress.

A–C. The vasodilation produced by the organic nitrates may result in reflex increases in heart rate and contractility and a decrease in left ventricular residual volume.

E. Organic nitrates will cause a decrease in venous pressure.

23. A. By definition, class I antiarrhythmic action is Na^+ channel blockade, which reduces membrane excitability or responsiveness.

24. B. Acute lupus erythematosus has been observed with procainamide; thus, this drug is contraindicated in patients with a history of SLE.

A, C–E. None of the other drugs will precipitate lupus erythematosus.

25. C. Class IB antiarrhythmic agents, such as mexiletine, are Na^+ channel blockers and act like local anesthetics, which is producing this patient's symptoms. The symptoms are most prominent as the drug levels peak at 2 to 3 hours after administration.

26. E. A β adrenergic receptor antagonist, propranolol is a class II antiarrhythmic agent that may help prevent ventricular fibrillation during the period following myocardial infarction.

A. Phenylephrine is an α adrenergic agonist.

B. Isoproterenol is a nonselective β adrenergic receptor agonist.

C. Norepinephrine is the endogenous postganglionic sympathetic neurotransmitter with both α and β agonist activity.

D. Nitroglycerin is indicated for acute relief of an angina pectoris attack.

27. B. Eptifibatide is a cyclic peptide that blocks the glycoprotein IIb/IIIa receptor to prevent platelet aggregation.

28. A. Protamine sulfate is an antidote for heparin and forms a 1:1 complex with the anticoagulant. Administration of this drug will return the patient's aPTT to a normal range.

B–E. The other drugs have no effect on aPTT.

29. A. Thrombocytopenia is one of the adverse effects that may be observed following heparin administration. It may be mild and transient, but it may become severe if antiplatelet antibodies are formed. Platelet counts should be performed to monitor for thrombocytopenia.

B–E. None of these have any relevance in heparin therapy.

30. B. Warfarin is an oral anticoagulant drug that antagonizes the hepatic synthesis of the vitamin K-dependent clotting factors II (prothrombin), VII, IX, and X. It increases a patient's INR. Green leafy vegetables are a good source of vitamin K. Vitamin K is a warfarin antagonist. Thus, the expected result would be a decreased INR.

31. A. Lovastatin competitively inhibits HMG-CoA reductase, the rate-limiting enzyme in cholesterol synthesis.

B. Cholestyramine is an insoluble resin that is not absorbed by the body, but binds bile acids in the gut, thus preventing bile acids from being absorbed. This necessitates an increase in the hepatic conversion of cholesterol to bile acids, thereby reducing the cholesterol available through the enterohepatic circulation for production of plasma lipids. This also lowers LDL and plasma cholesterol.

C. Nicotinic acid (niacin) inhibits hepatocyte diacylglycerol acyltransferase-2, a key enzyme for triglyceride synthesis, decreasing the secretion of VLDL and LDL-C. It also decreases the hepatic catabolism of apo A-I and increases the half-life and concentrations of HDL-C.

D. Clofibrate lowers VLDL and plasma triglycerides by stimulating lipoprotein lipase. It also lowers cholesterol by inhibiting its synthesis and enhancing excretion in the bile.

32. A. Because the patient was started on the initial recommended dose, the cholesterol-lowering response was not great enough, and adverse reactions to the drug were not reported, the next step should be to increase the dose.

B. Bile acid sequestrant may be added if the statin does not reach the desired goal, but an adequate dose of the statin should be tried first.

C. Niacin is especially useful in patients with both hypertriglyceridemia and HDL-C levels. This patient has normal triglycerides and borderline high HDL.

D. Clofibrate is useful in hypertriglyceridemia and hypercholesterolemia.

E. The patient's weight is near normal.

33. C. Flushing of the skin is a side effect of nicotinic acid (niacin). It results from the stimulation of prostaglandins D_2 and E_2 from subcutaneous Langerhans cells by a G protein-coupled niacin receptor.

A, B, D. Flushing is not associated with lovastatin, cholestyramine, or probucol.

34. D. Gemfibrozil is indicated for hypertriglyceridemia and hypercholesterolemia.

A, B, E. β blockers and verapamil (a calcium channel blocker) do not lower cholesterol levels.

C. Ezetimibe inhibits cholesterol absorption in the small intestine but it is not as effective at lowering cholesterol or triglyceride levels as gemfibrozil.

35. D. Spironolactone is a competitive antagonist to aldosterone and so inhibits the synthesis of Na$^+$ channel proteins and Na$^+$/K$^+$-ATPases, which promotes the reabsorption of Na$^+$, Cl-, and water.

A–C, E. The other drugs work independently of aldosterone.

36. D. Acetazolamide is a carbonic anhydrase inhibitor that acts in the proximal convoluted tubule to reduce the absorption of bicarbonate ions from the glomerular filtrate. The effectiveness of its diuretic action decreases as plasma bicarbonate is depleted. This causes metabolic acidosis.

A. Chlorothiazide is a thiazide diuretic.

B. Ethacrynic acid is a loop diuretic used to treat chronic heart failure, pulmonary edema due to left ventricular failure, hypertension, acute oliguria, and hypercalcemia.

C. Amiloride is a potassium-sparing diuretic used, in combination with a thiazide diuretic, to treat hypertension.

E. Spironolactone is a potassium-sparing diuretic used to treat hypertension, primary aldosteronism, hyperuricemia, hypokalemia, or glucose intolerance.

37. D. Triamterene is a potassium-sparing diuretic that decreases excretion of potassium and could lead to hyperkalemia.

A. Acetazolamide is a potassium-depleting diuretic.

B, C, E. The loop (furosemide, ethacrynic acid) and thiazide (chlorothiazide) diuretics increase potassium excretion and may cause hypokalemia.

38. A. These are effects seen with nonselective β-adrenergic receptor blocking agents such as propranolol. The normal physiological effects mediated by β-adrenergic receptors include increased heart rate and contractility and bronchodilation. Blocking these receptors may lead to bradycardia, bronchoconstriction, and heart failure.

B. Captopril is an angiotensin-converting enzyme inhibitor used in the treatment of heart failure. It does not cause bradycardia or bronchoconstriction.

C. Hydralazine is an arterial vasodilator used to treat hypertension. It may cause reflex tachycardia and will not cause bronchoconstriction or heart failure.

D. Diazoxide is an arterial vasodilator used to treat acute hypertensive emergencies. It does not cause bradycardia, bronchoconstriction, or heart failure.

E. Hydrochlorothiazide is a thiazide diuretic used to treat hypertension. It would be helpful, if anything, in heart failure and would not cause bradycardia or bronchoconstriction.

39. A. Of the drugs listed, hydralazine is the only one that acts directly on vascular smooth muscle to decrease peripheral resistance and decrease blood pressure.

B. Methyldopa is an α$_1$-adrenergic receptor blocking agent that reduces blood pressure by CNS reduction of sympathetic outflow.

C. Losartan blocks the binding of angiotensin II to the AT$_1$-type of angiotensin receptors.

D. Guanethidine is an adrenergic neuron blocker that reduces blood pressure by preventing norepinephrine release, depleting norepinephrine stores, and blocking its reuptake.

E. Enalapril is an angiotensin-converting enzyme inhibitor that reduces blood pressure by preventing the vasoconstrictive effects of angiotensin II on vascular smooth muscle.

40. D. Of the drugs listed, diazoxide, an arterial vasodilator, is the only one used for acute hypertensive emergencies.

A. Propranolol is a nonselective β-adrenergic receptor blocking agent used to treat hypertension, angina, and some arrhythmias.

B. Captopril is an angiotensin-converting enzyme inhibitor used in the treatment of heart failure and hypertension.

C. Clonidine is an agonist at central nervous system α$_2$-adrenoceptors, which, in turn, causes inhibition of sympathetic tone. It is not used for hypertensive emergencies.

E. Hydrochlorothiazide is a thiazide diuretic used to treat hypertension but not for hypertensive emergencies.

41. E. Prazosin is an α1-adrenergic receptor blocker. This inhibits the vasoconstriction produced by endogenous norepinephrine on vascular smooth muscle.

42. B. Lidocaine is a class IB antiarrythmic agent that inhibits the sodium conductance in cardiac cells.

A. Acetazolamide is a carbonic anhydrase inhibitor used to treat glaucoma.

C. Hydrochlorothiazide is a thiazide diuretic used to treat hypertension.

D. Digoxin is a cardiac glycoside that is now infrequently used in the treatment of heart failure.

E. Furosemide is a loop diuretic used to treat chronic heart failure, pulmonary edema due to left ventricular failure, hypertension, acute oliguria, and hypercalcemia.

43. D. Metoprolol is a β-blocker that decreases heart rate both at rest and in response to exercise.

A. Isoproterenol is a synthetic catecholamine that acts as a β-adrenergic receptor agonist and so will tend to increase heart rate.

B. Nitroglycerin is a vasodilator that may produce a small increase in heart rate.

C. Atropine is a muscarinic cholinergic receptor antagonist that will increase heart rate by blocking vagal (parasympathetic) slowing of the heart.

E. Nifedipine is a calcium channel blocker that acts predominantly on vascular smooth muscle causing vasodilation at therapeutic doses. It has little effect on heart rate.

44. A. Both the therapeutic and toxic effects of digitalis preparations such as digoxin are related to inhibition of the Na_+-K_+-ATPase. Inhibition of the Na^+-K^+ pump may lead to a significant reduction of intracellular K^+, which leads to some of the toxic effects. These toxicities are worsened by low potassium and reduced by correcting the K^+ deficiency.

B-D. These agents do not cause hypokalemia.

E. Triamterene is a potassium-sparing diuretic and so will prevent hypokalemia.

45. D. All drugs should be used with caution in pregnancy, but drugs that act directly on the renin-angiotensin system, including angiotensin-converting enzyme (ACE) inhibitors, angiotensin II receptor antagonists, and direct renin inhibitors can cause injury or death to the developing fetus, and their use in pregnancy should be avoided.

46. A. Aliskiren is a relatively new drug that produces a dose-dependent reduction in plasma renin activity by binding to the proteolytic site of renin and preventing cleavage of angiotensinogen.

B. Captopril is an angiotensin-converting enzyme inhibitor that inhibits the formation of angiotensin II from angiotensin I.

C. Candesartan is an angiotensin II receptor antagonist.

D. Angiotensinogen is the precursor to angiotensin I that is cleaved by renin.

E. Aldosterone is an endogenous mineralocorticoid that increases the reabsorption of sodium and water in the kidney.

47. E. Lidocaine and other class IB drugs have little effect on atrial tissues or atrioventricular nodal conduction and are thus not effective for most forms of supraventricular arrhythmias.

A-D. These agents delay conduction at the atrioventricular node and are therefore useful in treating supraventricular arrhythmias.

48. B. Dobutamine, a synthetic catecholamine used for short-term support in severe heart failure, stimulates the cardiac β_1 receptors to produce a positive inotropic action. It is not effective orally. Dobutamine is not used long term, as it may cause arrhythmias and increase oxygen consumption.

A. Digoxin is a cardiac glycoside which will increase cardiac contractility and its usefulness is limited by its toxicity. Otherwise digoxin does not fit the question criteria.

C. Prazosin is an α1-adrenergic receptor antagonist that causes vasodilation of vascular smooth muscle. It does not fit the question criteria.

D. Captopril is an angiotensin converting enzyme inhibitor that causes vasodilation of vascular smooth muscle. It does not fit the question criteria.

E. Lidocaine is a class IB antiarrythmic agent that inhibits the sodium conductance in cardiac cells. It does not fit the question criteria.

49. A. Although its main use is sublingually for treatment of angina pectoris, nitroglycerin is used for short-term intravenous treatment of severe heart failure. It dilates large capacitance veins and reduces preload.

B. Nitroglycerin will also reduce afterload but this is not the primary mechanism by which it relieves the symptoms of CHF.

C, D. Nitroglycerin does not relieve CHF by affecting myocardial contractility or ventricular automaticity.

50. B. Of the drug classes listed, the two that are indicated for treatment of both hypertension and angina are calcium channel blockers and β-adrenergic receptor blockers. However, β-adrenergic receptor blockers cause bronchoconstriction and are therefore contraindicated in asthma, leaving only calcium channel blockers as the drug class of choice.

A. Diuretics are used in the treatment of hypertension but not angina.

D. Angiotensin-converting enzyme (ACE) inhibitors are used in the treatment of hypertension and heart failure. They are not used in angina.

E. An α_1-adrenergic receptor blocking agent is used in the treatment of hypertension and heart failure. They are not used in angina.

51. C. Mexiletine is a class IB antiarrhythmic that acts by shortening the action potential duration and the QT interval but has little effect on myocardial contractility.

A. Procainamide is a class IA agent that prolongs the action potential duration and QT interval. It also depresses myocardial contractility.

B. Propranolol is a class II agent that depresses AV nodal conduction. It also depresses myocardial contractility.

D. Flecainide is a class IC agent that slows conduction in all cardiac tissues (including the AV node). It also depresses myocardial contractility.

E. Verapamil is a class IV agent that depresses AV nodal conduction. It also depresses myocardial contractility.

52. D. Class IC agents such as flecainide are sodium channel blockers that slow conduction in all cardiac tissues (including the AV node) and depress myocardial contractility. However, they are noted for not having an effect on the duration of the action potential.

A. Procainamide is a class IA sodium channel blocker that prolongs the action potential duration and QT interval and depresses myocardial contractility.

B. Propranolol is a class II β blocker agent that depresses AV nodal conduction and depresses myocardial contractility.

C. Mexiletine is a class IB sodium channel blocker that acts by shortening the action potential duration and the QT interval but has little effect on myocardial contractility.

53. A. Propranolol is a nonselective β-blocker that may be used in a patient with angina and high blood pressure, as it is also an antihypertensive agent.

B. Propranolol would be contraindicated in a patient with a first- or second-degree atrioventricular block, as it may further depress AV nodal conduction.

C. Dyspnea, wheezing, and eosinophilia in the sputum are symptoms of asthma, which also contraindicates the use of β-blockers.

D. The β-blocker agents that are useful in heart failure are bisoprolol, carvedilol, and metoprolol.

E. Beta-blockers decrease insulin sensitivity and are contraindicated in diabetes mellitus.

54. B. Cholestyramine binds bile acids in the gut, thus preventing bile acids from being absorbed and increasing their elimination.

A. Lovastatin competitively inhibits HMG-CoA reductase, the rate-limiting enzyme in cholesterol synthesis.

C. Nicotinic acid (niacin) inhibits hepatocyte diacylglycerol acyltransferase-2, a key enzyme for triglyceride synthesis, decreasing the secretion of very low density lipoprotein (VLDL) and low density lipoprotein cholesterol (LDL-C). It also decreases the hepatic catabolism of apo A-I and increases the half-life and concentrations of high density lipoprotein cholesterol (HDL-C).

D. Clofibrate lowers very low density lipoproteins (VLDL) and plasma triglycerides by stimulating lipoprotein lipase. It also lowers cholesterol by inhibiting its synthesis and enhancing excretion in the bile.

55. A. These are symptoms of rhabdomyolysis, the rapid breakdown of muscle fibers. It is a rare but serious side effect of lovastatin and other statins.

B–D. Rhabdomyolysis is not a side effect of the other agents.

56. B. Gallstones may occur with long-term use of clofibrate.

A, C, D. Gallstones are not associated with the other listed drugs.

57. A. Protamine sulfate is an antidote for heparin and forms a 1:1 complex with the anticoagulant.

B–E. Protamine sulfate will not counteract the other agents listed.

58. D. Heparin is not effective orally and must be given intravenously or subcutaneously.

A–C, E. The other drugs are effective when given orally.

59. C. Tissue plasminogen activator preferentially activates plasminogen bound to fibrin.

A. Heparin combines with, and catalytically activates, a plasma cofactor named antithrombin III. This complex neutralizes several activated clotting factors, particularly factors IIa (thrombin) and Xa.

B. Warfarin antagonizes the hepatic synthesis of the vitamin K-dependent clotting factors II (prothrombin), VII, IX, and X.

D. Streptokinase promotes the dissolution of thrombi by stimulating the conversion of endogenous plasminogen to plasmin (fibrinolysin).

E. Bivalirudin inhibits clot-bound and circulating thrombin.

60. D. Warfarin exerts its anticoagulant action by antagonizing the hepatic synthesis of the vitamin K-dependent clotting factors II (prothrombin), VII, IX, and X.

61. C. Aspirin acetylates platelet cyclooxygenase and irreversibly inhibits the enzyme. This in turn inhibits the formation of thromboxane A_2 from arachidonic acid and reduces platelet aggregation and activation.

62. E. Ticlopidine is indicated for patients who have experienced or are at risk for cerebrovascular or cardiovascular thrombotic events, and it is recommended for patients who cannot take aspirin.

A. Deferoxamine is a specific chelating agent for iron.

B. Desmopressin stimulates the release of clotting factor VIII from the vascular endothelium. It is used preoperatively in hemophilic patients with low circulating levels of this factor.

C. Ferrous sulfate is used to treat iron deficiency anemia.

D. Erythropoietin is a renal hormone which regulates the production of red blood cells in bone marrow.

63. A. The patient is exhibiting signs of pulmonary edema secondary to heart failure. Loop diuretics, such as furosemide, produce a strong diuresis by inhibiting the $Na^+/K^+/2Cl^-$ cotransporter in the thick ascending loop of Henle. Of the drugs listed, furosemide provides the most rapid relief and is the most potent.

B. Mannitol is an osmotic diuretic most commonly used to provide acute reduction of cerebrospinal or intraocular pressure.

C. Acetazolamide is a carbonic anhydrase inhibitor used to treat glaucoma.

D. Chlorothiazide is a thiazide diuretic used to treat hypertension.

E. Spironolactone is a potassium-sparing diuretic used to treat hypertension, primary aldosteronism, hyperuricemia, hypokalemia, or glucose intolerance.

64. B. Osmotic diuretics, such as mannitol, are used for acute reduction of intracranial pressure.

A. Labetalol blocks both α_1- and β-adrenergic receptors and is used in the treatment of hypertension.

C. Acetazolamide is a carbonic anhydrase inhibitor used to treat glaucoma.

D. Chlorothiazide is a thiazide diuretic used in the treatment of hypertension.

E. Spironolactone is a potassium-sparing diuretic used in hypertension, primary aldosteronism, hyperuricemia, hypokalemia, or glucose intolerance.

65. D. Nifedipine is a dihydropyridine calcium channel antagonist that acts by blocking L-type (long-lasting) calcium channels. This causes vasodilation of vascular smooth muscle and a reduction in blood pressure.

66. A. A vasodilator added to this treatment regimen has been shown to be effective in African-American patients with severe heart failure.

67. D. Of the antianginal drugs listed, isosorbide dinitrate would have a beneficial effect in angina and heart failure without worsening the pulmonary or diabetic symptoms.

A. Nonselective β-blockers may worsen pulmonary function (via inhibition of β_2-mediated bronchodilation) and diabetes.

B. β_1 selective adrenergic blockers are not appropriate as they can worsen asthma and should be used with caution in diabetic patients.

C, E. The calcium channel blockers diltiazem and verapamil decrease myocardial contractility and may worsen the heart failure.

68. B. Nitroglycerin is indicated for acute relief of an angina pectoris attack. It is given sublingually and rapidly absorbed through the oral mucosa. Therapeutic effects are observed within 2 to 4 minutes but last for only 1 to 2 hours.

A, E. The calcium channel blockers diltiazem and verapamil are more appropriate for variant or unstable angina due to coronary vasospasm.

C. Metoprolol is likely to have been the first drug given. Metoprolol is a β-adrenergic receptor antagonist useful for the prophylaxis of effort-induced angina, but it is not effective for the acute termination of effort-induced angina or for the treatment of coronary artery spasm.

69. B. On the EKG, the P wave indicates depolarization of the atria, and the QRS complex reflects ventricular depolarization. The P-R interval is the time between the onset of atrial depolarization and the onset of ventricular depolarization. Because verapamil slows phase 0 to decrease automaticity, it would be expected to increase the P-R interval.

70. D. Statins (HMG-CoA reductase inhibitors) may produce liver disease. Thus, liver enzymes such as serum alanine aminotransferase should be tested prior to and periodically during statin therapy.

A–C, E. The other tests are not specifically related to statin administration.

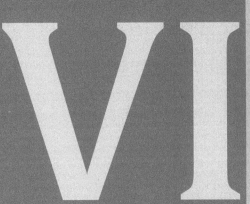

Unit VI

Drugs Acting on the Respiratory and Gastrointestinal Systems

26   Drugs Acting on the Respiratory System

Summary

The drugs acting on the respiratory system are used to treat lower respiratory tract disorders (asthma and chronic obstructive pulmonary disease [COPD]) and upper respiratory disorders (rhinitis and cough). The primary drugs used to treat asthma include inhaled corticosteroids (beclomethasone, budesonide, ciclesonide, flunisolide, fluticasone, mometasone, and triamcinolone) and short-acting (albuterol, levalbuterol, metaproterenol, and terbutaline) and long-acting (arformoterol, formoterol, and salmeterol) β$_2$ receptor agonists. Leukotriene modifiers (montelukast, zafirlukast, and zileuton) and low-dose theophylline are alternatives. Anticholinergics (ipratropium, tiotropium, aclidinium, and umeclidinium) and anti-immunoglobulin E (omalizumab) therapies are reserved for patients who remain refractory to the above treatments. For patients with COPD either antimuscarinics or β$_2$ receptor agonists may be used as primary bronchodilator therapy. Patients whose symptoms are not adequately controlled by one drug may receive both an antimuscarinic and a β$_2$ receptor agonist with inhaled corticosteroids as add-on therapy. Theophylline and roflumilast may be tried in refractory cases. For rhinitis, intranasal (phenylephrine, oxymetazoline, naphazoline) and oral (pseudoephedrine and phenylephrine) sympathomimetics are used as decongestants. H$_1$ antihistamines (azelastine, cetirizine, fexofenadine, loratadine, and olopatadine) and intranasal corticosteroids are used to treat allergic rhinitis. Mast cell stabilizers (cromolyn sodium and nedocromil) are alternatives. Antitussives (codeine and dextromethorphan), expectorants (guaifenesin), and mucolytic drugs (acetylcysteine) provide symptomatic relief of cough.

Keywords: asthma, COPD, allergies, cough

26.1   Introduction

The drugs acting on the respiratory system are used to treat upper respiratory disorders that affect the nose and nasal sinuses or lower respiratory tract disorders that affect the airways to the lungs. The lower respiratory tract disorders include asthma and chronic obstructive pulmonary disease (COPD). Upper respiratory disorders include rhinitis and cough which mainly result from allergies and the common cold.

26.2   Asthma and Chronic Obstructive Pulmonary Disease

26.2.1   Asthma

Asthma is predominantly an inflammatory disease with associated bronchospasm, mucosal swelling, and increased mucus production. There is episodic bronchial obstruction causing wheezing, dyspnea, cough, and mucosal edema. In children, the only sign of asthma may be a persistent cough.

The etiology and immunopathogenesis of asthma are illustrated in ▶ Fig. 26.1 and ▶ Fig. 26.2. The role of inflammatory autocoids (e.g., histamine and leukotrienes) in relation to asthma is discussed in Chapter 32.

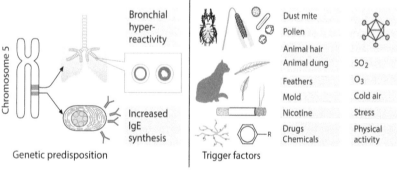

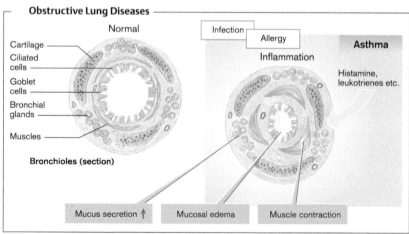

Fig. 26.1 Asthma: genetic predisposition and trigger factors.
Bronchial hyperreactivity and the tendency to increase interleukin-4 (IL-4)-dependent immunoglobulin E (IgE) production may be inherited through genes on chromosome 5 in patients with allergic asthma. This type of asthma is commonly triggered by animal hair, dust mites, feathers, pollen, and mold. In nonallergic asthma, the bronchial hyperreactivity is caused by the inhalation of chemicals, cigarette smoke, viral infections, cold air, exercise, and stress. Drugs (e.g., aspirin) can also cause an attack. In response to these triggers, mucus secretion is increased, vascular permeability is increased leading to edema, and the bronchial muscles contract. All of these lead to a decrease in the diameter of the airway and difficulty breathing.

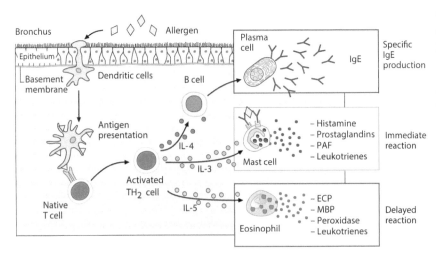

Fig. 26.2 Asthma: immunopathogenesis.
Allergens attach to, and are taken up by, dendritic cells that lie in the ciliated respiratory epithelium. The interaction of the allergen (antigen), antigen presenting cells, and native T cells leads to the differentiation of the T cells to T-helper (TH₂) cells, which release cytokines. Interleukin-4 (IL-4) activates B cells, which differentiate into plasma cells and release immunoglobulin E (IgE) that attaches to the surface of mast cells. The mast cells then degranulate when the allergens bridge two IgE molecules on their surface, especially when they are activated by IL-3. This cascade of events releases inflammatory mediators that are responsible for the bronchoconstriction/bronchospasm, mucosal swelling, and increased mucus production in allergic asthma. ECP, eosinophil cationic protein; MBP, major basic protein; PAF, platelet-activating factor.

26.2.2 Chronic Obstructive Pulmonary Disease

COPD is the term used to describe chronic obstructive bronchitis and emphysema which always coexist to varying degrees. The characteristic symptoms of COPD are persistent cough, sputum, dyspnea (shortness of breath), and wheezing.

Chronic bronchitis is defined clinically as sputum production on most days for 3 months of 2 consecutive years. Inflammation (most commonly caused by cigarette smoke) causes the bronchial tubes to thicken and scar and produce excess mucus. This mucus cannot be expectorated, given that cilia are destroyed as part of the disease process. These factors combine to cause narrowing of the airway lumen and obstruction.

Emphysema occurs when the walls of the alveoli are progressively destroyed. This decreases the surface area of the alveoli for oxygen exchange with the blood and causes the small airways to collapse during expiration, trapping air in the lungs. This may be caused by cigarette smoke or α₁ antitrypsin deficiency.

Clinical Correlation

Drugs Causing Respiratory Depression

Barbiturates, benzodiazepines, and opioids are all known to cause respiratory depression. Barbiturates and benzodiazepines act by facilitating the effects of γ-aminobutyric acid (GABA, the main inhibitory neurotransmitter in the central nervous system [CNS]) at the α subunit of the GABA$_A$ receptor. Opioids act at μ receptors throughout the body, the effects of which can be both excitatory and inhibitory. These drugs depress the response of the respiratory center in the medulla to hypercapnia (↑ CO_2) leading to respiratory depression.

Clinical Correlation

Atopy and Asthma

Atopy describes a hereditary predisposition for type I hypersensitivity reactions, which are mediated by immunoglobulin E (IgE). Atopic conditions include asthma, eczema, hay fever, and generalized allergies (e.g., to certain foods and dust). Gastroesophageal reflux disease (GERD) is also known to have a strong association with asthma, although the cause of this is unclear (see Chapter 27).

Clinical Correlation

Nonsteroidal Anti-inflammatory Drug-induced Bronchospasm

A significant proportion of adults with asthma experience bronchospasm after taking aspirin and other nonsteroidal anti-inflammatory drugs (NSAIDs). This can be serious and sometimes fatal. Aspirin and other NSAIDs are, therefore, contraindicated in patients with asthma who have a history of hypersensitivity reactions and should be used with caution in all asthmatics. Acetaminophen can be used by asthmatics to treat mild-to-moderate pain (see Chapter 33).

Clinical Correlation

Drug Delivery via an Endotracheal Tube

In an emergency situation, drugs are sometimes given via an endotracheal tube (e.g., epinephrine, naloxone, atropine, and lidocaine). They can exert local or systemic effects.

Notes

Alpha₁ Antitrypsin Deficiency

Alpha₁ antitrypsin is a glycoprotein protease inhibitor produced in the liver that plays a role in controlling inflammation and repairing tissues, as well as in blood coagulation. Deficiency of α₁ antitrypsin is a common inherited genetic disorder that causes uninhibited tissue breakdown by neutrophil elastase, mainly in the lungs (causing panacinar emphysema) and the liver.

VI

Clinical Correlation

Clinical Signs of Chronic Obstructive Pulmonary Disease

The clinical signs of COPD include observation that the patient is leaning forward with arms outstretched and palms on knees to assist breathing, pursed lips, use of accessory muscles of respiration (e.g., sternocleidomastoid, scalene, and intercostal muscles, which are not used during normal respiration), hyperinflation of the lungs, causing a barrel chest appearance, descended trachea, respiratory distress, crackles at the lung base, distant heart sounds, and wheezing. Cyanosis, hemoptysis (coughing up of blood), and finger clubbing (see below) are seen infrequently.

Clinical Correlation

Finger Clubbing

Finger clubbing is a clinical sign associated with numerous diseases and conditions, but it is most commonly associated with heart and lung diseases. It is characterized by softening of the nails and red, shiny skin next to the nail. This progresses to an increased convexity of the nail bed and a loss of the angle between the nail bed and the fold. The ends of the fingers also become larger. It has recently been found to be due to increased levels of prostaglandin E_2 (PGE_2) in the blood, which is a mediator of inflammation. The lung contains an enzyme that normally breaks this down, but in disease states where the lungs are compromised, it can build up, manifesting with finger clubbing.

Clinical Correlation

Pink Puffers and Blue Bloaters

Some patients with COPD increase their alveolar ventilation rate to try to cope with their shortness of breath. In this way, they manage to achieve a relatively normal O_2 level in the blood, and their carbon dioxide (CO_2) levels can be either normal or low. They are termed "pink puffers" because they are breathless and pink from the exertion. Other patients with COPD do not have the muscle or lung capacity to increase their ventilation rate. They have low blood O_2 levels and high CO_2 levels, and so appear blue. Right-sided heart failure may develop secondary to pulmonary hypertension (cor pulmonale), resulting in edema and "bloating." Oxygen should be used with caution in "blue bloaters." These patients rely on their hypoxic drive to breathe, as their respiratory centers have become used to the high level of CO_2 in the body. Oxygen therapy may remove this stimulus to breathe in these patients, causing hypoventilation or apnea. This resolves when oxygen therapy is ceased.

26.3 Treatment of Asthma and Chronic Obstructive Pulmonary Disease

Patients who experience intermittent asthma are typically treated with a short-acting β_2 receptor agonist (SABA) that is taken on an as-needed basis for the rapid relief of asthma symptoms. Patients with mild persistent asthma usually receive low-dose inhaled corticosteroids (ICS), with the dose being adjusted to the lowest level that maintains asthma control. Leukotriene modifiers or low-dose theophylline are alternatives. If asthma persists despite low-dose ICS, a long-acting β_2 receptor agonist (LABA) may be added or the dose of ICS increased, with ICS plus leukotriene modifier or theophylline as alternatives. Severe persistent asthma may require a higher dose of ICS along with a LABA, leukotriene modifier, or theophylline. Anticholinergics and anti-IgE therapies are reserved for patients who remain refractory to the above treatments (See ▶ Fig. 26.3).

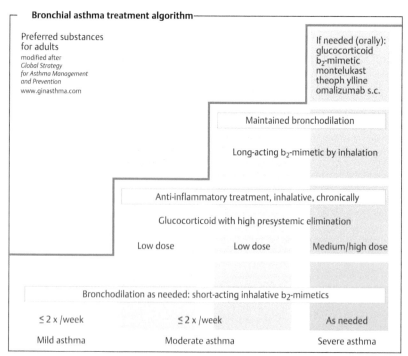

Bronchial asthma treatment algorithm

Preferred substances for adults
modified after
Global Strategy for Asthma Management and Prevention
www.ginasthma.com

If needed (orally):
glucocorticoid
b₂-mimetic
montelukast
theoph ylline
omalizumab s.c.

Maintained bronchodilation

Long-acting b₂-mimetic by inhalation

Anti-inflammatory treatment, inhalative, chronically

Glucocorticoid with high presystemic elimination

| Low dose | Low dose | Medium/high dose |

Bronchodilation as needed: short-acting inhalative b₂-mimetics

| ≤ 2 x /week | ≤ 2 x /week | As needed |
| Mild asthma | Moderate asthma | Severe asthma |

Fig. 26.3 Stepwise approach to asthma treatment.
Step 1. Medications of first choice for patients with mild intermittent asthma are inhaled short-acting β_2 receptor agonists taken on an as-needed basis for the rapid relief of asthma symptoms. Step 2. Patients with more frequent attacks receive low-dose inhaled corticosteroids with an inhaled short-acting β_2-receptor agonist available for the rapid relief of asthma symptoms. Step 3. If asthma persists despite low-dose ICS, a long-acting β_2 receptor agonist (LABA) is added. Step 4. Severe persistent asthma may require higher dose of ICS along with a LABA, leukotriene modifier, or theophylline. Anticholinergics and anti-immunoglobulin E therapies are reserved for patients who remain refractory to the above treatments.

Table 26.1 Summary of drugs used to treat asthma

	Drug class	Examples	Molecular target and effect
Bronchodilators (relievers)	β₂ agonists	*Short-acting:* albuterol, levalbuterol, metaproterenol, pirbuterol, and terbutaline *Long-acting:* salmeterol, formoterol, and vilanterol	Activate β₂ adrenergic receptors on airway smooth muscle to produce bronchodilation
	Anticholinergics	Tiotropium	Blocks muscarinic receptors on airway smooth muscle to prevent ACh-mediated bronchoconstriction
	PDE inhibitor	Theophylline	Inhibits the breakdown of cellular cAMP by PDE to produce bronchodilation
Anti-inflammatories (controllers)	Corticosteroids	Beclomethasone, budesonide, ciclesonide, fluticasone, flunisolide, mometasone, and triamcinolone	Anti-inflammatory effects are detailed in Chapter 16 (▶ Table 16.8, ▶ Fig. 16.10). These lead to decreased airway hyperreactivity and decreased mucus secretion
	Leukotriene modifiers	Montelukast Zafirlukast Zileuton	Montelukast and zafirlukast are leukotriene receptor antagonists and zileuton is a leukotriene synthesis inhibitor. These lead to decreased airway hyperreactivity and decreased mucus secretion (see ▶ Fig. 26.4)
	Anti-IgE antibody	Omalizumab	Blocks IgE binding to mast cells and basophils, inhibiting IgE-mediated release of mediators of the allergic response
	IL-5 antagonist antibodies	Mepolizumab Reslizumab	

Abbreviations: ACh, acetylcholine; cAMP, cyclic adenosine monophosphate; IgE, immunoglobulin E; IL-5, interleukin 5; PDE, phosphodiesterase.

For patients with COPD, occasional dyspnea can be treated with a short-acting bronchodilator while those with moderate or severe dyspnea can be treated with a long-acting bronchodilator drug. The main difference from asthma treatment is that in COPD either antimuscarinics or β₂ receptor agonists may be used. Patients whose symptoms are not adequately controlled by one drug may receive both an antimuscarinic and a β₂ receptor agonist. If symptoms still persist, an ICS may be added. Theophylline and roflumilast may be tried in refractory cases. All patients should undergo smoking cessation therapy and pulmonary rehabilitation. Oxygen therapy may improve quality of life of patients with hypoxemia (▶ Table 26.1).

26.3.1 Corticosteroids

Beclomethasone, Budesonide, Ciclesonide, Flunisolide, Fluticasone, Mometasone, and Triamcinolone

Mechanism of Action

These anti-inflammatory agents decrease bronchial hyperreactivity and the formation of mucus. They are the most effective antiasthmatic drugs available. They are less effective than bronchodilators for COPD and should not be used as monotherapy for COPD.

Pharmacokinetics

- These agents are inhaled through metered dose inhalers or dry powder inhalers. In severe persistent asthma, they may be given orally. In asthma emergencies (status asthmaticus), they may be given intravenously (IV).
- They should be used at the lowest dose that provides adequate control of symptoms.

Uses

- Moderate-to-severe asthma.
- Corticosteroids are generally not used in COPD patients unless bronchodilation cannot be achieved with β₂-adrenergic receptor agonists and anticholinergic drugs.

Side Effects

- Throat irritation and dysphonia (speech impairment and hoarseness) may limit compliance.
- Oral candidiasis (thrush) is possible as a result of inhibition of normal host defenses. The chances of developing thrush may be reduced by using spacer devices with the inhaler, rinsing the mouth after use of the inhaler, and/or decreasing the steroid dosing frequency.
- Endocrine effects have rarely been reported, but the growth of children should be monitored to ensure there is no suppression of the hypothalamic–pituitary axis (see Chapter 16).
- High doses inhaled or long-term systemic corticosteroid therapy for refractory asthma can lead to a Cushing-like response (see Chapter 16).

26.3.2 Beta₂ Adrenergic Receptor Agonists

These agents are also discussed in Chapter 6.

Albuterol, Levalbuterol, Metaproterenol, Terbutaline, Arformoterol, Formoterol, and Salmeterol

- Short-acting: albuterol, levalbuterol, metaproterenol, terbutaline.
- Long-acting: arformoterol, formoterol, salmeterol.

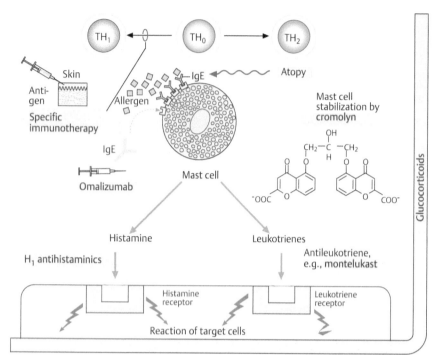

Fig. 26.4 Atopy and antiallergy therapy.
Atopy is thought to be linked to the differentiation of T-helper lymphocytes toward the TH$_2$ phenotype. Specific immunotherapy involves antigen injections that are intended to hyposensitize an individual by shifting T-helper cells toward TH$_1$. Monoclonal antibodies (e.g., omalizumab) inactivate immunoglobulin E and prevent it from binding to mast cells. Cromolyn prevents the release of inflammatory mediators from mast cells. H$_1$ antihistamines and antileukotrienes block their respective inflammatory mediator at receptors. Glucocorticoids have significant antiallergic activity and act at various stages of the allergic response.

Mechanism of Action

Beta$_2$ adrenergic receptor agonists relax bronchial smooth muscle, thereby reversing bronchoconstriction. They do not significantly decrease the bronchial hyperresponsiveness or the primary inflammatory reactions responsible for the persistence of asthma.

Pharmacokinetics

These agents are inhaled through metered dose inhalers or nebulizers.

Uses

- Short-acting agents act rapidly to provide symptomatic relief of acute asthma symptoms.
- Long-acting agents are used to treat asthma that is not well controlled by corticosteroids alone.
- These drugs form the cornerstone of bronchodilation therapy in COPD, often in combination with an anticholinergic drug.

Side Effects

Tremor, anxiety, and restlessness.

26.4 Anticholinergic Drugs

26.4.1 Ipratropium, Tiotropium, Aclidinium, Umeclidinium

Mechanism of Action

Anticholinergic drugs produce bronchodilation by blocking the bronchoconstrictive effects of acetylcholine released from parasympathetic neurons acting on muscarinic receptors on bronchial smooth muscle. They have the further advantage of reducing mucus production by inhibiting vagal stimulation of goblet cells.

Uses

These drugs have limited efficacy in asthma but are useful alone or as add-ons to β_2 agonists in moderate-to-severe COPD.

Side Effects

Dry mouth, blurred vision, tachycardia, urinary retention, and constipation.

26.4.2 Leukotriene Modifiers

Leukotrienes are potent bronchoconstrictors produced by cells involved in inflammatory responses, including mast cells and eosinophils (see Chapter 32).

Montelukast, Zafirlukast, and Zileuton

Mechanisms of Action

- Montelukast and zafirlukast are leukotriene receptor antagonists (▶ Fig. 26.4). They bind with high affinity to the cysteinyl leukotriene receptor 1 (Cys-LT$_1$) receptor, blocking the effects of the cysteinyl leukotrienes (LTC$_4$, LTD$_4$, and LTE$_4$).
- Zileuton is a leukotriene synthesis inhibitor. It inhibits the enzyme lipoxygenase and thus inhibits the formation of all lipoxygenase products, including the Cys-LTs and non-Cys-LTs (▶ Fig. 26.5).

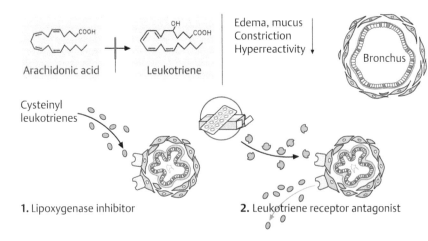

1. Lipoxygenase inhibitor   2. Leukotriene receptor antagonist

Fig. 26.5 Leukotriene antagonists.
Cysteine leukotriene synthesis can be blocked by inhibiting lipoxygenase, the enzyme responsible for converting arachidonic acid to leukotrienes. This can be achieved by drugs such as zileuton. Montelukast, on the other hand, blocks leukotriene receptors on target tissues.

VI

Clinical Correlation

Status Asthmaticus

Status asthmaticus is an acute, severe exacerbation of asthma characterized by a severe limitation of airflow and increased work of breathing, along with variable degrees of hypoxia (low tissue O_2). Treatment includes oxygen therapy, IV fluids for hydration and to thin mucus secretions, nebulized albuterol and ipratropium, and parenteral corticosteroids. Treatment may also include intramuscular or subcutaneous epinephrine (never IV) to induce rapid bronchodilation.

Clinical Correlation

Respiration and Acid–Base Balance

The lungs, along with the kidneys, regulate acid–base balance. They do this by modulating the CO_2 concentration in the blood. A respiratory alkalosis occurs as a result of hyperventilation: CO_2 levels are reduced (as the patient is breathing out more CO_2), and pH is increased. Causes of this include stroke, meningitis, COPD ("pink puffers"), anxiety, and hyperthyroidism. A respiratory acidosis ($\uparrow CO_2$; $\downarrow$ pH) is caused when CO_2 becomes trapped in the body due to a failure of respiration, which can be neuromuscular, physical, or respiratory (e.g., emphysema) in origin.

Pharmacokinetics

These drugs are administered orally and are well absorbed.

Uses

- Prophylaxis of asthma.
- Allergic rhinitis (see below).

Side Effects

Some patients experience headache with these drugs; otherwise, they are well tolerated.

26.5 Mast Cell Stabilizers

26.5.1 Cromolyn Sodium

Mechanism of Action

Cromolyn sodium inhibits mast cell degranulation and other allergy mediators by blocking Ca^{2+} channels in the cell membrane. This causes a reduction in bronchial hyperresponsiveness.

Uses

- Prophylaxis of asthma. It is not a bronchodilator and is of no use in acute asthma. It is not as effective as corticosteroids, but it has an excellent safety profile.
- Allergic rhinitis.

Side Effects

The side effects associated with cromolyn sodium are minimal.

26.6 Methylxanthines

26.6.1 Theophylline

Mechanism of Action

Theophylline has several molecular actions, although it is not clear which is responsible for the therapeutic effect in asthma. Classically, theophylline was categorized as a phosphodiesterase inhibitor. It has also been shown to have activity as a prostaglandin antagonist, an inhibitor of Ca^{2+} transport, a stimulator of endogenous catecholamine release, a β agonist, and an adenosine antagonist. All of these could contribute to its ability to relax the bronchial smooth muscle.

Pharmacokinetics

- Prolonged-release oral formulations are most commonly used.
- Monitoring of serum levels is essential because of large interindividual variability.

Uses

Theophylline is used infrequently in the maintenance therapy of moderate-to-severe asthma. May be used in COPD if other bronchodilators are ineffective, unavailable, or unaffordable.

Side Effects

- Life-threatening toxicity (seizures and cardiac arrhythmias) can occur at high doses without warning signs.
- Nausea, cramps, insomnia, and headache are common with loading doses.

26.7 Anti-immunoglobulin E Antibody

26.7.1 Omalizumab

Mechanism of Action

Omalizumab is a recombinant humanized monoclonal antibody directed against IgE that binds free IgE. This prevents IgE from binding to mast cells and basophils, thereby inhibiting IgE-dependent hypersensitivity reactions to allergens.

Pharmacokinetics

Given by subcutaneous injection, every 2 to 4 weeks.

Notes

Pulmonary Surfactant

Pulmonary surfactants are lipoproteins produced by alveolar cells (type II pneumocytes), starting at around 24 to 28 weeks gestation. By week 35, most babies have developed an adequate amount. Surfactant acts to reduce the surface tension of the lung, thus increasing compliance (the ability of the lungs to stretch when pressure is applied) and preventing atelectasis (collapsing of the lung) at the end of expiration. Premature neonates born before lung maturation can be given steroids to promote type II pneumocyte differentiation and the production of surfactant.

Clinical Correlation

Test for Fetal Lung Maturity

Fetal lung maturity can be tested by extracting a sample of amniotic fluid and measuring the lecithin:sphingomyelin ratio (L:S ratio). An L:S ratio less than 2:1 indicates surfactant deficiency and therefore lung immaturity.

Uses

Omalizumab is generally reserved for use in patients with severe, persistent, IgE-mediated allergic asthma that is inadequately controlled with the other medications discussed above.

It has also been proposed for use in other type I allergic reactions.

26.7.2 Roflumilast

Mechanism of Action

Roflumilast is a selective inhibitor of phosphodiesterase-4. It is not a bronchodilator but acts by reducing inflammation.

Pharmacokinetics

- Taken orally once per day.

Uses

Roflumilast is used to reduce exacerbations in patients with severe COPD, chronic bronchitis, and a history of exacerbations.

Side Effects

- Psychiatric reactions including insomnia, anxiety, depression, and suicidal ideation.
- Weight loss.

Contraindication

Decreased liver function.

26.7.3 Azithromycin

Mechanism of Action

Azithromycin is a macrolide antibiotic (see Chapter 29).

Pharmacokinetics

- Effective orally.

Uses

Azithromycin is approved for use in acute infective exacerbations of mild-to-moderate COPD. Off-label daily use has been shown to reduce the risk of COPD exacerbations, but resistance develops rapidly to macrolide antibiotics (see Chapter 29).

26.8 Alpha$_1$ Proteinase Inhibitors

26.8.1 Prolastin^{TM}, Zemaira^{TM}, and Aralast^{TM}

Note: There are no generic names for this type of drug.

Mechanism of Action

These agents are α_1 antitrypsin products that are derived from the plasma of blood donors.

Pharmacokinetics

- Given IV on a weekly basis.

Uses

- Indicated for patients with panacinar emphysema who have α_1 antitrypsin deficiency.

26.9 Neonatal Respiratory Distress Syndrome

Neonatal respiratory distress syndrome (NRDS) is a hyaline membrane disease often seen in premature infants that is caused by a deficiency in pulmonary surfactant.

26.9.1 Beractant, Calfactant, Lucinactant, and Poractant Alfa

Mechanism of Action

Beractant is a modified bovine lung extract (a natural surfactant). Calfactant is a bovine calf lung extract. Poractant is a purified porcine lung extract. Lucinactant is a synthetic surfactant.

Pharmacokinetics

These agents are given by tracheal instillation.

Uses

Used for prevention or treatment of neonatal respiratory distress syndrome.

26.10 Treatment of Rhinitis

Rhinitis is inflammation of the mucous membranes of the nasal cavity. Characteristic symptoms include sneezing, watery rhinorrhea, itching of the nose, eyes, ears, and throat, red and watering eyes, and nasal congestion. It can be caused by infection (usually viral) or allergy (▶ Fig. 26.6).

26.10.1 Decongestants

Phenylephrine, Oxymetazoline, Naphazoline, Pseudoephedrine, and Phenylephrine

- Intranasal decongestants: phenylephrine, oxymetazoline, naphazoline.
- Oral decongestants: pseudoephedrine, phenylephrine.

Mechanism of Action

Decongestants are sympathomimetics that decrease nasal blood flow by activating α_1 adrenergic receptors (▶ Fig. 26.7).

Pharmacokinetics

Intranasal agents have a more rapid onset of action and produce fewer systemic effects than oral agents, but oral agents have a longer duration of action.

Uses

Symptomatic treatment of rhinitis.

Side Effects

- Oral decongestants can cause systemic effects, such as CNS stimulation, tachycardia, hypertension, and urinary retention.
- Rebound nasal congestion may occur upon withdrawal of the drug if used for more than 5 days. This is more common with intranasal agents.

Contraindications

Hypertension, coronary artery disease, or in patients on monoamine oxidase inhibitors (MAOIs) (see Chapter 10).

26.11 H₁ Antihistamines

Note: Only H_1 antihistamine agents that are used for allergic rhinitis are discussed here. See Chapter 32 for a full discussion of histamines and antihistamines.

26.11.1 Azelastine, Cetirizine, Fexofenadine, Loratadine, and Olopatadine

- These are second-generation H_1 antihistamines.
- Related compounds include desloratadine, the active metabolite of loratadine, and levocetirizine, the active *R*-enantiomer of cetirizine.

Mechanism of Action

H_1 antihistamines block H_1 receptors and prevent histamine-induced reactions (e.g., increased vascular permeability,

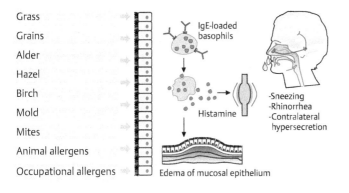

Grass
Grains
Alder
Hazel
Birch
Mold
Mites
Animal allergens
Occupational allergens

IgE-loaded basophils

Histamine

-Sneezing
-Rhinorrhea
-Contralateral hypersecretion

Edema of mucosal epithelium

Nasal allergen exposure

Prick test

Fig. 26.6 Allergic rhinitis.
Allergic rhinitis is triggered by the contact of an allergen with immunoglobulin E (IgE)-bearing mast cells in the nasal mucosa. The fact that mast cells have IgE attached suggests prior sensitization to the allergen. The mast cells release their mediators, causing sneezing, rhinorrhea, and contralateral hypersecretion in the unexposed nostril (due to a central reflex). The offending allergen can be identified by nasal allergen exposure or by a prick test.

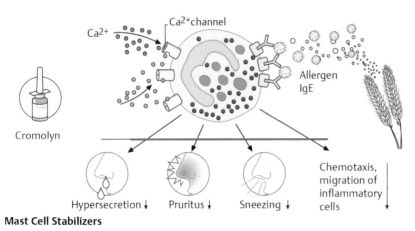

Fig. 26.7 Medications used in rhinitis.
Cromolyn inhibits mast cell degranulation of histamine and other allergy mediators by blocking Ca^{2+} channels in the cell membrane. α sympathomimetics are given by nasal spray or drops to reduce nasal swelling and congestion.

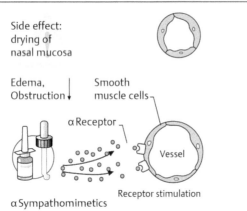

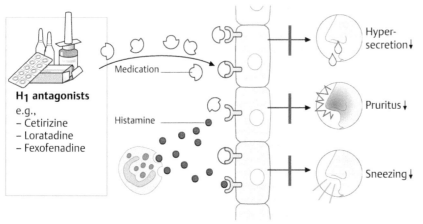

Fig. 26.8 Antihistamines for allergic rhinitis.
Antihistamines competitively inhibit histamine at its receptors. The newer second- and third-generation H_1 antihistamines (shown) are more effective and less sedative than older agents. They reduce hypersecretion, pruritus, and sneezing in patients with allergic rhinitis, allergic conjunctivitis, and urticaria (hives), but they do not have any effect on mucosal swelling.

smooth muscle contraction, mucus production, and pruritus [itching]). They also inhibit the "wheal and fare" response of the skin (▶ Fig. 26.8).

Pharmacokinetics

- Usually given orally but may be given topically into eye or nose (azelastine and olopatadine).
- These agents do not enter the brain as readily as first-generation H_1 antihistamines and so produce little, if any, sedation.

Uses

- First-line treatment for mild-to-moderate allergic rhinitis. In moderate-to-severe cases, intranasal corticosteroids are more effective than H_1 antihistamines.
- Also used for other allergic reactions, for example, urticaria.

Side Effects

- Mild sedation can occur with cetirizine at recommended doses and with loratadine in higher-than-recommended doses.

- Gastric effects: loss of appetite, constipation or diarrhea, nausea, and vomiting.

26.11.2 Mast Cell Stabilizer

Cromolyn Sodium

This drug, discussed in detail in 26.5.1 above, can be administered intranasally 3–4 times a day for the symptomatic treatment of allergic rhinitis (▶ Fig. 26.7).

26.11.3 Leukotriene Inhibitor

Montelukast

The leukotriene receptor antagonist montelukast (see above) is also approved for use in allergic rhinitis.

26.11.4 Intranasal Steroids

Beclomethasone, Budesonide, Ciclesonide, Flunisolide, Fluticasone, Mometasone, and Triamcinolone

These agents (see 26.3.1 and Chapter 16) are administered intranasally to provide a topical reduction of inflammation in allergic rhinitis. This method of delivery reduces the adverse effects associated with systemically administered corticosteroids (see Chapter 16).

26.12 Treatment of Cough

Antitussive medication, such as opiates, the opiate analogue dextromethorphan, antihistamines, and decongestants, may have beneficial effects in patients with an acute cough, depending on the cause. Persistent or chronic cough lasting more than 1 week may indicate an underlying infection (pertussis [whooping cough] or tuberculosis), a drug reaction (angiotensin-converting enzyme [ACE] inhibitors), another disorder (chronic bronchitis), or an environmental cause (smoke or occupational exposure).

The use and effectiveness of cough suppressants and over-the-counter cold medicines are controversial, especially in patients younger than 15 years. The risks of drug overdose, morbidity, and mortality may outweigh the benefits.

26.12.1 Opiates

Codeine and Dextromethorphan

- Codeine is available in some over-the-counter cold remedies.
- Dextromethorphan is an opiate analogue that is not analgesic or addictive; however, it is an antitussive (see Chapter 13).

Mechanism of Action

All opiates have central antitussive activity by acting on the cough center in the medulla to elevate the cough threshold.

26.12.2 Antihistamines and Decongestants

Diphenhydramine, Chlorpheniramine, Pseudoephedrine, and Phenylephrine

- First-generation antihistamines: diphenhydramine and chlorpheniramine.
- Decongestants: pseudoephedrine and phenylephrine.

Mechanism of Action

First-generation antihistamines possess anticholinergic drying activity and are used in combination with decongestants to decrease cough by decreasing postnasal drip, which stimulates the cough reflex.

Clinical Correlation

Cystic Fibrosis

Cystic fibrosis is an autosomal recessive disease in which there is a defect in the epithelial transport protein cystic fibrosis transmembrane conduction regulator (CFTR) found in the lungs, pancreas, liver, genital tract, intestines, nasal mucosa, and sweat glands. This alters Cl^- transport in and out of cells and inhibits some Na^+ channels. In the lungs, Na^+ and water are absorbed from secretions that then become thick and sticky. In the pancreas, secretions are thick and sticky because duct cells cannot secrete Cl^- via the CFTR and water normally follows this ion movement. Sweat is salty because Cl^- is not being absorbed via the CFTR and so Na^+ also remains in the duct lumen. Symptoms include cough, wheezing, repeated lung and sinus infections, salty taste to the skin, steatorrhea (foul-smelling, greasy stools), poor weight gain and growth, meconium ileus (in newborns), and infertility in men. Complications of this disease include bronchiectasis (abnormal dilation of the large airways), deficiency of fat-soluble vitamins (A, D, E, K), diabetes, cirrhosis, gallstones, rectal prolapse, pancreatitis, osteoporosis, pneumothorax, cor pulmonale, and respiratory failure. Treatment involves daily physical therapy to help expectorate secretions from the lungs, antibiotics to treat lung infections, mucolytics, and bronchodilators.

26.13 Treatment of Excess Mucus Production

26.13.1 Expectorants

Expectorants facilitate the removal of fluids from the lungs.

Guaifenesin

Mechanism of Action

Guaifenesin increases the volume and reduces the viscosity of bronchial secretions. This may make it easier for coughing to remove the secretions, but the effectiveness to reduce cough is questionable.

VI

Pharmacokinetics

- Given orally.

Uses

Although guaifenesin is found in over-the-counter medicines, its effectiveness in cough and colds is controversial. Its only approved use is to loosen phlegm in patients forming an abnormal amount of sputum (chronic bronchitis), but this usage is also of questionable efficacy.

26.13.2 Mucolytic Drugs

Mucolytic drugs decrease the viscosity of mucus.

Acetylcysteine

Mechanism of Action

Acetylcysteine has a free sulfhydryl group that opens the disulfide bonds in mucoproteins and lowers mucus viscosity.

Pharmacokinetics

- Given by inhalation or taken orally.

Uses

- Acetylcysteine is used to decrease mucus viscosity in acute and chronic bronchopulmonary diseases, during surgery, in cystic fibrosis, and in diagnostic bronchial procedures.
- Acetylcysteine is also given orally to treat acetaminophen overdose (see Chapter 33).

27 Drugs Acting on the Gastrointestinal System

Summary

These drugs are used to treat gastric acidity, peptic ulcers, gastroesophageal reflux disease (GERD), bowel motility disorders, nausea, vomiting, and appetite disorders. Proton pump inhibitors (omeprazole, esomeprazole, lansoprazole, pantoprazole, and rabeprazole) are used to treat peptic ulcers and GERD. Gastric antacids (calcium carbonate, magnesium hydroxide, aluminum hydroxide, and sodium bicarbonate) partially neutralize gastric acid, thus protecting the stomach mucosa. H_2 receptor antagonists (cimetidine, ranitidine, famotidine, and nizatidine) inhibit gastric acid secretion. Sucralfate and misoprostol are mucosal protective agents that accelerate the healing of duodenal ulcers. Antiemetic drugs include NK_1 receptor antagonists (aprepitant, netupitant, and rolapitant), dronabinol, scopolamine, and $5-HT_3$ receptor antagonists (ondansetron, granisetron, dolasetron, and palonosetron). Prokinetic drugs include metoclopramide and domperidone. Laxatives and cathartics include magnesium hydroxide, sodium phosphate, polyethylene glycol, docusate, castor oil, bisacodyl, cascara, aloe, senna, mineral oil, bran, methylcellulose, sodium carboxymethylcellulose, psyllium, lubiprostone, and linaclotide. Antidiarrheals include bismuth subsalicylate, kaolin, pectin, paregoric, diphenoxylate, and loperamide. Drugs used in inflammatory bowel disease include aminosalicylates (mesalamine, balsalazide, olsalazine, and sulfasalazine), tumor necrosis factor-α inhibitors (adalimumab, certolizumab pegol, golimumab, and infliximab), an integrin inhibitor (natalizumab), corticosteroids, immunosuppressants (cyclosporine), and antimetabolites (methotrexate, azathioprine, and mercaptopurine). Irritable bowel syndrome is treated with either antidiarrheals or laxatives. Central nervous system-acting appetite suppressants include amphetamine and its derivatives, phentermine and topiramate in combination, and lorcaserin. Orlistat is a peripherally acting weight-loss medication. Appetite enhancers include megestrol and dronabinol.

Keywords: GERD, antacids, gallstones, antiemetics, laxatives, diarrhea

27.1 Introduction to Drugs Acting on the Gastrointestinal System

The gastrointestinal (GI) tract includes the mouth, stomach, small intestine (duodenum, jejunum, and ileum), large intestine (cecum and colon), rectum, anus, and its accompanying exocrine glands (the salivary glands, the pancreas, and the gallbladder).

Drugs affecting the GI system are used in the treatment of gastric acidity, peptic ulcers, gastroesophageal reflux disease (GERD), bowel motility disorders (gastroparesis [delayed gastric emptying due to partial paralysis of the stomach muscles], constipation, and diarrhea), and for the treatment of nausea and vomiting.

27.2 Proton Pump Inhibitors

27.2.1 Omeprazole, Esomeprazole, Lansoprazole, Pantoprazole, and Rabeprazole

Mechanism of Action

Proton pump inhibitors inhibit the proton ($H^+–K^+–ATPase$) pump of the parietal cells in the stomach, thus inhibiting gastric acid (HCl) secretion into the lumen of the stomach (▶ Fig. 27.1).

Foundations

$H^+–K^+–ATPase$ (the Proton) Pump

$H^+–K^+–ATPase$ is an integral transmembrane protein that is present in gastric parietal cells. It functions to actively transport H^+ into the lumen of the stomach against its electrochemical gradient in exchange for K^+ (one H^+ is exchanged for one K^+). The energy required to drive this exchange is derived from the hydrolysis of adenosine triphosphate (ATP).

Foundations

Gastric Acid Production

Gastric acid is secreted from parietal cells when stimulated by the vagus nerve, histamine, and gastrin. CO_2 and H_2O react inside parietal cells, under the influence of carbonic anhydrase, to form bicarbonate (HCO_3^-) and H^+. H^+ is then pumped into the lumen of the stomach by $H^+–K^+–ATPase$. Cl^- is also secreted from parietal cells into the lumen by simple diffusion. H^+, Cl^-, and water combine in the lumen to form hydrochloric acid (HCl). The HCO_3^- produced is secreted into the bloodstream.

Clinical Correlation

Gastroesophageal Reflux Disease

GERD occurs when stomach acid continuously refluxes into the esophagus causing pain, heartburn, and inflammation because the esophagus lacks the protective lining of the stomach. The pain of GERD radiates to the back and is worsened by stooping and ingesting hot drinks. GERD is exacerbated by increased intra-abdominal pressure (obesity, big meals, and tight clothing), reduced lower esophageal sphincter (LES) tone (pregnancy, hiatus hernia, achalasia, fatty meals and smoking, and tricyclic and anticholinergic drugs). Treatment is with antacids (e.g., calcium carbonate), H_2 receptor antagonists (e.g., cimetidine), or proton pump inhibitors (e.g., omeprazole). Medication to strengthen the LES, known as prokinetic drugs (e.g., metoclopramide), may also be used. If medications alone do not control symptoms, surgery to tighten the LES may be necessary.

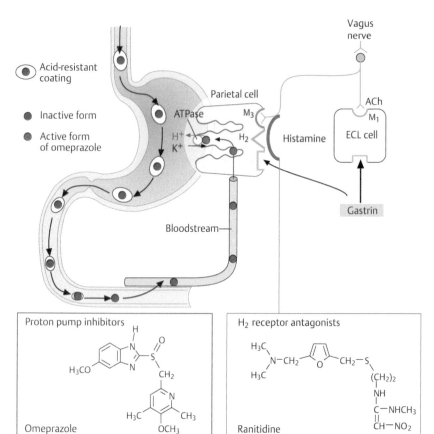

Fig. 27.1 Drugs used to lower gastric acid production.
Proton pump inhibitors block the H^+–K^+–ATPase pump on gastric parietal cells. H_2 receptor antagonists act to block histamine receptors on parietal cells. Both omeprazole and ranitidine ultimately lower gastric acid production. ACh, acetylcholine; ECL, enterochromaffin-like cell.

Foundations

Gastric pH and Mucosal Protection

Normal gastric pH is 2.0 to 3.0. Gastric mucosa is protected from this acidic environment by several mechanisms: the secretion of mucus provides a barrier between gastric acid and stomach mucosa; HCO_3^- ions secreted from the epithelium of the stomach neutralize H^+ ions; the epithelium itself is largely impenetrable to H^+ ions; and a rich mucosal blood supply ensures that if H^+ ions do penetrate the epithelium, then they are rapidly removed.

Uses

- Peptic ulcers.
- GERD.

Side Effects

There are minimal side effects. GI pain and diarrhea are the most common.

27.3 Gastric Antacids

27.3.1 Mechanism of Action

Gastric antacids (▶ Fig. 27.2) partially neutralize gastric acid and inhibit pepsin (a proteolytic enzyme) activity both directly and by increasing pH, thus protecting the stomach mucosa.

These agents must be taken frequently to maintain increased pH in the stomach.
- *Nonsystemic antacids* are compounds that are not absorbed into the systemic circulation. Their anionic group neutralizes the H^+ ions in gastric acid. This releases their cationic group which combines with HCO_3^- from the pancreas to form an insoluble basic compound that is excreted in feces. Thus these agents do not produce metabolic alkalosis.
- *Systemic antacids* are absorbed into the systemic circulation. They have a cationic group that does not form insoluble basic compounds with HCO_3^-. Thus the HCO_3^- can be absorbed producing a metabolic alkalosis.

Uses

- Peptic ulcers.
- Acid indigestion.
- Hyperchlorhydria (excess HCl in the stomach).

27.3.2 Nonsystemic Antacids

Calcium Carbonate

Side Effects

- Ca^{2+} salts have an unpleasant chalky taste and they precipitate in the GI tract to cause constipation. Rapid neutralization of gastric acid can also cause belching (CO_2 gas forms).
- Hypercalcemia can occur with chronic usage if large amounts of milk and dairy products are ingested ("milk-alkali syndrome").
- May cause a rebound acid secretion.

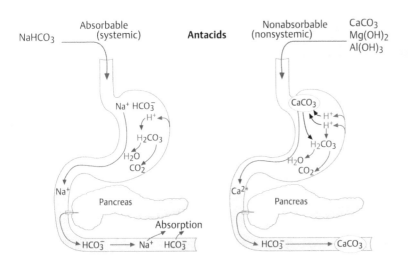

Fig. 27.2 Drugs used to neutralize gastric acid. Antacids have an anionic group that combines with H^+ in gastric acid, neutralizing it. The anion that is released in this reaction either remains in solution and is absorbed in the duodenum with HCO_3^- (from the pancreas) or it combines with HCO_3^- to form an insoluble precipitate that is excreted in feces.

Magnesium Hydroxide (Milk of Magnesia)

Effects

- Mg^{2+} salts act as both antacids and laxative agents.
- The laxative effect is lessened by concomitant use with calcium carbonate or aluminum hydroxide, both of which tend to produce constipation.

Side Effects

Some absorption and retention of Mg^{2+} (if renal function is impaired) could produce neurologic or cardiovascular toxicity.

Aluminum Hydroxide

Mechanism of Action

Aluminum salts remain in the stomach for long periods and slowly react with stomach acid to form aluminum chloride. Aluminum hydroxide may inhibit the action of pepsin and stimulate stomach mucus secretion.

Side Effects

- Constipation.
- Osteomalacia (by interfering with PO_4^{3-} absorption).
- Decreased absorption of some drugs (e.g., tetracyclines and other antibiotics).

Note: Because some antacids have constipating effects and others laxative effects, a mixture of these salts are combined in over-the-counter and prescription preparations to negate and, thus, avoid these unwanted effects.

27.3.3 Systemic Antacid

Sodium Bicarbonate

Side Effects

Sodium bicarbonate ($NaHCO_3$) is a highly soluble agent that rapidly neutralizes acid, producing lots of CO_2 and causing episodes of belching. Severe distention of the stomach by CO_2 gas may be dangerous if a gastric ulcer that could perforate is present.

27.4 Histamine (H_2) Receptor Antagonists

See Chapter 32 for a full discussion of histamine and antihistamines.

27.4.1 Cimetidine, Ranitidine, Famotidine, and Nizatidine

Mechanism of Action

H_2 receptor antagonists act specifically to competitively block the H_2 histamine receptors of parietal cells (▶ Fig. 27.1). They inhibit both basal and stimulated gastric acid secretion.

Pharmacokinetics

These drugs have a more rapid onset of action than the proton pump inhibitors and can be used for acute relief of symptoms.
- Ranitidine is several times more potent than cimetidine and thus requires less frequent dosing.
- Cimetidine inhibits cytochrome P-450 enzymes, possibly leading to drug interactions.

Uses

- Promotion of healing of peptic ulcers.
- Prophylaxis of recurrent peptic ulcers.
- GERD.

Side Effects

Headache, nausea, and skin rash.

Clinical Correlation

Peptic Ulcers

An ulcer is a lesion extending through the mucosa and submucosa into deeper structures of the wall of the GI tract. Ulcers are the result of breakdown of the mucosal barrier (mucus and HCO_3^-) that normally protects the lining of the GI tract and/or increased secretion of H^+ or pepsin. There are two types of peptic ulcers: gastric ulcers and duodenal ulcers. Gastric ulcers are commonly found on the lesser curvature between the corpus and antrum of the stomach. They are often caused by *Helicobacter pylori,* a gram-negative spiral bacillus that secretes cytotoxins that disrupt the mucosal barrier causing inflammation and destruction. High levels of membrane urease are secreted by *H. pylori*, which converts urea to NH_3. NH_3 neutralizes gastric acid around the bacterium, allowing it to survive in the acidic lumen of the stomach. Duodenal ulcers are the most common ulcers and are often associated with increased gastric H^+ secretion (but not necessarily). Duodenal ulcers also frequently occur due to *H. pylori* that inhibits somatostatin secretion leading to increased gastric H^+ secretion. There is also decreased HCO_3^- secretion in the duodenum which impedes neutralization of the excess H^+ delivered from the stomach.

Clinical Correlation

Zollinger–Ellison Syndrome

Zollinger–Ellison syndrome is a condition caused by gastrin-secreting pancreatic adenomas that lead to multiple ulcers in the stomach and duodenum. These ulcers are frequently drug resistant and accompanied by diarrhea and steatorrhea (as well as all of the usual peptic ulcers' symptoms, such as burning abdominal discomfort, heartburn, nausea and vomiting, and weight loss). Tests for the condition will show raised serum gastrin and gastric acid levels. Treatment involves the use of proton pump inhibitors to heal the ulcers and surgical resection of the offending tumor if this is possible. If surgery is not an option or if full resection is not possible, then chemotherapy may be employed to slow tumor growth. The 5-year survival rate is low (20%) if the tumor metastasizes (usually to the liver).

Foundations

Exudates and Transudates

Exudates are fluids that accumulate in tissues as a result of vascular leakiness in inflammatory states (e.g., in ulcers). They are composed of water, plasma proteins, and blood cells. Transudates are fluid accumulations caused by changes in colloid oncotic pressure, not by inflammation. They have a low protein content. It is important to distinguish between exudates and transudates in conditions such as pleural effusion (fluid accumulation in the pleural space). Exudate fluid suggests a local cause (e.g., cancer or pneumonia), whereas transudate fluid suggests the involvement of systemic factors (e.g., liver failure or renal failure).

Clinical Correlation

Gastric Ulcer Formation with NSAIDs

Aspirin and other nonsteroidal anti-inflammatory drugs (NSAIDs) inhibit cyclooxygenase-1 (COX-1), an enzyme needed to produce prostaglandins which stimulate protective mucus formation in mucus neck cells in the epithelium of the stomach. They also decrease the formation of HCO_3^- in these cells. Diminished mucus and HCO_3^- production leaves the mucosa unprotected from the effects of gastric acid and more prone to gastric ulcer formation.

27.5 Mucosal Protective Agents

27.5.1 Sucralfate

Sucralfate is a complex of sulfated sucrose and polyaluminum hydroxide.

Mechanism of Action

Sucralfate is thought to accelerate the healing of duodenal ulcers by forming a protective barrier over the ulcer base. It forms an ulcer-adherent complex with the proteinaceous exudate at the ulcer site. It is also thought to protect ulcers from pepsin (▶ Fig. 27.3). Sucralfate is not absorbed and does not inhibit acid secretion or neutralize acid.

Pharmacokinetics

It may bind digoxin or tetracyclines, decreasing their absorption.

Uses

It is used to treat peptic ulcers.

Side Effects

Constipation may occur.

27.5.2 Misoprostol

Mechanism of Action

Misoprostol is a prostaglandin derivative that acts to promote protective mucus secretion from epithelial cells in the stomach and inhibit gastric acid secretion for gastric parietal cells (▶ Fig. 27.4).

Uses

It is used to treat peptic ulcers.

Side Effects

May cause diarrhea and abdominal cramping.

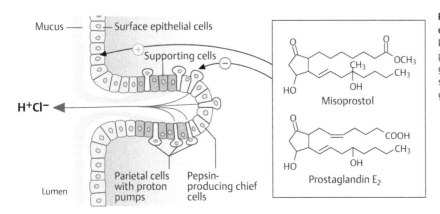

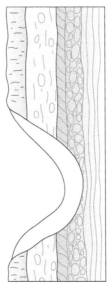

Fig. 27.3 Chemical structure and protective effect of sucralfate.
Sucralfate contains numerous aluminum hydroxide residues. When sucralfate is acted upon by gastric acid, it undergoes cross-linking and forms a paste that is able to adhere to the mucosal defect and exposed deeper layers. This coating of the ulcer protects it from acids and pepsin, allowing it to heal more rapidly.

Fig. 27.4 Chemical structure and protective effect of misoprostol.
Locally released prostaglandins promote mucus production from surface epithelial cells and inhibit gastric acid secretion from parietal cells in the stomach. Misoprostol is a semisynthetic prostaglandin derivative and mimics these effects.

27.5.3 Bismuth Subsalicylate

Bismuth subsalicylate ($C_7H_5BiO_4$) is found in over-the-counter preparations such as Pepto-Bismol which is a suspension of trivalent bismuth and salicylate in magnesium aluminum silicate clay.

Mechanism of Action

The mechanism of action is unclear.

Uses

- Heartburn.
- Diarrhea.
- It is included in combination drug regimens for *H. pylori*.

27.6 Drugs to Eradicate *H. pylori*

H. pylori is a gram-negative spiral bacillus that is found in the gastric epithelium of 70 to 90% of patients with peptic ulcers. It increases mucosal cell inflammation and destruction.

27.6.1 Treatment of *H. pylori*

Combination drug regimens are recommended for patients who test positive for *H. pylori*.
- Triple therapy: Bismuth plus metronidazole plus tetracycline, or H$_2$ antagonist plus metronidazole, or clarithromycin plus tetracycline, or proton pump inhibitor plus clarithromycin plus metronidazole, or amoxicillin for 2 weeks.
- Quadruple therapy: Proton pump inhibitor plus metronidazole plus bismuth plus tetracycline for 2 weeks.

27.7 Drugs to Dissolve Gallstones

27.7.1 Ursodiol

Ursodiol is a naturally occurring bile acid found in high amounts in bear bile and in small amounts in human bile.

Mechanism of Action

Ursodiol decreases secretion of cholesterol into bile by reducing cholesterol absorption and suppressing liver cholesterol synthesis. This alters bile composition and allows reabsorption of cholesterol-containing gallstones. Because reabsorption is slow, therapy must continue for at least 9 months.

Note: Ursodiol will not dissolve pigment stones or stones containing Ca^{2+}.

Clinical Correlation

Diagnosis of *H. pylori* Infection

H. pylori can be diagnosed by the carbon-13-urea breath test. This involves fasting for about 6 hours and then drinking a solution of ^{13}C-urea in water. Breath samples are then taken at intervals. If *H. pylori* is present, ^{13}C-urea is broken down to $^{13}CO_2$ by urease and will be measurable in the expired breath.

Clinical Correlation

Gallstones

The majority of gallstones (75%) are formed when the amount of cholesterol in bile exceeds the ability of bile salts and phospholipids to emulsify it, causing cholesterol to precipitate out of solution. Gallstones may also be caused by an increased amount of unconjugated bilirubin (often in the form of calcium bilirubinate) in the bile ("pigment stones"). Gallstones may be asymptomatic or they can cause obstruction of a duct causing severe pain, vomiting, and fever. Nondrug treatment includes lithotripsy (shock wave obliteration of gallstones that allow the stone fragments to be excreted) or surgical removal of the gallbladder (cholecystectomy).

Clinical Correlation

Chronic Pancreatitis

Chronic pancreatitis is ongoing inflammation of the pancreas. It is most commonly caused by alcohol abuse, but it may also occur with conditions such as gallstones, due to blockage of the pancreatic duct by the gallstone, or cystic fibrosis, due to blockage of the pancreatic duct by thick, viscous secretions. Typically, a patient with chronic pancreatitis falls ill for a prolonged period and has abdominal pain that radiates to the back, has diabetes mellitus, steatorrhea (increased fat content of stools), and weight loss. Treatment involves pancreatic enzyme replacements, lifestyle changes, and surgery if necessary.

Clinical Correlation

Steatorrhea

Steatorrhea is the production of feces that have a high content of fat. They are often oily and foul smelling, and they tend to float. Steatorrhea occurs when fat digestion or absorption is impaired. This can occur due to pancreatic disease (e.g., cystic fibrosis, chronic pancreatitis) where there is a deficiency of pancreatic lipase that would normally digest fats. It may also occur in conditions that cause hypersecretion of gastrin (e.g.,

Zollinger–Ellison syndrome) where gastrin increases H^+ secretion which lowers duodenal pH, inactivating pancreatic lipase. It may also occur due to liver disease which causes a deficiency of bile acids. Ileal resection will impair fat absorption due to impairment of bile recirculation to the liver. Treatment for steatorrhea due to pancreatic disease is pancreatic enzyme replacement (e.g., pancrelipase).

Pharmacokinetics

- Administered orally.
- It is conjugated in the liver to glycine or taurine and excreted in the bile. Conjugated ursodiol undergoes extensive enterohepatic recirculation and has a long serum half-life. Thus, with long-term daily administration, ursodiol will eventually comprise 30 to 50% of the circulating bile acid pool.

Uses

- Treatment of gallstones.
- It is also given prophylactically for the prevention of gallstones in obese patients undergoing rapid weight loss.

Side Effects

Side effects associated with ursodiol are rare.

Contraindications

Gallstones with a radiopaque component.

27.8 Pancreatic Enzyme Replacements

27.8.1 Pancrelipase

Pancrelipase is the first pancreatic enzyme preparation approved by the U.S. Food and Drug Administration (FDA).

Mechanism of Action

It is a combination of lipases, proteases, and amylases derived from porcine pancreas. It acts to replace the normal endogenous pancreatic enzymes.

Pharmacokinetics

- Enteric-coated microspheres in capsules withstand gastric acid and disintegrate at pH > 6.
- Administered with meals and snacks to treat malabsorption.

Uses

- Chronic pancreatitis.
- Cystic fibrosis (see Chapter 26).
- Steatorrhea.

27.9 Antiemetic Drugs

Nausea and vomiting (emesis) are mechanisms to remove toxic or noxious substances after ingestion. However, they also may occur in response to motion, pregnancy, or disease. Vomiting is controlled by the vomiting center in the medulla, which receives inputs from the nearby chemoreceptor trigger zone (CTZ), the vestibular apparatus of the inner ear, the cerebral cortex, and the GI tract. ▶ Table 27.1 summarizes the drugs that are most effective in treating different causes of nausea and vomiting and indicates their sites of action. Each class of drug includes a chapter reference to where these drugs are discussed in detail. The drugs that are not discussed in other sections are included below.

27.9.1 NK₁ Antagonists

Aprepitant, Netupitant, and Rolapitant

Mechanism of Action

NK_1 receptor antagonists block the actions of substance P at NK_1 receptors. The antiemetic action is mainly due to blockade of NK_1 receptors in the brain.

Pharmacokinetics

- Given orally.
- Extensively metabolized in the liver (via cytochrome P-450 3A4 [CYP3A4]).

Uses

Chemotherapy-induced nausea and vomiting.

Side Effects

- Constipation, diarrhea, and loss of appetite.
- Headache, hiccups, and fatigue.

Drug Interactions

Interactions may occur due to induction of cytochrome P-450 enzymes in the liver.

27.9.2 Cannabinoid Agonists

Dronabinol

This agent is a derivative of marijuana.

Mechanism of Action

Dronabinol acts on the vomiting center of the brain to prevent emesis, but the mechanism is unknown.

Pharmacokinetics

- Given orally.

Uses

Chemotherapy-induced emesis that is unresponsive to other drugs.

Side Effects

- Sympathomimetic activity that leads to heart palpitations and tachycardia.
- Marijuana-like central nervous system (CNS) effects, such as euphoria, somnolence, dizziness, and disturbances in thinking.
- Abdominal pain, nausea, and vomiting.
- Xerostomia (dry mouth) is very common.

27.9.3 Anticholinergic Drugs

Scopolamine

Mechanism of Action

Scopolamine is a competitive antagonist at muscarinic receptors.

Pharmacokinetics

It can be given via transdermal patch to reduce the side effects.

Table 27.1 Summary of drugs used to treat different causes of nausea and vomiting

Etiology of nausea or vomiting	Drug class	Examples	Site of action
Motion sickness (inner ear disease)	Antihistamine (Chapter 32)	Diphenhydramine, dimenhydrinate	Vestibular, GI
	Anticholinergic (Chapter 5)	Scopolamine	CTZ, vestibular, GI
Medication-, toxin-, or metabolic-induced vomiting	D₂ dopamine antagonist	Prochlorperazine, thiethylperazine	CTZ, GI
Chemotherapy- and radiation-induced vomiting Postoperative vomiting Pregnancy	5-HT₃ antagonist (Chapter 7)	Ondansetron, dolasetron, granisetron, palonosetron	CTZ, GI
Chemotherapy-induced nausea and vomiting	NK₁ antagonist	Aprepitant, netupitant, rolapitant	GI
Chronic idiopathic nausea Functional vomiting Cyclic vomiting syndrome	Tricyclic antidepressant (Chapter 10)	Amitriptyline, nortriptyline	Cortex
Chemotherapy-induced vomiting unresponsive to other drugs	Cannabinoid agonist	Dronabinol	Vomiting center

Abbreviations: CTZ, chemoreceptor trigger zone; GI, gastrointestinal.

VI

Uses

- Motion sickness.
- Inner ear disease (vertigo).

Side Effects

Side effects include dry mouth, blurred vision, urinary retention, palpitations, and headache.

27.9.4 Antihistamines

These agents are also discussed in Chapter 32.

Diphenhydramine and Dimenhydrinate

Mechanism of Action

These agents act in the vestibular apparatus of the inner ear and the GI tract to prevent emesis, probably via their anticholinergic actions.

> #### Clinical Correlation
>
> #### Vertigo
>
> Vertigo is the illusion of movement (e.g., that the room is spinning). It is most commonly caused by disorders of the inner ear, such as Meniere disease (a syndrome characterized by vertigo, tinnitus, and deafness), vestibular neuronitis, lesions involving cranial nerve VIII, head injury causing vestibular damage, benign postural vertigo (vertigo occurs when certain positions are adopted, or movements made), and by drugs (e.g., gentamicin, barbiturates, and alcohol). Other causes of vertigo are migraine, epilepsy, multiple sclerosis, and tumors. Treatment depends on the cause, but anticholinergic drugs and antihistamines are often used to prevent nausea and vomiting. Note that dizziness is a distinct entity from vertigo and is used to describe a feeling of lightheadedness or weakness.

> #### Foundations
>
> #### The Vomiting Reflex
>
> The vomiting reflex begins with a single retrograde peristaltic contraction beginning in the middle of the small intestine that propels intestinal contents through a relaxed gastroduodenal junction into the stomach. Inspiration occurs against a closed glottis, lowering intraesophageal pressure. The duodenum and antrum contract to prevent movement of chyme back into the small intestine. The abdominal muscles then forcibly contract (Valsalva maneuver), increasing intra-abdominal pressure which creates more pressure in the stomach than in the esophagus. This forces gastric contents into the esophagus. The larynx and hyoid bone are drawn forward, decreasing the tone of the upper esophageal sphincter (UES) leading to the gastric and esophageal contents being expelled via the oral cavity.

Uses

- Motion sickness.
- Inner ear disease (vertigo).

Side Effects

Sedation and the usual anticholinergic side effects (listed above for scopolamine).

27.9.5 Dopamine Antagonists

Prochlorperazine and Promethazine

Mechanism of Action

These agents prevent vomiting by blocking D_2 dopamine receptors in the medullary chemoreceptor trigger zone.

Uses

Medication-, toxin-, or metabolic-induced emesis.

Side Effects

Anticholinergic: orthostatic (postural) hypotension, dry mouth, constipation, and blurred vision.

Contraindications

Parkinson disease.

27.9.6 5-Hydroxytryptamine type 3 (5-HT$_3$) Receptor Antagonists

Ondansetron, Granisetron, Dolasetron, and Palonosetron

Mechanism of Action

These agents block 5-HT$_3$ receptors in the CNS and GI tract. Activation of these receptors normally triggers vomiting.

Uses

- Chemotherapy- and radiation-induced emesis.
- Postoperative emesis.
- Pregnancy.

Side Effects

Constipation, diarrhea, headache, and fatigue are the side effects.

27.9.7 Tricyclic Antidepressants

Amitriptyline and Nortriptyline

Mechanism of Action

These agents act in the cortex of the brain to inhibit the reuptake of norepinephrine and serotonin (see Chapter 10).

Uses

- Chronic idiopathic nausea.
- Functional vomiting.
- Cyclic vomiting syndrome.

27.10 Prokinetic (Gastric Motility Promoting) Drugs

Gastroparesis, also known as delayed gastric emptying, is a disorder in which the stomach takes too long to empty its contents. The most frequent cause is diabetes mellitus, but it can also be caused by smooth muscle or nervous system disorders or, in many cases, is idiopathic.

27.10.1 Metoclopramide and Domperidone

Mechanism of Action

Metoclopramide and domperidone (not approved in the United States) are D_2 dopamine receptor antagonists that increase release of acetylcholine from nerve endings in the GI tract, leading to increased GI motility and rate of gastric emptying. They also increase lower esophageal tone.

Uses

- Gastroparesis.
- Reflux esophagitis.
- Antiemetic.

Side Effects

- Metoclopramide may produce extrapyramidal side effects similar to those seen with typical antipsychotics, including parkinsonism, dystonia, and, with longer-term use, tardive dyskinesia (see Chapter 12). Domperidone does not readily cross the blood–brain barrier and does not produce these CNS effects.
- Sedation.
- Prolactin secretion is increased.

27.10.2 Erythromycin

See Chapter 29 for a full discussion of this agent.

Mechanism of Action

Erythromycin stimulates motilin receptors and increases GI motility. Motilin is an endogenous peptide that produces contraction of the upper GI tract via motilin receptors on smooth muscle cells and enteric neurons.

Side Effects

Nausea, vomiting, and abdominal cramps.

27.11 Laxative and Cathartic Drugs

Laxatives and cathartics are drugs that promote defecation. Laxatives promote the excretion of a soft, formed stool, and

Table 27.2 Uses and contraindications of laxatives and cathartics

Uses	Contraindications
Radiologic exams of gastrointestinal tract	Colic (attacks of severe abdominal pain), nausea, and cramps
Bowel surgery	Undiagnosed abdominal pain
Proctologic exam	Patients with symptoms of appendicitis
Useful in patients with a hernia or cardiovascular disease (to avoid straining at stool)	
Anorectal disorders (e.g., hemorrhoids)	
Useful after antihelmintic therapy or poisoning by drugs or foods	

cathartics promote fluid evacuation. The uses and contraindications for these laxatives and cathartics are included in ▶ Table 27.2.

Foundations

Peristaltic Reflex

Stretching of the intestinal wall during the passage of a bolus triggers a reflex that simultaneously contracts the circular muscles behind the bolus and relaxes the circular muscles in front of it. At the same time, longitudinal muscles behind the bolus are relaxed and in front of it are contracted. This propels the bolus in an aboral direction.

Foundations

Electrolytes

Electrolytes are ions that can conduct electricity when in solution (as acids or bases). The main body electrolytes are Na^+, K^+, Ca^{2+}, Mg^{2+}, Cl^-, HPO_4^{2-}, and HCO_3^-. Osmotic gradients exist across cell membranes in the body such that the movement of ions can regulate water balance, acid–base balance (blood pH), nerve conductance, and muscle contractility. Pharmacological causes of electrolyte disturbances include cathartics, thiazide diuretics, spironolactone, and alcohol abuse. Pathophysiological causes include renal disease and malignancy of endocrine glands.

27.11.1 Saline (Osmotic) Cathartics

Mechanism of Action

Saline cathartics act by causing water to be retained through an osmotic effect. Stretching of the bowel lumen by this increase in water stimulates peristalsis.

Magnesium Hydroxide, Sodium Phosphate, and Polyethylene Glycol

Pharmacokinetics

- Poorly and slowly absorbed from the GI tract.
- Water retention indirectly increases peristalsis, with watery evacuation occurring in < 3 hours.

VI

• Approximately 20% of magnesium is absorbed, but it is rapidly excreted if renal function is normal. Mg^{2+} intoxication can occur if renal function is impaired, resulting in weakness, nausea, vomiting, and respiratory depression.

Side Effects

• Electrolyte imbalance.
• Cerebral failure can occur with sodium phosphate.

Lactulose

Mechanism of Action

Intestinal bacteria hydrolyze the drug, which leads to more acidic pH of the colon. This reduces the ability of bacteria to form ammonia.

Pharmacokinetics

Given orally, but not absorbed.

Uses

Lactulose is a specialized laxative for chronic liver disease or hepatic coma to decrease plasma levels of ammonia.

27.11.2 Stool Softeners

Mechanism of Action

Stool softeners act by keeping feces soft so tenesmus (straining at stool) is avoided. There is no direct or reflex stimulation of peristalsis with these agents.

Docusate

Mechanism of Action

Docusate induces stool softening by lowering surface tension to promote water penetration into feces.

Pharmacokinetics

Effects are seen within 1 to 2 days.

Uses

The main use of this agent is to limit straining, as it has minimal laxative effects.

27.11.3 Contact (Stimulant-Irritant) Cathartics

Mechanism of Action

Contact cathartics increase intestinal motor activity (peristalsis) and stimulate water and electrolyte accumulation in the colon (▶ Fig. 27.5).

Castor Oil

Castor oil is derived from the seeds of *Ricinus communis*.

Pharmacokinetics

Pancreatic lipases hydrolyze castor oil to the active irritant agent ricinoleic acid that acts on the small intestine in 1 to 3 hours.

Side Effects

Castor oil has a disagreeable taste and should not be used just prior to bedtime.

Bisacodyl

Pharmacokinetics

Bisacodyl given orally acts in 6 to 8 hours; thus, it is often given at bedtime to produce effects by morning. Rectal suppositories are effective within 1 hour.

Anthraquinones: Cascara, Aloe, and Senna

Pharmacokinetics

They act on the large intestine in 6 to 8 hours.

Side Effects

Electrolyte imbalance from excessive catharsis.

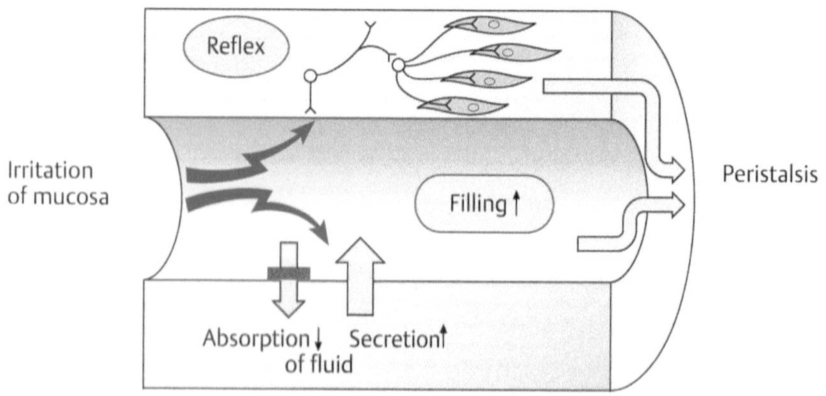

Fig. 27.5 Stimulation of peristalsis by mucosal irritation.
Irritant laxatives exert an irritant action on the intestinal mucosa. This causes less fluid to be absorbed than is secreted. This filling of the intestinal lumen stimulates reflex peristalsis. Peristalsis is also directly simulated by the irritant action.

27.11.4 Lubricant Laxatives

Mechanism of Action

Lubricant laxatives act by retarding reabsorption of water.

Mineral Oil

Mineral oil is a mixture of liquid hydrocarbons obtained from petroleum.

Side Effects

- Lipid pneumonia in elderly or debilitated patients if oil is aspirated.
- Foreign-body reactions in mesenteric lymph nodes, liver, spleen, and intestinal mucosa may occur.
- Absorption of essential fat-soluble substances (vitamins A, D, and K, and carotene) may be blocked.

Foundations

Effects of Fiber

In the stomach, fiber binds water which enlarges the particle size so that fiber passes the pyloric sphincter later, delaying gastric emptying. In the ileum and colon, in particular, the water-binding (swelling) capacity of fiber lowers transit time. Fiber may bind mineral and trace elements as well as fat-soluble vitamins thus not allowing them to be absorbed. The binding of steroids leads to an increased excretion of bile acids and cholesterol, which may be helpful in people with fat metabolism disorders. Glucose absorption is also delayed by high-fiber intake, improving glucose control in diabetics. Stool volume is increased and the consistency of stool is softer with fiber intake. However, intestinal bacteria ferment the polysaccharides in fiber-producing methane and CO_2. During fermentation, short-chain fatty acids are produced that positively affect the composition of the intestinal flora and the intestinal pH. Finally, the binding of ammonia by fiber increases fecal nitrogen excretion thereby unburdening the liver and kidneys.

27.11.5 Bulk-forming Laxatives

Mechanism of Action

Bulk-forming laxatives act by absorbing and retaining water, causing fecal material to become hydrated and soft. They may also act to reflexively stimulate peristalsis (▶ Fig. 27.6 and ▶ Fig. 27.7).

Bran (and Other Dietary Fiber), Methylcellulose, Sodium Carboxymethylcellulose, and Psyllium Preparations

These are naturally occurring or synthetic polysaccharides.

Pharmacokinetics

- Action is within 1 to 3 days.
- Some drug absorption may be reduced because of binding to these agents.

Side Effects

Intestinal obstruction has been reported.

27.11.6 Chloride Channel Activators

Mechanism of Action

Both of these drugs increase chloride, accompanying ions, and water in lumen of the small intestine to produce a laxative effect. Lubiprostone directly activates ClC-2 chloride channels in the small intestine. Linaclotide activates guanylate cyclase of intestinal epithelial cells which then activates cystic fibrosis transmembrane conductance regulator chloride channels.

Side Effects

- Minimal systemic absorption of these drugs leads to minimal systemic side effects.

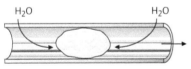
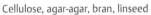

H₂O   H₂O

Cellulose, agar-agar, bran, linseed

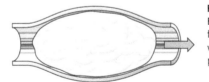

Fig. 27.6 Bulk laxatives.
Bulk laxatives are insoluble and nonabsorbable from the intestine. They absorb water and expand within the intestinal lumen; this stimulates peristalsis.

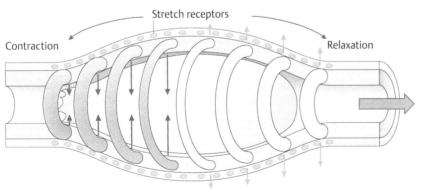

Stretch receptors

Contraction   Relaxation

Fig. 27.7 Stimulation of peristalsis by an intraluminal bolus.
Distention of the intestinal wall by fecal matter activates mechanoreceptors that induce a neuronally mediated ascending reflex contraction of intestinal smooth muscle (*red*) and a descending relaxation (*blue*). This propulsive movement of the intestinal musculature (peristalsis) allows fecal matter to move in the direction of the anus for evacuation.

VI

- GI side effects are the most common and include abdominal pain, flatulence, and excessive diarrhea.
- Despite the lack of systemic absorption, an increase in fetal deaths has been observed in animal studies with lubiprostone, so it is not recommended for use in pregnancy.

Uses

- Chronic constipation.
- Irritable bowel syndrome (IBS) with constipation.

27.12 Antidiarrheal Agents

Antidiarrheal therapy aims to prevent the dehydration and electrolyte imbalance that can quickly occur in severe diarrhea, as well as preventing excessive bowel movements.

Note: Antibacterial agents are useful only if bacteria are the cause of the diarrhea (which is uncommon). They cause depletion of the normal intestinal bacterial flora, which, in turn, may cause proliferation of pathogenic bacteria, leading to diarrhea.

27.12.1 Adsorbents

Bismuth Subsalicylate, Kaolin, and Pectin

- Bismuth subsalicylate.
- Kaolin (hydrated aluminum silicate).
- Pectin (a purified carbohydrate from acid extracts of apples or the rinds of citrus fruits).

Mechanism of Action

These agents absorb bacterial toxins and fluid in the gut.

Pharmacokinetics

- Bismuth subsalicylate is given as chewable tablets or in an aqueous suspension.
- Kaolin is often given in a mixture with pectin.

Uses

- Diarrhea and dysentery.

Side Effects

These drugs are not absorbed, so they do not have systemic side effects. Constipation may occur.

27.12.2 Opioids

See Chapter 13 for a full discussion of these drugs.

Mechanism of Action

These agents decrease propulsion and peristalsis. GI contents are delayed in passage, allowing time for feces to become desiccated. This further retards passage through the colon.
- Opioids are effective in acute diarrheal states, but they should not be used for enteric infections.

- Opium alkaloids are effective for controlling severe diarrhea or dysentery, but with chronic therapy, there is a risk of dependence.

Paregoric

Paregoric is a camphorated tincture of opium.

Uses

Used to treat infantile diarrhea.

Codeine and/or Morphine

These are purified opium alkaloids.

Pharmacokinetics

They exert a local action in the GI tract.

27.12.3 Diphenoxylate

Diphenoxylate is a congener of meperidine. It is often given in combination with atropine.

Side Effects

High or chronic doses lead to euphoria and physical dependence.

27.12.4 Loperamide

Loperamide is a derivative of haloperidol that resembles meperidine. This agent appears to be as effective as diphenoxylate, with few side effects reported.

Uses

- Prophylaxis and treatment of travelers' diarrhea.
- IBS.

Antidiarrheal agents and their site of action are summarized in ▶ Fig. 27.8.

27.13 Drugs Used in Inflammatory Bowel Disease

There are two types of inflammatory bowel disease (IBD): Crohn disease and ulcerative colitis (▶ Fig. 27.9). Crohn disease is a chronic inflammatory disease that can affect the entire GI tract but most commonly affects the terminal ileum and colon. It causes ulcers, fistulas (abnormal communications), and granulomata, producing symptoms such as fever, diarrhea, weight loss, and abdominal pain. Ulcerative colitis is a recurrent inflammatory disease of the colon and rectum that causes bloody diarrhea, weight loss, fever, and abdominal pain. The goal of therapy for IBDs is to reduce the inflammatory response by using drugs such as steroids and sulfasalazine.

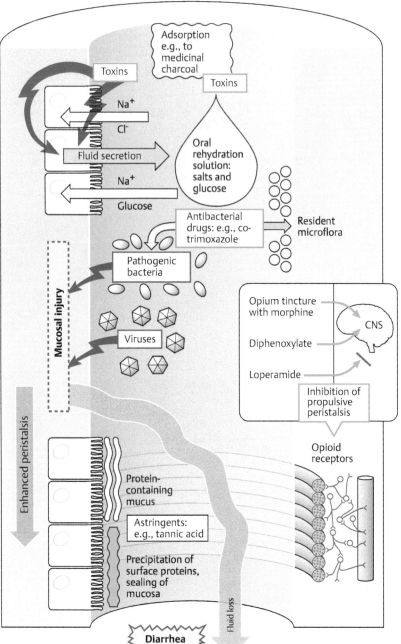

Fig. 27.8 Antidiarrheals and their site of action. Bacteria can secrete toxins that inhibit the ability of enterocytes to absorb sodium chloride (NaCl) and water. They also stimulate fluid secretion into the intestinal lumen. Bacteria and viruses also cause mucosal inflammation, which further causes luminal fluid loss. This increase in luminal fluid stimulates peristalsis. Adsorbents bind to toxins and promote their evacuation. As a consequence, more salt and water are able to be reabsorbed. Opioids activate enteric nerves, resulting in inhibition of propulsion and peristalsis. Loperamide is pumped back into the body by the endothelial cells of the blood–brain barrier, so it does not produce the unwanted central nervous system effects of morphine and diphenoxylate. Oral rehydration solutions contain glucose, which is absorbed into intestinal cells, drawing water along with it.

27.13.1 Aminosalicylates

Mesalamine, Balsalazide, Olsalazine, and Sulfasalazine

- Mesalamine is 5-aminosalicylic acid (5-ASA), the active moiety of all the aminosalicylates used to treat IBD.
- Balsalazide, olsalazine, and sulfasalazine are prodrugs that are metabolized to 5-ASA.

Mechanism of Action

5-ASA acts within the intestinal tract (mainly the terminal ileum and colon) to inhibit prostaglandin and leukotriene synthesis, thus reducing the inflammatory reaction (▶ Fig. 27.10 and ▶ Fig. 27.11).

Uses

For treatment of mild-to-moderate ulcerative colitis.

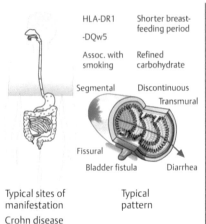
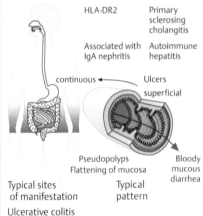

HLA-DR1 Shorter breast-feeding period

-DQw5

Assoc. with smoking / Refined carbohydrate

Segmental / Discontinuous

Transmural

Fissural

Bladder fistula / Diarrhea

Typical sites of manifestation

Typical pattern

Crohn disease

HLA-DR2 Primary sclerosing cholangitis

Associated with IgA nephritis / Autoimmune hepatitis

continuous / Ulcers / superficial

Pseudopolyps / Bloody mucous diarrhea
Flattening of mucosa

Typical sites of manifestation

Typical pattern

Ulcerative colitis

Fig. 27.9 Crohn's disease and ulcerative colitis.
The typical pattern of Crohn's disease is segmental inflammation that affects all layers of the intestinal wall, producing fistulae, abscesses, and perforation. Inflammatory conglomerate tumors develop in adjacent structures due to fistulae and abscess formation. Crohn's disease is associated with human leukocyte antigens DR1 and DQw5. Patients were often not breastfed for a long period as infants, and have a history of smoking and high intake of refined carbohydrates. In ulcerative colitis, there is relapsing and remitting inflammation of the colon, as well as superficial ulcerations that spread proximally. This leads to fattening of the intestinal mucosa and destruction of goblet cells. Hyperregeneration causes pseudopolyp production. Ulcerative colitis is thought to be autoimmune and is associated with immunoglobulin A nephritis and autoimmune hepatitis, among other conditions.

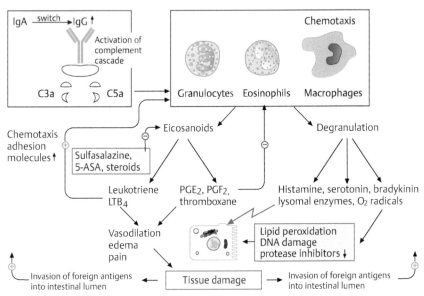

Fig. 27.10 Drug treatment of Crohn's disease and ulcerative colitis.
Acute attacks of Crohn's disease and ulcerative colitis are treated with sulfasalazine and 5-aminosalicylic acid (see also ▶ Fig. 27.11). Crohn's disease also may involve treatment with steroids. These drugs inhibit prostaglandin and leukotriene synthesis and intervene late in the inflammatory cascade.

Side Effects

- Nausea, vomiting, diarrhea, headache, and abdominal pain.
- Bone marrow suppression.

27.13.2 Tumor Necrosis Factor-α Inhibitors

Adalimumab, Certolizumab Pegol, Golimumab, and Infiximab

Mechanism of Action

These agents are monoclonal antibodies or antibody fragments that bind and neutralize tumor necrosis factor-α (TNF-α), a principal cytokine that mediates IBD.

Pharmacokinetics

These drugs must be given by injection.

Uses

- Moderate-to-severe Crohn's disease unresponsive to other therapies (adalimumab, certolizumab pegol, and infiximab).
- Moderate-to-severe ulcerative colitis not responsive to other drugs (adalimumab, golimumab, infiximab).

Side Effects

- Reactivation of tuberculosis.
- Increased respiratory infections.

27.13.3 Integrin Inhibitor

Natalizumab

Mechanism of Action

Monoclonal antibody to the α4-subunit of integrins on the surface of leukocytes, thus inhibiting leukocyte migration and activation in the GI tract.

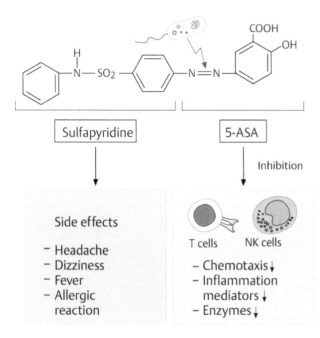

Fig. 27.11 Sulfasalazine.
Sulfasalazine is converted to its active forms sulfapyridine and 5-aminosalicylic acid by intestinal bacteria. These active forms inhibit the inflammatory reaction in intestinal mucosa.

Pharmacokinetics

Given by IV injection once every 4 weeks.

Uses

In select patients with moderate-to-severe Crohn's disease unresponsive to other therapies.

Side Effects

Progressive multifocal leukoencephalopathy (PML) due to reactivation of a human polyomavirus (JC virus), which is present in latent form in over 80% of adults.

Drug Interactions

Should not be used in combination with immunosuppressants or inhibitors of TNF-α.

27.13.4 Corticosteroids

These agents are also discussed in Chapters 16, 26, 32, and 34.

Prednisone and Budesonide

Uses

Corticosteroids are effective in both ulcerative colitis and Crohn's disease in inducing a remission in acute persistent disease. They are used systemically until adequate control of inflammation is achieved, then the dose is tapered and discontinued to avoid the side effects seen with long-term systemic steroid use (see Chapter 16).

▶ Fig. 27.12 provides a summary of the effects and side effects of corticosteroids.

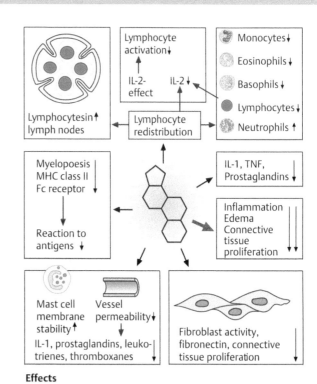

Side effects

Fig. 27.12 Corticosteroids: effects and side effects.
Corticosteroids act to decrease inflammation and reduce connective tissue proliferation by the mechanisms shown. Short-term side effects are edema and weight gain. Gastric ulceration, hypertension, steroid-induced diabetes mellitus, and increased susceptibility to infections may also occur. Longer-term use may lead to more serious side effects, such as Cushing syndrome, skin atrophy, osteoporosis, and seizures. IL-1, interleukin-1; IL-2, interleukin-2; MHC, major histocompatibility complex; TNF, tumor necrosis factor.

27.13.5 Immunosuppressants

These agents are also discussed in Chapter 34.

Cyclosporine

Mechanisms of Action

Cyclosporine decreases interleukin-2 (IL-2) synthesis in T helper cells.

Uses

This agent is sometimes used in patients unresponsive to steroids or in chronic cases of moderate-to-severe IBD, although it is not approved by the FDA for this purpose.

27.13.6 Antimetabolites

These agents are discussed further in Chapters 33 and 34.

Methotrexate, Azathioprine, and Mercaptopurine

Mechanisms of Action

- Methotrexate inhibits dihydrofolate reductase, which reduces purine and pyrimidine synthesis in lymphocytes and so dampens the immune response (▶ Fig. 27.13).
- Azathioprine is converted to 6-mercaptopurine. Mercaptopurine is a purine analogue that causes pseudofeedback inhibition of the first step in purine biosynthesis and inhibition of purine intraconversions.

Pharmacokinetics

The onset of action of these drugs takes several weeks.

Uses

Moderate-to-severe IBD (mainly Crohn's disease).

Side Effects

Bone marrow depression.

Clinical Correlation

Irritable Bowel Syndrome

IBS is a chronic idiopathic condition. Symptoms include abdominal pain, bloating, and cramps, which are associated with bowel habit alteration in the form of constipation or diarrhea. Treatment is guided by the symptoms and their severity. Mild IBS may respond to dietary changes. Drugs may be called in for patients with moderate-to-severe symptoms. Drugs used to treat IBS are shown in ▶ Table 27.3.

Note: IBS is not associated with pathophysiological changes in gut structure and is diagnosed only when all else has been excluded.

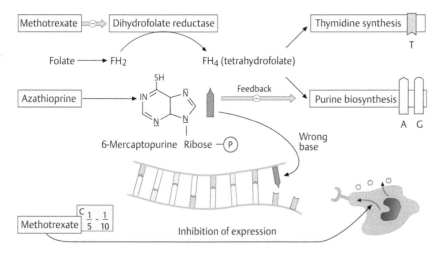

Fig. 27.13 Antimetabolites.
Methotrexate inhibits purine and thymidine synthesis. It does this by inhibiting the formation of tetrahydrofolate by binding to dihydrofolate reductase, the enzyme that catalyzes its formation from folate. Methotrexate also inhibits cell growth in rapidly proliferating tissues (e.g., bone marrow). Azathioprine is converted to 6-mercaptopurine, which is a false substrate for purine biosynthesis. It is also incorporated in DNA and RNA, where it acts as a "wrong" base and damages the cell.

Table 27.3 Drugs used to treat irritable bowel syndrome

IBS type	Drug	Drug class	Other
With diarrhea (IBS-D)	Rifaximin	Antibiotic	Not absorbed systemically
	Loperamide	Antidiarrheal	See text above
	Alosetron	5-HT$_3$ antagonist	Reserved for severe cases. May cause serious constipation complications
	Dicyclomine	Anticholinergic	Anticholinergic side effects including nausea, dry mouth, blurred vision, dizziness
With constipation (IBS-C)	Psyllium	Bulk-forming laxative	See text above
	Polyethylene glycol	Osmotic cathartic	See text above
	Lubiprostone	Chloride channel activator	See text above
	Linaclotide	Chloride channel activator	See text above

27.14 Drugs Used in Irritable Bowel Syndrome

See Clinical Box and ▶ Table 27.3.

27.15 Appetite-suppressing and Appetite-enhancing Drugs

Finding safe and effective pharmacotherapies for obesity has been elusive, for several reasons. For many agents, weight loss returns when the drug is stopped. Some agents have been subject to recreational use and abuse. Others have been withdrawn from the market due to adverse side effects. Primary therapy of obesity involves lifestyle changes (diet and exercise). Surgery may also be considered. Failed drugs and currently available therapies are discussed below.

27.15.1 CNS-acting Appetite Suppressants

Amphetamine and Its Derivatives: Methylphenidate, Ephedrine, and Phenylpropanolamine

Mechanism of Action

These sympathomimetic agents are effective in suppressing appetite; however, any weight lost while on the drug is rapidly regained upon cessation.

Uses

These agents are unsuitable for the treatment of obesity due to their CNS-stimulating and other side effects (see Chapter 15).

Fenfluramine and Dexfenfluramine

Dexfenfluramine is the D-isomer of fenfluramine.

These agents were previously used as appetite suppressants, but they were shown to cause pulmonary hypertension and valvular heart disease, which led to their withdrawal from the market.

Sibutramine

Sibutramine is a serotonin and norepinephrine reuptake inhibitor that was approved for long-term use in patients with obesity. It was withdrawn from the market due to increased risk of serious cardiac complications.

27.15.2 Agents Approved for Short-Term Use in Obesity

Phendimetrazine, Phentermine, Diethylpropion

Mechanism of Action

These drugs are centrally acting sympathomimetics, similar to amphetamine, that are still approved for short-term therapy.

Side Effects

Sympathomimetic side effects include increased blood pressure, cardiac effects, and CNS stimulation (see Chapter 15).

27.15.3 Agents Approved for Long-Term Use in Obesity

Phentermine/Topiramate Combination

Mechanism of Action

As discussed above, phentermine is a sympathomimetic. Topiramate is an antiepileptic drug (see Chapter 11) whose exact mechanism to decrease appetite is unknown.

Dosing

The dosage of these drugs in combination is lower than either drug when used alone.

Contraindication

Pregnancy, as there is an increased risk of cleft palate.

Side Effects

Increased heart rate, paresthesias, headache, insomnia, dry mouth, and constipation.

Lorcaserin

Mechanism of Action

It is a $5\text{-}HT_{2C}$ receptor agonist. Decreases appetite by activating $5\text{-}HT_{2C}$ receptors on pro-opiomelanocortin neurons in the hypothalamus.

Contraindication

Pregnancy, as weight loss may harm fetus.

Side Effects

Nausea, headache, fatigue.

27.15.4 Peripherally Acting Weight Loss Medication

Orlistat

This agent is available over-the-counter.

Mechanism of Action

Orlistat is an inhibitor of the pancreatic and gastric lipases that hydrolyze dietary fat into fatty acids and monoacylglycerols. This prevents ~ 30% of dietary fat from being absorbed. Orlistat produces a weight loss of ~ 9 to 10% in 12 months.

Pharmacokinetics

Not absorbed from the GI tract.

Side Effects

No systemic side effects are seen; however, adverse GI effects are common and include flatulence, fecal urgency, fatty/oily stools, and increased frequency of defecation. These side effects can be minimized by decreasing dietary fat intake.

27.15.5 Appetite Enhancers

Megestrol

Megestrol is a synthetic form of progesterone.

Mechanism of Action

The mechanism to affect the appetite is unknown.

Uses

Megestrol is used to enhance appetite in patients with human immunodeficiency virus/acquired immunodeficiency syndrome (HIV/AIDS) and cancer.

Dronabinol

Dronabinol is synthetic δ-9-tetrahydrocannabinol, the main active ingredient in marijuana.

Mechanism of Action

Dronabinol stimulates the appetite by acting on cannabinoid receptors in the CNS (see above).

Uses

In states where it is available, medicinal marijuana is used by patients with AIDS and cancer as an appetite enhancer and to prevent chemotherapy-induced nausea and vomiting.

Unit VI Review Questions

1. Bronchodilation is best accomplished via
   A. Activation of α_1 adrenergic receptors.
   B. Activation of α_2 adrenergic receptors.
   C. Activation of β_1 adrenergic receptors.
   D. Activation of β_2 adrenergic receptors.
   E. Activation of muscarinic receptors.

2. Which of the following agents is used for treatment of persistent asthma to decrease inflammation, decrease the formation of mucus, and decrease the hyperreactivity of bronchial smooth muscle?
   A. Inhaled corticosteroid.
   B. Systemic corticosteroid.
   C. Inhaled β_2 adrenergic selective agonist.
   D. Systemic β_2 adrenergic selective agonist.
   E. Systemic phosphodiesterase inhibitor.

3. A patient with a history of asthma presents with severe respiratory distress and hypoxemia because of an acute, severe asthma attack. A β adrenergic receptor agonist is administered immediately by inhalation. A systemic drug is then administered to treat the inflammatory component of the acute asthma. Which of the following was administered?
   A. Cromolyn.
   B. A parenteral corticosteroid.
   C. Oral theophylline.
   D. An inhaled corticosteroid.
   E. Antibiotics.

4. A 12-year-old girl is being treated for asthma. The drug treatment has resulted in abdominal discomfort, difficulty sleeping, and a persistent headache. These are common side effects of which agent?
   A. Atropine.
   B. Beclomethasone.
   C. Cromolyn sodium.
   D. Ipratropium.
   E. Theophylline.

5. A 62-year-old woman has just been diagnosed with mild chronic obstructive pulmonary disease (COPD). Which of the following options would be the most appropriate initial therapy for this patient?
   A. Budesonide.
   B. Cromolyn sodium.
   C. Ipratropium.
   D. Propranolol.
   E. Scopolamine.

6. A 67-year-old man is being treated for COPD, osteoarthritis, and hypercholesterolemia. He complains about his mouth and throat always feeling dry and having to constantly sip on water to alleviate it. This complaint is most likely to be caused by which of the following drugs?
   A. Budesonide.
   B. Naproxen.
   C. Simvastatin.
   D. Tiotropium.

7. Which of the following inhibits acid secretion by direct interaction with the H^+–K^+–ATPase in the parietal cell?
   A. Ursodiol.
   B. Omeprazole.
   C. Ranitidine.
   D. Sucralfate.
   E. Calcium carbonate.

8. Prostaglandins present in the gastric mucosa are believed to
   A. Increase capillary permeability when aspirin damages the gastric mucosal barrier to ion diffusion.
   B. Block the binding of acetylcholine on parietal cell muscarinic receptors.
   C. Inhibit parietal cell hydrochloric acid production.
   D. Block the entry of calcium into the parietal cell.
   E. Inhibit gastric bicarbonate secretion.

9. Which of the following is an H_2-histamine receptor antagonist?
   A. Cimetidine.
   B. Ondansetron.
   C. Lactulose.
   D. Docusate.
   E. Sodium bicarbonate.

10. A 58-year-old woman has rheumatoid arthritis. The patient's symptoms have responded favorably to treatment with a nonsteroidal anti-inflammatory agent. To decrease the potential of a gastric ulcer, the patient is instructed to take misoprostol simultaneously with the anti-inflammatory agent. What is misoprostol?
    A. A prostaglandin E_1 analogue that inhibits gastric acid secretion.
    B. An antacid that decreases the pH of gastric secretions.
    C. An NSAID-binding agent that prevents absorption in the stomach.
    D. An H_2-histamine receptor blocker that inhibits gastric acid secretion.
    E. A proton pump inhibitor that inhibits gastric acid secretion.

11. A 59-year-old man with metastatic squamous non-small-cell lung cancer is undergoing cisplatin/pemetrexed chemotherapy. Which of the following drugs, used in combination with dexamethasone and ondansetron, would be an effective antiemetic for this patient?
    A. Aprepitant.
    B. Bismuth subsalicylate.
    C. Diphenhydramine.
    D. Milk of magnesia.
    E. Scopolamine.

12. Use of a laxative would be contraindicated in a patient with which of the following?
    A. Appendicitis.
    B. Hemorrhoids.
    C. Inguinal hernia.
    D. IBS-C.

13. Which of the following is a long-acting, selective β_2 adrenergic receptor agonist that is not effective in the treatment of

acute relief of asthma symptoms but is used for chronic treatment of patients not well-controlled by a steroid alone?

A. Dopamine.
B. Albuterol.
C. Prazosin.
D. Pindolol.
E. Salmeterol.

14. Montelukast and zafirlukast are alternative agents for the treatment of mild persistent asthma. The mechanism of action of these agents is

A. Activation of β_2-adrenergic receptors.
B. Activation of cholinergic receptors.
C. Blockade of leukotriene receptors.
D. Blockade of steroid receptors.
E. Stabilization of mast cells.

15. Which of the following is a therapeutic agent for chronic obstructive pulmonary disease (COPD)?

A. Methyltestosterone.
B. Montelukast.
C. Propranolol.
D. Oxygen.
E. Cromolyn.

16. Many antacids are marketed as combinations of magnesium and aluminum hydroxide because

A. Aluminum hydroxide alone tastes very bad.
B. Magnesium minimizes the absorption of aluminum.
C. The laxative effect of magnesium is counteracted by the constipating effect of aluminum.
D. Magnesium hydroxide alone neutralizes gastric acid too slowly.
E. The "acid rebound" induced by aluminum hydroxide can be minimized.

17. Which of the following aids ulcer healing by forming a protective barrier over the ulcer?

A. Sucralfate.
B. Ranitidine.
C. Misoprostol.
D. Cimetidine.
E. Calcium carbonate.

18. Which of the following frequently induces a significant "acid rebound" of gastric pH?

A. Sucralfate.
B. Omeprazole.
C. Misoprostol.
D. Cimetidine.
E. Calcium carbonate.

19. Which of the following cathartics or laxatives is a bulk-forming agent?

A. Castor oil.
B. Magnesium hydroxide.
C. Milk of magnesia.
D. Methyl or carboxymethylcellulose.
E. Phenolphthalein.

20. A variety of stimuli can produce nausea and vomiting, and a variety of drugs can act as antiemetics. A mechanism of action for the most common agent for motion sickness is to block

A. D_2 dopamine receptors.
B. 5-HT_3 serotonin receptors.
C. NK_1 receptors.
D. Muscarinic receptors.
E. Cannabinoid receptors.

21. An 8-year-old boy is experiencing wheezing and coughing. The parents report that he experienced the same problem last spring, but the symptoms seem worse this spring. You consider treatment with an albuterol inhaler. Which of the following is a side effect that may be observed with albuterol?

A. Bradycardia.
B. Diarrhea.
C. Restlessness.
D. Sedation.
E. Tinnitus.

22. An 8-year-old boy is experiencing wheezing and coughing. The parents report that he experienced the same problem last spring, but the symptoms seem worse this spring. You consider treatment with an albuterol inhaler. The patient is started on albuterol but experiences restlessness. The parents feel that this side effect is unacceptable. If your primary concern is to minimize side effects, which agent would be most appropriate?

A. Beclomethasone.
B. Montelukast.
C. Theophylline.
D. Ipratropium.
E. Albuterol.

23. A 58-year-old male patient has moderate chronic obstructive pulmonary disease. He was initially treated with albuterol but continues to experience dyspnea. He is told to add an inhaler containing ipratropium bromide four times per day. What is the purpose of this additional drug?

A. To block the effects of the sympathetic nervous system on bronchial smooth muscle.
B. To block the effects of the parasympathetic nervous system on bronchial smooth muscle.
C. To mimic the effects of the sympathetic nervous system on bronchial smooth muscle.
D. To mimic the effects of the parasympathetic nervous system on bronchial smooth muscle.
E. To inhibit acetylcholinesterase and increase the half-life of acetylcholine released from neurons that innervate the bronchi.

24. A patient diagnosed with peptic ulcer disease is started on a regimen of antacids (a magnesium-plus-aluminum combination product) and an H_2 receptor blocker. Assuming the patient is otherwise healthy and typical, which of the following responses is most likely to cause premature

cessation of therapy (noncompliance) unless the patient is explicitly instructed to anticipate it?

A. Prompt relief of ulcer pain.
B. Dry mouth and blurred vision.
C. Orthostatic hypotension and fainting.
D. Skeletal muscle tremor.
E. Wheezing and dyspnea.

25. It was determined that a 50-year-old, slightly obese patient had reflux esophagitis. The patient's symptoms were heartburn, reflux of bloody material, and waking up at night coughing and choking with a mouthful of fluid. This patient's condition could be relieved by which of the following agents?

A. Propranolol.
B. Hydrochloric acid.
C. Omeprazole.
D. Progesterone.
E. Chlorpromazine.

26. An 82-year-old patient is taking a laxative. The possible side effects include the possibility of pneumonia from aspirating the substance and interference with the absorption of fat-soluble vitamins. Which laxative is the patient most likely taking?

A. Mineral oil.
B. Magnesium hydroxide.
C. Phenolphthalein.
D. Psyllium.
E. Milk of magnesia.

27. A 45-year-old man recently diagnosed with Crohn disease received sulfasalazine for weeks. The symptoms persisted so prednisone was added for another week, but improvement was still negligible. The gastroenterologist decided to add a biological drug that is an integrin inhibitor to the therapy. Which of the following drugs was administered?

A. Mesalamine.
B. Sulfasalazine.
C. Adalimumab.
D. Natalizumab.
E. Azathioprine.

28. A 30-year-old man went to his physician complaining of intermittent abdominal pain, bloating, diarrhea, and rectal bleeding over the past month. Sigmoidoscopy showed erythematous mucosa in the rectum, sigmoid colon, and distal descending colon. The mucosa had areas of fine granular appearance with some focal hemorrhage and ulcerations. Biopsies demonstrated abnormal crypt abscesses. A diagnosis of mild ulcerative colitis was made, and a therapy was prescribed. Which of the following drugs would be most appropriate for the patient at this time? (Select all that apply.)

A. Metronidazole.
B. Natalizumab.
C. Cyclosporine.
D. Sulfasalazine.
E. Budesonide.

Unit VI Answers and Explanations

1. D. Activation of β_2 adrenergic receptors on bronchial smooth muscle produces smooth muscle relaxation and bronchodilation.

A. α_1 adrenergic receptors may be present on the vasculature of the lung and regulate vasoconstriction.

B. α_2 adrenergic receptors may be found on presynaptic terminals of sympathetic neurons and regulate neurotransmitter release.

C. β_1 adrenergic receptors are found mainly in the heart. Activation of these receptors causes increased heart rate and force and velocity of contraction.

E. Activation of muscarinic cholinergic receptors causes bronchoconstriction.

2. A. Decreased inflammation, decreased formation of mucus, and decreased hyperreactivity of bronchial smooth muscle are all effects of corticosteroids. They are administered by inhalation to minimize systemic side effects that would be seen if given systemically (B).

C, D. β_2 adrenergic receptor selective agonists do not produce these effects, but they do produce bronchodilation.

E. Theophylline is a systemic phosphodiesterase inhibitor that mainly produces bronchodilation, but it may also have some anti-inflammatory actions. It does not decrease the formation of mucus or decrease hyperreactivity of bronchial smooth muscle.

3. B. For acute, severe asthma attacks, parenteral steroids are used.

A, C. Cromolyn, a mast cell stabilizer, and theophylline, a systemic phosphodiesterase inhibitor, are not used for acute asthma attacks.

D. Inhaled corticosteroids are used for the chronic treatment of asthma.

E. Antibiotics are not effective for treating asthma.

4. E. These side effects are produced by theophylline, which is a systemic phosphodiesterase inhibitor.

A, D. Atropine and ipratropium produce anticholinergic side effects, such as dry mouth, blurred vision, tachycardia, urinary retention, and constipation.

B. Beclomethasone may cause throat irritation, dysphonia, oral candidiasis, and growth disturbances in children (rarely).

C. Cromolyn sodium, a mast cell stabilizer, does not produce these side effects.

5. C. Ipratropium is an antimuscarinic that may be used as initial therapy for COPD.

A. Budesonide is a corticosteroid.

B. Cromolyn sodium is a mast cell stabilizer used for prophylaxis of asthma.

D. Propranolol is a β adrenergic receptor antagonist. Its use would be contraindicated in COPD.

E. Scopolamine is a centrally acting anticholinergic used to treat motion sickness and to prevent emesis.

6. D. This side effect is a characteristic of muscarinic anticholinergic drugs. Tiotropium is an antimuscarinic that may be used as initial therapy for COPD. None of the other drugs would be expected to produce the dry mouth.

A. Budesonide is a corticosteroid.

B. Naproxen is a NSAID used for arthritis.

C. Simvastatin is an HMG CoA reductase inhibitor used to treat hyperlipidemia.

E. Scopolamine is a centrally acting anticholinergic used to treat motion sickness and to prevent emesis.

7. B. Omeprazole inhibits the proton pump (H^+–K^+–ATPase) of the parietal cells in the stomach, thereby inhibiting gastric acid secretion.

A. Ursodiol decreases the secretion of cholesterol into bile by reducing cholesterol absorption and suppressing cholesterol synthesis in the liver. It is used to treat cholesterol-containing gallstones.

C. Ranitidine is an H_2-histamine receptor antagonist that blocks the H_2-histamine receptors of parietal cells, thereby inhibiting both basal and stimulated gastric acid secretion.

D. Sucralfate forms an ulcer-adherent complex with the proteinaceous exudate at the ulcer site.

E. Calcium carbonate is a nonsystemic antacid.

8. C. Prostaglandins inhibit parietal cell hydrochloric acid production in the gastric mucosa. They also increase mucus production.

9. A. Cimetidine is an H_2-histamine receptor antagonist that blocks the H_2-histamine receptors of parietal cells, thereby inhibiting both basal and stimulated gastric acid secretion.

B. Ondansetron is an antiemetic drug that blocks 5-HT_3 receptors in the CNS and gastrointestinal tract.

C. Lactulose is a specialized laxative for chronic liver disease or hepatic coma as it decreases plasma levels of ammonia formed by intestinal bacteria.

D. Docusate is a stool softening agent that lowers surface tension and promotes water absorption into feces.

E. Sodium bicarbonate is a systemic antacid.

10. A. Misoprostol is a prostaglandin derivative that has both cytoprotective and antisecretory actions. It does not act by any of the other listed mechanisms.

11. A. Aprepitant is an NK_1 receptor antagonist used to prevent chemotherapy-induced nausea and vomiting.

B. Bismuth subsalicylate is used to treat heartburn and diarrhea. It is also used in combination drug regimens for *H. pylori*.

C. Diphenhydramine has antihistamine and anticholinergic actions. It is used to treat motion sickness and vertigo.

D. Milk of magnesia is a gastric antacid.

E. Scopolamine is a centrally acting anticholinergic used to treat motion sickness and to prevent emesis.

12. A. Appendicitis. Administration of a laxative to a patient with an inflamed appendix may cause it to rupture.

B, C, D. Laxatives may be useful to treat hemorrhoids in patients with an inguinal hernia and in patients with IBS-C.

13. E. Salmeterol is a long-acting β_2 agonist used in the treatment of chronic asthma symptoms.

A. Dopamine is an endogenous neurotransmitter.

B. Albuterol is a short-acting β_2 agonist for acute relief of asthma symptoms.

C. Prazosin is an $\alpha1$ receptor blocker used to treat hypertension.

D. Pindolol is a nonselective β-adrenergic blocking agent used to treat hypertension. It may worsen asthma symptoms (via blockage of β_2-mediated bronchodilation).

14. C. Montelukast and zafirlukast are leukotriene receptor antagonists.

15. D. Supplemental oxygen is the only therapeutic agent that has been shown to decrease mortality in patients with COPD.

A. Methyltestosterone is a testosterone analogue used mainly for hypogonadism.

B, E. Montelukast, a leukotriene antagonist, and cromolyn, a mast cell stabilizer, are used to treat asthma.

C. Administration of propranolol, a nonselective β-blocker, could worsen lung function.

16. C. Magnesium salts have a laxative effect whereas calcium or aluminum salts tend to produce constipation. The combination is used to achieve a balance of these side effects.

17. A. Sucralfate forms an ulcer-adherent complex with the proteinaceous exudate at the ulcer site. It is not absorbed and does not inhibit acid secretion or neutralize acid.

B, D. Ranitidine and cimetidine are H_2-histamine receptor antagonists that block the H_2-histamine receptors of parietal cells, thereby inhibiting both basal and stimulated gastric acid secretion.

C. Misoprostol is a prostaglandin derivative that acts to promote protective mucus secretion from epithelial cells in the stomach and inhibit gastric acid secretion for gastric parietal cells.

E. Calcium carbonate is an antacid.

18. E. Calcium salts, such as calcium carbonate, may cause a rebound acid secretion.

A. Sucralfate forms an ulcer-adherent complex with the proteinaceous exudate at the ulcer site.

B. Omeprazole inhibits the proton pump (H^+-K^+-ATPase) of the parietal cells in the stomach, thus inhibiting gastric acid secretion.

C. Misoprostol is a prostaglandin derivative that acts to promote protective mucus secretion from epithelial cells in the stomach and inhibit gastric acid secretion for gastric parietal cells.

D. Cimetidine is an H_2-histamine receptor antagonist that blocks the H_2-histamine receptors of parietal cells, thereby inhibiting both basal and stimulated gastric acid secretion.

19. D. Bulk-forming agents include bran and other dietary fiber, methylcellulose, sodium carboxymethylcellulose, and psyllium preparations.

A, E. Castor oil and phenolphthalein are contact (stimulant-irritant) cathartics.

B. Magnesium hydroxide is a saline (osmotic) cathartic.

C. Milk of magnesia is a saline (osmotic) cathartic.

20. D. Drugs having central nervous system (CNS) muscarinic receptor blocking actions, such as scopolamine and benztropine, or antihistamines with CNS anticholinergic effects, such as diphenhydramine, cyclizine, and dimenhydrinate, are commonly used to treat motion sickness.

A. D_2 dopamine receptor blockers, such as prochlorperazine, act on the chemoreceptor trigger zone in the medulla and are used less commonly in motion sickness.

B, C. 5-HT_3 receptor blockers, such as ondansetron, and NK_1 receptor antagonists, such as aprepitant, are used for chemotherapy-induced nausea and vomiting.

E. Cannabinoids, the psychoactive ingredients in marijuana, are appetite stimulants and antiemetics. Dronabinol, a synthetic δ-9-tetrahydrocannabinol, is used clinically for the prevention of chemotherapy-induced nausea and vomiting.

21. C. Of the side effects listed, the one most likely to be seen with albuterol is restlessness.

22. B. Montelukast has the most favorable side effect profile of the agents listed.

23. B. Ipratropium is an antagonist of muscarinic cholinergic receptors. Postganglionic parasympathetic neurons release acetylcholine that interacts with muscarinic cholinergic receptors on smooth muscle. Thus, ipratropium blocks the effects of the parasympathetic nervous system on bronchial smooth muscle.

A, C–E. The other choices are invalid.

24. A. By decreasing acid secretions, these agents can provide rapid symptomatic relief of gastric ulcers. A patient may associate relief of symptoms with a cure. It takes several weeks, however, for repair of the gastric mucosa to occur.

B–E. The other side effects are not likely to occur with this therapeutic regimen.

25. C. The patient is experiencing gastroesophageal reflux disease. Of the agents listed, the only one approved for such use is omeprazole.

A. Propranolol is a nonselective β-adrenergic receptor blocker used to treat hypertension.

B. Hydrochloric acid is an endogenous acid secreted by gastric parietal cells.

D. Progesterone is a hormone that supports female reproductive tissues and processes, especially maintaining pregnancy.

E. Chlorpromazine is an antipsychotic and antiemetic drug.

26. A. The side effects are possible with mineral oil, a lubricant laxative, but not the other agents listed.

B. Magnesium hydroxide is a saline (osmotic) cathartic. It may produce neurological or cardiovascular toxicity if renal function is impaired.

C. Phenolphthalein is a contact (stimulant-irritant) cathartic. It may turn feces and urine red.

D. Psyllium is a bulk-forming laxative.

E. Milk of magnesia is a saline (osmotic) cathartic. It may produce electrolyte disturbances.

27. D. Natalizumab is a monoclonal antibody to the α4-subunit of integrins on the surface of leukocytes, thus inhibiting leukocyte migration and activation in the GI tract. It may be used in select patients with moderate-to-severe Crohn's disease unresponsive to other therapies.

A, B. Mesalamine is 5-aminosalicylic acid (5-ASA), the active moiety of the aminosalicylates used to treat IBD. Sulfasalazine is a prodrug that is metabolized to 5-ASA.

C. Adalimumab is a humanized monoclonal antibody to TNF-α that may be used to treat moderate-to-severe Crohn disease unresponsive to other therapies.

E. Azathioaprine is an antimetabolite used to treat moderate-to-severe Crohn disease.

28. D and E. Sulfasalazine is a prodrug that is metabolized to 5-aminosalicylic acid (5-ASA). Budesonide is a corticosteroid. Both of these may be used to treat mild ulcerative colitis.

A. Metronidazole is an antibiotic used to treat pseudomembranous colitis, an inflammation of the colon due to superinfection with *C. difficile*.

B. Natalizumab is a monoclonal antibody to the α4-subunit of integrins on the surface of leukocytes, thus inhibiting leukocyte migration and activation in the GI tract. It may be used in select patients with moderate-to-severe Crohn disease unresponsive to other therapies.

C. Cyclosporine decreases interleukin-2 (IL-2) synthesis in T helper cells. It is sometimes used in patients unresponsive to steroids or in chronic cases of moderate-to-severe IBD, although it is not approved by the FDA for this purpose.

Unit VII

Antimicrobial Drugs

By Katharina Brandl

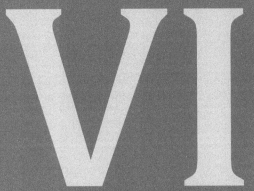

28 Principles of Antimicrobial Therapy

Summary

Before initiating an antimicrobial therapy, several considerations need to be made including patient-specific as well as pathogen-specific characteristics. In addition, the pharmacodynamic and pharmacokinetic properties of drugs, the mode of administration, and different dosing regimens have an influence on antimicrobial selection. Antibiotics can be given alone or in combination, and as empiric or as prophylactic therapy. Several tests are available to determine bacterial sensitivity to antimicrobial agents allowing for optimal selection. In this chapter, we discuss several considerations that need to be made before initiating an antibiotic therapy. In addition, mechanisms underlying antibacterial resistance will be introduced.

Keywords: antibiotics, antibacterial, resistance

28.1 Introduction

Infectious diseases are caused by microbes or microbial products. Antimicrobial drugs are intended to eliminate foreign organisms from healthy tissues of the patient without comparable effects on the normal tissue cells of the host. This essential property of these drugs is called *selective toxicity*. In this chapter, we will introduce some important characteristics of antibiotic therapy.

28.2 Classification of Antimicrobial Agents

28.2.1 Chemical Structure and Mechanism of Action

The main classification of antimicrobial agents is based on their chemical structure (e.g., β-lactams and aminoglycosides) and their mechanism of action (see ▶ Table 28.1).

Table 28.1 Mechanism of action of antimicrobial agents

Mechanism of action	Drugs
Inhibition of bacterial cell wall synthesis	β-lactams: penicillins, cephalosporins, monobactams, and carbapenems Others: vancomycin and bacitracin
Cell membrane active agents	Daptomycin and telavancin
Inhibition of protein synthesis	Bacteriostatic: tetracyclines, macrolides, clindamycin, streptogramins, and oxazolidinones Bactericidal: aminoglycosides
Inhibition of nucleic acid metabolism by inhibiting RNA polymerase	Rifampin
Inhibition of nucleic acid metabolism by inhibiting DNA gyrase or topoisomerase	Fluoroquinolones
Inhibition of essential enzymes of folate metabolism (antimetabolites)	Trimethoprim and sulfonamides

28.2.2 Bacteriostatic or Bactericidal

Antimicrobial agents are also classified on the basis of their bacteriostatic or bactericidal activity (▶ Fig. 28.1).

Foundations

Anatomy of Bacteria

Bacteria are single-cell organisms 0.3 to 5 μm in size that are typically spherical (cocci), straight (bacilli), curved, or spiral rods. They lack a nuclear membrane and have no true nucleus. The chromosome in bacteria is typically a single, closed circle DNA that is concentrated in a nucleoid region. Some bacteria possess smaller extrachromosomal pieces of DNA called plasmids. The cytoplasmic membrane is surrounded by a cell wall. The cell wall of gram-negative bacteria has an outer membrane that is absent in gram-positive bacteria.

Foundations

Oxygen Levels and Bacterial Growth

Different bacteria require different oxygen levels for optimal growth and cell division. There are obligate aerobes that require a high level of oxygen for growth, microaerophiles that require oxygen but at a reduced level, facultative anaerobes that can grow in the presence or absence of oxygen, aerotolerant anaerobes that can tolerate some oxygen, and obligate anaerobes that grow only in the absence of oxygen.

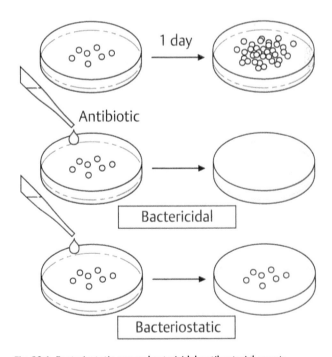

Fig. 28.1 Bacteriostatic versus bactericidal antibacterial agents. Bacteria are able to multiply in vitro in a growth medium if conditions are favorable. If the growth medium contains an antibiotic, the bacteria may be killed (bactericidal effect) or the bacteria may survive but do not multiply (bacteriostatic effect).

VII

Superinfections

Antibiotic drugs alter the normal microbial population of the intestinal, upper respiratory, and genitourinary tracts. This alteration of the normal flora may lead to the development of a superinfection which is defined as the appearance of a new infection during therapy of the primary infection. This phenomenon is relatively common and may be dangerous because the superinfecting microbes are frequently drug resistant. Superinfections are more likely to occur with broad-spectrum antibiotics and longer treatment durations.

Foundations

Gram Staining

Gram staining is a laboratory test that allows bacteria to be classified in two groups, i.e., gram-positive and gram-negative bacteria, based on the composition of their cell walls. Cell walls of gram-positive bacteria are rich in proteoglycan but have no lipopolysaccharide and stain purple, whereas gram-negative bacteria have little proteoglycan in cell walls but are rich in lipopolysaccharide and stain pink. Gram staining is an important tool in helping to determine the species of bacteria responsible for infections so that the most appropriate antimicrobial agent is selected for treatment.

- **Bacteriostatic agents** primarily inhibit bacterial growth. Killing of the organism is then dependent upon host defense mechanisms. The disadvantage of these agents is that in the setting of inadequate host defense mechanisms (e.g., immunocompromised patients), any partially inhibited organisms may survive, replicate, and produce recurrent disease when the antibiotic is discontinued.
- **Bactericidal agents** are capable of killing the bacteria and are preferred if the patient has neutropenia or immunosuppression.

28.2.3 Spectra of Antimicrobial Agents

Antimicrobial agents are further classified into spectra depending on the range of microorganisms on which they act:
- **Narrow-spectrum agents** are effective against a limited range of microorganisms.
- **Extended-spectrum agents** are principally effective against gram-positive bacteria, but they are also effective against a significant range of gram-negative bacteria.
- **Broad-spectrum agents** are effective against a wide range of microorganisms.

The use of broad-spectrum antibiotics should be limited, as they predispose patients to superinfection (the appearance of a new infection during treatment) by disrupting the body's natural bacterial flora.

28.3 Selection of Antimicrobial Agents

The selection of antimicrobial agents involves the consideration of many factors relating to the microorganisms involved, patient (host) factors, and pharmacology of the agents themselves.

28.3.1 Microorganism Factors

Species of Microorganism

Successful treatment of an infection requires knowledge of the pathogen(s) involved. Rapid tests are available to confirm the presence of some common infections prior to the initiation of antibiotic therapy. Examples include a dipstick test for the presence of bacteria in the urine and a throat swab for strep throat. In more severe infections, especially if the pathogen has shown antibiotic resistance, definitive identification of the infectious microorganism and its susceptibility to various antibiotics by laboratory testing is required.

Bacterial identification typically involves characterization by gram staining, cell shape, and media requirements for growth. More advanced tests involve binding of specific antibodies and genetic analysis by polymerase chain reaction (PCR) or gene sequencing.

Susceptibility to Antimicrobial Agents

Bacterial strains, even of the same species, may vary widely in antibiotic sensitivity. Several tests are available for determination of bacterial sensitivity to antimicrobial agents to allow for optimal selection. The standard tests are disk diffusion tests and agar or broth dilution tests. Other quantitative tests are used to determine minimal inhibitory concentration (MIC) and minimal bactericidal concentration (MBC). The MIC is the concentration of an antibiotic necessary to inhibit microbial growth under standardized conditions whereas the MBC is the concentration of antibiotic required to kill the microorganism. The results of these tests can then be used to determine the antibiotic dose required.

Resistance to Antimicrobial Agent

Bacterial resistance to an antimicrobial agent may be intrinsic or acquired (▶ Fig. 28.2). Acquired resistance can occur due to spontaneous mutations or by the transfer of drug-resistant genes.

Spontaneous Mutations

Spontaneous DNA mutations are rare, occurring in one in 10^6 to one in 10^8 base pairs. The chance that a given mutation will lead to antibiotic resistance is even less likely. On the other hand, the fast replication rate of bacteria, as well as the large numbers of cells attained, increases the chance that a spontaneous mutation will lead to antibiotic resistance. The antibiotic provides selective pressure on the organisms, killing the non-mutant cells while the resistant mutants proliferate.

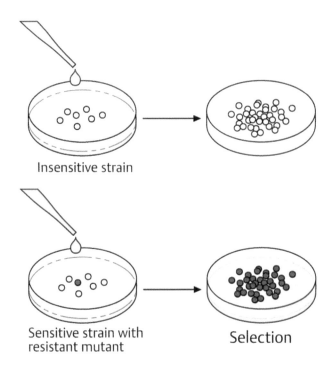

Fig. 28.2 Bacterial resistance.
Some bacteria are naturally insensitive to antibacterial drugs and can grow and multiply in their presence. Other bacteria that are normally sensitive to antibacterial agents may develop mutant strains such that when an antibacterial agent is given, the sensitive bacteria are killed, but the mutant bacteria are able to multiply unimpeded.

Table 28.2 Mechanisms of acquired antibiotic resistance

Mechanism of resistance	Example
Inactivation of the drug	Bacterial β-lactamases (penicillinases) inactivate penicillins and cephalosporins by cleaving the β-lactam ring of the drug
Mutation of the target	Bacteria synthesize modified targets against which the drug has no effect (e.g., group B *Streptococcus*, which is frequently responsible for peripartum maternal and neonatal infections, can develop resistance to erythromycin via genes that modify the ribosomal target of the drug)
Prevention of the drug from entering the cell by decreasing permeability of the cell	Changes in porins in the outer cell membrane can reduce the amount of antibiotic that can enter the bacterium
Actively transporting the drug out of the cell	The multidrug resistance pump exports a variety of foreign molecules, including some antibiotics, and imports protons in an exchange reaction

Transfer of Drug-Resistant Genes

Bacteria are able to transfer genes that confer resistance to each other. This usually occurs via plasmids, which are small, circular, extrachromosomal pieces of DNA; or via transposons, which are small pieces of DNA that can hop from DNA molecule to DNA molecule. Once in a chromosome or a plasmid, the transposons can be integrated stably. They then act by the four main mechanisms described in ► Table 28.2 to achieve resistance.

► Table 28.2

Clinical Correlation

Disk Diffusion Test

Sensitivity to various antibiotics can be determined with the disk diffusion method. Microorganisms are cultured over paper disks on an agar surface. The disks contain antibiotic drugs. After 18 to 24 hours of incubation, the inhibition of bacterial growth around the disk, termed the "zone of inhibition," is measured. The diameter of the zone depends on the activity of the drug against the test strain. Newer methods measure bacterial gene expression by the PCR to identify specific pathogens.

Clinical Correlation

Broth Dilution Tests

In dilution tests, the concentration of antibiotics is serially diluted in either solid agar or liquid broth containing a culture of the test microorganism. The lowest concentration of the agent that prevents growth after 18 to 24 hours of incubation is known as the MIC. Automated systems also use a broth dilution method. Bacterial growth is measured as the optical density of culture of the organism in liquid (broth) in various concentrations of drug. The MIC is the concentration at which the optical density remains below a threshold.

Foundations

Bacterial Enzymes

Enzymes are produced by many organisms and serve to promote or enhance the infection by breaking down tissues to produce foodstuffs and allowing the spread of the organism within tissue. Mucinase is produced by *Entamoeba histolytica* and acts to dissolve the protective mucoid coating on intestinal epithelial cells. Many clostridial organisms, including *Clostridium perfringens*, produce collagenase that dissolves collagen in connective tissue. The connective tissue between cells, hyaluronic acid, is degraded by many bacteria (e.g., *Streptococci*, *Clostridia*, and *Staphylococci*) that produce hyaluronidase. Streptokinase and staphylokinase are examples of enzymes that break down blood clots. Other enzymes include phospholipase C, proteases, DNase, lipases, and lysins.

Foundations

Bacterial Toxins

Many bacteria produce toxins that may cause damage to the host. Diseases such as diphtheria, tetanus, staphylococcal scalded skin syndrome, and cholera are caused by the production of a toxin at the site of the infection. Despite efforts to classify toxins, many are labeled by the site on which they act; for example, neurotoxins act on the nervous system, hemotoxins lyse erythrocytes, hepatotoxins affect the liver, and enterotoxins act on the intestine. These differences in cell site are related to receptor specificity and ability of the toxin to bind to a host cell membrane receptor.

VII

Foundations

Exotoxins and Endotoxins

Toxins that are released from the bacterial cell are termed *exotoxins* and can be released from both gram-positive and gram-negative bacteria. They can be single proteins or polymeric toxins composed of A and B subunits. The B component of subunit toxins bind to specific receptors on the host cell membrane, causing the release of the A or active subunit. Examples of A-B toxins include tetanus toxin, *Pseudomonas* exotoxin A, Shiga toxin, botulinum toxin, cholera toxin, and diphtheria toxin. The genes for exotoxin production may be located on the bacterial genome or encoded on a plasmid or lysogenic bacteriophage. In the gram-negative organism, part of the cell envelope is an endotoxin (lipopolysaccharide). Importantly, the toxic moiety of endotoxin is lipid A, which is released when the organism lyses. It can activate several cells of the immune system by binding to the TLR4/MD2 receptor complex. After binding to its receptor on the cell membrane, for example, interleukin-1 (IL-1), tumor necrosis factor-α (TNF-α), prostaglandins, and IL-6 are released triggering fever and inflammation.

Foundations

Superantigens

In some instances, organisms produce superantigens that are capable of activating T cells by specific binding to the T cell and linkage to a class II major histocompatibility complex moiety on another cell type. Such linkage causes T cell activation and the release of several pyrogenic cytokines. Superantigens are produced by *Staphylococcus aureus* that results in toxic shock syndrome, *Streptococcus pyogenes* (erythrogenic toxins), and staphylococcal enterotoxins.

Foundations

Antibiotics in Abscesses

Antibiotics affect the growth and replication of bacteria; as such, they are most effective against actively growing bacterial cultures. When infection becomes more stagnant (e.g., in abscesses), antibiotics alone are often not sufficient, as they are unable to penetrate the capsule that forms around the abscess, and they tend to be less effective in low pH environments. In these cases, the abscess should be incised and drained to allow most of the pus to be evacuated and promote better penetration of the antibiotic to any residual bacteria.

Resistance is more likely in cases of hospital-acquired infections because widespread antibiotic use in hospitals selects for resistant organisms. Furthermore, hospital strains are often resistant to multiple antibiotics. This resistance is usually due to the acquisition of plasmids carrying several genes that encode the enzymes that mediate resistance. Multidrug resistance (MDR) occurs when microorganisms develop resistance to multiple classes of antibiotics, either by use of the MDR pump or by acquiring various resistance genes.

28.3.2 Patient Factors

When selecting an antimicrobial agent, the mode of administration, dosing regimen, and patient's acute health status, as well as his or her overall health, need to be considered with regard to the factors listed in ▶ Table 28.3.

28.3.3 Drug Factors

The pharmacokinetics of drugs has an influence on antimicrobial selection. ▶ Table 28.4 lists the factors that should be considered.

Table 28.3 Patient factors affecting selection of antimicrobial agents

Factor	Explanation
Renal disease	Drugs that are eliminated by the kidneys may accumulate in renal disease, causing toxicity. This may necessitate a dose reduction of any antibiotic given
Hepatic disease	A dose reduction may also be necessary for antibiotics that are extensively metabolized and excreted by the liver. Some antibiotics are contraindicated in liver disease
Pregnancy	Most antibiotics are able to cross the placenta, so the risk of teratogenesis must be considered
Lactation	The potential for a toxic accumulation of drug in the infant via breast milk must be considered
Immune status	Patients with compromised immune systems (e.g., those undergoing cancer chemotherapy or with HIV) will generally require higher doses and longer courses of treatment
Age	Older patients tend to have decreased renal function; infants have poorly developed drug detoxification mechanisms

Abbreviation: HIV, human immunodeficiency virus.

Table 28.4 Drug factors affecting selection of antimicrobial agents

Factor	Explanation
Site of infection	Access of the antimicrobial agent to the site of infection determines whether or not an adequate drug concentration can be achieved. • Drugs that are extensively bound to plasma proteins may not penetrate the site of infection to the same extent as those that show less protein binding • If the infection involves the central nervous system, the drug must penetrate the blood–brain barrier (lipid-soluble and low-molecular-weight drugs)
Mode of administration	• Many agents are rapidly and completely absorbed after oral administration and can be given by mouth. Sometimes an initial injection will be followed by a course of oral therapy • In patients with severe acute infections, drugs may be given intravenously or intramuscularly, so that effective therapeutic levels of antibiotics can reach the site of infection more rapidly

28.4 Empiric Treatment of Infectious Diseases and Combination Therapy

28.4.1 Empiric Treatment

The selection of an antimicrobial agent for a patient who is diagnosed with an infectious disease can be empirical, that is, initiated with a drug that is most likely to treat the case at hand. The choice of an antibiotic with which to initiate empiric therapy is based on the most likely pathogen for a given infection and the susceptibility profile of the suspected pathogen. The site and severity of the infection, as well as patient factors also have an important influence on the choice of agent. With empiric therapy, an otherwise healthy outpatient with a mild infection caused by a pathogen with known antibiotic susceptibility can be treated immediately, successfully, and without further testing. In more severe or prolonged infections, in patients who are hospitalized or have other illnesses, or when the causative pathogen exhibits antibiotic resistance, empiric factors may be used to initiate therapy without a delay. Once the infectious microorganism is identified by laboratory testing and its susceptibility to antibiotics determined, definitive therapy can be continued with a different agent if the empiric choice was not optimal.

28.4.2 Combination Therapy

In cases of superinfection or resistance, combinations of antibiotics may be warranted. The resultant anti-infective activity of two drugs may be:
- **Indifferent** (the addition of the second drug makes no difference).
- **Additive** (the total effect of the two drugs is equal to the sum of the effect of each drug given individually).
- **Synergistic** (the effect of the two drugs given together is greater than the sum of the two drugs given individually). These interactions are the most important clinically, and several types can be exploited to achieve better therapeutic results. For example, two drugs may sequentially block a microbial metabolic pathway, one drug may enhance the entry of a second drug into bacteria or fungi, or one drug may prevent the inactivation of a second drug by microbial enzymes.
- **Antagonistic** (the effect of the drugs given together is less than the sum of the drugs given individually). Antagonism is rarely observed clinically, but it could occur if a bacteriostatic drug, which inhibits protein synthesis, is given with a bactericidal drug that depends on cell growth to be effective.

28.4.3 Prophylaxis of Infection with Antimicrobial Agents

Antibiotics may be used prophylactically to prevent infection in individuals exposed to contagious pathogens or to prevent recurrent infections. Because of the potential for the development of antibiotic resistance and the potential to cause superinfections, specific guidelines have been developed for the prophylactic uses of antibiotics. Prophylaxis is recommended for patients undergoing procedures that will cause bacteremia (e.g., dental, upper gastrointestinal, or respiratory tract procedures) and for patients in whom the complications of infection could be fatal.

This includes the following:
- Patients with a history of bacterial endocarditis.
- Patients with prosthetic heart valves.
- Cardiac transplantation patients who have developed valve problems.

Specific guidelines are also in place for surgical patients and for the treatment of wounds.

28.5 Reference Tables

▶ Table 28.5 and ▶ Table 28.6 have been included for reference when discussing the spectra of agents in the chapters that follow.

VII

Table 28.5 Selected examples of gram-positive and gram-negative bacteria

Gram-positive		Gram-negative	
Cocci	**Bacilli**	**Cocci**	**Bacilli**
Staphylococcus	Bacillus	Neisseria	Enterobacteriaceae
S. aureus	B. cereus	N. gonorrhoeae	Escherichia
S. epidermidis	B. anthracis	N. meningitides	Yersinia
Streptococcus	Listeria		Proteus
S. pyogenes	Actinomyces		Serratia
S. viridans	Clostridium		Salmonella
S. pneumoniae	C. difficile		Shigella
Enterococcus	C. perfringens		Morganella
E. faecalis	C. tetani		Enterobacter
E. mutans	C. botulinum		Citrobacter
			Klebsiella
			Campylobacter
			Legionella
			Vibrio
			Pseudomonas
			Helicobacter
			H. pylori
			Bacteroides

Table 28.6 Miscellaneous microorganisms

Mycobacterium
M. tuberculosis
M. leprae
Spirochetes
Treponema
Leptospira
Borrelia

Mycoplasma

Chlamydia

Rickettsia

29 Antibacterial Drugs

Summary

Antibacterial drugs are a large group of molecules with different chemical structures that act on bacteria in order to inhibit their growth or survival. The targets of antibacterial drugs are unique to prokaryotic cells and therefore serious toxicity is rare. This makes antibiotics one of the most commonly prescribed drugs.

In this chapter, the different classes of antibacterial drugs will be discussed along with their mechanisms of action, common adverse effects, and their major therapeutic uses. Antibiotics are classified on the basis of their mechanism of action: agents can act on the bacterial cell wall or interfere with bacterial metabolism. Another important target of antibacterial drugs are bacterial ribosomes as they differ in size and chemical composition from eukaryotic ribosomes.

Keywords: antibiotics, antibacterials, antituberculosis, antifungals

29.1 Introduction

The discoveries of antibiotics provide one of the most important success stories of modern medicine. While certain infectious diseases were fatal before the discovery of antibiotics, they can be easily treated now with a few tablets. However, the development of microbial resistance is a common challenge to the use of antibacterial drugs. Many providers overuse antibiotics in patients that are unlikely to have a bacterial infection. Some providers use broad-spectrum antibiotics when not needed; others use antibiotics over a prolonged time. Selection needs to be carefully considered in order to avoid the development of antibiotic resistant bacteria. This chapter will introduce the most common antibiotics and their major uses. Antibacterial agents act on the bacterial cell to disrupt the integrity of the cell structure or its metabolism (▶ Fig. 29.1).

29.2 Inhibitors of Bacterial Cell Wall Synthesis

Antibacterial drugs that act as inhibitors of cell wall synthesis include the β-lactam antibiotics (listed in ▶ Table 29.1 with their structures shown in ▶ Fig. 29.2) and vancomycin. These agents have a high degree of selective toxicity against bacteria because mammalian cells do not have cell walls. Another category of agents, β-lactamase inhibitors, has been included in this section, as they augment the action of β-lactam antibiotics.

29.2.1 Penicillins

Mechanism of Action

The β-lactam antibiotics bind covalently to penicillin-binding proteins (PBPs) of bacterial cell membranes and inhibit their activity. As a consequence, enzymes such as transpeptidase, carboxypeptidase, and transglycosylase are inhibited. Various strains of bacteria have different types of PBPs which may account for their differential sensitivity to antibiotics. Incubation of susceptible bacteria with β-lactam antibiotics leads to morphological abnormalities and cell death. These drugs are bactericidal. Although the mechanism leading to cell death is not completely understood, the activation of an autolytic system and the disruption of cell wall morphogenesis might be involved (▶ Fig. 29.3).

Table 29.1 β-lactam antibiotics

β-lactam antibiotics	Individual drugs
Penicillins	*Narrow spectrum:* penicillin G, penicillin V *Penicillinase resistant:* nafcillin, oxacillin, dicloxicillin *Extended spectrum:* amoxicillin, ampicillin, piperacillin
Cephalosporins	*First generation:* cefazolin, cephalexin, cefadroxil *Second generation:* cefuroxime, cefoxitin, cefotetan *Third generation:* cefotaxime, ceftriaxone, ceftazidime, cefixime, and cefpodoxime *Fourth generation:* cefepime *Advanced (fifth) generation:* ceftaroline, ceftolozane/tazobactam
Monobactams	aztreonam
Carbapenems	imipenem/cilastatin, meropenem, doripenem, ertapenem

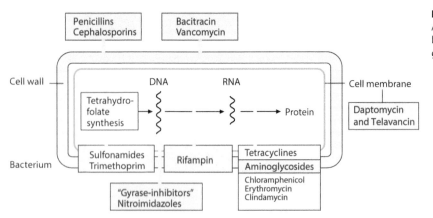

Fig. 29.1 Site of action of antibacterial agents. Antibacterial agents act at different sites in the bacterial cell to promote cell lysis or inhibition of growth.

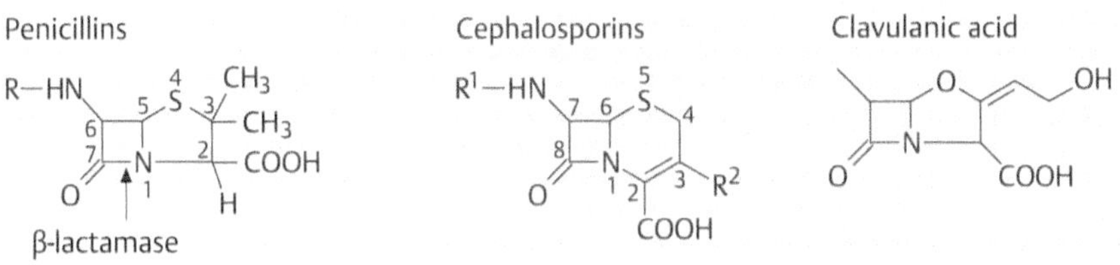

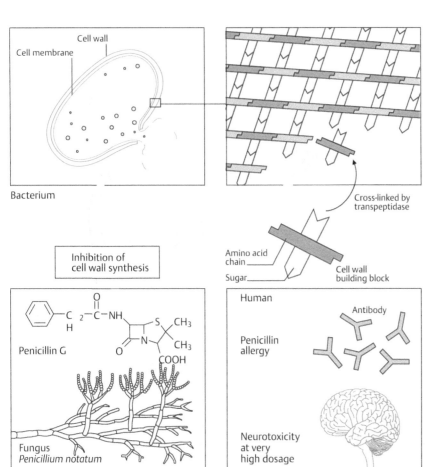

Penicillins

β-lactamase

Cephalosporins

Clavulanic acid

Fig. 29.2 Chemical structure of β-lactam antibiotics.
The structural core of the β-lactam antibiotics is shown. The arrow points to the β-lactam ring that the compounds have in common. This is also the site at which resistant bacterial strains with β-lactamase activity can cleave the β-lactam ring and inactivate the antibiotics.

Fig. 29.3 Penicillin G: structure, origin, and mechanism of action of penicillins.
Bacteria possess a cell wall composed of peptidoglycan molecules cross-linked to form a lattice. The enzyme transpeptidase is responsible for this cross-linkage. Penicillins disrupt cell wall synthesis by inhibiting transpeptidase. When bacteria are in their growth and replication phase, penicillins are bactericidal. Hypersensitivity (type I) is the most common adverse effect of penicillins.

Cell membrane

Cell wall

Bacterium

Cross-linked by transpeptidase

Inhibition of cell wall synthesis

Amino acid chain

Sugar

Cell wall building block

Penicillin G

Fungus
Penicillium notatum

Human

Antibody

Penicillin allergy

Neurotoxicity at very high dosage

Foundations

Structure of the Bacterial Cell Wall

The peptidoglycan of the bacterial cell wall is composed of alternating units of polymers N-acetylglucosamine (NAG) and N-acetylmuramic acid (NAM). The polymers contain tetrapeptides that extend from the NAM residues. A pentaglycine bridge crosslinks the tetrapeptides. In gram-positive bacteria, the cytoplasmic membrane is surrounded by a thick cell wall containing many layers of peptidoglycan and teichoic acids. In contrast, the cytoplasmic membrane of gram-negative bacteria is surrounded by a thin cell wall consisting of a few layers of peptidoglycan and an outer lipid bilayer containing polysaccharides and lipoproteins.

Foundations

Gram-Negative Cell Walls

The outer layer of gram-negative bacteria is a lipoprotein–polysaccharide complex termed *lipopolysaccharide* or *endotoxin*. This component is composed of several polysaccharides linked to lipid A. The outermost portion of lipopolysaccharide is referred to as the *O antigen* and "flaps in the wind." The lipid A moiety is responsible for the toxic portion of lipopolysaccharide. An area referred to as the *periplasmic space* is located between the cell wall and cell membrane. The "space" contains several proteins, including those that inactivate antibiotics (e.g., β-lactamase). The outer membrane of the cell wall of gram-negative microbes is not as permeable to antibiotics as is the cell wall of gram-positive organisms. Hydrophilic antibiotics are dependent on porins to gain access to the periplasmatic space.

VII

Foundations

Penicillin-Binding Proteins

The PBPs are transpeptidases and similar enzymes involved in bacterial cell wall synthesis. They were named on the basis of their ability to bind penicillin before their functional roles were discovered. A single type of bacterium may contain 3 to 10 different PBPs. PBPs are located in the cytoplasmic membrane and catalyze several reactions involved in cross-linking the peptidoglycan of the cell wall. The major activity is transpeptidase, but some also have carboxypeptidase and endopeptidase activity. They all have active sites that bind to β-lactam antibiotics.

Notes

Hypersensitivity

Hypersensitivity results from immune responses against a normally innocuous antigen. These responses fall into the following two major categories:

1. *Immediate hypersensitivity:* Type I hypersensitivity is an allergic reaction to an antigen. It is mediated by immunoglobulin E that attaches to mast cells and basophils, which degranulate upon subsequent exposure to the same antigen, releasing substances such as histamine, leukotrienes, and prostaglandins. These substances are responsible for allergic symptoms, for example, tissue swelling and itching. Type II hypersensitivity produces antibodies that bind to antigens on the surface of the patient's own cells. This activates an immune response against the antigen, for example, via the complement cascade. Alternatively, cells to which antibodies attach are killed by natural killer cells and macrophages (cytotoxicity). Type III hypersensitivity reactions occur when antigens and antibodies bind forming immune complexes. Deposition of these immune complexes in tissues (e.g., joints blood vessels, renal glomeruli) produces inflammation.

2. *Delayed-type hypersensitivity:* Type IV hypersensitivity occurs days after exposure to the antigen. In this case, the antigen forms a complex with type I or II major histocompatibility complex (MHC), which then activates cytotoxic T cells (CTLs), T helper (Th)1, and Th17 cells. Th cells secrete cytokines, triggering inflammation, and CTLs kill target cells.

Side Effects

- Hypersensitivity (allergic) reactions are the most common toxic complication. There is a small incidence (5–10%) of cross-reactivity among the penicillins and cephalosporins.
- Neurologic reactions (lethargy, confusion, and seizures) may occur with high blood and cerebrospinal fluid (CSF) levels.
- Diarrhea is a frequent nonspecific reaction of antibiotic therapy. Within the penicillins it is most common with amoxicillin and ampicillin.

Resistance

Bacteria may acquire genes (usually via plasmids) to produce β-lactamase enzymes (e.g., penicillinase), which open the β-lactam ring and destroy the activity of the antibiotic (▶ Fig. 29.4).

Natural Penicillins

Penicillin G and Penicillin V

Spectrum

- Narrow (mainly gram-positive organisms).
- Effective against *Streptococcus pyogenes, Streptococcus pneumoniae, Streptococcus viridans, Listeria monocytogenes, Treponema pallidum, Neisseria meningitides,* and *Enterococcus faecalis.*
- Penicillin G is the treatment of choice for all stages of syphilis.

Pharmacokinetics

- Penicillin G should be given parenterally because oral absorption is erratic due to instability in gastric acid.

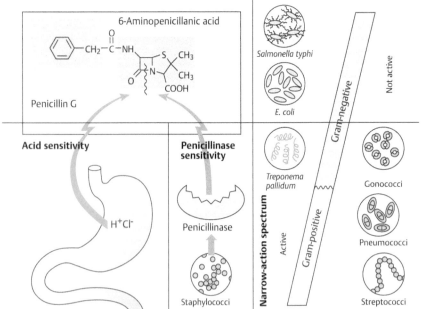

Fig. 29.4 Disadvantages of penicillin G. Penicillin G is inactivated by gastric acid, which cleaves the β-lactam ring. This can be circumvented by parenteral administration of the drug. The β-lactam ring is also opened by β-lactamases (e.g., penicillinase), which are produced by some staphylococcal strains rendering them resistant to penicillins. Penicillin G has a narrow spectrum of action. It is active against many gram-positive bacteria, gram-negative cocci, and spirochetes but is inactive against most gram-negative pathogens.

- Penicillin G benzathine and penicillin G procaine are long-acting forms for intramuscular injection.
- Penicillin V is acid stable and can be given orally (▶ Fig. 29.5).
- Neither penicillin G nor penicillin V penetrates CSF.

Uses

- Treatment of streptococcal pharyngitis.
- Treatment of syphilis.
- Treatment of infections with penicillin-susceptible strains of *Listeria*, *Streptococcus*, and *Enterococcus*.

Penicillinase-Resistant Penicillins (Also Known as Anti-Staphylococcal Penicillins)

Oxacillin, Dicloxacillin, and Nafcillin

- *Parenteral agents:* oxacillin, nafcillin.
- *Oral agent:* dicloxacillin.

Spectrum

- Very narrow (mainly gram-positive organisms that produce penicillinase; ▶ Fig. 29.5).
- Effective against methicillin-sensitive *Staphylococcus aureus* (MSSA), *S. pyogenes*, *S. pneumoniae*.

Uses

Treatment of *S. aureus* (MSSA) infections (endocarditis, osteomyelitis).

Clinical Correlation

Endocarditis

Endocarditis is an infection of the endocardium of the heart. It occurs when bacteria from any source, for example, dental procedures or periodontal tissues, gain entry to the blood and colonize the heart valves causing "vegetations." This is more likely to occur with damaged or artificial heart valves. Causative bacteria include *S. viridans*, *E. faecalis*, and *S. aureus*. Symptoms include fever, changing heart murmur, fatigue, weight loss, night sweats, hematuria, and splenomegaly (enlarged spleen). Complications of endocarditis include stroke (from embolic vegetations), heart failure, renal failure, and abscesses. Treatment involves an extended course (4–6 weeks) of IV antibiotic therapy, the choice of which is directed by blood culture of the causative bacteria.

Clinical Correlation

Methicillin-Resistant *Staphylococcus aureus*

Methicillin-resistant *S. aureus* (MRSA) is an infection caused by *S. aureus* exposure that is resistant to treatment by β-lactam antibiotics (e.g., oxacillin, penicillin, and amoxicillin). It mostly occurs in hospitals (nosocomial) and other treatment centers. It tends to affect people with weakened immune systems. Staphylococcal infections, including MRSA, usually start with a boil on the skin, which can progress to form deep abscesses that enable the bacteria to penetrate into the bloodstream and bone. Treatment involves surgical drainage of abscesses and vancomycin therapy.

Aminopenicillins

Ampicillin and Amoxicillin

Spectrum

- Extended spectrum.
- These agents are active against some important gram-positive (e.g., *S. pneumoniae*, *S. pyogenes*, *E. faecalis*) and gram-negative pathogens (e.g., *Haemophilus influenzae*).
- When combined with a β-lactamase inhibitor, they are also active against MSSA and more gram-negative bacteria such as *Proteus mirabilis*, *Escherichia coli*, *Klebsiella*, and *H. influenzae*). In addition, they can be used for the anaerobic bacteria *Bacteroides fragilis*.

Pharmacokinetics

Normally, these agents do not penetrate CSF, but they may penetrate CSF if the meninges are inflamed. Ampicillin penetrates CSF in neonates with meningitis.

Uses

Ampicillin is used for treatment of enterococcus infections. Amoxicillin is used for treatment of the following:

- Uncomplicated upper respiratory infections (e.g., pharyngitis, sinusitis, otitis media).
- Lower respiratory infections (acute exacerbations of chronic bronchitis and pneumonia)
- Treatment of *Helicobacter pylori* infections (part of the triple therapy including clarithromycin and a proton pump inhibitor).

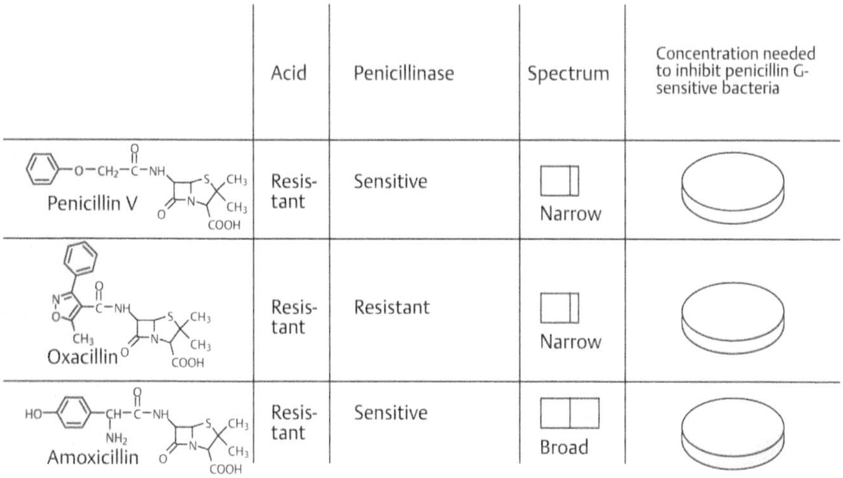

VII

	Acid	Penicillinase	Spectrum	Concentration needed to inhibit penicillin G-sensitive bacteria
Penicillin V	Resistant	Sensitive	Narrow	
Oxacillin	Resistant	Resistant	Narrow	
Amoxicillin	Resistant	Sensitive	Broad	

Fig. 29.5 Derivatives of penicillin G.
The derivatives of penicillin G have some advantages over their predecessor. Penicillin V has similar antibacterial properties to penicillin G but is stable in gastric acid and so can be given orally (as can the other derivatives shown). Oxicillin is one of the penicillins that are penicillinase resistant and is therefore useful in treating penicillinase-producing staphylococci infections. Amoxicillin has a broader spectrum of action than penicillin G, as it is active against more gram-negative pathogens.

Antipseudomonal Penicillins

Piperacillin/Tazobactam

Spectrum

- Broad
- These agents are active against a variety of gram-positive (e.g., *S. pneumoniae, S. pyogenes, E. faecalis, MSSA*) and gram-negative pathogens (e.g., *P. mirabilis, E. coli, Klebsiella, Enterobacter, Serratia, H. influenzae,* and *Pseudomonas*).

Pharmacokinetics

Piperacillin penetrates CSF, particularly when the meninges are inflamed, but it is not used for meningitis.

Uses

- Treatment of nosocomial infections (e.g., pneumonia, intra-abdominal infections, and urinary tract infection [UTI]).
- Treatment of neutropenic fever.

Clinical Correlation

Otitis Media

Otitis media is a bacterial or viral infection of the middle ear, usually in children. It tends to occur following an upper respiratory tract infection, such as the common cold, which causes congestion and swelling of the nasal passages, throat, and eustachian tubes. Blockage of the eustachian tubes causes fluid accumulation in the middle ear. Symptoms include ear pain, hearing deficits, purulent discharge from the ear, balance problems, headache, loss of appetite, vomiting, and diarrhea. Otitis media is usually self-resolving in 1 to 2 weeks, so no treatment may be indicated. Nonsteroidal anti-inflammatory drugs may be taken for ear pain. Amoxicillin is usually the antibiotic of choice when antibiotics are indicated.

Clinical Correlation

Antibiotic Penetration into Cerebrospinal Fluid

The ability of antibiotics to enter the brain depends on their plasma protein binding properties, molecular size, lipid solubility, and degree of local inflammation. Penetration is greater for small, nonprotein-bound, lipid-soluble drugs. Drug penetration is also enhanced if the meninges are inflamed. Penicillin G, ampicillin, cefuroxime, ceftriaxone, cefotaxime, and metronidazole are useful in meningitis and brain abscesses.

29.2.2 Cephalosporins

Mechanism of Action

Same as for penicillins.

Side Effects

Like the penicillins, cephalosporins are relatively free of severe adverse reactions. The most common adverse effects are hypersensitivity reactions, most commonly observed as a maculo-papular rash after several days of therapy. Specific side effects of certain cephalosporins are discussed within the different generations.

First-Generation Cephalosporins

Cefazolin, Cephalexin, and Cefadroxil

- Parenteral agents: cefazolin.
- Oral agents: cephalexin and cefadroxil.

Spectrum

- First-generation cephalosporins are effective against many gram-positive cocci (*S. pneumoniae, S. pyogenes,* MSSA) and some gram-negative pathogens (e.g., *P. mirabilis, E. coli, Klebsiella*).
- These agents are all susceptible to β-lactamase inactivation and are not effective for infections due to enterococci or MRSA (▶ Table 29.2).

Pharmacokinetics

- Cefazolin has the longest half-life, reaches the highest plasma levels after injection, and is least irritating of the parenteral agents, making it the best choice for intramuscular injection.
- These agents do not penetrate the CSF and cannot be used to treat meningitis.

Uses

- Simple skin and soft tissue infections.
- MSSA infection (endocarditis, osteomyelitis).
- Surgical prophylaxis.

Second-Generation Cephalosporins

Cefuroxime, Cefoxitin, and Cefotetan

- *Parenteral agents:* cefuroxime, cefoxitin, and cefotetan.
- *Oral agent:* cefuroxime.

Spectrum

- The second-generation cephalosporins retain some activity against gram-positive bacteria (*S. pneumoniae, S. pyogenes,* MSSA) and have a greater activity against gram-negative organisms, especially *H. influenza, P. mirabilis, E. coli, Klebsiella, Enterobacter,* and *Serratia.*
- They are also more resistant to β-lactamase. However, first-generation agents are preferred for most gram-positive indications, and third-generation agents are usually more active against gram-negative pathogens.
- Cefoxitin and cefotetan have additional activity against anaerobic bacteria.

Pharmacokinetics

Cefuroxime is the only second-generation agent that penetrates the CSF.

Uses

- Treatment of upper and lower respiratory tract infections.
- Treatment of UTIs.

Table 29.2 Summary of the treatment of microorganisms

Microorganisms	Primary antimicrobial drugs	Secondary antimicrobial drugs
Gram-positive cocci		
Staphylococcus aureus or *S. epidermidis*	Penicillinase-resistant penicillins: Nafcillin, oxacillin, dicloxicillin	Vancomycin
Enterococcus faecalis	Ampicillin ± gentamicin	Vancomycin ± gentamycin
Streptococcus pyogenes	Penicillin G or penicillin V	Clindamycin or macrolide
Streptococcus pneumonia	Ceftriaxone or ampicillin	Macrolide or doxycycline
Gram-positive bacilli		
Bacillus anthracis	Fluoroquinolone	
Listeria monocytogenes	Ampicillin ± gentamicin	
Gram-negative cocci		
Neisseria gonorrhoeae	Ceftriaxone	
N. meningitides	Penicillin G	
Gram-negative bacilli		
Enterobacteriaceae		
Escherichia coli	Third-generation cephalosporin	
Yersinia pestis	Streptomycin	
Proteus mirabilis	Ampicillin	
P. vulgaris	Third-generation cephalosporin	
Salmonella typhi	Ceftriaxone or a fluoroquinolone	
Shigella	Fluoroquinolone	
Enterobacter	Trimethoprim-sulfamethoxazole	
Klebsiella pneumoniae	Third-generation cephalosporin	
Campylobacter jejuni	Fluoroquinolone or erythromycin	
Legionella	Fluoroquinolone	
Vibrio cholera	Macrolides, fluoroquinolones, or tetracyclines	
Helicobacter pylori	Amoxicillin + clarithromycin + omeprazole or tetracycline + metronidazole + bismuth subsalicylate + omeprazole	
Anaerobes		
Bacteroides fragilis	Metronidazole	
Clostridium difficile	Metronidazole or vancomycin	
Miscellaneous		
Mycobacterium tuberculosis	Isoniazid + rifampin + pyrazinamide ± ethambutol	
Mycobacterium leprae	Dapsone + rifampin	
Spirochetes		
Treponema pallidum	Penicillin G	
Leptospira	Doxycycline	
Borrelia burgdorferi	Doxycycline	
Mycoplasma pneumoniae	Macrolide or fluoroquinolone	
Chlamydia trachomatis	Doxycycline	
Chlamydia pneumoniae	Doxycycline	
Rickettsia	Doxycycline	

- Surgical prophylaxis.
- Treatment of uncomplicated gonorrhea.

Side Effects

- Concurrent use of ethanol with cephalosporins that contain a methyltetrazolethiol side chain (cefotetan) may result in a disulfiram-like reaction, including flushing, tachycardia, headache, sweating, thirst, nausea, and vomiting, due to inhibition of acetaldehyde metabolism.
- Competitive inhibition between the methyltetrazolethiol group and vitamin K-dependent carboxylase, which is responsible for converting clotting factors II, VII, IX, and X to their active forms, may lead to hypoprothrombinemia (low blood prothrombin levels). The reaction is preventable and reversible by supplementing vitamin K.

Third-Generation Cephalosporins

Cefotaxime, Ceftriaxone, Ceftazidime, Cefixime, and Cefpodoxime

- *Parenteral agents:* cefotaxime, ceftriaxone, ceftazidime, and cefixime.
- *Oral agents:* cefixime, cefpodoxime.

Spectrum

- Third-generation cephalosporins are less active than first-generation agents against gram-positive organisms (e.g., *S. pneumoniae, S. pyogenes,* MSSA) but have further increased activity against gram-negative organisms including *H. influenza, P. mirabilis, E. coli, Klebsiella, Enterobacter,* and *Serratia.*
- All third-generation cephalosporins are resistant to hydrolysis by β-lactamases.
- Their activity is variable against anaerobes (e.g., *B. fragilis*).
- Ceftazidime has antipseudomonal activity.

Clinical Correlation

Meningitis

Meningitis is an inflammation of the meninges of the brain (pia mater and arachnoid), usually due to a viral infection but can also be caused by a bacterial or fungal infection. Symptoms include headache, stiff neck on passively moving chin toward chest, photophobia (sensitivity to light), irritability, drowsiness, vomiting, fever, seizures, and rashes (viral or meningococcal meningitis). Predisposing factors for meningitis include head injury (especially basal skull fracture), otitis media, sinusitis, mastoiditis, and a compromised immune system (e.g., carcinoma, HIV infection, diabetes, splenectomy, or immunosuppressant drugs). A lumbar puncture often provides a definitive diagnosis of meningitis. Empiric treatment with a broad-spectrum antibiotic is required for bacterial meningitis. For viral meningitis, treatment includes bed rest and fluids, but this normally resolves on its own in a week or two.

Pharmacokinetics

- Penetration into CSF (ceftazidime, ceftriaxone, and cefotaxime).
- Long half-life (ceftriaxone).
- Eliminated via the bile (ceftriaxone).

VII

Uses

- Treatment of community-acquired meningitis (ceftriaxone, first-line drug).
- Treatment of community-acquired pneumonia (ceftriaxone and cefotaxime).
- Treatment of hospital-acquired pneumonia (ceftazidime).
- Treatment of gonorrhea (ceftriaxone).
- Treatment of UTIs (ceftriaxone, cefotaxime, and ceftazidime).

Fourth-Generation Cephalosporins

Cefepime

Spectrum

- Cefepime is an extended-spectrum agent that has a similar spectrum of activity to third-generation cephalosporins; however, it also has excellent activity against *Pseudomonas aeruginosa*.
- It also exhibits activity against some anaerobes (*Clostridium* spp.) and has greater resistance to β-lactamases than third-generation cephalosporins.

Spectrum

- Treatment of community-acquired and nosocomial pneumonia.
- Treatment of UTIs.
- Treatment of meningitis.
- Treatment of neutropenic fever.

Advanced Generation of Cephalosporins

Ceftaroline

Spectrum

- Ceftaroline is an advanced (or fifth) generation cephalosporine that was developed to treat resistant gram-positive infections including MRSA and multi-drug resistant pneumococcus.
- Similar activity as third-generation cephalosporins, but no activity against *P. aeruginosa* and anaerobes.

Uses

- Treatment of skin and skin structure infections (including MRSA).
- Treatment of community-acquired pneumonia.

Ceftolozane/Tazobactam

Spectrum

- Ceftolozane/tazobactam is an advanced (or fifth) generation cephalosporine that was developed to treat resistant gram-negative infections including bacteria that produce extended spectrum beta-lactamases (ESBL) and AmpC beta-lactamases (AMPCES), and *P. aeruginosa* infections.
- Minimal activity against gram-positive organisms and anaerobes.

Uses

- Treatment of complicated UTIs and pyelonephritis.
- Treatment of complicated intra-abdominal infections.
- Treatment of hospital-acquired pneumonia.

29.2.3 Monobactams

Aztreonam

Mechanism of Action

Same as for penicillins.

Spectrum

- Narrow.
- Mainly active against gram-negative aerobes, including *H. influenza, P. mirabilis, E. coli, Klebsiella, Enterobacter, Serratia*, and *P. aeruginosa*.
- It is highly stable to β lactamases.
- Limited cross-reactivity with other β-lactam antibiotics and is generally considered safe to administer to patients with a penicillin allergy.

29.2.4 Carbapenems

Imipenem/cilastin, Meropenem, Doripenem, and Ertapenem

Mechanism of Action

- Same as for penicillins.
- Cilastatin prevents renal enzymes from breaking down imipenem and prolongs its effects.

Spectrum

- Broadest spectrum of all β-lactam antibiotics.
- Activity against most gram-positive and gram-negative organisms, including anaerobes.
- Ertapenem has no activity against pseudomonas.

Pharmacokinetics

- All carbapenems are administered systemically.
- Imipenem is metabolized by a renal peptidase. To circumvent this, cilastatin, a specific inhibitor of the renal enzyme, is administered with imipenem. Cilastatin also prevents renal toxicity sometimes observed with imipenem alone.
- Penetration into CSF is highly variable. It is not used for meningitis.

Uses

Used to treat serious infections in which a mixture of gram-positive, gram-negative, and anaerobic bacteria may be involved.

Resistance

Resistance can develop to these agents, especially in *Pseudomonas* species.

Side Effects

Like other β-lactam antibiotics, carbapenems have a low incidence of serious adverse reactions, but imipenem may trigger seizures.

29.3 β-Lactamase Inhibitors

Many bacteria produce β-lactamase enzymes (e.g., penicillinase) that open the β-lactam ring and destroy the activity of the antibiotic. To combat this, β-lactamase inhibitors can be combined with β-lactam antibiotics (amoxicillin and piperacillin) to further extend their usefulness. Many cephalosporins are resistant to β-lactamase enzymes.

29.3.1 Clavulanic Acid

Mechanism of Action

- Clavulanic acid is an irreversible inhibitor of many bacterial β-lactamases.
- It is marketed in combination with amoxicillin.

29.3.2 Sulbactam and Tazobactam

The properties of these drugs are similar to clavulanic acid.
- Sulbactam is marketed in combination with ampicillin.
- Tazobactam is marketed in combination with piperacillin and ceftolozane.

29.3.3 Glycopeptide Antibiotic

Vancomycin

Mechanism of Action

Vancomycin binds to the terminal D-alanine-D-alanyl peptide portion of the peptidoglycan precursor and inhibits bacterial cell wall synthesis. This is at a different step from β-lactam antibiotics. Bacterial autolysins subsequently cause cell wall lysis. Vancomycin is usually bactericidal.

Spectrum

- Active only against gram-positive bacteria (e.g., *S. pneumoniae*, *S. pyogenes*, MSSA, MRSA, and *E. faecalis*).

Pharmacokinetics

- Oral vancomycin is not absorbed (used for *Clostridium difficile* infections).
- When given intravenously, it must be administered slowly as a dilute solution to minimize thrombophlebitis, as well as flushing reactions associated with histamine release.
- Vancomycin is able to penetrate CSF in the presence of inflammation.

Uses

- Treatment of skin and soft tissue infections.
- Treatment of sepsis.
- Treatment of severe MRSA infections.
- Treatment of *C. difficile* infections.

Clinical Correlation

Antibiotic-Associated Pseudomembranous Colitis

Pseudomembranous colitis is an inflammation of the colon due to superinfection with *C. difficile*, a gram-positive bacillus. It typically occurs following a course of antibiotic treatment in which the normal gut commensal bacteria are eradicated, allowing *C. difficile* to colonize the gut unimpeded. The most common antibiotics that cause this condition are the penicillins, cephalosporins, fluoroquinolones, and clindamycin. Symptoms of pseudomembranous colitis include diarrhea, fever, and abdominal pain. It is treated with metronidazole or vancomycin.

Clinical Correlation

Necrotizing Fasciitis

Necrotizing fasciitis is a rare infection that penetrates into deeper layers of the skin and subcutaneous tissue and is able to spread along fascial planes. It can be caused by a variety of bacteria, including group A streptococci, *S. aureus*, *Clostridium perfringens*, and *B. fragilis*. Signs and symptoms include intense pain, signs of inflammation (although these may be absent if the infection is in deep tissues), diarrhea, vomiting, and fever. The skin will blister and undergo necrosis. Treatment for this condition involves giving antibiotics such as penicillin, vancomycin, or clindamycin early in the process, often before the diagnosis has been confirmed. Necrotic tissue will require surgical debridement or amputation.

Foundations

Protein Synthesis

The first stage in protein synthesis involves unzipping of the DNA double helix by RNA polymerase, followed by transcription of DNA to messenger RNA (mRNA). This process occurs in the nucleus. mRNA (codon) migrates into the cytoplasm and attaches to a ribosome. Translation of mRNA into a protein occurs when transfer RNA (tRNA) and its accompanying amino acid bind to mRNA by forming complementary base pairs (anticodon). The amino acids join to form a polypeptide chain. Protein synthesis is stopped when a termination codon is translated, and the polypeptide chain is released from the ribosome.

29.4 Other Inhibitors of Cell Wall Synthesis

29.4.1 Bacitracin

Mechanism of Action

Bacitracin is a polypeptide antibiotic that inhibits the formation of bacterial cell walls. It interferes with the dephosphorylation step in the lipid carrier that transfers peptidoglycan subunits to the growing cell wall.

Spectrum

Active against gram-positive organisms.

Pharmacokinetics

This agent is not absorbed after oral administration. It is administered topically and systemically.

Uses

- Topical treatment of gram-positive infections on the skin or in the eye.
- Renal toxicity limits its usefulness to topical application, but it may be used in infants with staphylococcal pneumonia and empyema that are resistant to safer antibiotics.

Side Effects

Renal toxicity when given systemically.

29.5 Cell Membrane Active Agents

29.5.1 Daptomycin

Mechanism of Action

Daptomycin interferes with the inner membrane and creates channels through which bacterial electrolytes leak, leading to membrane depolarization. This is followed by arrest of DNA, RNA, and protein synthesis, resulting in cell death.

Spectrum

Active against a variety of gram-positive organisms including *S. pneumoniae*, *S. pyogenes*, MSSA, MRSA, *E. faecalis*, and *Enterococcus faecium*.

Uses

- Treatment of skin and soft tissue infections (particularly with MRSA).
- Treatment of serious MRSA infections (e.g., endocarditis and osteomyelitis).
- Not used in pneumonia as daptomycin is inactivated by pulmonary surfactant.

Side Effects

- Musculoskeletal effects such as muscle pain and muscle weakness (weekly monitoring of creatine phosphokinase is recommended).

29.5.2 Telavancin

Mechanism of Action

Telavancin has a dual mechanism of action and inhibits cell wall synthesis (by binding to D-Ala-D-Ala and preventing the cross-linking) and also interferes with the inner cell membrane similar to daptomycin.

Spectrum

- Developed for the treatment of gram-positive organisms including MRSA, multi-drug resistant *pneumococcus*, and vancomycin-resistant *enterococcus (VRE)*.
- No activity against gram-negative organisms and anaerobes.

Uses

- Treatment of skin and skin structure infections.
- Treatment of nosocomial pneumonia.

Side Effects

- Nephrotoxic.
- Teratogenic.

29.6 Inhibitors of Protein Synthesis

These agents inhibit bacterial protein synthesis. They exhibit selective toxicity for bacterial cells by binding to bacterial ribosomal subunits (50S and 30S), which differ in structure from the mammalian ribosomal subunits (60S and 40S).

29.6.1 Macrolide Antibiotics

Macrolide antibiotics are characterized by the presence of a 14- or 15-member lactone ring. Erythromycin is the prototype of these antibiotics, but newer macrolides possess improved pharmacokinetic properties and modest changes in the antibacterial spectrum.

Mechanism of Action

Macrolides bind to the P site of the 50S bacterial ribosomal subunit. They block protein synthesis when a large amino acid or a polypeptide is in the P site (▶ Fig. 29.6).

Erythromycin, Azithromycin, Clarithromycin, and Telithromycin

Spectrum

- Narrow-spectrum agents.
- Active against gram-positive bacteria (*S. pneumoniae*, *S. pyogenes*).
- Active against pathogens causing atypical pneumonia: *Legionella pneumonia*, *Chlamydia* spp., *Mycoplasma pneumonia*, and *Mycobacterium avium* (MAC) infection.
- Telithromycin was developed to overcome resistance issues and has increased activity to *S. pneumonia* (compared to other macrolide antibiotics).

Pharmacokinetics

- Oral absorption is variable (erythromycin is destroyed by stomach acid; therefore, enteric coating is necessary).
- Wide tissue distribution, but poor penetration into CSF.
- Primarily hepatic and biliary elimination (exception is clarithromycin, mainly renally eliminated).

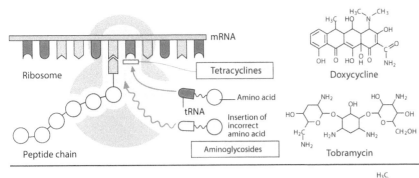

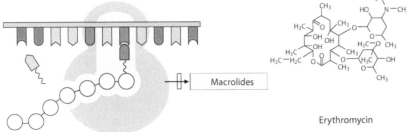

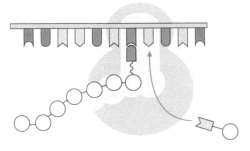

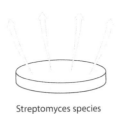

Streptomyces species

Fig. 29.6 Protein synthesis and modes of action of antibacterial drugs.

Protein synthesis involves the translation of genetic sequences in messenger RNA (mRNA), transcribed from DNA. Peptide synthesis occurs in the ribosome, where transfer RNA (tRNA) delivers amino acids to mRNA. Adjacent amino acids are linked into a peptide chain by the enzyme peptidyltransferase. Tetracyclines inhibit the binding of amino acyl-tRNA complexes and have a bacteriostatic effect. They have a broad spectrum of action. Aminoglycosides induce the binding of wrong amino acyl-tRNA complexes, resulting in the synthesis of false proteins. These agents are bactericidal and act mainly against gram-negative pathogens. Macrolides prevent the ribosome from moving along the mRNA to "read" it. They are bacteriostatic against mainly gram-positive pathogens.

Uses

- Treatment of community-acquired pneumonia.
- Treatment of gonorrhea.
- Treatment of *M. avium* complex infection.

Side Effects

- Gastrointestinal (GI) adverse effects (mainly with erythromycin as it acts as a motilin receptor agonist in the GI tract).
- Cholestatic jaundice.
- QT prolongation.

Resistance

- Develops rapidly.
- Most common mechanism involves the methylation of 50S bases in ribosomal RNA. The methylated rRNA remains active in protein synthesis, but no longer binds the drug.

29.6.2 Lincosamides

Clindamycin

Mechanism of Action

Clindamycin attaches to the 50S ribosomal subunit at or near the macrolide attachment site.

Spectrum

- Narrow.
- Active against a variety of gram-positive bacteria including *S. pneumoniae*, *S. pyogenes*, MSSA, and MRSA.
- Excellent activity against anaerobic bacteria including *B. fragilis*.

Pharmacokinetics

- Orally well absorbed.
- Wide tissue distribution in the body, no significant concentrations in CSF.
- Concentration in bone has high clinical value (osteomyelitis).
- Metabolized extensively and excreted primarily in bile and feces.

Clinical Correlation

Jaundice

Jaundice refers to the yellow pigmentation of the skin, sclerae, and mucous membranes due to raised plasma bilirubin.

Prehepatic (or hemolytic) jaundice: Excess bilirubin (e.g., from hemolysis) or an inborn failure of bilirubin metabolism results in unconjugated bilirubin remaining in the bloodstream.

Unconjugated bilirubin is water-insoluble and so does not appear in urine.

Hepatocellular (or hepatic) jaundice: In hepatocellular jaundice, there is diminished hepatocyte function leading to an increased amount of both conjugated and unconjugated bilirubin. Diminished hepatocyte function may follow cirrhosis, autoimmune diseases, drug damage (e.g., acetaminophen, barbiturates), or viral infections (e.g., hepatitis A, B, C; Epstein–Barr virus).

Posthepatic (obstructive) jaundice: This form of jaundice usually occurs following blockade of the common bile duct by gallstones. In this case, plasma conjugated bilirubin rises. Conjugated bilirubin is water-soluble and appears in urine (making it dark). At the same time, less conjugated bilirubin passes into the gut and is converted to stercobilin; therefore, feces appear paler.

Uses

- Treatment of skin and skin structure infection.
- Treatment of intra-abdominal infections (e.g., peritonitis, intra-abdominal abscesses) and gynecologic infections.
- Treatment of sepsis and anaerobic infections.

Side Effects

- Diarrhea is the most common adverse effect. Clindamycin is the antibiotic that most frequently causes antibiotic-associated pseudomembranous colitis.
- Skin rashes and reversible changes in hepatic enzymes in serum may also occur.

29.6.3 Tetracyclines

Tetracycline, Doxycycline, Minocycline, and Tigecycline

Mechanism of Action

Tetracyclines preferentially bind to the 30S subunit of the microbial ribosome, interfere with binding of amino acyl-tRNA, and inhibit chain termination (▶ Fig. 29.6). Tetracyclines are usually bacteriostatic.

Spectrum

- Broad spectrum.
- Effective against a variety of gram-positive (e.g., *S. pneumoniae*, MSSA, MRSA) and gram-negative bacteria (e.g., *H. influenza*).
- Tigecycline is also active against additional gram-positive (e.g., *E. faecalis* and *E. faecium*) and gram-negative bacteria (e.g., *H. influenza, P. mirabilis, E. coli, Klebsiella, Enterobacter,* and *Serratia*)
- Also active against *Moraxella catarrhalis, Chlamydia trachomatis, Borrelia, Rickettsia, H. pylori,* and *Plasmodium* spp.

Pharmacokinetics

- Well absorbed after oral administration.
- Absorption is delayed by food, calcium salts, and aluminum salts (▶ Fig. 29.7).

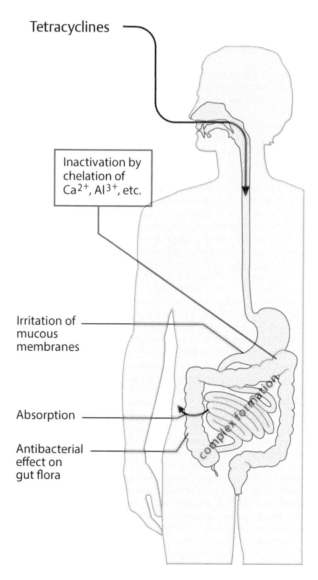

Fig. 29.7 Aspects of the therapeutic use of tetracyclines. Tetracyclines are absorbed to varying degrees in the gastrointestinal (GI) tract. They tend to cause irritation to mucous membranes, and they alter the natural flora of the gut, which allows pathogenic bacteria to proliferate. These factors account for the GI upset that often accompanies tetracycline use. Tetracyclines also form insoluble complexes with cations, such as Ca^{2+} and Al^{3+}, which causes them to be unable to be absorbed, to be unable to exert their antibacterial effects, and to lose their irritant properties.

- Wide tissue distribution.
- Doxycycline and tigecycline (in contrast to other tetracyclines) are eliminated by nonrenal mechanisms.
- No penetration into CSF.

Uses

- Treatment of community-acquired pneumonia.
- Treatment of skin and skin structure infections.
- Treatment of rickettsial infections, chlamydial infections, sexually transmitted diseases, acne, and brucellosis.
- Malaria prophylaxis.

Side Effects

- Allergic reactions including rash, urticaria, and anaphylaxis.
- Tooth enamel dysplasia.
- Irregularities in bone growth.
- GI distress.
- Altering normal GI flora → superinfection with *C. difficile.*
- Phototoxicity.
- Avoid in pregnancy due to discoloration of teeth and interference with skeletal growth.

Clinical Correlation

Tetracycline Staining of Teeth

Tetracycline that is ingested is incorporated into developing enamel, causing intrinsic tooth discoloration. It appears as a yellow-brown band on the teeth that were forming at the time of the tetracycline therapy. It is not harmful to teeth but is unsightly and typically camouflaged by porcelain veneers.

Clinical Correlation

Cholera

Cholera is an infectious disease caused by *Vibrio cholerae*, a gram-negative bacteria. It is spread via the fecal–oral route. *V. cholerae* toxin increases cAMP concentrations in intestinal mucosal cells, causing the opening of Cl⁻ channels and massive secretion of Cl⁻. This results in the production of a profuse amount of watery diarrhea which causes severe dehydration. This can lead to kidney failure, shock, coma, and death. Treatment requires rapid replacement of lost body fluids with oral or IV solutions containing salts and sugar. Tetracycline reduces fluid loss and diminishes transmission of the bacteria.

29.6.4 Aminoglycosides

Streptomycin, Tobramycin, Gentamicin, and Amikacin

Mechanism of Action

All aminoglycosides inhibit bacterial protein synthesis. The initial binding step involves binding to negatively charged phosphates in LPS and a "cracking" of the membrane that results in membrane damage. Aminoglycosides are actively transported across the cell membrane in an oxygen-dependent process. Inside the cell, they inhibit the formation of the initiation complex on 30S subunit. This leads to misreading of mRNA and the incorporation of wrong amino acids into the peptide. As a consequence, nonfunctional or toxic proteins are accumulating (► Fig. 29.6). These agents are bactericidal.

Spectrum

- Narrow spectrum.
- As monotherapy these are only active against gram-negative bacteria.
- When combined with a cell-wall-active agent, they may provide synergistic killing of gram-positive organisms.

- Because aminoglycosides are actively transported into a bacterial cell by an oxygen-dependent enzyme system, only aerobic bacteria are sensitive to these drugs.

Pharmacokinetics

- Aminoglycosides are not absorbed from the GI tract but are readily absorbed from intramuscular or subcutaneous sites (► Fig. 29.8).
- They are distributed to extracellular water, but penetrate CSF poorly, even when the meninges are inflamed.
- They are excreted in the urine after glomerular filtration of the parent compound.

Uses

- Treatment of serious systemic infections including UTI pyelonephritis, pneumonia, bacteremia, septicemia, bone and joint infections due to gram-negative pathogens.
- Combined with a cell-wall-active agent: treatment for severe infection due to a gram-positive pathogen (e.g., endocarditis).

Side Effects

- Renal toxicity.
- Ototoxicity (agents may damage both vestibular and auditory functions of the vestibulocochlear nerve).
- Allergic reactions occasionally occur.

29.7 Other Inhibitors of Protein Synthesis

29.7.1 Oxazolidinones

Linezolid and Tedizolid

Mechanism of Action

Linezolid inhibits protein synthesis by binding to the 50S subunit and preventing the formation of the ribosome complex that initiates protein synthesis.

Spectrum

- Narrow spectrum.
- Effective against most gram-positive bacteria including, e.g., *S. pneumoniae, S. pyogenes*, MSSA, MRSA, *E. faecalis*, and *E. faecium.*
- No activity against gram-negative organisms and most anaerobes.

Pharmacokinetics

- Linezolid and tedizolid are well absorbed after oral administration and can be administered orally and systemically.
- These agents are widely distributed including penetration into CSF.

Uses

- Treatment of community acquired and hospital acquired pneumonia.
- Treatment of skin and skin structure infections.
- Treatment of serious MRSA and VRE infections.

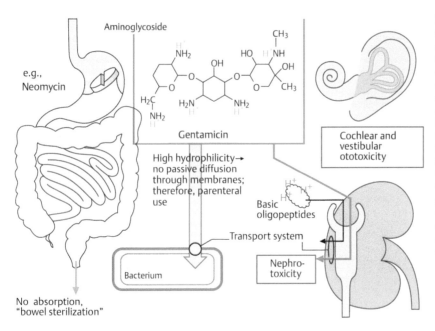

Fig. 29.8 Aspects of the therapeutic use of aminoglycosides.
Aminoglycosides consist of glycoside-linked amino sugars. They contain numerous hydroxyl and amino groups that can bind protons; hence, they are highly polar. This renders them unable to diffuse through membranes, and thus unable to be adsorbed enterally. This lack of absorption is used by giving neomycin orally to eradicate intestinal bacteria (e.g., prior to bowel surgery) or to reduce NH_3 formation by gut bacteria in hepatic coma. Otherwise, aminoglycosides are given by injection for serious infections. Aminoglycosides gain access to the bacterial interior via bacterial transport systems. In the kidney, they enter the proximal tubule via an uptake system for oligopeptides and cause damage to tubular cells. They can also cause damage to the vestibular apparatus and organ of Corti in the ear.

Side Effects

- GI adverse effects.
- Mitochondrial toxicities including hematologic effects (neutropenia, anemia, thrombocytopenia), peripheral neuropathy, and lactic acidosis.

Interactions

- Inhibit monoamine oxidase (MAO): risk of serotonin syndrome when used together with other serotonergic drugs (e.g., SSRIs, TCAs, or triptans).

Clinical Correlation

Notifiable Diseases

Certain diseases must be reported by clinicians to the National Notifiable Diseases Surveillance System (NNDSS), operated by the Centers for Disease Control and Prevention (CDC). Examples of such diseases are human immunodeficiency virus/acquired immunodeficiency syndrome (HIV/AIDS), measles, mumps, pertussis, hepatitis C, meningococcal disease, typhoid fever, TB, polio, rubella, malaria, syphilis, and gonorrhea.

29.7.2 Streptogramins

Quinupristin/Dalfopristin

Mechanism of Action

The streptogramins quinupristin/dalfopristin act synergistically. They share the same ribosomal binding site as clindamycin and the macrolides and therefore inhibit protein synthesis in a similar manner. The drug seems to be bactericidal for some pathogens (e.g., *Staphylococcus* spp. and *Streptococcus* spp.) and bacteriostatic for others (e.g., *Enterococcus* spp.).

Spectrum

- Narrow spectrum.
- Effective against many gram-positive bacteria including, e.g., *S. pneumoniae, S. pyogenes,* MSSA, MRSA, *E. faecium).*
- No activity against *E. faecalis.*
- No activity against gram-negative organisms and most anaerobes.

Pharmacokinetics

- Quinupristin/dalfopristin are not absorbed orally and can be only given systemically.
- No penetration into CSF.

Uses

- Treatment of skin and skin structure infections.
- Treatment of MRSA and VRE infections.

Side Effects

- Pain at the infusion site.
- Musculoskeletal adverse effects: arthralgias/myalgias.

Interactions

Major CYP450 interactions as quinupristin/dalfopristin are potent CYP450 inhibitors.

29.8 Inhibitors of Nucleic Acid Metabolism

29.8.1 Gyrase Inhibitors: Fluoroquinolones (Quinolones)

Ciprofloxacin, Gemifloxacin, Levofloxacin, Moxifloxacin, and Ofloxacin

Fluoroquinolones are chemically derived from the urinary antiseptic nalidixic acid and are all fluorinated compounds.

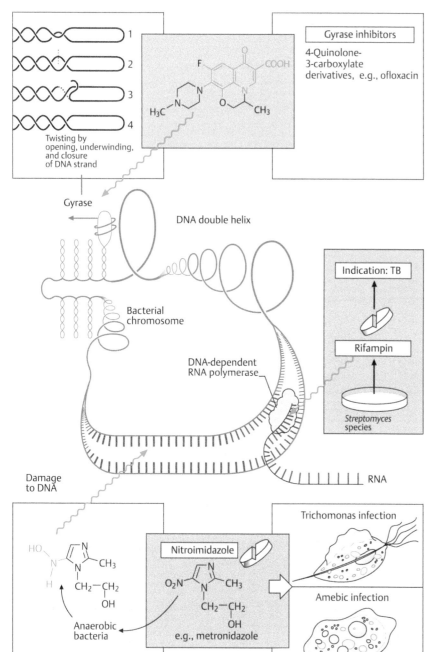

Fig. 29.9 Antibacterial drugs acting on DNA. Antibacterial drugs act on bacterial DNA, preventing the reading of the genetic information at the DNA template, thus damaging the regulatory center of cell metabolism. Gyrase (topoisomerase II) catalyzes the supercoiling of DNA strands. It does this by opening, underwinding, and closing the DNA strand such that the full loop need not be rotated. Gyrase inhibitors (green portion of ofloxacin formula) seem to act to prevent the resealing of opened strands. Metronidazole damages DNA by complex formation or strand breakage. Anaerobic bacteria are able to convert metronidazole to reactive metabolites that attack DNA; thus, it is effective only in this group of bacteria. Rifampin inhibits DNA-dependent RNA polymerase, the enzyme that catalyzes RNA transcription from the DNA template.

Mechanism of Action

Fluoroquinolones inhibit bacterial DNA gyrase (also known as topoisomerase II), an enzyme involved in DNA nicking and supercoiling, and are bactericidal drugs (▶ Fig. 29.9).

Spectrum

Fluoroquinolones are broad-spectrum agents.
- Active against a wide variety of gram-negative bacteria (e.g., *H. influenza, P. mirabilis, E. coli, Klebsiella, Enterobacter, Serratia*).

- Gram-positive organisms are usually less susceptible, but *S. pyogenes, S. pneumonia,* and *S. aureus* are susceptible.
- Ciprofloxacin and levofloxacin are highly active against *Pseudomonas* species.
- Moxifloxacin and gemifloxacin are active against anaerobic bacteria (e.g., *B. fragilis*).

Pharmacokinetics

- Well-absorbed after oral administration and widely distributed in the body.

- Modest CSF penetration and not used for meningitis.
- Renal excretion (exception: moxifloxacin).

Uses

- Treatment of urinary tract infections.
- Treatment of community-acquired pneumonia.
- Treatment of gram-negative infections.
- Treatment of traveler's diarrhea.
- Prophylaxis and treatment of anthrax (ciprofloxacin).

Side Effects

- Fluoroquinolones are usually well tolerated. The most common adverse effects are nausea, vomiting, and diarrhea.
- Irreversible damage to developing cartilage has been observed in studies with young animals; therefore, fluoroquinolones are not recommended for patients younger than 18 years or for use in pregnancy.
- All fluoroquinolones can lead to QT prolongation.
- Dermatologic reactions (photosensitivity, rashes) can occur.

29.9 Inhibitors of Folate Metabolism (Antimetabolites)

Antimetabolites are substances that have structural similarity to substrates used in intermediary metabolism of the cell and that compete for enzymatic binding sites. Examples include purine and pyrimidine analogues used in cancer or antiviral chemotherapy, as well as the sulfonamide antibacterial drugs that are discussed in this section. The ultimate effects of these antimetabolites may be exerted on nucleic acids, proteins, and cell walls.

29.9.1 Sulfonamides

Sulfamethoxazole/Trimethoprim and Sulfadiazine

Mechanism of Action

Sulfonamides are structurally similar to *p*-aminobenzoic acid (PABA). They inhibit the synthesis of dihydrofolic acid in microbes that must synthesize dihydrofolic acid from PABA (▶ Fig. 29.10). Dihydrofolic acid is then reduced to form tetrahydrofolic acid by dihydrofolate reductase. This is required for the synthesis of purines and pyrimidines and amino acids. They are bacteriostatic at concentrations achieved in most body tissues and fluids, but bactericidal concentrations may be found in the urine.

Trimethoprim is used in combination with sulfamethoxazole. It causes selective inhibition of bacterial dihydrofolate reductase.

Spectrum

- Broad spectrum.
- Effective against most gram-positive bacteria (e.g., MRSA, MSSA, *E. faecalis, E. faecium*) and many gram-negative bacteria (e.g., *H. influenza, P. mirabilis, E. coli, Klebsiella, Enterobacter, Serratia*).
- No activity against anaerobes.
- Sulfamethoxazole in combination with trimethoprim is also active against *Nocardia* spp., *Pneumocystis jiroveci*, and *L. monocytogenes*.

Pharmacokinetics

- Sulfonamides are readily absorbed after oral administration.
- Sulfonamides are widely distributed in the body and have a good CNS penetration.
- Sulfonamides are eliminated in the urine.

Uses

- Treatment of urinary tract infections.
- Treatment of pneumocystis pneumonia.
- Treatment of uncomplicated respiratory infections.

Side Effects

- The most common adverse effects of sulfonamides are nausea and vomiting and hypersensitivity reactions (rash and pruritus).
- Severe dermatologic reactions such as Steven–Johnson syndrome are more common in HIV-infected patients and older adults.
- Toxicity to the hematopoietic system (neutropenia, anemia, thrombocytopenia) due to the antifolate effect on fast dividing cells.

29.10 Miscellaneous Antibacterial Drugs

29.10.1 Polymyxin B

Mechanism of Action

Binds to the phospholipids of the gram-negative cell wall. A detergent-like mechanism disturbs the integrity of the cell wall. Polymyxin B is bactericidal.

Spectrum

Primarily active against gram-negative organisms, particularly *P. aeruginosa*.

Pharmacokinetics

These agents do not penetrate CSF but can be used topically or intravenously for life-threatening infections.

Uses

Treatment of urinary tract infection and sepsis caused by sensitive strains of *P. aeruginosa* or by other sensitive organisms when other antibiotics are ineffective or contraindicated.

Side Effects

Renal damage and various neurologic changes limit the usefulness of this drug to mainly topical applications.

29.10.2 Metronidazole

Mechanism of Action

Metronidazole has a cytotoxic effect on bacteria by generating free radicals and damaging DNA, but the precise mechanism of action is unclear (▶ Fig. 29.9). Metronidazole is a prodrug and requires reduction. This only occurs in anaerobic bacteria (due to the presence of electron transport proteins).

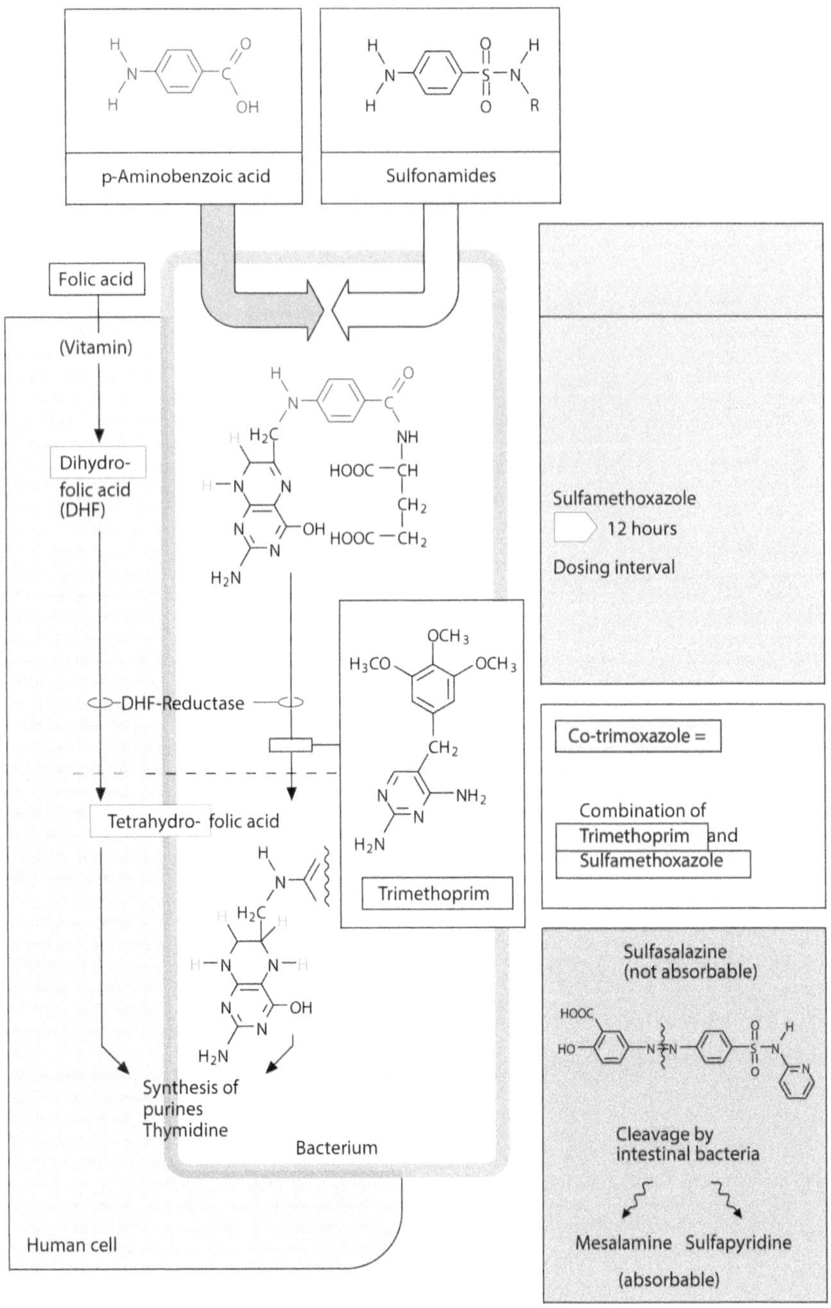

Fig. 29.10 Inhibitors of tetrahydrofolate synthesis.
Bacteria, unlike humans, are able to synthesize dihydrofolic acid (DHF), which is converted to tetrahydrofolic acid (THF) by the enzyme dihydrofolate reductase. THF is then used to synthesize purines and thymidine. Sulfonamides structurally resemble p-aminobenzoic acid (PABA), a precursor in DHF synthesis. They act as a false substrate and competitively inhibit the utilization of PABA, and hence DHF synthesis. Trimethoprim inhibits bacterial DHF-reductase. The human enzyme is less sensitive to trimethoprim and therefore it is relatively selective for bacteria. Co-trimoxazole is a combination of trimethoprim and sulfamethoxazole. THF synthesis is inhibited on two sites. Sulfasalazine, a drug used in inflammatory bowel disease (e.g., Crohn disease and ulcerative colitis), is cleaved by intestinal bacteria to mesalamine and sulfapyridine. Mesalamine exerts its anti-inflammatory effects on the gut mucosa when present in high concentrations. Coupling to sulfonamide prevents premature absorption in the upper small bowel, but it can be absorbed following cleavage and may exert adverse effects.

Spectrum

Active against many anaerobic bacteria including *C. difficile* and *B. fragilis* and against several protozoae.

Pharmacokinetics

Well absorbed after oral administration.

Side Effects

Neurologic effects, disulfiram-like inhibition of aldehyde dehydrogenase, and various GI symptoms including nausea, diarrhea, and metallic taste.

Notes

Anaerobic Bacteria

The mucosal surfaces of the upper respiratory tract, GI tract, and genitourinary tract are colonized with a large number of anaerobic microbes. The infections are usually not transmissible and are polymicrobic (they involve several different species). Infections with nonspore-forming anaerobes lead to necrosis and abscess formation and are chronic. Specific clinical syndromes include skin and soft tissue infections, gynecologic infections, respiratory tract infections, brain abscesses, bacteremia, and intra-abdominal infections.

Anaerobic Infections

Clues for anaerobic infection are as follows:
- Clinical setting influence (i.e., infection following bowel surgery).
- Proximity to a mucosal surface.
- Discharge that is foul-smelling.
- Presence of gas in tissue (palpable masses that move may be gas).
- Dead and necrotic tissue, or the presence of intestinal pseudomembrane.
- Bite wound infections from humans or animals.
- Malignancy-associated infections.
- Presence of septic thrombophlebitis.
- Presence of sulfur granules (actinomycosis).
- Laboratory cultures that are negative under aerobic culture.
- Polymicrobial gram stain assessment.

29.11 Antimycobacterial Drugs

Tuberculosis is an infection spread by inhalation of *Mycobacterium tuberculosis* that mainly affects the lungs. Most infected individuals have asymptomatic latent infections. Active tuberculosis occurs in ~ 10% of untreated individuals with latent infections, particularly in response to decreased immune function caused by stress, malnutrition, or other diseases. Most cases (75%) are pulmonary, with a chronic cough accompanied by malaise, anorexia, fever, chills, and night sweats. When the infection moves outside the lungs, it is known as extrapulmonary tuberculosis (▶ Table 29.3).

Antimycobacterial drugs are used to treat tuberculosis caused by *M. tuberculosis*; *M. avium-intracellulare* complex caused by several different species including *M. avium-intracellulare*; and leprosy (also known as Hansen disease) caused by *Mycobacterium leprae*. Therapy for active mycobacterial infections includes at least two drugs to prevent failure due to emergence of resistant strains and continues for approximately 6 months.

29.11.1 Antituberculosis Drugs

Isoniazid (Isonicotine Hydrazine [INH])

Mechanism of Action

Isoniazid, or isonicotine hydrazine (INH), inhibits cell wall synthesis by interfering with mycolic acid synthesis. It can be either tuberculostatic or tuberculocidal, depending on its concentration (▶ Fig. 29.11).

Table 29.3 Protocol for the treatment of tuberculosis

Treatment type	Antimicrobial protocol
Treatment of active tuberculosis	Until susceptibility tests are available, treatment with 4 drugs (isoniazid, rifampin, pyrazinamide, and ethambutol) for 6 months. When susceptibility to isoniazid, rifampin, and pyrazinamide is proved, ethambutol can be discontinued
Treatment of latent tuberculosis	Isoniazid for 9 months or combination of isoniazid and rifapentine for 12 weeks or rifampin for 4 months

Spectrum

INH is effective only against mycobacteria.

Pharmacokinetics

- INH is readily absorbed after oral administration and is widely distributed in the body, including into CSF and tissues.
- Fast acetylators metabolize the drug more rapidly than slow acetylators.

Uses

Used for prophylaxis as well as for treatment of mycobacterial infections.

Side Effects

- INH is usually well tolerated in most patients.
- INH elevates liver enzymes and some patients may develop isoniazid-induced hepatitis during the first 3 months of therapy.
- Excretion of pyridoxine is enhanced by INH, resulting in decreased pyridoxine levels. Pyridoxine deficiency can present as peripheral neuropathy. However, coadministration of vitamin B_6 prevents these symptoms.

Ethambutol

Mechanism of Action

Ethambutol is a bacteriostatic agent that inhibits bacterial cell wall synthesis. The exact mechanism is unknown.

Spectrum

Ethambutol is effective only against mycobacteria.

Pharmacokinetics

Ethambutol is readily absorbed after oral administration and is widely distributed in the body, including into CSF and tissues.

Uses

Used in combination therapy for the treatment of mycobacterial infections.

Side Effects

Ethambutol is usually well tolerated, but visual disturbances (retrobulbar neuritis) have been reported.

Retrobulbar Neuritis

Retrobulbar neuritis is a form of optic neuritis in which the optic nerve becomes inflamed behind the eyeball. It is most commonly caused by drugs, multiple sclerosis, meningitis, syphilis, and tumors. Symptoms include pain on moving the eyes, blurred vision or loss of vision, and tenderness of the eye to pressure. This condition may resolve without the need for treatment, or prednisone may be required.

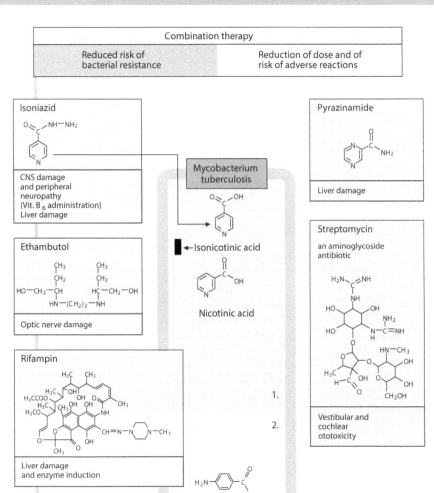

Fig. 29.11 Drugs used to treat infections with mycobacteria (1. tuberculosis, 2. leprosy). Antitubercular drugs of choice are shown (1). Their mechanisms of action are unclear, but isoniazid is converted to isonicotinic acid in the bacterium. This substance is unable to diffuse through cell membranes and so accumulates intracellularly. Antileprotic drugs shown (2) are frequently combined with rifampin. Dapsone inhibits dihydrofolate (DHF) synthesis.

VII

Clinical Correlation

Antibiotics and the Contraceptive Pill

Antibiotics are thought to reduce the efficacy of the contraceptive pill, although the extent to which they do this is subject to debate. Rifampin and griseofulvin are known to induce hepatic enzymes and enhance the metabolism of the contraceptive pill. Other broad-spectrum antibiotics affect the absorption of estrogen from the gut by eradicating the bacterial flora responsible for this. Patients are advised to use barrier methods of contraception, in addition to using the contraceptive pill, while taking antibiotics and for 1 week after.

Rifampin

Mechanism of Action

Rifampin inhibits bacterial and mycobacterial RNA synthesis by binding to the DNA-dependent RNA polymerase. It acts bacteriostatic or bactericidal, depending on the concentration (▶ Fig. 29.1).

Spectrum

Active against *Mycobacterium* spp. and other microbes (including *Staphylococcus* spp., *N. meningitides*).

Pharmacokinetics

- Well absorbed orally.
- Wide tissue distribution and penetrates CSF well.
- Metabolized in the liver and induces its own metabolism over time.

Uses

- Used alone or in combination therapy for the treatment of mycobacterial infections.
- Prophylaxis of meningococcal infections.

Side Effects

- Gives a harmless orange color to body fluids, including contact lenses.
- Induces most CYP450 enzymes, which enhances elimination of warfarin, phenytoin, estrogen, and other drugs.

Pyrazinamide

Mechanism of Action

The mechanism of action is uncertain.

Spectrum

Pyrazinamide is effective only against mycobacteria.

Pharmacokinetics

Well absorbed orally and widely distributed into body tissues and fluids including CSF.

Uses

Used alone or in combination therapy for the treatment of mycobacterial infections.

Side Effects

Patients must be monitored for signs of hepatotoxicity.

29.11.2 Antileprotic Drugs

Dapsone (Diaminophenylsulfone [DDS])

Mechanism of Action

Dapsone's mechanism of action is similar to that of sulfonamides.

Pharmacokinetics

Its long half-life permits once-weekly administration.

Uses

For treatment of leprosy.

Side Effects

Dose-related hematologic effects are most common.

29.12 Antiseptics and Disinfectants

29.12.1 Urinary Antiseptics

Urinary antiseptics are defined as substances that can be given orally but provide significant antibacterial effects only in the urine.

Nitrofurantoin

Mechanism of Action

This agent has bacteriostatic activity against several urinary tract pathogens. Nitrofurantoin is reduced by bacterial proteins to reactive metabolites. These can inactivate bacterial ribosomal proteins, leading to inhibition of protein synthesis, DNA, RNA, and cell wall synthesis.

Uses

Treatment of urinary tract infections.

Clinical Correlation

Urinary Tract Infections

UTIs are common, especially in women due to the proximity of the urethra to the vagina (allowing easier spread of sexually transmitted infections and diseases) and due to the relative length of the urethra compared to men (men have longer urethras). UTIs present with any of the following symptoms: frequency of urination, urgency, strangury (frequent, painful expulsion of small amounts of urine despite urgency), hematuria (blood in the urine), cloudy urine, incontinence, fever with diarrhea and vomiting, and pain (usually suprapubic pain in women and anal pain in men). Trimethoprim and sulfamethoxazole are given to treat uncomplicated UTIs caused by susceptible bacteria (*E. coli, Staphylococci, Streptococci, Pseudomonas,* and *Proteus*). In addition, patients are advised to drink plenty of fluids and urinate often.

Side Effects

Hypersensitivity reactions, nausea, and vomiting are limitations to its usefulness, but a crystalline form of nitrofurantoin has a reduced incidence of GI intolerance.

29.12.2 External Antiseptics and Disinfectants

Antiseptics that are too toxic for internal use may be effective for removal of microbes from the skin (disinfectants) or surgical instruments (antiseptics). They have important roles in medicine or dentistry. Some examples are included in ▶ Table 29.4.

Table 29.4 External antiseptics and disinfectants

Class of substance	Examples
Detergents	Anionic: ordinary soaps Cationic: benzalkonium chloride
Phenols (probably also act as detergents)	Phenol: hexylresorcinol Cresol: hexachlorophene
Alcohols	Ethanol and isopropyl alcohol
Halogens	Chlorine, chloramines, and iodine
Metals	Silver (used in combination with sulfadiazine) and mercury (thimerosal)
Oxidants	Hydrogen peroxide, permanganate, sodium peroxide, and perborate

VII

30 Antiviral Drugs

Summary

Viruses are small parasites that require the metabolic processes and activities of the host cell. Therefore, virus reproduction requires the virus particle to infect a cell and use the cytoplasmic machinery to synthesize the macromolecules necessary for the assembly of new virus particles. Viruses contain DNA or RNA, not both, and range in size from 20 (parvoviruses) to 300 nm (poxviruses); the largest virus approximates the size of the smallest bacterial cells (chlamydia and mycoplasma).

Viral replication begins with attachment whereby specific ligands on the virus recognize and bind to specific receptors on the host cell surface. Once inside the host cell, there is viral uncoating that is the removal of the viral nucleic acid from the capsid. The last stage in viral replication is genome expression. Viruses adapt host cell machinery to transcribe viral RNA from a viral DNA template, producing key proteins for new virus synthesis. Release of daughter viruses results in the spread of the virus, both within and outside the host (▶ Fig. 30.1).

Antiviral drugs are used to treat susceptible viral infections, which include herpes simplex virus, varicella zoster virus, cytomegalovirus (CMV), influenza viruses, respiratory syncytial virus (RSV), hepatitis B, hepatitis C, and human immunodeficiency virus (HIV). Antiviral drugs target an essential viral enzyme or protein to inhibit a pathway unique to the virus but not the cell (▶ Table 30.1).

Keywords: herpes, cytomegalovirus, influenza, HIV

30.1 Introduction

In contrast to antibiotic drugs that cover a wide variety of pathogens, antiviral drugs only act against a specific virus. The lack of "broad-spectrum" antivirals is probably due to very few viral-specific targets. Once inside a cell, the virus uses the host machinery to replicate and is therefore "hidden" for most of its life cycle. Antivirals are available, for example, to treat influenza viruses, hepatitis B and C, and CMV. Today, most antiviral drugs are available to treat HIV, converting this deadly disease to a chronic condition with a "once-a-day" tablet regimen.

30.2 Agents to Treat Herpes Simplex Virus and Varicella Zoster Virus Infections

30.2.1 Acyclovir, Famciclovir, Penciclovir, and Valacyclovir

Mechanism of Action

These agents are nucleoside analogues that must be phosphorylated intracellularly to exert their antiviral effects. They inhibit DNA polymerase and, once incorporated into viral DNA, terminate chain elongation. Due to their action on virus-specific thymidine kinase and viral DNA polymerase, these agents exhibit remarkable selective toxicity (▶ Fig. 30.2 and ▶ Fig. 30.3).

Spectrum

Herpes simplex virus (HSV) and varicella zoster virus (VZV).

Pharmacokinetics

Although oral bioavailability of acyclovir is low, this compound is effective after oral administration, by injection, or topical application. The other agents are available for oral administration and have longer half-lives that require one or two doses daily.

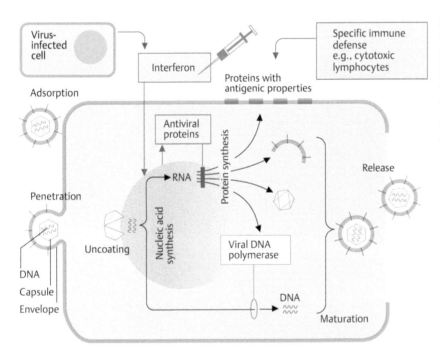

Fig. 30.1 Viral multiplication and mechanism of action of antiviral agents. Viruses can be destroyed by cytotoxic T lymphocytes, which are part of the specific immune response. These lymphocytes detect the virus via proteins on the viral membranes. They may also be inactivated by antibodies. Interferons are glycoproteins that are released from virus-infected cells. They stimulate the production of antiviral proteins in neighboring cells, which destroy or suppress viral DNA and thus prevent viral protein synthesis.

Table 30.1 Selected viruses

Family	Typical example(s)	Nucleic acid polarity and structure	Envelope
DNA viruses			
Parvoviridae	Human parvovirus	ssDNA (+ or −)	No
Hepadnaviridae	Hepatitis B	dsDNA/ss portions	Yes
Papovaviridae	JC virus	dsDNA circular	No
Adenoviridae	Human adenovirus	dsDNA	No
Herpesviridae	Herpes simplex 1 (α), Herpes simplex 2 (α), CMV (β), Epstein–Barr (γ)	dsDNA	Yes
Poxviridae	Vaccinia virus	dsDNA closed ends	Yes
RNA viruses			
Togaviridae	Rubella virus	ssRNA (+)	Yes
Picornaviridae	Poliovirus	ssRNA (+)	No
Flaviviridae	Yellow fever virus (hepatitis C virus)	ssRNA (+)	Yes
Rhabdoviridae	Rabies virus	ssRNA (−)	Yes
Coronaviridae	Coronaviruses	ssRNA (+)	Yes
Paramyxoviridae	Measles virus	ssRNA (−)	Yes
Orthomyxoviridae	Influenza virus	ssRNA (−) segments	Yes
Bunyaviridae	Encephalitis virus	ssRNA (− circular)	Yes
Arenaviridae	Lymphocytic choriomen	ssRNA (− circular)	Yes
Retroviridae	HIV	ssRNA (+ identical)	Yes
Reoviridae	Rotaviruses	dsRNA (segments)	No
Caliciviridae	Norwalk virus	ssRNA (+)	No
Filoviridae	Ebola, Marburg	ssRNA	Yes

Abbreviations: CMV, cytomegalovirus; ds, double-stranded; HIV, human immunodeficiency virus; ss, single-stranded.

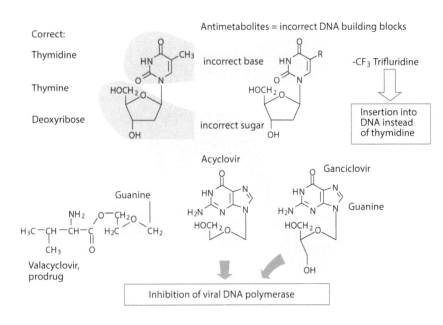

Fig. 30.2 Chemical structure of virustatic antimetabolites.
Nucleosides consist of a base (e.g., thymine) and deoxyribose. Virustatic antimetabolites act as false nucleosides or sugars. In the body, they are incorporated into viral DNA and terminate replication. Acyclovir and ganciclovir also inhibit viral DNA polymerase.

Clinical Correlation

Herpes Simplex Virus

HSV type 1 is the most common HSV infection and usually produces cold sores and other blisters around the mouth, lips, and face. These may be accompanied by fever, sore throat, and lymphadenopathy. It spreads via saliva. HSV type 2 is usually responsible for genital herpes and is sexually transmitted. Symptoms include blisters around the vagina, anus, buttocks, penis shaft/glans, or scrotum that may be accompanied by itching, pain, dysuria (difficult or painful urination), and fever. Complications of HSV infections include herpetic whitlow (vesicles develop on an infected digit), herpetic simplex keratitis (corneal ulcers), herpetic simplex meningitis (rarely occurs but is usually due to HSV type 2), and herpetic simplex encephalitis (usually HSV type 1). Treatment of HSV may include the use of antiviral medications, such as acyclovir and analgesics. Herpes simplex encephalitis has a high risk of mortality and requires urgent care.

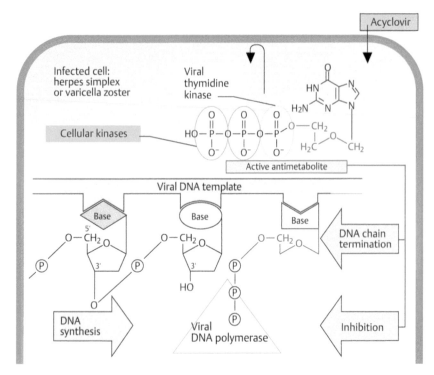

Fig. 30.3 Activation of acyclovir and inhibition of viral DNA synthesis.
In an infected cell, viral thymidine kinase performs the initial phosphorylation step; then cellular kinases attach the remaining phosphate residues. The activation of acyclovir occurs only in infected cells, which gives it high specificity and tolerability. Furthermore, the polar phosphate residues render acyclovir unable to diffuse across cell membranes and cause it to accumulate in infected cells. Acyclovir triphosphate is a preferred substrate of viral DNA polymerase and inhibits its activity. Following incorporation of acyclovir triphosphate into viral DNA, it induces strand breakage because it lacks the 3′-OH group of deoxyribose that is required for the attachment of additional nucleotides.

Uses

- Treatment and prophylaxis of herpes genitalis.
- Treatment of viral encephalitis.
- Treatment of complicated herpes simplex infections.

Clinical Correlation

Herpes Zoster (Shingles)

Chickenpox is the primary infection with VZV. Following the initial infection, the virus remains dormant in the dorsal root ganglia. Reactivation of the virus causes shingles. Shingles starts with pain, tingling, or burning in a dermatomal distribution (often the ophthalmic division of the trigeminal nerve and lower thoracic dermatomes are affected). This is accompanied by fever and malaise. Later, a vesicular rash develops involving the same dermatome. Complications of shingles include postherpetic neuralgia of the affected dermatome. This pain can range from mild to very severe and can persist for months or years. Treatment of shingles may involve the early use of antiviral medications, such as acyclovir, to shorten the course of the infection and reduce pain and complications. Pain may also be treated with oxycodone (a narcotic analgesic), amitriptyline (a tricyclic antidepressant), gabapentin (an anticonvulsant), or lidocaine (a local anesthetic). Postherpetic neuralgia can be treated with carbamazepine or phenytoin and prednisone. If these are unsuccessful, surgical ablation of the appropriate ganglion may be tried but is often unsuccessful and may leave the patient with numbness of the dermatome supplied.

30.3 Agents to Treat Cytomegalovirus

30.3.1 Ganciclovir and Valganciclovir

Mechanism of Action

The mechanism of action is similar to acyclovir.

Spectrum

CMV infections.

Pharmacokinetics

Ganciclovir has poor bioavailability and is therefore administered by intravenous (IV) infusion or as an intravitreal implant (for CMV retinitis). Valganciclovir is an orally active prodrug.

Uses

Treatment and prophylaxis of CMV infections.

Side Effects

Bone marrow suppression.

30.3.2 Foscarnet

Foscarnet is a pyrophosphate analogue.

Mechanism of Action

Foscarnet directly inhibits viral DNA polymerases without requiring activation by phosphorylation.

Spectrum

CMV infections resistant to other drugs.

Pharmacokinetics

Foscarnet is infused IV or by intravitreal injection (for retinitis).

Uses

Treatment of CMV infections resistant to other drugs or in patients with HIV.

Toxicity

Renal toxicity leading to electrolyte imbalances.

30.3.3 Cidofovir

Cidofovir is a cytosine analogue.

Mechanism of Action

Cidofovir directly inhibits viral DNA polymerases without requiring activation by phosphorylation.

Spectrum

CMV infections resistant to other drugs.

Pharmacokinetics

Cidofovir is administered IV or by intravitreal injection.

Uses

Treatment and prophylaxis of CMV retinitis.

Toxicity

Renal toxicity and neutropenia.

Clinical Correlation

Cytomegalovirus

CMV is an infection that is often asymptomatic and therefore goes unnoticed. It is spread by a variety of routes such as saliva, blood, semen, urine, and breast milk. Like HSV, it lies dormant after the initial infection and may become reactivated. Symptoms, if any, are similar to mononucleosis and include fever, fatigue, weakness, sore throat, swollen glands, muscle and joint aches, and a feeling of generally being unwell. Treatment with ganciclovir is generally reserved for immunocompromised patients.

30.4 Agents to Treat Respiratory Syncytial Virus

30.4.1 Ribavirin

Mechanism of Action

Ribavirin is phosphorylated to mono-, di-, and triphosphate forms and interferes with purine metabolism by inhibiting inosine monophosphate dehydrogenase.

Spectrum

RSV infection and hepatitis C.

Pharmacokinetics

Ribavirin is administered by aerosol for RSV to prevent systemic toxicity. It is given orally for hepatitis C.

Uses

For RSV, its use is limited to infants and children with severe lower respiratory tract infections. For hepatitis C, it is used in combination therapy with interferon alfa.

Toxicity

Hemolytic anemia (if taken systemically).

Clinical Correlation

Respiratory Syncytial Virus

RSV is a virus that causes infections of the respiratory tract and lungs. It gains entry to the body through the eyes, nose, or mouth and is typically spread by droplets via coughing or sneezing or direct contact (e.g., shaking hands). Symptoms are usually mild and include congested or runny nose, cough, sore throat, headache, fever, and a general feeling of being unwell. Treatment is usually limited to over-the-counter drugs, such as acetaminophen, to reduce fever. Treatment with ribavirin is reserved for infants and children with severe RSV infections.

30.5 Other Antiviral Agents

30.5.1 Trifluridine

Mechanism of Action

Trifluridine is an analogue of thymidine that acts by inhibiting viral DNA polymerase.

Uses

Herpes simplex keratitis (applied topically to the cornea of infected eyes).

Side Effects

Local stinging and irritation around the eyes.

30.6 Agents to Treat Influenza

30.6.1 Oseltamivir and Zanamivir

Mechanism of Action

These agents are analogues of sialic acid and inhibit the influenza neuraminidase. Without neuraminidase, the hemagglutinin of the virus binds to sialic acid, forming clumps and preventing virus release (▶ Fig. 30.4).

Spectrum

Influenza A and B.

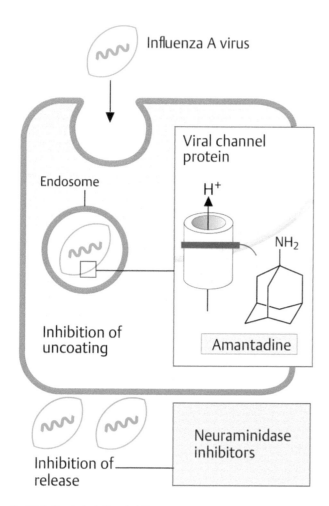

Fig. 30.4 Prophylaxis for viral flu.
Amantadine specifically prevents uncoating of influenza A viruses. Influenza A is endocytosed into cells, but they require protons, supplied by the endosome, to penetrate the virus and allow it to release its RNA. Amantadine prevents this influx of protons into the virus. Neuraminidase inhibitors are effective against influenza A and B. Normally, viral neuraminidase splits off N-acetylneuraminic (sialic) acid residues on the cellular cell surface coat, thereby enabling newly formed virus particles to be detached from the host cell.

Pharmacokinetics

Oseltamivir is an orally administered prodrug. Activation occurs via hepatic enzymes and the drug is widely distributed throughout the body. Zanamivir is administered by inhalation.

Uses

Treatment and prophylaxis of influenza A and B infection.

Side Effects

• Nausea and vomiting (oseltamivir).
• Cough, and nasal and throat symptoms (zanamivir).

30.6.2 Amantadine and Rimantadine

Mechanism of Action

These agents are highly selective antiviral drugs that inhibit the growth of influenza A viruses by acting as ion channel blockers of the viral M_2 protein, thus preventing viral uncoating (▶ Fig. 30.4).

Spectrum

Influenza A.

Pharmacokinetics

Completely absorbed from the gastrointestinal (GI) tract and excreted unchanged in the urine.

Uses

Prophylaxis and treatment of influenza A virus infections.

Side Effects

Nausea and anorexia are the most common adverse effects. Central nervous system side effects (nervousness, confusion, insomnia, dizziness, and hallucinations) are less common.

Clinical Correlation

Influenza

Influenza (or "flu") is a viral infection that affects the respiratory tract and lungs. The virus has three types: A, B, and C. It is spread by droplets that are either inhaled following coughing or sneezing, or directly transferred from an infected person. Symptoms of flu may mimic the common cold initially with nasal congestion or runny nose, sneezing, and sore throat. However, these symptoms rapidly become worse and progress to include fever, chills and sweats, aching muscles, headache, fatigue, weakness, and a general feeling of being unwell. Complications include pneumonia, otitis media, sinusitis, and bronchitis. Treatment for influenza usually involves bed rest, fluids, and nonsteroidal anti-inflammatory drugs. However, antiviral medications such as oseltamivir and zanamivir may sometimes be used to shorten the course of the infection.

30.7 Drugs for Hepatitis B and Hepatitis C

30.7.1 Interferon Alfa

Several forms of interferon, including alfa-2a and alfa-2b, are available.

Mechanism of Action

Interferons are endogenous cytokines that demonstrate antiviral and immunomodulatory properties.

Pharmacokinetics

- Injected subcutaneously (SC).
- Peginterferons, interferon formulated with polyethylene glycol, have longer half-lives, and can be given once weekly. These agents have largely replaced standard interferons.

Uses

- Hepatitis B therapy.
- Hepatitis C therapy when used in combination with ribavirin.

Side Effects

Flulike syndrome with headache, chills, fever, and muscle pain is common within hours of injection. Adverse effects on all systems may be observed with chronic use, including
- Alopecia, pruritus (itching), and rash.
- Weight loss.
- Bone marrow suppression.
- GI upset.
- Joint and muscle pain.
- Dizziness, headache, and insomnia.
- Anxiety, irritability, and depression.

30.7.2 Adefovir Dipivoxil, Entecavir, Lamivudine, Telbivudine, and Tenofovir

Mechanism of Action

These agents are nucleoside/nucleotide analogues that inhibit viral DNA polymerase.

Pharmacokinetics

Well absorbed after oral administration.

Uses

Treatment of chronic hepatitis B.

Side Effects

- Dizziness, fatigue, headache, and nausea are the most common adverse effects of all these agents.
- Renal toxicity including a Fanconi-like syndrome (tenofovir).
- Asthenia and dose-dependent nephrotoxicity (adefovir dipivoxil).

- Myalgia and myopathy, and increased serum creatine kinase levels (telbivudine).

30.7.3 Boceprevir, Simeprevir, and Telaprevir

Mechanism of Action

These agents bind to the NS3/4A protease and inhibit the replication of hepatitis C virus.

Pharmacokinetics

Well absorbed after oral administration.

Uses

Used in the therapy of hepatitis C in combination with interferon alfa.

Side Effects

- Fatigue, nausea, headache, and anemia.
- Rash, pruritus (telaprevir).

30.7.4 Sofosbuvir

Mechanism of Action

Sofosbuvir inhibits the NS5B polymerase which is essential for viral replication. The drug acts as a chain terminator.

Pharmacokinetics

Well absorbed after oral administration.

Uses

Used in the therapy of hepatitis C in combination with other antiviral drugs.

Side Effects

Fatigue, nausea, headache, pruritus, and anemia.

30.7.5 Ribavirin

See discussion under Agents to treat Respiratory Syncytial Virus (RSV).
▶ Table 30.2 summarizes the drugs used to treat non-HIV viral infections.

Table 30.2 Drugs used to treat viral infections (non-HIV)

Agents	Antiviral activity
Amantadine/rimantadine	Influenza A
Neuraminidase inhibitors	Influenza A and B
Acyclovir and analogues	Herpes viruses
Ganciclovir and valganciclovir	CMV in HIV patients
Foscarnet	CMV, HSV (resistant)
Ribavirin	RSV, hepatitis C
Interferon	Hepatitis B, C; papillomavirus

Abbreviations: CMV, cytomegalovirus; HIV, human immunodeficiency virus; HSV, herpes simplex virus; RSV, respiratory syncytial virus.

Clinical Correlation

Hepatitis A, B, and C

Hepatitis is a viral infection that causes inflammation and dysfunction of the liver. The three main types are hepatitis A, B, and C (although D and E also exist). Hepatitis A is spread by the fecal–oral route, often via contaminated food or water. Symptoms tend to appear 1 month following the initial infection and include nausea and vomiting, loss of appetite, fever, abdominal pain, muscle aches, fatigue, itching, and jaundice. Hepatitis A usually resolves with no treatment. Hepatitis B is spread via blood, semen, or saliva. Symptoms are the same as hepatitis A but itching and joint pain are more prominent. Chronic infection with hepatitis B may lead to cirrhosis and/or liver cancer. Antiviral drugs, such as interferon alfa, may be used to slow liver damage but treatment is usually limited to supportive measures. Hepatitis C is spread in the same manner as hepatitis B. It is typically asymptomatic initially and may remain so for many years. Symptoms, when they do occur, are the same as those listed for hepatitis A and B but are generally milder. Like hepatitis B, chronic hepatitis C may lead to cirrhosis and liver cancer. Treatment may involve the use of interferon alfa. If hepatitis B or C lead to liver failure, then liver transplantation may be indicated.

30.8 Management of Human Immunodeficiency Virus

HIV is a retrovirus transmitted by free viral particles or infected immune cells (e.g., CD4 T cells, macrophages, and dendritic cells) in blood, semen, vaginal fluid, preejaculate, and breast milk. The goal of HIV therapy is to increase CD4 cell counts, suppress viral load, and reconstitute the immune system. Six classes of drugs are available to treat HIV. These include the nucleoside/nucleotide reverse transcriptase inhibitors (NRTIs), the nonnucleoside reverse transcriptase inhibitors (NNRTIs), protease inhibitors, integrase strand transfer inhibitors (INSTIs), fusion inhibitors, and agents that prevent the entry of HIV.

30.8.1 Nucleoside/Nucleotide Reverse Transcriptase Inhibitors

Abacavir (ABC), Didanosine (ddI), Emtricitabine (FTC), Lamivudine (3TC), Stavudine (d4T), Tenofovir (TDF), and Zidovudine (Azidothymidine, AZT)

AZT is the first antiretroviral drug approved by the U.S. Food and Drug Administration for the treatment of HIV.

Mechanism of Action

NRTIs are nucleoside or nucleotide analogues (▶ Fig. 30.5). These agents competitively inhibit HIV reverse transcriptase

Table 30.3 Side effects of nucleoside reverse transcriptase inhibitor drugs

Agent	Side effects
Abacavir (ABC)	Hypersensitivity, liver disease
Didanosine (ddI)	Pancreatitis
Emtricitabine (FTC)	Nausea, vomiting, headache, fatigue
Lamivudine (3TC)	Nausea, vomiting, headache, fatigue
Stavudine (d4T)	Peripheral neuropathy, diarrhea, nausea, vomiting
Tenofovir (TDF)	Rash, mild GI upset
Zidovudine (AZT)	Anemia, headache, fatigue, insomnia, nausea, vomiting

Abbreviations: GI, gastrointestinal; NRTI, nucleoside reverse transcriptase inhibitor.

and incorporation into the growing DNA strand causes chain termination.

Pharmacokinetics

Orally effective.

Side Effects

All NRTIs are associated with mitochondrial toxicity due to inhibition of mitochondrial DNA polymerase gamma. Therefore, adverse effects such as pancreatitis, fatty liver, lactic acidosis, and peripheral neuropathy can occur.

See ▶ Table 30.3 for the side effects of individual agents.

30.8.2 Nonnucleoside Reverse Transcriptase Inhibitors

Delavirdine, Efavirenz, Etravirine, Nevirapine, Relpivirine

Mechanism of Action

NNRTIs also interfere with viral DNA synthesis but bind near the active site of the viral reverse transcriptase to inhibit its activity (▶ Fig. 30.5).

Side Effects

- Headache, insomnia, dizziness, and nausea are common adverse effects of NNRTIs.
- All NNRTIs can lead to a rash (which may progress to Steven–Johnson syndrome).
- Other specific adverse effects for each agent are listed below.

Pharmacokinetics

- Orally effective.
- These drugs are substrates of CYP450 enzymes and may induce or inhibit the metabolism of other drugs metabolized by the liver. Numerous drug–drug interactions can occur.

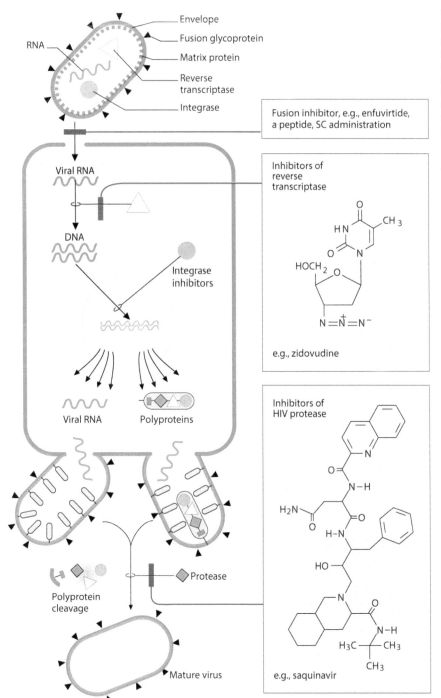

Fig. 30.5 HIV drugs.
Inhibitors of reverse transcriptase (RT) are nucleosides containing an abnormal sugar moiety and require phosphorylation for activation. As triphosphates, they inhibit RT and induce strand breakage following incorporation into DNA. Nonnucleoside inhibitors inhibit RT without requiring prior activation. Protease inhibitors prevent polyprotein cleavage, which is necessary for the maturation of viral cells. Fusion inhibitors prevent the change in conformation of viral fusion proteins that allows them to attach to host CD4 cells. SC, subcutaneous.

Notes

CD4 and CD8 Cells

CD4 cells (T helper cells) play an important role in the immune system by alerting other immune cells—B cells and cytotoxic T cells (CD8)—to kill pathogens or tumor cells. The normal range for CD4 cells in a blood sample is 500 to 1500; for CD8 cells, it is ~ 1,200.

Delavirdine

Side Effects

A rash develops on the upper body and arms within the first 1 to 3 weeks after taking the medication. This rash usually goes away within ~ 2 weeks. Other side effects include

- Elevated hepatic enzymes.
- Hepatic failure.
- Acute renal failure (rare).

Foundations

Replication of the HIV Virus

There are several steps involved in the replication of the HIV virus:

1. Proteins (gp120 protein) on the surface of the HIV virus cell are fused to CD4 + receptors (glycoproteins) found on the surface of helper T cells, monocytes, and macrophages.
2. HIV RNA, reverse transcriptase, HIV integrase, and other viral proteins are released into the host cell.
3. Single-stranded viral RNA is transcribed to double-stranded DNA in the cytoplasm by the action of reverse transcriptase.
4. New viral DNA migrates into the nucleus and becomes spliced into host DNA by the action of HIV integrase.
5. DNA is transcribed into new viral RNA, which is then translated into viral proteins.
6. New viral RNA and proteins congregate near the cell membrane and become enclosed in the membrane, forming immature (not yet infective) HIV virus cells, which bud off from the host cell.
7. The virus is cleaved by proteases into its mature, infective form.

Efavirenz

Side Effects

- Neuropsychiatric adverse effects: abnormal thinking, confusion, difficulty concentrating, sleep disturbances, vivid dreams, nightmares, suicidal tendencies.
- Hyperlipidemia.
- Potentially teratogenic.

Etravirine

Side Effects

- Generally well tolerated.
- Hypercholesterolemia.
- Hyperglycemia.

Nevirapine

Side Effects

- Hypercholesterolemia.
- Hepatotoxicity, hepatic failure.

Rilpivirine

Side Effects

- Depression, drowsiness, and headache.

- Hypercholesterolemia.

30.8.3 Protease Inhibitors

Saquinavir, Ritonavir, Lopinavir, Indinavir, Nelfinavir, Atazanavir, Tipranavir, and Darunavir

Mechanism of Action

Protease inhibitors inhibit the cleavage of protein precursors essential for viral assembly and viral release from the host cells (▶ Fig. 30.5).

Pharmacokinetics

Oral absorption can vary among the different agents. These drugs are substrates for CYP3A4, and interactions with other drugs that are CYP3A4 substrates may occur.

Side Effects

The general side effects of these drugs include the following:
- Changes in body fat distribution (central obesity, buffalo hump, gynecomastia).
- High sugar levels in the blood; onset or worsening of diabetes.
- Increased bleeding in patients with hemophilia.

The additional side effects of individual drugs are listed in ▶ Table 30.4.

30.8.4 Integrase Strand Transfer Inhibitor

Raltegravir, Dolutegravir, and Elvitegravir

Mechanism of Action

INSTIs inhibit the activity of viral integrase. This enzyme integrates the newly synthesized viral DNA into host cell DNA and

Table 30.4 Side effects of protease inhibitor drugs

Agent	Side effects
Atazanavir	Hyperbilirubinemia, nephrolithiasis
Darunavir	Rash, hepatoxicity
Indinavir	Nephrolithiasis
Lopinavir	Elevated liver enzymes, GI adverse effects
Nelfinavir	GI adverse effects
Saquinavir	GI adverse effects
Ritonavir	Abdominal pain, asthenia, fatigue, hyperbilirubinemia
Tipranavir	Hepatoxicity, rash

Abbreviations: GI, gastrointestinal.

is required for viral replication.

Pharmacokinetics

All INSTIs are well absorbed orally. Elvitegravir is only available with the pharmacokinetic booster cobicistat. Cobicistat is a CYP3A4 inhibitor and enhances systemic levels of elvitegravir allowing once-daily administration.

Side Effects

INSTIs are generally well tolerated and GI adverse effects and headache are most commonly reported.

30.8.5 Entry (Fusion) Inhibitor

Enfuvirtide

Mechanism of Action

Enfuvirtide binds to the transmembrane glycoprotein subunit (gp41) of the viral envelope and prevents the fusion of viral envelope and cell membrane (▶ Fig. 30.5).

Pharmacokinetics

Enfuvirtide is administered SC.

Side Effects

Local injection site reactions have been reported with enfuvirtide.

30.8.6 Chemokine Coreceptor Antagonist

Maraviroc

Mechanism of Action

Maraviroc blocks HIV from binding to chemokine receptor type 5 (CCR5), thus preventing the virus from entering target cells. This agent can only be used when the virus is CCR5-tropic. If the patient's virus is chemokine receptor type 4 (CCR4)-tropic or has a mixed population, as seen in later stages of the disease, maraviroc will not be effective.

Pharmacokinetics

Maraviroc is a substrate of CYP3A4 and p-glycoprotein and significant drug interactions may occur.

Side Effects

Increased cough and GI adverse effects were among the most common adverse effects reported with maraviroc use.

VII

31 Antifungal and Antiparasitic Drugs

Summary

Fungi are eukaryotic, but their cell membrane contains ergosterol instead of cholesterol that is present in the mammalian cell membrane. It is this unique cell membrane that allows for the selective toxicity of antifungal agents. In contrast to antibacterial agents that target a variety of unique characteristics of cells, antifungals have a very limited number of targets, the major one being ergosterol. Most of the antifungal agents discussed in this chapter either bind directly to ergosterol and change membrane permeability or inhibit its ergosterol synthesis.

Antiparasitic drugs have also a limited number of targets, as parasites are eukaryotes as well. Many of the antiparasitic drugs have widely unknown mechanisms and most likely create oxidative damage to the parasite.

This chapter describes important human fungal and protozoal infections including malaria and the drugs used to treat them.

Keywords: fungus, amoeba, malaria, roundworm, flatworm

31.1 Introduction

Fungal infections are becoming more common, particularly in immunocompromised and HIV patients. Antifungal medications include medications that target ergosterol, some cell wall components, or nucleic acid synthesis.

Parasitic infections are a worldwide health problem and the burden of disease is mainly found in tropics and subtropics. Many of the drugs used to treat parasitic diseases have been used for decades; however, their exact mechanism is not known. New drug discoveries within antiparasitic drugs are rare, and during the past few decades only one new antimalarial drug was brought to the market.

31.2 Drugs Used in the Treatment of Fungal Infections

31.2.1 Polyene Antifungals

Mechanism of Action

Polyene antifungals are named after large numbers of unsaturated bonds in their chemical structures. These drugs permeate into ergosterol-rich membranes (characteristic of fungi) and produce a detergent-like effect (▶ Fig. 31.1).

Nystatin

Pharmacokinetics

- Nystatin is used topically and orally (swish and swallow).
- It is highly toxic and is not used parenterally.

Uses

Treatment of cutaneous, mucocutaneous, and oral cavity *Candida* infections.

Side Effects

Intestinal upset when swallowed.

Amphotericin B

Pharmacokinetics

This agent has no oral bioavailability. Only administered intravenously.

Spectrum

Amphotericin B has a broad antifungal spectrum and is useful for most systemic fungal infections.

Uses

Serious systemic fungal infections (use limited by toxicity).

Side Effects

- Infusion-related reactions including flushing, chills, fever, and headache are common.
- Renal toxicity.
- Anemia (probably due to suppression of erythropoietin).

31.2.2 Azole Antifungal Agents

Fluconazole, Itraconazole, Voriconazole, Posaconazole, Isavuconazonium, Miconazole, Clotrimazole, and Ketoconazole

Mechanism of Action

Imidazole antifungal agents interfere with cytochrome P-450-dependent biosynthesis of ergosterol, causing disorganization of the fungal cell membrane (▶ Fig. 31.1). These agents have a broad spectrum of activity against pathogenic fungi. They may also inhibit several cytochrome P-450-dependent drug oxidations in patients, leading to drug interactions.

Fluconazole

Pharmacokinetics

Administered orally and systemically.

Uses

- Treatment of *Candida* infections.
- Treatment of cryptococcal meningitis.
- Antifungal prophylaxis in bone marrow transplant recipients, solid-organ transplant recipients, and ICU patients.

Itraconazole

Pharmacokinetics

Administered orally.

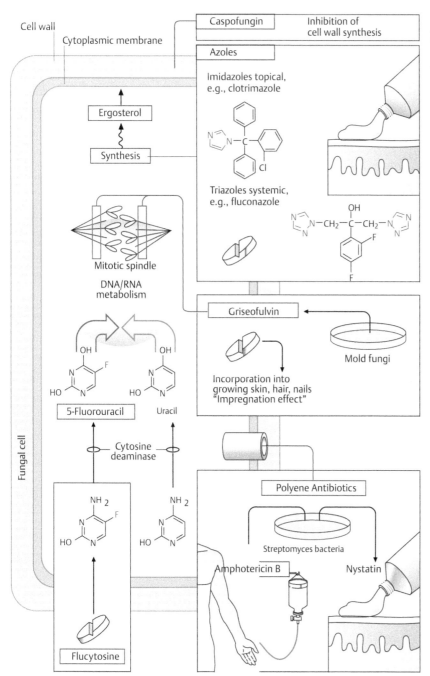

Fig. 31.1 Antifungal drugs.
Azole antifungals inhibit the synthesis of ergosterol, an integral component of fungal cell membranes. Polyene antifungals insert themselves into fungal cell membranes and produce a detergent-like effect. Flucytosine is an antimetabolite that is converted to 5-fluorouracil in fungi by fungal cytosine deaminase. Flucytosine is then incorporated into fungal DNA, causing disruption of DNA and RNA synthesis. Caspofungin inhibits fungal cell wall synthesis. Griseofulvin is active only against dermatophytes. It seems to inhibit fungal mitosis by acting as a spindle poison.

VII

Uses

Treatment of aspergillosis, blastomycosis, histoplasmosis, and onychomycosis.

Voriconazole

Pharmacokinetics

Administered orally and systemically.

Uses

- Treatment of *Candida* infections.
- Treatment of invasive aspergillosis.

Posaconazole

Pharmacokinetics

Administered orally and systemically.

Uses

- Prophylaxis of aspergillosis and candidiasis in patients with severe immunosuppression.
- Treatment of oropharyngeal candidiasis.

Isavuconazonium

Pharmacokinetics

Administered orally and systemically.

Uses

Treatment of invasive aspergillosis and mucormycosis.

Miconazole and Clotrimazole

Pharmacokinetics

Topical use only.

Uses

- Superficial tinea (ringworm) infections and vulvovaginal candidiasis.
- Treatment of oropharyngeal candidiasis.

Foundations

Pathogenic Fungal Forms

Pathogenic fungi are able to grow in two forms: filamentous and yeasts, depending on the growth conditions. Filamentous, or mold, grow as branching, threadlike filaments called hyphae. Several hyphae are collectively referred to as a mycelium. The hyphae may be septate, that is, divided by partitions or coeno-cytic with no partitions but a multinucleate hyphal structure. Yeasts grow as single cells that are ovoid or spherical and divide by budding or, rarely, by binary fission like bacteria. The ability to switch from one form to another is termed *dimorphism* and, with some fungi, correlates to a switch from free living to infectious organism.

Foundations

Fungal Reproduction

Fungi generally are capable of reproduction by asexual or sexual means. Asexual reproduction usually refers to the formation of spores, which show resistance to environmental conditions. Spores may be thallospores, which are produced from cells of the body of the fungus or conidia that are produced from specialized structures. Sexual reproduction occurs when two haploid nuclei come together in a single cell. The nuclei are combined to become diploid. Meiosis occurs and results in genetic exchange. Division then results in four haploid progeny nuclei.

Side Effects

Vaginal preparations may cause vaginal or stomach discomfort.

Ketoconazole

Pharmacokinetics

Ketoconazole has erratic oral absorption. It is dependent on gastrointestinal (GI) pH.

Uses

Rarely used for treatment or prophylaxis of fungal infections. Other azoles are preferred.

Side Effects

- GI adverse effects.
- Rash, pruritus, skin irritation.
- Gynecomastia and impotence in men as well as menstrual irregularities in women have been reported (ketoconazole inhibits testosterone synthesis).

31.2.3 Echinocandins

Caspofungin, Micafungin, and Anidulafungin

Mechanism of Action

These agents block the synthesis of β (1,3)-D-glucan, a polysaccharide component of the cell wall in many pathogenic fungi.

Pharmacokinetics

Oral bioavailability is low. These agents are only administered systemically.

Spectrum

Effective for *Candida* and *Aspergillus* species.

Uses

- Treatment of candidiasis.
- Treatment of invasive aspergillosis in patients that are refractory or intolerant of other antifungal medications.

Side Effects

These agents are generally well tolerated, but side effects may include elevation of liver enzymes.

31.2.4 Other Antifungals

Flucytosine

Mechanism of Action

Fungi metabolize the drug to its active form, 5-fluorouracil (▶ Fig. 31.1), which inhibits fungal DNA and RNA synthesis.

Pharmacokinetics

Administered orally.

Uses

Treatment of systemic *Candida* or *Cryptococcus* infections, often in combination with amphotericin B.

Side Effects

Hematologic toxicities including anemia, leukopenia, and thrombocytopenia due to bone marrow suppression.

Griseofulvin

Mechanism of Action

Griseofulvin inhibits fungal cell mitosis.

Pharmacokinetics

Given orally.

Uses

Treatment of tinea pedis and onychomycosis.

Side Effects

May include GI disturbances, peripheral neuropathies, and skin rashes.

Terbinafine

Mechanism of Action

This agent inhibits squalene epoxidase, a key enzyme in sterol biosynthesis.

Pharmacokinetics

Given orally or topically.

Uses

Treatment of onychomycosis of the toenail and fingernail due to dermatophytes.

Side Effects

May include GI disturbances, elevated hepatic enzymes, headache, and taste disturbances.

31.3 Drugs Used in the Treatment of Protozoan Infections

31.3.1 Amebicidal Drugs (Entamoeba histolytica)

Entamoeba histolytica is an intestinal protozoan. Most infections are asymptomatic but may lead to clinical syndromes ranging from dysentery to abscesses of the liver or other organs.

Metronidazole

Mechanism of Action

Metronidazole has a direct amebicidal effect and acts by inhibiting a unique electron transfer system of a variety of anaerobic organisms.

Pharmacokinetics

Orally effective.

Uses

- Treatment of amebiasis, trichomoniasis, and giardiasis.
- Treatment of anaerobic bacterial infections as discussed in Chapter 29.6.

Side Effects

- GI adverse effects including nausea, vomiting, diarrhea, and metallic taste.
- Peripheral neuropathy.
- Alcohol intolerance (disulfiram-like reaction) has been reported.

Contraindications

- Pregnancy.

Iodoquinol (Diiodohydroxyquinoline)

Spectrum

Iodoquinol is directly amebicidal to trophozoites and cysts.

Uses

Treatment of noninvasive or asymptomatic amebiasis.

Side Effects

- GI adverse effects.
- Thyroid gland enlargement.

Paromomycin

Paromomycin is a poorly absorbed aminoglycoside antibiotic.

Spectrum

In addition to eliminating intestinal bacteria, paromomycin directly kills trophozoites and intestinal cestodes.

Uses

- Treatment of intestinal amebiasis.
- Treatment of tapeworm infections (cestodiasis).
- Treatment of cryptosporidiosis.

Protozoan organisms, the diseases they cause, and the drugs of choice are included in ▶ Table 31.1.

31.3.2 Antimalarial Drugs

Malaria is one of the most common protozoan infections. It is caused by *Plasmodium* species that are transferred into the bloodstream via the bite of infected mosquitoes. Symptoms include interspersed bouts of fever and chills. The disease is most commonly found in tropical and subtropical climate regions.
  The *Plasmodium* species involved are
- *Plasmodium vivax* and *P. ovale,* which have erythrocytic and tissue (exoerythrocytic) cycles.
- *P. falciparum* and *P. malariae* which have only erythrocytic cycles.

Quinoline Derivatives

Chloroquine

Mechanisms of Action

Growth of malarial parasites in host erythrocytes requires digestion of hemoglobin in their acidic food vacuoles. This

Table 31.1 Treatment of protozoan infections

Organism	Disease	Drug(s) of choice
Entamoeba histolytica	Amebiasis	Metronidazolev followed by iodoquinol
Cryptosporidium parvum	Cryptosporidiosis	Nitazoxanide
Giardia lamblia (Giardia duodenalis)	Giardiasis	Metronidazole
Leishmania braziliensis, L. mexicana, and other species	Leishmaniasis	Sodium stibogluconate
Pneumocystis jiroveci	Pneumocystosis	Trimethoprim + sulfamethoxazole
Trichomonas vaginalis	Trichomoniasis (a sexually transmitted protozoan infection)	Metronidazole
Toxoplasma gondii	Toxoplasmosis	Pyrimethamine + sulfadiazine
Trypanosoma	South American trypanosomiasis (Chagas disease)	Nifurtimox
	African sleeping sickness	Early stage: Pentamidine Late stage: Eflornithine

produces heme, which is normally crystallized to a nontoxic form. Free heme is highly reactive and toxic to the parasite. Chloroquine accumulates in the digestive vacuoles and prevents detoxification of heme, leading to increased free heme and parasite death (▶ Fig. 31.2).

Spectrum

Chloroquine kills erythrocytic forms of *P. vivax, P. ovale, P. malariae,* and sensitive *P. falciparum.* It is not effective on liver forms.

Pharmacokinetics

- Well absorbed orally.
- Chloroquine is slowly excreted with a half-life of 3 to 5 days.

Uses

Treatment and prophylaxis of malaria.

Side Effects

- GI adverse effects are most common.
- Ocular effects including blurred vision and retinal changes.
- Methemoglobinemia and hemolytic anemia can occur in individuals with a genetic deficiency of glucose-6-phosphate dehydrogenase (G6PD).

Primaquine
Mechanism of Action

The mechanism of action of primaquine is unclear.

Spectrum

- Active against hepatic stages of *P. vivax* and *P. ovale.*
- Highly gametocidal against all four malaria species.

Pharmacokinetics

Rapidly absorbed after oral administration and metabolized to active forms by the liver.

Side Effects

- GI effects are most common.
- In individuals with G6PD deficiency, methemoglobinemia and hemolytic anemia can occur. Patients should be tested for G6PD deficiency.

Quinine and Quinidine

Quinine and quinidine are both alkaloids from the cinchona tree. Quinidine is a stereoisomer of quinine and more potent as well as more toxic than quinine.

Mechanism of Action

Quinine and quinidine act similarly to chloroquine (▶ Fig. 31.2).

Spectrum

- Effective against erythrocytic forms of all four *Plasmodium* species. No effect on liver stages.

Uses

Quinine is a traditional agent now largely replaced by newer drugs, but it is still useful in drug-resistant strains of *P. falciparum.* Quinidine is used for the treatment of severe malaria.

Clinical Correlation

Methemoglobinemia

Methemoglobinemia is a condition in which there are higher levels of methemoglobin in the blood than normal. It occurs when the ferrous ion (Fe^{2+}) is oxidized to the ferric state (Fe^{3+}) in red blood cells when they are exposed to exogenous oxidizing drugs and their metabolites. Methemoglobin does not bind oxygen, and people with this condition will show signs of hypoxia, including dyspnea (shortness of breath), dizziness, cyanosis, fatigue, and mental changes. It is treated by giving oxygen therapy and methylene blue, which is a substance that is able to reduce the iron in hemoglobin to its normal, oxygen-carrying state.

Pharmacokinetics

- Quinine is well absorbed orally.
- Quinidine is administered intravenously to critically ill patients.

Side Effects

- GI adverse effects are most common.
- Cinchonism is the most distinctive toxicity. It is a syndrome including headache, tinnitus, and diplopia.

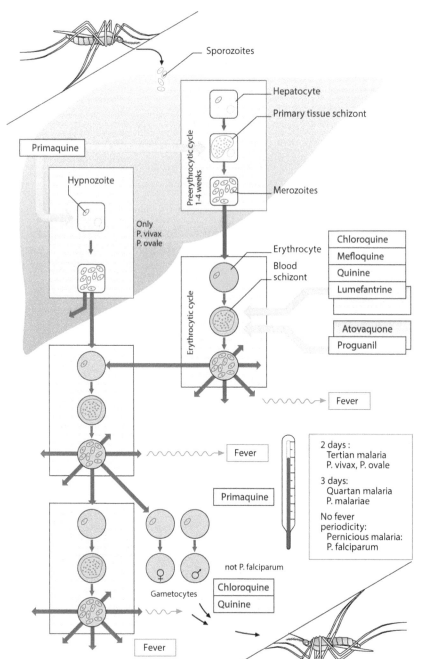

Fig. 31.2 Malaria: stages of the *Plasmodium* life cycle and therapeutic options.

A mosquito carrying malaria feeds on human blood and injects a parasite in the form of sporozoites into the bloodstream. The sporozoites travel to the liver and invade liver cells. Sporozoites mature into forms known as schizonts, which divide to form haploid twins called merozoites. Merozoites exit the liver and enter the bloodstream, where they invade erythrocytes and undergo asexual replication. Some merozoites develop into sexual forms of the parasite, called male and female gametocytes, that circulate in the bloodstream. When a mosquito bites an infected human, it ingests the gametocytes, which eventually form sporozoites. Different antimalarials selectively kill different developmental forms of parasites. Chloroquine and quinine accumulate within the acidic vacuoles of blood schizonts and inhibit the polymerization of heme released from digested hemoglobin. Free heme is toxic to schizonts. Atovaquone suppresses the synthesis of pyrimidine bases, probably by interfering with mitochondrial electron transport.

- Hemolysis can occur, particularly in individuals with G6PD deficiency.
- QT prolongation (due to quinidine's inhibitory effect on K-channels).

Mefloquine

Mechanisms of Action

Similar to chloroquine.

Spectrum

Effective against erythrocytic forms of all four *Plasmodium* species. No effect on liver stages.

Pharmacokinetics

- Mefloquine has a long half-life (10–14 days) and is taken as a single dose to treat mild-to-moderate malaria and once per week as prophylaxis.
- It crosses the blood–brain barrier.

Uses

Treatment and prophylaxis of chloroquine-resistant *P. falciparum.*

Side Effects

- GI distress is the most common.

- Central nervous system (CNS) symptoms including vivid dreams (common), headache, anxiety, psychosis, and seizures can occur. This drug is contraindicated in patients with history of seizure disorder, depression, generalized anxiety disorder, psychosis, schizophrenia, or any other major psychiatric disorder.

Antifolates

Atovaquone/Proguanil

Mechanisms of Action

- Atovaquone disrupts mitochondrial electron transport in parasite and inhibits nucleotide synthesis.
- Proguanil inhibits dihydrofolate reductase.

Spectrum

Effective against erythrocytic forms of all four *Plasmodium* species. No effect on liver stages.

Pharmacokinetics

Administered orally.

Uses

Treatment and prophylaxis of chloroquine-resistant *P. falciparum*.

Side Effects

- GI effects are the most common.
- Mild and reversible elevation of liver enzymes.

Artemisinin Derivatives

Artemether/Lumefantrine

Mechanisms of Action

Artemether binds iron and breaks down peroxide bridges. This leads to the production of free radicals and damages the parasite. The mechanism of lumefantrine is less clear.

Spectrum

Effective against erythrocytic stages of *P. falciparum* and *P. vivax*.

Pharmacokinetics

Well absorbed orally; short half-life: 1 to 3 hours.

Uses

Treatment and prophylaxis of uncomplicated infections due to *P. falciparum*.

Side Effects

- GI effects are common.
- CNS effects: dizziness.

31.4 Drugs Used in the Treatment of Metazoan Infections

31.4.1 Treatment of Nematode Infections (Roundworm)

Albendazole

Mechanism of Action

Albendazole inhibits microtubule synthesis and interferes with microtubule-dependent glucose uptake in the worm.

Pharmacokinetics

Largely unabsorbed; absorption can be enhanced with fatty meals.

Side Effects

Side effects are uncommon and include occasional abdominal distress and diarrhea.

Contraindications

Pregnancy.

31.4.2 Pyrantel Pamoate

Mechanism of Action

Pyrantel pamoate is a noncompetitive, depolarizing neuromuscular blocking agent that causes worm paralysis.

Side Effects

Some mild and transient GI effects and an elevation in liver enzymes may occur.

31.4.3 Ivermectin

Mechanism of Action

Ivermectin binds to glutamate-gated chloride channels on invertebrate nerve and muscle cells. This increases the permeability of cell membranes to chloride ions and hyperpolarizes the nerve or muscle cell, resulting in paralysis and death of the parasite.

Side Effects

GI effects and pruritus have been reported.

31.4.4 Treatment of Cestode Infections (Flatworm)

Praziquantel

Mechanism of Action

Praziquantel increases the permeability of cell membranes to Ca^{2+}, causing marked contraction initially and then a paralysis of worm.

Pharmacokinetics

Well absorbed.

Side Effects

Neurologic effects such as dizziness and headache have been reported.

Unit VII Review Questions

1. Bacteria are able to transfer genes that confer resistance to each other. This usually occurs via which of the following?
   A. Liposomes.
   B. DNA gyrase.
   C. Plasmids.
   D. Proteins.

2. Which of the following antibiotics have the *least* activity against *Pseudomonas aeruginosa*?
   A. Ciprofloxacin.
   B. Doxycycline.
   C. Gentamicin.
   D. Meropenem.
   E. Piperacillin.

3. A patient needs treatment for her "strep throat." She tells you that she developed a rash when she was treated with ampicillin for bronchitis a couple of years ago. Which of the following antibiotics would you recommend?
   A. Aztreonam.
   B. Cefazolin.
   C. Amoxicillin.
   D. Penicillin V.
   E. Vancomycin.

4. A patient with bloody diarrhea needs immediate treatment. Which of the following antibiotics would you recommend for empiric treatment?
   A. Ampicillin.
   B. Vancomycin.
   C. Ciprofloxacin.
   D. Linezolid.

5. A 15-day-old infant has a fever and has been crying nonstop overnight. He vomited after breastfeeding. He was born by vaginal delivery after an uncomplicated pregnancy to a healthy mother with no history of infectious diseases. The infant's nasopharynx was inflamed and mild nuchal rigidity was noticed. The infant's white blood count is elevated and urinalysis is normal. Gram stain of the cerebrospinal fluid reveals small gram-positive bacilli. Which of the following would be the best empiric therapy for this patient?
   A. Ampicillin.
   B. Aztreonam.
   C. Cephalexin.
   D. Gentamicin.
   E. Metronidazole.

6. Which of the following antibiotics cause flushing, tachycardia, nausea, and vomiting when taken with a glass of wine?
   A. Cefepime.
   B. Cefotetan.
   C. Ceftaroline.
   D. Ceftriaxone.
   E. Cefuroxime.

7. Which antibiotic inhibits terminal cross-linking of cell wall glycopeptides?
   A. Streptomycin.
   B. Cephalexin.
   C. Tigecycline.

D. Sulfamethoxazole.
E. Clindamycin.

8. An antibiotic that causes strong GI distress by stimulating motilin receptors causes which of the following additional side effects?
   A. Arthropathy.
   B. Enamel dysplasia.
   C. QT prolongation.
   D. Renal toxicity.
   E. Seizures.

9. A patient with penicillin-resistant *Streptococcus pneumoniae* requires an antibiotic therapy. Which of the following agents would be the best choice?
   A. Cefotaxime.
   B. Penicillin G.
   C. Daptomycin.
   D. Tobramycin.

10. An antibiotic leading to increased risk of tendon rupture has which of the following other side effects?
    A. Anemia.
    B. Lactic acidosis.
    C. Pancreatitis.
    D. Peripheral neuropathy.
    E. QT prolongation.

11. A patient develops severe bacteremia. The lab results reveal the presence of gram-positive cocci in clusters and the *lack* of the mecA plasmid. Which of the following antibiotics would you prescribe?
    A. Amoxicillin.
    B. Aztreonam.
    C. Dicloxacillin.
    D. Penicillin G.
    E. Vancomycin.

12. A 38-year-old woman noticed a small pimple on her left finger that increased in size within 3 hours. She reports to a medical clinic that drains it and does a bacterial culture of the fluid. Empiric antibiotic therapy is started with a cephalosporin. The culture indicates the presence of methicillin-resistant *Staphylococcus aureus* (MRSA). Which of the following antibiotics should be prescribed?
    A. Cephalexin.
    B. Oxacillin.
    C. Penicillin G.
    D. Vancomycin.

13. Which of the following antibiotics is a β-lactam antibiotic and acts predominantly on gram-negative organisms?
    A. Amoxicillin.
    B. Aztreonam.
    C. Erythromycin.
    D. Piperacillin.
    E. Vancomycin.

14. A relatively high incidence of pseudomembranous colitis occurs with
    A. Clindamycin.

B. Sulfamethoxazole.
C. Nitrofurantoin.
D. Tobramycin.
E. Metronidazole.

15. An antibiotic-resistant plasmid enters a *Pseudomonas aeruginosa* cell. This plasmid carries a β-lactamase gene and an aminoglycoside phosphotransferase gene. Which one of the following would be an effective antimicrobial agent against this cell?
   A. Levofloxacin.
   B. Gentamicin.
   C. Neomycin.
   D. Ampicillin.
   E. Cephalexin.

16. A woman presents with urethritis. A culture has revealed the organism to be *Neisseria gonorrhoeae*, which was sensitive to penicillin G, ceftriaxone, ampicillin, doxycycline, and azithromycin. The patient is 4 months pregnant and has previously had a severe hypersensitivity reaction to oxacillin. Which of the following drugs would be indicated for this patient?
   A. Ceftriaxone.
   B. Doxycycline.
   C. Azithromycin.
   D. Ampicillin.
   E. Penicillin G.

17. Which of the following may cause erosion of cartilage?
   A. Ciprofloxacin.
   B. Cefazolin.
   C. Gentamicin.
   D. Penicillin G.
   E. Azithromycin.

18. A 29-year-old woman has dysuria, increased frequency of urination, and urgency to urinate. A urine sample is yellow and cloudy. Dipstick urinalysis gives a pH of 5.0 and is positive for leukocyte esterases, nitrites, and blood. What is the rationale for prescribing a combination drug containing sulfamethoxazole and trimethoprim?
   A. Neither drug alone has an antibacterial action.
   B. The combination has a synergistic antibacterial effect.
   C. Trimethoprim prevents the development of sulfa drug allergies.
   D. Sulfamethoxazole traps trimethoprim in the urine.
   E. Sulfamethoxazole has a short half-life, and trimethoprim has a longer duration of action.

19. A 24-year-old woman with a history of epilepsy presents with a cough, weight loss, and night sweats. Her chest radiograph (X-ray) shows cavitary lesions in the upper left lobe of her lung. A sputum smear reveals many acid-fast bacilli. She is admitted to the hospital, put in a negative pressure room, and placed on a combination of isoniazid, rifampin, pyrazinamide, ethambutol, and vitamin B_6. What would be the reason for including B_6 in her regimen?
   A. To increase bacterial uptake of the drugs.
   B. To prevent central nervous system effects of isoniazid.
   C. To inhibit gastrointestinal side effects of the drugs.

D. To inhibit bacterial resistance.
E. To decrease the night sweats.

20. What is the usual dose-limiting adverse effect of the antitubercular drug ethambutol?
   A. Hepatotoxicity.
   B. Bone marrow depression.
   C. Loss of visual acuity.
   D. Central nervous system toxicity.
   E. Nephrotoxicity.

21. An HIV-positive patient develops acute pancreatitis. Which of the following medications is most likely responsible for this?
   A. Atazanavir.
   B. Didanosine.
   C. Maraviroc.
   D. Enfuvirtide.
   E. Raltegravir.

22. A 63-year-old man had a sharp, burning, intermittent pain in his left lower back for 3 days. He has now developed a rash in the area that was painful. The rash consists of rose-colored macules with clusters of vesicles and is restricted to a band along his back. There are no symptoms suggesting genitourinary or gastrointestinal involvement. Which of the following agents might be useful for treating this patient's symptoms?
   A. Acyclovir.
   B. Amantadine.
   C. Penicillin V.
   D. Cefazolin.
   E. Rifampin.

23. Which of the following, when administered to susceptible individuals, will reduce the incidence and/or severity of influenza types A and B disease?
   A. Trifluridine.
   B. Ribavirin.
   C. Oseltamivir.
   D. Interferon-α.
   E. Gancyclovir.

24. A 28-year-old man has a fever, headache, and chills, accompanied by joint and muscle aches and pains. Because seasonal influenza has been prevalent in the area, he is given zanamivir for inhalation. How does this drug prevent virus particle aggregation and release?
   A. Inhibits influenza neuraminidase.
   B. Inhibits influenza DNA polymerase.
   C. Acts as an ion channel blocker of the influenza M_2 protein.
   D. Inhibits influenza reverse transcriptase.
   E. Inhibits influenza protease.

25. Ribavirin inhibits the replication of which of the following viruses?
   A. Rubella viruses.
   B. Adenoviruses.
   C. Respiratory syncytial virus.
   D. Human immunodeficiency virus.
   E. Cytomegalovirus.

VII

26. Which of the following is most likely to impair renal function?
    A. Flucytosine.
    B. Griseofulvin.
    C. Amphotericin B.
    D. Ketoconazole.
    E. Terbinafine.

27. Which one of the following is the drug of choice in acute amebic dysentery?
    A. Chloroquine.
    B. Ivermectin.
    C. Metronidazole.
    D. Praziquantel.

28. Which of the following is administered for 2 weeks after patients leave an endemic malarial area to eradicate hepatic forms of the parasite?
    A. Mefloquine.
    B. Chloroquine.
    C. Quinine.
    D. Primaquine.
    E. Atovaquone/proguanil.

29. A 29-year-old woman being treated for cystitis with a combination drug containing sulfamethoxazole and trimethoprim has a vaginal discharge with itching. Although her dysuria has improved, she now has a thick, curdlike, white discharge from her vagina. There is no cervical discharge or tenderness, and the uterus and adnexa are normal. Which of the following agents may be useful for treatment of this patient?
    A. Topical miconazole.
    B. Oral penicillin.
    C. Oral metronidazole.
    D. Oral terbinafine.
    E. Topical terbinafine.

30. A woman who was born in the United States travels frequently to Pakistan to visit friends and relatives. Her last visit there was 9 months ago. She has had a fever with sweating, malaise, joint pain, and severe headache. Thin-film Giemsa-stained blood smear shows *Plasmodium vivax* schizonts. The patient is given a drug that accumulates within the acidic vacuoles of blood schizonts and inhibits the polymerization of heme released from digested hemoglobin. Which of the following drugs was she given?
    A. Atovaquone.
    B. Chloroquine.
    C. Artemether.
    D. Tetracycline.

31. Trimethoprim is selectively toxic to bacterial versus mammalian cells because
    A. Mammalian cells do not synthesize folic acid.
    B. Mammalian cells do not take up trimethoprim.
    C. Mammalian cells do not reduce dihydrofolic acid to tetrahydrofolic acid.
    D. Trimethoprim reacts only with the bacterial dihydrofolate reductase to inactivate it in a noncompetitive manner.

E. The mammalian dihydrofolate reductase is much less sensitive to competitive inhibition by trimethoprim than the bacterial enzymes.

32. The selective toxicity of flucytosine is due to the fact that
    A. Only the fungus can take up the drug.
    B. Mammalian cells have a different thymidylate synthetase that is not inhibited by the drug.
    C. Mammalian cells do not incorporate the drug into RNA.
    D. Mammalian cells cannot convert 5-fluorocytosine to 5-fluorouracil.
    E. Mammalian cells do not phosphorylate the drug to the active form.

33. Which of the following is considered to be the drug of choice for treatment of rickettsial infections?
    A. Erythromycin.
    B. Penicillin G.
    C. Doxycycline.
    D. Aztreonam.
    E. Amikacin.

34. Which of the following can cause permanent dental staining in children?
    A. Clindamycin.
    B. Streptomycin.
    C. Quinolones.
    D. Chloramphenicol.
    E. Tetracyclines.

35. A disulfiram-like reaction may occur with
    A. Oxacillin.
    B. Cefotaxime.
    C. Piperacillin.
    D. Cefoperazone.
    E. Chloramphenicol.

36. Mulitple drugs given in combination are used to treat *M. tuberculosis*. The main reason for this is to decrease the incidence of which of the following?
    A. Long-term side effects of the drugs.
    B. Development of bacterial resistance to the drugs.
    C. Patient noncompliance.
    D. Communicability of the disease.
    E. The number of patients who cannot afford therapy.

37. Useful treatment for serious *Bacteroides fragilis* infections outside the central nervous system includes
    A. Clindamycin.
    B. Sulfonamides.
    C. Nitrofurantoin.
    D. Tobramycin.
    E. Nalidixic acid.

38. Crystalluria is most commonly associated with
    A. Clindamycin.
    B. Sulfonamides.
    C. Nitrofurantoin.
    D. Tobramycin.
    E. Nalidixic acid.

39. Which of the following is administered alone to prevent the development of tuberculosis (TB) in individuals at risk?
   A. Pyrazinamide.
   B. Ethambutol.
   C. Rifampin.
   D. Isoniazid.
   E. Streptomycin.

40. Which of the following is indicated only for the treatment of uncomplicated gonorrhea?
   A. Nalidixic acid.
   B. Nitrofurantoin.
   C. Tetracycline.
   D. Spectinomycin.
   E. Minocycline.

41. Which of the following is stable in the presence of gastric acid and penicillinase-producing *Staphylococcus aureus*?
   A. Methicillin.
   B. Ampicillin.
   C. Oxacillin.
   D. Penicillin G.
   E. Phenoxymethyl penicillin.

42. Trimethoprim is an effective inhibitor of
   A. Protein synthesis.
   B. Folic acid synthesis.
   C. DNA gyrase.
   D. Penicillin-binding proteins.
   E. Membrane permeability.

43. Which antibiotic targets para-aminobenzoic acid (PABA)?
   A. Isoniazid.
   B. Chloramphenicol.
   C. Cycloserine.
   D. Sulfonamide.
   E. Rifampin.

44. Amantadine is an antiviral drug effective against
   A. Influenza A viruses.
   B. Influenza B viruses.
   C. Rubella viruses.
   D. Adenoviruses.

45. Acquired immunodeficiency syndrome (AIDS) is the result of an infection by
   A. Rubella virus.
   B. Adenovirus.
   C. Influenza A virus.
   D. Influenza B virus.
   E. Human immunodeficiency virus (HIV).

46. Which of the following is used to treat cytomegalovirus infection in a patient with human immunodeficiency virus (HIV)?
   A. Ganciclovir.
   B. Famciclovir.
   C. Penciclovir.
   D. Amantadine.
   E. Zanamivir.

47. Which of the following is useful in the treatment of systemic mycoses when administered orally?
   A. Miconazole.

   B. Clotrimazole.
   C. Metronidazole.
   D. Flucytosine.
   E. Cytarabine.

48. Which of the following inhibits ergosterol synthesis?
   A. Polyene antifungals.
   B. Imidazole antifungal agents.
   C. Flucytosine.
   D. Griseofulvin.
   E. Caspofungin.

49. The drug of choice for the treatment of tapeworm infestations is
   A. Mebendazole.
   B. Pyrantel pamoate.
   C. Thiabendazole.
   D. Praziquantel.
   E. Piperazine.

50. Which of the following causes a spastic paralysis of roundworms (*Ascaris*) and pinworms (*Enterobius*)?
   A. Mebendazole.
   B. Pyrantel pamoate.
   C. Thiabendazole.
   D. Niclosamide.
   E. Piperazine.

51. Which of the following treats the symptoms of malaria by killing erythrocytic forms of the parasite and causes a set of adverse effects referred to as cinchonism?
   A. Quinine.
   B. Chloroquine.
   C. Pyrimethamine.
   D. Primaquine.
   E. Pyribenzamine.

52. Which of the following binds to sterols, altering fungal cell wall permeability?
   A. Quinine.
   B. Chloroquine.
   C. Pyrimethamine.
   D. Primaquine.
   E. Pyribenzamine.

53. Bone marrow depression is most commonly associated with
   A. Flucytosine.
   B. Griseofulvin.
   C. Penciclovir.
   D. Amantadine.
   E. Zanamivir.

54. Which of the following drugs is effective against roundworm infestation?
   A. Chloroquine.
   B. Griseofulvin.
   C. Mebendazole.
   D. Amantadine.
   E. Ethambutol.

55. A 24-year-old man has a nonpruritic skin rash that first appeared on his abdomen weeks ago and has now spread to his entire body. He has a generalized lymphadenopathy but no fever or pain. Blood pressure and heart rate are normal.

VII

He is not taking any medications and denies illicit drug use, but he does drink alcohol. He admits to having unprotected sex with a woman he met at a party months ago. He also says he was concerned that he may have "caught something" because he had a pimple on his penis a "couple of weeks" later, but it "went away." He reports an allergy to penicillin. Otherwise, his medical history is unremarkable. A venereal disease research laboratory (VDRL) test followed by a fluorescent treponemal antibody absorption (FTA-ABS) test are positive. This patient should be treated with which of the following?

A. Amikacin.
B. Amoxicillin.
C. Doxycycline.
D. Cephalexin.
E. Dicloxacillin.

56. A high school student has a fever, sore throat, lymphadenopathy, and headache. A throat culture is negative for group A β-hemolytic streptococcus (GABS). The patient's parents insist that he be given amoxicillin, as this cured his sore throat the last time. Why would amoxicillin be ineffective in this case?

A. The patient is likely to become allergic to amoxicillin.
B. The patient is unlikely to be compliant.
C. The patient has Epstein-Barr virus (EBV) mononucleosis, which is caused by a virus.
D. Most strains of GABS are penicillin-resistant.
E. Previous exposure to amoxicillin has led to the development of resistant strains.

57. A 32-year-old man has weight loss, white plaques on the pharynx, and purple lesions on the abdomen, which on biopsy reveals Kaposi sarcoma. With which virus is this patient most likely infected?

A. Herpes simplex virus (HSV).
B. Human immunodeficiency virus (HIV).
C. Respiratory syncytial virus (RSV).
D. Varicella zoster virus (VZV).

58. A 63-year-old man had a sharp, burning, intermittent pain in his left lower back for days. He has now developed a rash in the area that was painful. The rash consists of rose-colored macules with clusters of vesicles and is restricted to a band along his back. There are no symptoms suggesting genitourinary or gastrointestinal involvment. The patient is given a drug that acts by which of the following mechanisms of action?

A. Inhibits viral neuraminidase.
B. Inhibits viral DNA polymerase.
C. Acts as an ion channel blocker of the viral M_2 protein.
D. Inhibits viral reverse transcriptase.
E. Inhibits viral protease.

59. A 32-year-old man has been diagnosed as infected with human immunodeficiency virus (HIV). Why does treatment of this disease require multiple drug therapy?

A. Resistance develops to monotherapy.
B. Different drugs affect different stages of viral replication.
C. Side effects in combined regimens are more tolerable.
D. Rashes are less common.
E. Multiple drugs are required in immunocompromised patients.

60. A woman who was born in the United States travels frequently to Pakistan to visit friends and relatives. She has had a *Plasmodium vivax* infection that was successfully treated with a drug that is effective on the erythrocytic form but is not effective on liver forms. Before administering a drug to treat the liver form, a test should be performed to check for which of the following?

A. Variegate porphyria.
B. Coinfection with human immunodeficiency virus (HIV).
C. Cytochrome P-3A(CYP3A4) isoforms.
D. Glucose-6-phosphate deficiency.
E. Serum alanine aminotransferase level.

61. A 7-year-old refugee has the eggs of *Trichuris* (whipworm), *Ascaris* (roundworm), and *Ancylostoma* (hookworm) in his stool. His hands and feet are not red or itching. He also has a microcytic anemia with a low serum iron. Which of the following drugs would be the best treatment for this patient?

A. Pyrantel orally and ferrous sulfate orally.
B. Pyrantel orally and thiabendazole orally.
C. Ferrous sulfate orally and thiabendazole orally.
D. Ferrous sulfate orally and mebendazole orally.
E. Thiabendazole orally and mebendazole orally.

Unit VII Answers and Explanations

1. C. Transfer of drug-resistant genes usually occurs via plasmids.

2. B. *Pseudomonas aeruginosa* is a gram-negative rod that can be treated with aminoglycosides (gentamicin), fluoroquinolones (ciprofloxacin has best activity), the carbapenems (meropenem), and the pseudomonas-penicillins (fourth-generation penicillins: piperacillin).

The major mechanisms of resistance to antibiotics of *Pseudomonas* are the low number of porin channels in the cell wall (therefore, earlier generation penicillins have no activity) and efflux pumps (tetracyclines). In fact, doxycycline is intrinsically resistant against pseudomonas (and proteus mirabilis) as both are substrates for their efflux pumps.

3. B. For "strep-throat" the drug of choice would be amoxicillin or penicillin (if the strain is sensitive). However, as the patient mentioned a "rash" after ampicillin treatment, the recommendation would be to switch to a cephalosporin (e.g., first generation). The cross-allergenicity is very low and therefore justifiable if the patient only had a "rash." The cross-allergenicity from penicillins to aztreonam is nearly 0%; however, aztreonam works only for gram-negatives. There would be no reason to prescribe vancomycin—this antibiotic should be reserved for more severe allergic reaction due to penicillins and for other life-threatening infections.

4. C. Bloody diarrhea can be caused by a variety of enteroinvasive pathogens like *Campylobacter*, *Salmonella*, *Shigella*, *Yersinia*, and *E. coli*. Therefore, an antibiotic used to treat gram-negative bacteria (all bacteria causing bloody diarrhea are gram-negative) would be indicated: Ampicillin has only poor gram-negative coverage, vancomycin and linezolid only work against gram-positive bacteria (mainly used for MRSA, VRE, VRSA). Empiric treatment for enteroinvasive diarrhea is ciprofloxacin.

5. A. The most common causes of meningitis in neonates are *Listeria* and group B *Streptococcus*. The symptoms with either bacteria are similar. When the disease presents 2 to 3 weeks postpartum, it is most likely to result from exposure to *Listeria* during or shortly after delivery. As cerebral fluid analysis reveals gram-positive bacilli, an infection with *Listeria* is very likely. Treatment of *Listeria* meningitis is with ampicillin plus or minus gentamicin because of the resistance of *Listeria* to cephalosporins, which are commonly chosen as empiric therapy for streptococcal meningitis in children. Aztreonam is only effective against gram-negative infections and metronidazole is mainly used for anaerobic infections.

6. B. The clinical presentation describes a disulfiram reaction caused by the inhibition of the aldehyde dehydrogenase. If ethanol is ingested and the aldehyde dehydrogenase is inhibited, acetaldehyde accumulates. The symptoms are flushing, nausea, vomiting, and headache (acetaldehyde is a potent vasodilator). Cefotetan can inhibit the aldehyde dehydrogenase and can cause a disulfiram reaction. Another antibiotic that can cause a disulfiram reaction is metronidazole.

7. B. Cephalosporins (e.g., cephalexin) inhibit bacterial cell wall synthesis in a manner identical to that of penicillin.

Streptomycin, tigecycline, and clindamycin inhibit bacterial protein synthesis.

Sulfamethoxazole, a sulfonamide, is structurally related to *p*-amino benzoic acid (PABA). It blocks folic acid synthesis in microbes that must synthesize folic acid from PABA.

8. C. Erythromycin enhances gut motility via stimulation of motilin receptors (erythromycin is also used for patients with gastroparesis). Other side effects of the macrolides are hepatotoxicity and QT prolongation.

Arthropathy is a typical side effect of the fluoroquinolones, and renal toxicity is important for the aminoglycosides (and also for β-lactam antibiotics, vancomycin, and for amphotericin). Administration of imipenem/cilastin can lead to CNS effects (e.g., seizures).

9. A. Third-generation cephalosporins have excellent activity against most strains of *S. pneumoniae*, including the vast majority of those resistant to penicillin.

Daptomycin is inactivated by pulmonary surfactant and is therefore not indicated for the treatment of pneumonia. Tobramycin (when used as monotherapy) is only active against gram-negative bacteria and therefore has no activity against streptococci.

10. E. Tendon rupture is an important side effect of fluoroquinolones. Fluoroquinolones have been known to cause direct toxicity to collagen and promote collagen degradation. Important side effects of fluoroquinolones are QT prolongation (as they block potassium channels), arthropathy (damage to the growing cartilage), dermatologic reactions (photosensitivity, rashes), and GI distress.

Lactic acidosis, peripheral neuropathy, and pancreatitis are typical side effects of nucleoside/nucleotide reverse transcriptase inhibitors (NRTIs; mitochondrial toxicity).

11. C. The major mechanism of antibiotic resistance of *S. aureus* (*MSSA*, as the mecA plasmid is lacking) is the production of β-lactamases. Therefore, any β-lactamase-resistant antibiotic can be used: Oxacillin, dicloxacillin, nafcillin (all second generation) OR amoxicillin + clavulanic acid OR ticarcillin + clavulanic acid, all cephalosporins, etc. Amoxicillin alone would have no activity as it is β-lactamase sensitive. Aztreonam has only activity against gram-negatives. Penicillin G is also β-lactamase sensitive. Vancomycin would *not* be indicated for MSSA (only for MRSA).

12. D. Once the lab results indicate MRSA, any β-lactam antibiotic is not effective any more. The resistance of MRSA depends on its changed penicillin-binding proteins (PBPs). As all β-lactam antibiotics share the same mechanism of action, namely binding to PBPs and inhibiting cell wall synthesis, an antibiotic must be chosen that acts independently from PBPs. First-line antibiotic for the treatment of MRSA is vancomycin.

VII

13. B. From the drugs listed, only amoxicillin, aztreonam, and piperacillin, are β-lactam antibiotics. Amoxicillin is mainly active against gram-positive organisms. Piperacillin has activity against gram-positive organisms as well as gram-negative organisms. Aztreonam is mainly active against gram-negative bacteria.

14. A. Clindamycin, like many antibacterial agents, alters the normal flora of the colon, which may lead to overgrowth of *Clostridium difficile*. Proliferation of drug-resistant *C. difficile* produces two toxins that may cause pseudomembranous colitis. The antibiotics that most commonly produce pseudomembranous colitis are ampicillin and clindamycin. The disease is treated by discontinuing ampicillin or clindamycin and giving either metronidazole or vancomycin.

B–E. The other agents listed typically do not produce pseudomembranous colitis.

15. A. β-lactam and aminoglycoside antibiotics would be ineffective against this cell. Levofloxacin is the only agent listed that is not a β-lactam or aminoglycoside. Levofloxacin is highly active against *Pseudomonas* infections.

16. C. Ceftriaxone is the drug of choice for uncomplicated urogenital gonococcal infections. Second-line agents are azithromycin and doxycycline. As the patient experienced severe penicillin allergy, penicillins and cephalosporins should be avoided. Doxycycline is contraindicated in pregnancy; therefore, azithromycin should be recommended.

17. A. Fluoroquinolones are associated with an increased risk of erosion of cartilage.

B–E. The other drugs are not typically associated with cartilage damage.

18. B. The combination is used because the drugs exert synergistic antibacterial activity. Sulfamethoxazole inhibits bacterial folic acid synthesis by competing with *p*-aminobenzoic acid, and trimethoprim inhibits dihydrofolate reductase, thus blocking two consecutive steps in the synthesis of nucleic acids and proteins essential to bacteria. Each drug alone does have some antibacterial activity. Trimethoprim does not prevent the development of sulfa drug allergies and sulfamethoxazole does not trap trimethoprim in the urine. The half-lives of the drugs are about equal.

19. B. Isoniazid reacts chemically with pyridoxal and can cause neuropathy and convulsions. This is usually not a problem in patients receiving adequate vitamin B_6 in the diet, but this patient has a history of seizures. Thus, coadministration of vitamin B_6 is used to avoid potential adverse neurologic effects.

20. C. Ethambutol is usually well tolerated, but retrobulbar neuritis (a visual field defect) is seen occasionally at high doses. The other conditions are not associated with ethambutol administration.

21. B. A "class" toxicity of NRTIs is mitochondrial toxicity (anemia, peripheral neuropathy, pancreatitis, and lactic acidosis) as reverse transcriptase inhibitors have some affinity for DNA polymerase gamma (mitochondrial enzyme). Didanosine belongs to the NRTIs with high mitochondrial toxicity, specifically pancreatitis. Didanosine is absolutely contraindicated in patients with pancreatitis. None of the other drugs belong to the NRTIs.

22. A. The symptoms are indicative of a herpes zoster flare-up or shingles. Acyclovir is an antiviral drug that is effective in the treatment of herpes.

Amantadine is an antiviral drug used in the prophylaxis and treatment of influenza. Penicillin V is a β-lactam antibiotic that is effective in mild-to-moderate streptococcal, staphylococcal, and pneumococcal infections such as skin, ear, and respiratory infections. Cefazolin is a first-generation cephalosporin that is effective against many gram-positive cocci. Rifampin is active against tuberculosis and other microbes.

23. C. Oseltamivir is an inhibitor of influenza neuraminidase and acts on both influenza types A and B. Without neuraminidase, the hemagglutinin of the virus binds to sialic acid, forming clumps and preventing virus release. Trifluridine is effective against herpes simplex keratitis. Ribavirin is effective against respiratory syncytial virus and hepatitis C. Interferon-α is used to treat hepatitis B and hepatitis C (in combination with ribavirin). Ganciclovir is used to treat cytomegalovirus infection in immunocompromised patients.

24. A. Zanamivir inhibits influenza neuraminidase. Without neuraminidase, the hemagglutinin of the virus binds to sialic acid, forming clumps and preventing virus release.

25. C. Ribavirin is administered by aerosol to treat lower respiratory tract infections caused by respiratory syncytial virus.

26. C. Of the drugs listed, amphotericin B is the one most likely to have renal side effects. Flucytosine is most likely to have hematological side effects. Griseofulvin may cause GI disturbances, CNS abnormalities, and skin rashes. Ketoconazole may cause fatal hepatic toxicity and terbinafine may cause rash and increased liver enzymes.

27. C. Metronidazole is used to treat systemic and intestinal forms of amebiasis. Chloroquine is an antimalarial agent. Ivermectin and praziquantel are drugs used to treat infections with helminths.

28. D. Primaquine can destroy exoerythrocytic forms of the parasite and is gametocidal. All other drugs mentioned are only active against the erythrocytic forms and do not act on liver forms of the parasite.

29. A. The patient has vulvovaginal candidiasis. Alteration of the normal flora by the systemic antibiotics likely contributed to the emergence of the *Candida* infection. Usually a topical antifungal agent such as miconazole is effective. Penicillin and metronidazole are antibiotic agents that are unsuitable for fungal infections. Terbinafine is used to treat onychomycosis (nail infections).

30. B. Chloroquine accumulates within the acidic vacuoles of blood schizonts and inhibits the polymerization of heme released from digested hemoglobin.

31. E. Trimethoprim inhibits bacterial dihydrofolate reductase. The human enzyme is less sensitive to trimethoprim, so it is relatively selectively toxic to bacteria.

32. D. Fungi susceptible to flucytosine are capable of deaminating it to 5-fluorouracil, an antimetabolite used in cancer chemotherapy. Mammalian cells lack cytosine deaminase, so flucytosine is not metabolized to fluorouracil.

33. C. *Rickettsiae* are intracellular parasites that transmit typhus, spotted fevers, and Q fever. In the United States, the two rickettsial diseases of significance are Rocky Mountain spotted fever (*Rickettsia rickettsii*) and Q fever (*Coxiella burnetii*). The tetracyclines are effective against these organisms. Doxycycline is the only tetracycline listed and is the drug of choice of many practitioners.

34. E. Tetracyclines are incorporated into enamel during tooth development (last half of pregnancy, infancy, and childhood to 8 years old) and may cause permanent discoloration of the teeth.

35. D. Concurrent use of ethanol with cephalosporins that contain a methyltetrazolethiol side chain (e.g., cefamandole, cefotetan, cefmetazole, and cefoperazone), may result in a disulfiram-like reaction, including flushing, tachycardia, headache, sweating, thirst, nausea, and vomiting, due to inhibition of acetaldehyde metabolism.

A. Oxacillin is a penicillinase-resistant penicillin. It does not cause a disulfiram-like reaction with ethanol.

B. Cefotaxime is a third generation cephalosporin. It does not contain a methyltetrazolethiol side chain and therefore does not cause a disulfiram-like reaction with ethanol.

C. Piperacillin is an extended spectrum penicillin. It does not cause a disulfiram-like reaction with ethanol.

E. Chloramphenicol is an inhibitor of bacterial protein synthesis. It does not cause a disulfiram-like reaction with ethanol.

36. B. Antituberculosis drugs must be used in combination to avoid the occurrence of rapid resistance which occurs when a single drug is given.

37. A. Clindamycin is effective against *Bacteroides fragilis*.

B. Sulfonamides are effective against most gram-positive bacteria, many gram-negative bacteria, Nocardia, Actinomyces, Chlamydia, and Plasmodium. They are not effective against *Bacteroides fragilis*.

C, E. Nitrofurantoin and nalidixic acid are urinary antiseptic agents.

D. Tobramycin is effective against gram-positive and gram-negative bacteria. Because aminoglycosides, such as tobramycin, are actively transported into a bacterial cell by an oxygen-dependent enzyme system, only aerobic bacteria are sensitive to these drugs. Thus they are not effective against *Bacteroides fragilis* (anaerobic).

38. B. Sulfonamides may form crystals and precipitate, particularly in acidic urine; thus, patients taking sulfonamides must maintain adequate fluid intake during therapy to prevent crystalluria and stone formation.

A, C–E. Crystalluria is not typically associated with the other drugs listed.

39. D. Isoniazid is used for prophylaxis as well as for treatment of active TB infections.

A–C, E. The other agents listed would not be administered alone to prevent the development of TB.

40. D. Spectinomycin is used exclusively for treatment of gonorrhea.

A, B. Nalidixic acid and nitrofurantoin are used as urinary antiseptic agents.

C, E. Tetracycline and minocycline are used for rickettsial infections, chlamydial infections, sexually transmitted diseases, acne, and brucellosis. They are also an alternative therapy in penicillin-allergic patients.

41. C. Oxacillin is effective orally and is resistant to penicillinases. It is also effective against gram-positive organisms.

A. Methicillin is ineffective orally and therefore must be given parentally.

B, D, E. These agents are sensitive to penicillinases.

42. B. Trimethoprim inhibits bacterial dihydrofolate reductase, thus inhibiting folic acid synthesis.

43. D. Sulfonamides are structurally similar to PABA and block folic acid synthesis in microbes that must synthesize folic acid from PABA.

44. A. Amantadine is a highly selective antiviral drug that inhibits the growth of influenza A viruses by blocking the viral M2 ion channel protein, which prevents viral uncoating.

B–D. Amantadine is not used in the treatment of influenza B, rubella, or adenoviruses.

45. E. HIV is a retrovirus that causes AIDS.

46. A. Ganciclovir is used to treat cytomegalovirus infection in immunocompromised patients, such as those with HIV.

B, C. Famciclovir and penciclovir are used in herpes infections.

D, E. Amantadine is for treatment of influenza A and zanamivir for influenza types A and B.

47. D. Flucytosine is an orally effective antifungal useful in systemic *Candida* or *Cryptococcus* infections.

A, B. Miconazole and clotrimazole are topical antifungals.

C. Metronidazole is an amebicidal drug.

E. Cytarabine is an anticancer drug.

48. B. Imidazole antifungal agents interfere with cytochrome P-450–dependent biosynthesis of ergosterol.

VII

A. Polyene antifungals permeate into ergosterol-rich membranes and produce a detergent-like effect.

C. Flucytosine is metabolized by fungus to fluorouracil.

D. Griseofulvin inhibits fungal mitosis by disrupting the mitotic spindle.

E. Caspofungin blocks the synthesis of β (1,3)-D-glucan, a polysaccharide component of the fungal cell wall.

49. D. Praziquantel is an orally effective agent for the treatment of cestode, or tapeworm, infections.

A–C, E. Mebendazole, pyrantel, thiabendazole, and piperazine are used to treat nematode, or roundworm, infections.

50. B. Pyrantel is a noncompetitive depolarizing neuromuscular blocking agent that causes worm paralysis.

A, C. Mebendazole and thiabendazole bind to and inhibit tubulin synthesis and also inhibit glucose uptake and larval development.

D. Niclosamide is an obsolete anthelmintic effective against cestodes, or tapeworms.

E. Piperazine produces competitive block of acetylcholine on worm muscle. Worms are paralyzed and eliminated alive.

51. A. Quinine poisoning is called cinchonism. The name derives from the fact that the natural source of quinine is cinchona bark. Headache, tinnitus, and diplopia are signs of mild cinchonism.

52. A. Amphotericin B is a polyene antifungal that permeates into ergosterol-rich membranes and produces a detergent-like effect.

B. Ketoconazole is an imidazole antifungal agent that interferes with cytochrome P-450–dependent biosynthesis of ergosterol.

C. Flucytosine is metabolized by fungus to fluorouracil.

D. Griseofulvin inhibits fungal mitosis by disrupting the mitotic spindle.

E. Caspofungin blocks the synthesis of β (1,3)-d-glucan, a polysaccharide component of the fungal cell wall.

53. A. Of the drugs listed, flucytosine is the one most likely to have hematological side effects.

B. Griseofulvin may cause gastrointestinal disturbances, central nervous system abnormalities, and skin rashes.

C. Amphotericin B may cause renal toxicity.

D. Ketoconazole may cause fatal hepatic toxicity, and adverse cardiac events when taken with terfenadine, astemizole, or cisapride.

E. Terbinafine may cause a hypersensitivity rash, increased liver enzymes, or liver failure (rarely).

54. C. Of the drugs listed, mebendazole is effective against nematode, or roundworm, infestation.

A. Chloroquine is an antimalarial agent.

B. Griseofulvin is an antifungal agent.

D. Amantadine is an antiviral agent.

E. Ethambutol is an antituberculosis drug.

55. C. The drug of choice for the treatment of syphilis is benzathine penicillin G. Patients who are allergic to penicillin can be treated with doxycycline, ceftriazone, or tetracycline.

A. Amikacin is an aminoglycoside antibiotic that is effective against gram-negative and gram-positive aerobic bacteria.

B, E. Amoxicillin and dicloxacillin are penicillins, to which the patient is allergic.

D. Patients that are allergic to pencillin are often also allergic to cephalosporins, such as cephalexin.

56. C. Amoxicillin is an antibacterial drug. Although previously the patient likely had a strep throat that was cured by amoxicillin, the symptoms in this case are not consistent with GABS, and the throat culture is negative. The patient most likely has EBV mononucleosis, which is caused by a virus and would not be susceptible to amoxicillin.

57. B. Although Kaposi sarcoma can occur in elderly men in the United States and endemically in Africa, in the United States Kaposi sarcoma is usually seen in men with HIV infection.

58. B. These are symptoms of shingles, a flare-up of herpes zoster. Treatment is with an antiviral drug such as acyclovir that acts to inhibit viral DNA polymerase.

59. A. In the treatment of acquired immunodeficiency syndrome (AIDS) with highly active antiretroviral therapy (HAART), combination therapy is used to decrease the development of resistance. It usually involves using three agents from two different classes.

B-E. The other choices are invalid.

60. D. Primaquine may result in methemoglobinemia and hemolytic anemia in individuals with a genetic deficiency of glucose-6-phosphate dehydrogenase.

61. D. This patient requires antiparasitic treatment and treatment for his anemia. For the latter, oral ferrous sulfate is indicated. Either thiabendazole or mebendazole will kill the worms, but thiabendazole has greater systemic toxicity. Because the patient has no systemic symptoms, mebendazole, which is not absorbed but will kill worms in the gut, is recommended.

Unit VIII

Autocoids and Analgesic, Antipyretic, and Anti-inflammatory Drugs

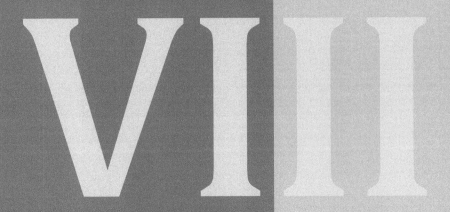

32 Autocoids and Related Drugs

Summary

The autocoids include serotonin, bradykinin, histamine, and eicosanoids. The triptans are serotonin agonist drugs (sumatriptan, zolmitriptan, naratriptan, rizatriptan, eletriptan, frovatriptan, and almotriptan) used to treat migraine headaches. Bradykinin, a potent vasodilator, is formed by the action of the plasma enzyme kallikrein. Icatibant is an antagonist of the B_2 subtype of bradykinin receptors. Ecallantide is an inhibitor of plasma kallikrein. These drugs are used to treat hereditary angioedema. H_1 antihistamines include the first-generation, diphenhydramine, promethazine, and chlorpheniramine, with significant sedative, anticholinergic, and antiemetic effects. Second-generation, nonsedating H_1 antihistamines are loratadine, fexofenadine, and cetirizine. H_1 antihistamines are used for relief of allergic rhinitis, allergic conjunctivitis, and the common cold. H_2 antihistamines, such as cimetidine, famotidine, nizatidine, and ranitidine, inhibit gastric acid secretion and are used to treat peptic ulcers and gastroesophageal reflux disease (GERD). Cromolyn sodium inhibits mast cell degranulation. It is used prophylactically for asthma and for seasonal allergic rhinitis. Omalizumab is an antibody to IgE. It can be used to treat IgE-mediated allergic asthma. The eicosanoids are derived from arachidonic acid and include the prostaglandins, prostacyclins, thromboxanes, and leukotrienes. Prostaglandin analogues have a variety of specialized uses: to maintain the patency of ductus arteriosus in neonates; treat erectile dysfunction; treat ocular hypertension or open-angle glaucoma or hypotrichosis of the eyelashes; as abortifacients or to induce labor at term; for prophylaxis of nonsteroidal anti-inflammatory drug (NSAID)-induced gastric ulcers (as it is a potent inhibitor of gastric secretion of acid). Aspirin and corticosteroids exert their anti-inflammatory effects by blocking the synthesis of prostaglandins.

Keywords: serotonin, bradykinin, histamine, prostaglandin, leukotrienes

32.1 Introduction to Autocoids and Related Drugs

Autocoids are biologically active molecules that are locally acting hormones. They are synthesized and released in a paracrine fashion and play a role in vasoconstriction, vasodilation, and inflammation. The autocoids include serotonin, bradykinin, histamine, and eicosanoids.

Foundations

Autocrine, Paracrine, and Endocrine Signaling

Autocrine signaling occurs when a cell secretes a hormone that binds to receptors and produces an effect on that same cell.

Paracrine signaling occurs when a cell secretes a hormone that acts on nearby cells.

Endocrine signaling occurs when a cell secretes a substance that enters the bloodstream, is transported to distant tissues, and acts on cells in that tissue.

32.2 Serotonin and Related Drugs

32.2.1 Serotonin

Serotonin is also discussed in Chapter 10.

Synthesis

Serotonin (5-hydroxytryptamine [5-HT]) is synthesized from tryptophan by tryptophan hydroxylase.

Location

High concentrations of serotonin are found in enterochromaffin cells of the gastrointestinal (GI) tract. They are also found in platelets and in the central nervous system (CNS).

Metabolism

Metabolism is by oxidative deamination via monoamine oxidase (MAO).

Receptors

Serotonin receptors are found in the CNS, GI tract, and on smooth muscle. They are grouped into four major groups: $5\text{-}HT_1$, $5\text{-}HT_2$, $5\text{-}HT_3$, and $5\text{-}HT_{4\text{-}7}$. Each of these families has numerous members.

- The $5\text{-}HT_1$ (G_i), $5\text{-}HT_2$ (G_q), and $5\text{-}HT_{4\text{-}7}$ (G_s) receptor families are G protein-coupled receptors.
- The $5\text{-}HT_3$ receptor is a ligand-gated ion channel.

Effects

- CNS: ascending systems are involved in the promotion of sleep, in determining mood, and in mental illness (through interactions in limbic areas); descending systems may be involved in modulating pain perception.
- GI tract: increases contractility of the gut.
- Smooth muscle: vasoconstriction.

32.2.2 Serotonin Agonist Drugs: Triptans

Almotriptan, Eletriptan, Rizatriptan, Sumatriptan, Zolmitriptan, Frovatriptan, and Naratriptan

Mechanism of Action

These agents are selective $5\text{-}HT_{1B/1D}$ receptor agonists. Their mechanism to decrease migraine may result from the ability of these drugs to

- Directly produce constriction of pial and dural blood vessels.
- Inhibit the release of vasodilator and proinflammatory peptides (calcitonin gene-related peptide [cGRP], substance P, and vasoactive intestinal peptide [VIP]).

- Activate presynaptic inhibitory serotonin receptors of trigeminal nerve afferents innervating intracranial vessels.

Pharmacokinetics

- Administered by subcutaneous (SC) injection, as a nasal spray, or orally.
- Agents vary in speed of onset and duration of action.
- Effective at any time during the attack but more effective if given earlier (during the aura preceding migraine onset).
- Also help to relieve nausea and vomiting which accompany the attack.

Clinical Correlation

Carcinoid Tumors and Serotonin Syndrome

Carcinoid tumors are neuroendocrine tumors of the GI tract, urogenital tract, or the pulmonary bronchioles. Carcinoid tumors can contain and secrete numerous autocoids, including prostaglandins and serotonin, causing symptoms such as flushing and diarrhea. Cardiac diseases due to fibrosis of the endocardium and valves, as well as asthma-like symptoms, are also common. Flushing may be precipitated by stress, alcohol, certain foods, and drugs, particularly selective serotonin reuptake inhibitors (SSRIs), so these should be avoided. Heart failure, wheezing, and diarrhea are treated with diuretics, bronchodilators, and antidiarrheal agents (e.g., loperamide and diphenoxylate), respectively. If patients remain symptomatic, serotonin receptor antagonists, antihistamines, and somatostatin analogues are the drugs of choice. 5-HT$_3$ receptor antagonists (ondansetron, tropisetron, dolasetron, granisetron, palonosetron, ramosetron, alosetron, and cilansetron) can control diarrhea and nausea, and occasionally ameliorate the flushing. A combination of histamine H$_1$ and H$_2$ receptor antagonists (diphenhydramine and cimetidine or ranitidine) may control flushing in patients with upper GI or pulmonary carcinoids. Synthetic analogues of somatostatin (octreotide and lanreotide) are the most widely used agents to control the symptoms of patients with carcinoid syndrome.

Uses

- Acute migraine.
- Cluster headaches.

Side Effects

- Chest pain, flushing, nausea, weakness, and dizziness.
- In rare cases, serious cardiac events (coronary artery vasospasm, transient myocardial ischemia, myocardial infarction, ventricular tachycardia, and fibrillation) and hypertensive episodes have occurred.

Contraindications

Coronary, cerebrovascular, or other arterial disease; uncontrolled hypertension.

Drug Interactions

- Hypertensive crisis (see Chapter 10) may occur if patient has used MAO inhibitors (MAOIs) within 2 weeks.
- Serotonin syndrome (see Chapter 10) may occur if these agents are combined with SSRIs.

32.2.3 Mixed Serotonin Drugs: Ergot Alkaloid Derivatives

Ergot alkaloids are also discussed in Chapter 17.

Ergotamine

Mechanism of Action

Ergotamine causes intense vasoconstriction. It also has partial agonist or antagonist activity against serotonergic, dopaminergic, and α adrenergic receptors.

Pharmacokinetics

- Variable absorption after oral administration.
- May be given via sublingual, rectal, and intramuscular routes.
- Caffeine enhances both the absorption and the peripheral action of ergotamine.
- Limitations have been placed on the total dose of ergotamine that can be taken per attack and per week to prevent ergot poisoning.

Uses

Acute migraine.

Side Effects

Nausea, vomiting, weakness, and paresthesias.

Toxicity

The most serious toxic effects result from sustained vasoconstriction that can lead to brain or cardiac ischemia.

Contraindications

Pregnancy.

32.2.4 Dihydroergotamine Mesylate

Dihydroergotamine mesylate is an ergot alkaloid derivative.

Pharmacokinetics

Given by intramuscular injection, SC injection, or nasal spray.

Uses

Acute migraine.

Note: Dihydroergotamine mesylate is less effective than ergotamine but has a lower incidence of vomiting when injected.

VIII

Clinical Correlation

Migraine

Migraines are characterized by a severe, unilateral throbbing headache, which is often preceded by an aura (usually visual), and may be accompanied by nausea, vomiting, and photophobia. They are caused by the dilation of blood vessels in the pia mater and dura mater surrounding the brain. This triggers the release of neuropeptides, such as cGRP and substance P from parasympathetic nerve fibers approximating these vessels, and excites nociceptive fibers, which travel in the trigeminal nerve back to the brain. The involvement of 5-HT in migraine is suggested by the finding that blockade of 5-HT receptors can prevent or stop migraine attacks. A nonopiate analgesic (e.g., aspirin, acetaminophen, or NSAID) may be effective for acute treatment of mild-to-moderate migraine. Treatment of moderate-to-severe acute migraine includes triptans and ergot alkaloid derivatives. Drugs used for migraine prophylaxis include the β blockers, anticonvulsants, and antidepressants, although the mechanisms of action of these agents in migraine are not understood.

Clinical Correlation

Cluster Headaches

Cluster headaches (migrainous neuralgia) are severe, unilateral, nonpulsatile, periorbital headaches that occur frequently throughout the day for several weeks, followed by a pain-free period that can last several months. Like migraine headaches, cluster headaches have an unknown etiology but appear to result from changes in brain blood flow. Drugs that are effective in terminating migraine are usually effective in terminating cluster headaches, including the triptans and dihydroergotamine. Approximately 50 to 70% of cluster headaches can be terminated by inhalation of 100% oxygen.

▸ Table 32.1 lists other serotonin agonists and antagonists, noting their uses and where they have been discussed in other chapters.

32.3 Bradykinin and Related Drugs

32.3.1 Bradykinin

Synthesis

Bradykinin is formed from the α_2 globulin precursor bradykininogen by the plasma enzyme kallikrein. Kallikrein is activated by kinins, trypsin, plasmin, factor XIIa, and pepsin.

Location

Bradykinin is found in plasma and tissues.

Metabolism

Bradykinin exists in plasma in an inactive form and has a half-life of ~ 15 seconds. A single passage through the pulmonary vascular bed destroys 80 to 90% of the kinins. The principal catabolizing enzymes in the lung are kininase I (carboxypeptidase) and kininase II (angiotensin-converting enzyme).

Table 32.1 Serotonin agents and uses

Serotonin agents	Receptor subtype	Uses(s)	Chapter reference(s)
Agonists			
Triptans	5-HT_{1D}	Migraine	Chapter 32
Partial agonist			
Buspirone	5-HT_{1A}	Anxiety	Chapter 9
Antagonists			
Ondansetron, dolasetron, and palonosetron	5-HT_3	Nausea and vomiting	Chapter 27
Trazadone	5-HT_{2A}	Antidepressant	Chapter 10
Clozapine and other atypical antipsychotic agents	5-HT_{2A}	Antipsychotic	Chapter 12
Reuptake inhibitors			
Fluoxetine and other SSRIs[a]	–	Antidepressant	Chapter 10

[a]These agents are thought to act by decreasing neuronal serotonin uptake. Abbreviations: 5-HT, 5-hydroxytryptamine; SSRI, selective serotonin reuptake inhibitor.

Receptors

There are two types of bradykinin receptors: B_1 and B_2. B_2 receptors mediate the majority of bradykinin effects, including vasodilation, stimulation of pain, smooth muscle contraction, and increased capillary permeability.

Effects

- Cardiovascular: bradykinin is a potent vasodilator (10 times more potent than histamine). It causes vasodilation of blood vessels in the muscle, kidney, viscera, heart, and brain. Plasma kinins increase capillary permeability, which leads to edema.
- Renal function and blood pressure: bradykinin may be involved in the local regulation of renal function. The kinin system may be activated to blunt the effects of pressor agents.
- Smooth muscle: bradykinin is a potent constrictor of uterine, bronchiolar, and GI smooth muscle.
- Nerve endings: bradykinin is a potent inducer of pain.
- Inflammation: kinins mimic the manifestations of inflammation.

Clinical Correlation

Sepsis

Sepsis is a potentially life-threatening condition in which there is a widespread inflammatory state caused by the release of inflammatory mediators, including cytokines and kinins. These inflammatory mediators are released in response to infection and cause damage to the endothelium of blood vessels, which allows them to leak fluid. This causes tissue edema, hypotension, and hypoperfusion of organs. It also activates the clotting cascade, which leads to disseminated intravascular coagulation (DIC). The hypoperfusion of organs (from hypotension or DIC) may result in multiple organ failure and death.

Clinical Correlation

Disseminated Intravascular Coagulation

DIC is a pathologic activation of coagulation mechanisms. Events such as malignancy, infection, trauma, and obstetric complications trigger the release of kinins, which leads to the formation of small blood clots in blood vessels, which in turn consumes clotting factors and platelets (hence, DIC is known as a consumption coagulopathy). The fibrin strands in these blood clots also hemolyze passing red blood cells. Patients with DIC are acutely ill and show signs of shock. There is bleeding at any site in the body, including any old venipuncture site or wound. The patient may also have renal failure. Treatment mainly involves treating the underlying cause of the DIC, but other supportive measures, such as the administration of fresh frozen plasma, platelets, and blood, may be needed.

32.3.2 B_2 Bradykinin Antagonist and Kallikrein Inhibitor

Icatibant is an antagonist of the B_2 receptor. Ecallantide is an inhibitor of plasma kallikrein.

Pharmacokinetics

Given by SC injection.

Uses

For treatment of acute attacks of hereditary angioedema.

32.4 Histamine and Related Drugs

32.4.1 Histamine

Synthesis

Histamine is synthesized from histidine by histidine decarboxylase.

Location

Histamine is found in basophils within the blood, in mast cells in tissues, and in some neurons. It is also found in high concentrations in the skin, mucosa of the bronchi, and intestinal mucosa.

Metabolism

The breakdown of histamine involves two main pathways:
- Ring methylation, which is catalyzed by histamine-N-methyltransferase, followed by oxidative deamination by MAO.
- Oxidative deamination, which is catalyzed by diamineoxidase.
- The metabolites are excreted in urine.

Receptors

- H_1 receptors are coupled to G_q, leading to activation of phospholipase C and the phosphatidylinositol (PIP_2) signaling pathway. H_1 receptors mediate bronchoconstriction, contraction of the gut, and vascular dilation.
- H_2 receptors are coupled to G_s and these activate adenylate cyclase and stimulate cyclic adenosine monophosphate production. H_2 receptors are present in gastric parietal cells. They mediate gastric secretion and vascular dilation.
- H_3 and H_4 receptors have also been identified, but there are no therapeutic agents that selectively interact with these receptors. H_3 receptors are found mainly in the CNS, whereas H_4 receptors are found in bone marrow and white blood cells.
- Release: Tissue release and production of histamine are stimulated by damage to cells and tissues (▶ Fig. 32.1). Antigen–antibody reactions, snake venoms, and drugs (e.g., curare and morphine) can also liberate histamine from tissue stores.

Effects

- Cardiovascular system (effects are mediated by both H_1 and H_2 receptors): dilation of small blood vessels results in flushing and decreased systemic pressure. Increased capillary permeability results in edema.
- CNS: histamine acts as a neurotransmitter.
- Smooth muscle: with the exception of vascular smooth muscle (which is relaxed), most other smooth muscles are stimulated to constrict by histamine. Constrictor effects (H_1) are most prominent in the bronchi and uterus. Responses of intestinal muscle vary, and there are few effects on the bladder, gallbladder, ureter, or iris.
- Glands: histamine stimulates secretions via H_2 receptors from the salivary, bronchial, and gastric glands.
- Nerve endings: histamine stimulates nerve endings via H_1 receptors, causing pain and pruritus (itching).
- Inflammation: intradermally injected histamine elicits the following triple response: a localized red spot forms followed by a brighter red flush or flare extending ~ 1 cm beyond the original red spot, then a wheal that develops in 1 to 2 minutes.

32.4.2 H_1 Antihistamines

Chlorpheniramine, Diphenhydramine, Promethazine, Cetirizine, Fexofenadine, and Loratadine

- First-generation H_1 antihistamines: Diphenhydramine, promethazine, and chlorpheniramine. These agents have significant sedative, anticholinergic, and antiemetic effects.
- Second-generation H_1 antihistamines: Loratadine, fexofenadine, and cetirizine. These agents are nonsedating antihistamines.

Foundations

Nitric Oxide

Nitric oxide (NO) is a transmitter substance that is synthesized as required from arginine under the influence of the enzyme NO synthase. NO synthase is activated by Ca^{2+}/calmodulin in neurons and endothelial cells. NO diffuses into neighboring cells, where it activates guanylate cyclase. This, in turn, activates protein kinase G which blocks the nuclear IP_3 receptor. This cascade of events results in decreased cytosolic Ca^{2+} concentration and vasodilation. Histamine promotes vasodilation by causing the vascular endothelium to release NO.

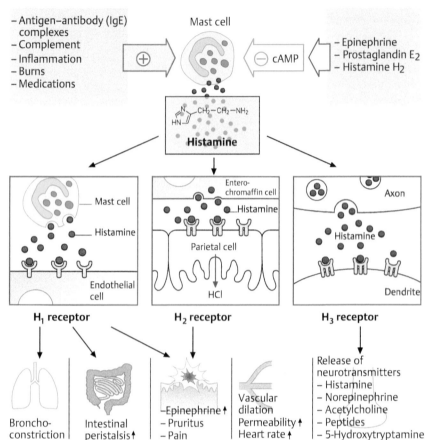

Fig. 32.1 Histamine.
Histamine is formed by tissue mast cells and basophils. Its release is stimulated by immuno-globulin E (IgE) complexes (type 1 hypersensitivity), activated complement, burns, inflammation, and some drugs. Its release is inhibited by epinephrine, prostaglandin E_2, and feedback inhibition from histamine itself. The effects of histamine via its different receptors are shown here.

Clinical Correlation

Histamine and Allergy

Allergy (also known as hypersensitivity [type I]) is an immune reaction to an allergen (e.g., pollen, dust, or insect stings) that would not elicit such a response in most people. When an allergen is encountered for the first time, it stimulates the production of immunoglobulin E (IgE). IgE attaches to mast cells and sensitizes these cells to this allergen, so that when it is next encountered, mast cells are stimulated to produce histamine and other inflammatory mediators (e.g., prostaglandins, interleukins, cytokines, and leukotrienes). The inflammatory mediators released are then responsible for producing all of the classic signs of allergy, such as rhinorrhea (runny nose), itch, swelling, and difficulty breathing. Anaphylactic shock is a severe type I hypersensitivity reaction characterized by generalized vasodilation, marked fall in blood pressure, and severe bronchoconstriction. Mediators other than histamine are also involved in the anaphylactic response, so the most effective treatment is epinephrine (given intramuscularly). Antihistamines and glucocorticoids decrease the magnitude of the late-occurring response (e.g., hives or itching).

Mechanism of Action

H_1 antihistamines block H_1 receptors and prevent histamine-induced reactions such as increased vascular permeability, smooth muscle contraction, mucus production, and pruritus. They also inhibit the "wheal and flare" response of the skin.

Pharmacokinetics

- These agents are well absorbed following oral administration.
- They are widely distributed and extensively metabolized. They induce hepatic microsomal enzymes and may facilitate their own metabolism.
- First-generation agents can penetrate the CNS, whereas second-generation agents show poor CNS penetration.
- Metabolites are eliminated in the urine (they are frequently eliminated more rapidly by children).

Effects

- Smooth muscle: these agents antagonize the constrictor action of histamine on respiratory and vascular smooth muscle. They also antagonize the changes in capillary permeability produced by histamine that results in edema.
- CNS: CNS depression, characterized by sedation and decreased alertness, is common with first-generation agents. Paradoxical restlessness, nervousness, and insomnia are occasionally observed. These agents may possess antiemetic effects and are effective against motion sickness.
- Autonomic nervous system: anticholinergic effects.
- Allergic reactions: antagonizes normal hypersensitivity symptoms.
- Local anesthetics (promethazine): this effect is thought to be due to Na^+ channel blockage in nervous tissue.

Uses

- Used for symptomatic relief of allergic rhinitis, allergic conjunctivitis, and the common cold.
- Over-the-counter sedative drugs (diphenhydramine).
- Motion sickness, vertigo, and emesis (dimenhydrinate, meclizine, prochlorperazine, promethazine).
- Appetite suppressants.

Side Effects

- Sedation is the most common adverse effect and often is responsible for poor compliance.
- Loss of appetite, constipation or diarrhea, nausea, and vomiting.
- Anticholinergic effects: dry mouth, cough, palpitations, and headache.
- Allergic dermatitis (with topical application).

Toxicity

Initially, there are central excitatory effects, including hallucinations, excitement, ataxia, and convulsions. This can progress to coma, respiratory collapse, and death within 1 to 2 hours. Treatment is supportive, that is, it involves treatment to prevent, control, or relieve side effects and complications.

32.4.3 H$_2$ Antihistamines

These agents are also discussed in Chapter 27.

Cimetidine, Famotidine, Nizatidine, and Ranitidine

Mechanism of Action

H$_2$ antihistamines are competitive antagonists at the H$_2$ receptor. They inhibit gastric acid secretions elicited by histamine.

Pharmacokinetics

- Well absorbed orally and eliminated in the urine.
- Cimetidine inhibits cytochrome P-450 in the liver, which metabolizes many drugs, thus potentiating the effects of such drugs.

Uses

- Treatment of peptic ulcers.
- Treatment of GERD.

Side Effects

These include diarrhea, nausea and vomiting, dizziness, headaches, and skin rashes. Cimetidine may also cause loss of libido, impotence, and gynecomastia.

32.4.4 Inhibitor of Histamine and Leukotriene Release from Mast Cells

Cromolyn Sodium

This drug is also discussed in Chapter 26.

Mechanism of Action

Cromolyn sodium inhibits mast cell degranulation of histamine and other inflammatory mediators. It also reduces bronchial hyperresponsiveness.

Uses

- Used prophylactically for asthma.
- Seasonal allergic rhinitis.

Side Effects

Its side effects are minimal.

32.4.5 Other Histamine-Related Drug: Anti-IgE Antibody

Omalizumab

Mechanism of Action

Omalizumab is a recombinant humanized monoclonal antibody directed against IgE. It binds to free IgE, thus preventing activation of mast cells and basophils.

Uses

IgE-mediated allergic asthma and has been proposed for use in other type I allergic reactions.

Notes

Gastric Acid and Histamine

Histamine is one of the main regulators of gastric acid secretion. It is released from enterochromaffin-like cells in response to stimulation by the vagus nerve and gastrin hormone. Once released, histamine acts on parietal cells to increase the activity of H$^+$–K$^+$–ATPase (the proton pump) which pumps H$^+$ ions out of parietal cells in exchange for K$^+$. The H$^+$ ions cause an osmotic gradient across the membrane, resulting in an outward diffusion of water. The water then combines with H$^+$ and Cl$^-$ ions to form gastric acid (See callout boxes in Chapter 27).

▶ Table 32.2 summarizes the effects of serotonin, bradykinin, and histamine.

32.5 Eicosanoids and Related Drugs

32.5.1 Eicosanoids

Eicosanoids (*eicosa* = Greek for 20) are a group of autocoids derived from the 20-carbon fatty acid, arachidonic acid, and include the prostaglandins, prostacyclins, thromboxanes, and leukotrienes.

VIII

Table 32.2 Summary of effects of serotonin, bradykinin, and histamine

System	Serotonin	Bradykinin	Histamine
Smooth muscle			
Vascular	Direct vasoconstriction and endothelial-mediated	Vasodilation	Vasodilation
Bronchial	dilation	Contraction	Contraction
Uterine	Mild contraction	Contraction	Contraction
Gastrointestinal	Contraction	Contraction	Contraction
	Contraction		
Inflammation	Mediator	Mediator	Mediator
Platelet aggregation	Enhances	Inhibits	Enhances
Gastrointestinal system	Stimulates smooth muscle to increase peristalsis		Stimulates gastric acid secretion
Cardiovascular system	Direct vasoconstriction of pulmonary and lung vessels. Endothelial-mediated vasodilation in heart and skeletal muscle	Vasodilation, lowering blood pressure	Vasodilation, lowering blood pressure. Increases capillary permeability, leading to edema
Central nervous system	Ascending systems: • Sleep • Determining mood Descending systems: • Modulating perception of pain		Acts as a neurotransmitter
Peripheral nervous system	Sensitizes sensory nerve endings, causing pain and itching	Sensitizes sensory nerve endings to pain	Sensitizes sensory nerve endings, causing pain and itching

Synthesis

Eicosanoids are generated from cell membrane phospholipids. Phospholipase A_2 is activated by hormones or other stimuli to form arachidonate, which is then metabolized by cyclooxygenases (COX-1, COX-2, and COX-3) to form prostaglandin H_2 (PGH_2). Alternatively, arachidonate is metabolized by lipoxygenase to form the leukotrienes. PGH_2 is further converted to prostacyclin, other prostaglandins, and thromboxanes (▶ Fig. 32.2). The eicosanoids bind to specific G protein-coupled receptors.

Effects

The major effects of prostaglandin, prostacyclin, and thromboxanes are summarized in ▶ Table 32.3.

32.5.2 Prostaglandin Agonists

Alprostadil

Mechanism of Action

Alprostadil is a prostaglandin E_1 (PGE_1) analogue that relaxes vascular smooth muscle, causing vasodilation.

Uses

- Maintaining the patency of ductus arteriosus in neonates who are dependent on the patent ductus for survival while they are awaiting surgery to repair the congenital heart defect. It is administered intravenously (IV).
- Treatment of erectile dysfunction in patients not responding to other therapies (behavioral therapy, vacuum constriction devices, or selective phosphodiesterase type 5 inhibitors). It is administered by intracavernosal injection or intraurethral suppository.

Side Effects

No side effects have been noted.

Bimatoprost, Latanoprost, and Travoprost

Mechanism of Action

These agents are prostaglandin F_{2a} analogue agonists.

Uses

- Ocular hypertension or open-angle glaucoma. These agents are believed to reduce intraocular pressure by increasing uveoscleral outflow. They are administered as eye drops.
- Hypotrichosis (reduced amount of hair) of the eyelashes (bimatoprost).

Dinoprostone and Carboprost Tromethamine

Mechanism of Action

- Dinoprostone is a synthetic form of prostaglandin E_2 (PGE_2).
- Carboprost tromethamine is a synthetic form of 15-methyl PGF_{2a}.

Notes

Ductus Arteriosus

PGE_2 is responsible for keeping the ductus arteriosus open during fetal development. The ductus arteriosus is the vascular connection between the pulmonary artery and aorta that allows blood to bypass the fetus's lungs in utero. It begins to close shortly after birth. If it fails to close, the condition is known as patent ductus arteriosus. This can be closed surgically or by using indomethacin, an NSAID which inhibits prostaglandin synthesis.

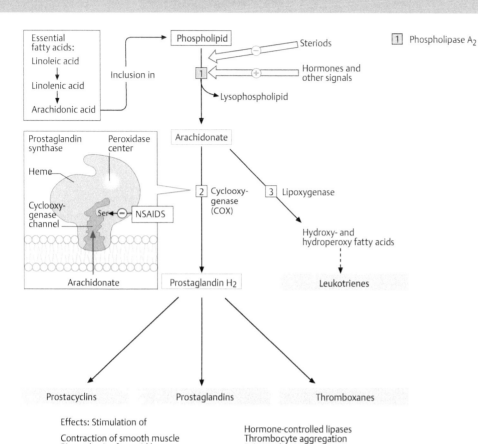

Fig. 32.2 Eicosanoid synthesis.
Arachidonic acid, a polyunsaturated fatty acid found in membrane phospholipids, is the starting material for eicosanoids. The arachidonate moiety is released from the phospholipids by the action of the enzyme phospholipase A$_2$ (1). Phospholipase A$_2$ is activated by hormones and other signals (via G proteins), and it is inactivated by steroids. Arachidonic acids may then form prostaglandin H$_2$ (PGH$_2$) when acted upon by cyclooxygenase (COX) (2). PGH$_2$ is the parent substance for prostacyclins, prostaglandins, and thromboxanes. In a different pathway, PGH$_2$ may be acted upon by lipoxygenase (3), forming hydroxy- and hydroperoxy fatty acids, which then form leukotrienes. Aspirin (acetylsalicylic acid) and related nonsteroidal anti-inflammatory drugs (NSAIDs) inhibit the COX activity of prostaglandin synthase, so the formation of most eicosanoids is blocked. This explains their analgesic, antipyretic, and antirheumatic effects.

VIII

Table 32.3 Actions of prostaglandins (PGs), prostacyclin, and thromboxanes

System	PGEs	PGFs	Prostacyclin	Thromboxanes
Smooth muscle				
Vascular	Vasodilation	Vasoconstriction	Dilation	Constriction
Bronchial	Relaxation	Contraction		Contraction
Uterine	Contraction	Contraction		
Gastrointestinal	Contraction	Contraction		
Inflammation	Mediator	Mediator	Mediator	Mediator
Platelet aggregation	Inhibits		Inhibits	Stimulates
Gastric acid secretion	Decreases		Decreases	
Central nervous system	Fever and sedation			
Peripheral nervous system	Sensitizes nerve endings to pain		Sensitizes nerve endings to pain	
Kidneys	Increased renal blood flow, renin secretion, and natriuresis			

Notes

Prostaglandins in Sperm

Sperm is rich in prostaglandins. Prostaglandins help to soften and ripen the cervix, which is why sexual intercourse is advocated as a natural way to induce labor around the time of the due date.

Uses

• Abortifacients (second trimester).
• Induction of labor at term.

Misoprostol

Mechanism of Action

Misoprostol is a synthetic PGE$_1$ methyl ester.

Uses

• Abortifacient (in combination with mifepristone; see Chapter 17).
• Prophylaxis of NSAID-induced gastric ulcers (as it is a potent inhibitor of gastric secretion of acid).

Contraindications

Do not administer any of the above synthetic prostaglandin agents to pregnant women, as they can cause abortion, premature birth, or birth defects.

32.5.3 Prostaglandin Antagonists: Nonsteroidal Anti-inflammatory Drugs

Aspirin (Acetylsalicylic Acid)

Mechanism of Action

NSAIDs (including aspirin) block the synthesis of prostaglandins by inhibiting COX and the formation of both PGG_2 and PGH_2, the precursors of all other prostaglandins. This mechanism is discussed in more detail in Chapter 33.

32.5.4 Prostaglandin Antagonists: Corticosteroids

Prednisone

Mechanism of Action

Corticosteroids block the synthesis of prostaglandins by inhibiting the enzyme phospholipase A_2, which blocks the conversion of membrane phospholipids into arachidonic acid, the precursor of all of the eicosanoids.

32.6 Leukotrienes and Related Drugs

32.6.1 Leukotrienes

Synthesis

See section 32.5.1 and ▶ Fig. 32.2.

Location

Leukotrienes are produced in cells involved in inflammatory responses: mast cells, basophils, and eosinophils.

Effects

- Leukotrienes are involved in the development of the inflammatory responses by promoting endothelial cell adherence of inflammatory mediators, leukocyte chemotaxis (movement in response to the influence of chemical stimulation), and chemokine (a family of chemotactic cytokines) production at the site of inflammation.
- Leukotrienes are potent bronchoconstrictors.

32.6.2 Leukotriene Modifier Agents

These agents are discussed in Chapter 26 for the treatment of asthma.

33 Analgesic, Antipyretic, and Anti-inflammatory Drugs

Summary

Nonsteroidal anti-inflammatory drugs (NSAIDs) are analgesic, antipyretic, and anti-inflammatory. NSAIDs inhibit the cyclooxygenase enzymes COX-1 and COX-2, with COX-2 inhibition thought to be the major mechanism for the analgesic, antipyretic, and anti-inflammatory effects. The NSAIDs include indomethacin, diclofenac, etodolac, ketorolac, sulindac, tolmetin, ibuprofen, fenoprofen, flurbiprofen, ketoprofen, naproxen, oxaprozin, piroxicam, meloxicam, and nabumetone. Aspirin (acetylsalicylic acid) irreversibly inhibits COX-1 and COX-2. Other NSAIDs are competitive inhibitors of COX-1 and COX-2. Other salicylic acid derivatives that do not irreversibly inhibit COX enzymes include mesalamine, olsalazine, and sulfasalazine. Other salicylates include choline magnesium salicylate, salsalate, and diflunisal. Celecoxib is a selective inhibitor of COX-2. Acetaminophen is unique in that it does not have significant anti-inflammatory activity, although it is analgesic and antipyretic.

Disease-modifying antirheumatic drugs (DMARDs) are the drugs that slow the progression of rheumatoid arthritis (RA), reducing both symptoms and joint damage. DMARDs include methotrexate, hydroxychloroquine, sulfasalazine, gold salts, and leflunomide. There are also numerous antibody-based DMARDs. Tumor necrosis factor-α (TNF-α) inhibitors include adalimumab, certolizumab pegol, etanercept, golimumab, and infliximab. Other biological DMARDs include anakinra, tocilizumab, abatacept, rituximab, and tofacitinib.

The therapy of gout involves treatment of acute attacks with colchicine and NSAIDs, and chronic treatment for hyperuricemia. Probenecid and sulfinpyrazone block the reabsorption of uric acid in the kidney. Allopurinol reduces the synthesis of uric acid by inhibiting xanthine oxidase. Febuxostat is a newer xanthine oxidase inhibitor. Pegloticase catalyzes the conversion of serum uric acid to an inert metabolite. Lesinurad inhibits uric acid transporters in the kidney.

Keywords: pain, fever, arthritis, gout

33.1 Introduction to Analgesic, Antipyretic, and Anti-inflammatory Drugs

Inflammation is usually the result of a noxious stimulus that results in the destruction of or injury to tissue. Inflammation functions to remove noxious agents from the site of injury, repair damage, and return tissue function to normal. The clinical features of inflammation are swelling, redness, heat, and pain. Anti-inflammatory drugs are used to reduce the symptoms of inflammation.

33.2 Nonsteroidal Anti-inflammatory Drugs

Nonsteroidal anti-inflammatory drugs (NSAIDs) are analgesic, antipyretic, and anti-inflammatory drugs, thus named to distinguish them from the glucocorticosteroids, the other major class of anti-inflammatory drugs. The NSAIDs include some commonly used over-the-counter agents, as well as many prescription-only agents.

33.2.1 Indomethacin, Diclofenac, Etodolac, Ketorolac, Sulindac, Tolmetin, Ibuprofen, Fenoprofen, Flurbiprofen, Ketoprofen, Naproxen, Oxaprozin, Piroxicam, Meloxicam, Nabumetone

Mechanism of Action

- *Anti-inflammatory:* NSAIDs inhibit the cyclooxygenase (COX) enzymes COX-1 and COX-2 (▶ Fig. 33.1). These enzymes catalyze the formation of prostaglandin H$_2$, which is the precursor

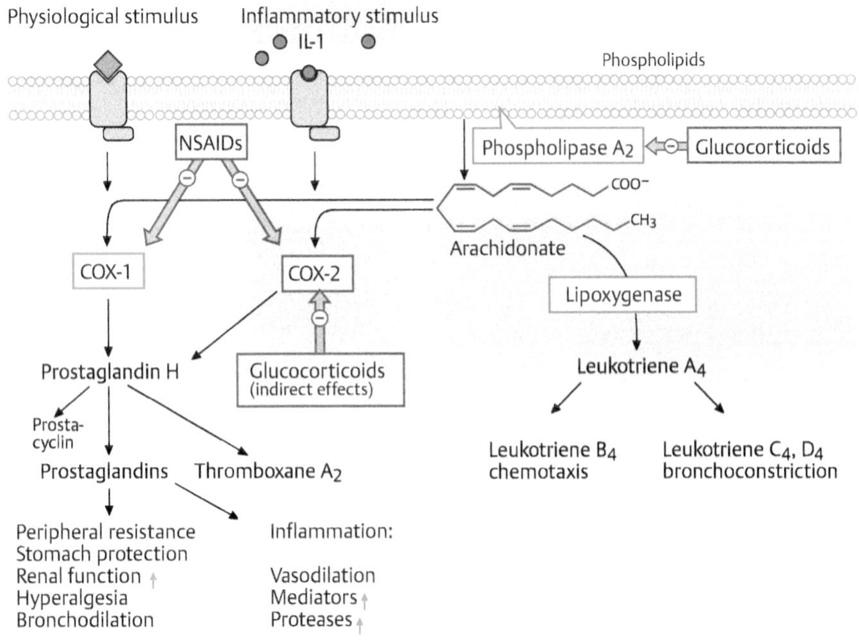

Fig. 33.1 Nonsteroidal anti-inflammatory drugs (NSAIDs).
Most NSAIDs inhibit prostaglandin metabolism by inhibiting both forms of the enzyme cyclooxygenase (COX-1 and COX-2). Celecoxib is a selective inhibitor of COX-2. COX catalyzes the formation of prostaglandin H$_2$ which is the most important step in prostaglandin production. The normal physiological effects of COX-1 and COX-2 are shown. Because NSAIDs block these actions, they have an anti-inflammatory effect (wanted), but they also block the physiological effects of COX-1, which are the main cause of NSAID side effects (unwanted). Glucocorticoids also inhibit prostaglandin (and leukotriene) production by inhibiting phospholipase A$_2$ and COX-2 (indirectly).

VIII

for prostaglandin, prostacyclin, and thromboxane synthesis. COX-1 is present in most tissues. In the gastrointestinal (GI) tract it maintains the normal lining of the stomach. It is also involved in kidney and platelet function. COX-2 is induced by inflammation. COX-2 inhibition is thought to be the major mechanism for the analgesic, antipyretic, and anti-inflammatory effects of aspirin and the other NSAIDs.

- Aspirin inhibits the COX enzymes by acetylating a single serine residue. This is an irreversible covalent modification that inactivates both COX-1 and COX-2. Other NSAIDs are competitive inhibitors of the COXs.
- *Analgesic*: NSAID analgesic effects occur as a result of decreased prostaglandin formation.
- *Antipyretic*: Antipyretic effects are the result of decreasing prostaglandins in the temperature control center in the hypothalamus.

Uses

- Mild-to-moderate pain (e.g., dental, muscle, joint, and postoperative).
- Inflammation and accompanying pain associated with diseases, such as rheumatoid arthritis (RA) (high doses).
- Reduction of fever.
- Aspirin is also used for the treatment and prophylaxis of thrombosis (low doses). It is widely used to prevent myocardial infarction (MI), stroke, and peripheral vascular thrombosis. It is also used after angioplasty, placement of stents, or bypass surgery to prevent thrombosis and restenosis.

Side Effects

Many of the adverse effects of aspirin and the other NSAIDs result from inhibition of COX-1 (▶ Fig. 33.2). These include

- Acute renal failure.
- Skin rash or hypersensitivity reactions. These require immediate discontinuation of the drug.
- Gastric distress, occult gastric bleeding, and acute hemorrhage. These effects may be worsened with concomitant use of ethanol and selective serotonin reuptake inhibitors (SSRIs).
- Bronchospasm in NSAID-sensitive asthmatics (see Chapter 26).

Notes

Inflammatory Mediators

Cytokines, which are secreted primarily by activated macrophages, are important mediators of inflammation. The most important inflammatory mediators are interleukin-1 (IL-1), interleukin-6 (IL-6), and tumor necrosis factor-α (TNF-α). Local effects include induction of adhesion molecule expression on vascular endothelium (promoting cell adherence), increased vascular permeability (promoting influx of serum components), and activation of lymphocytes. Systemic effects include increased leukocyte production, fever, and induction of acute phase response. Other important cytokines include interleukin-8 (IL-8), a potent chemotactic factor for recruitment of neutrophils, basophils, and T cells, and interleukin-12 (IL-12), which activates natural killer cells and promotes differentiation of T cells into T helper (TH) cells.

Notes

Set Point Temperature and Temperature Regulation

The preoptic region and adjacent anterior nuclei of the hypothalamus contain a thermostat for establishing the set point temperature. The set point temperature (~37 °C) is the body core temperature that the system attempts to maintain. If core temperature falls below the set point, then the following mechanisms may be induced by the posterior hypothalamus: somatic nervous system activation induces shivering, generating heat by causing ATP hydrolysis in the contractile apparatus of skeletal muscle; thyroid hormones may be released generating heat by increasing the activity of Na^+–K^+–ATPase; and sympathetic nervous system activation causes vasoconstriction of blood vessels to the skin, resulting in heat conservation. If core temperature rises above the set point, then the following mechanisms may be induced by the anterior hypothalamus: sympathetic cholinergic activation of sweat glands (via muscarinic receptors) increases heat loss by evaporation of water from the skin; and lowered sympathetic adrenergic activity causes dilation of blood vessels to the skin, resulting in heat loss by convection and radiation.

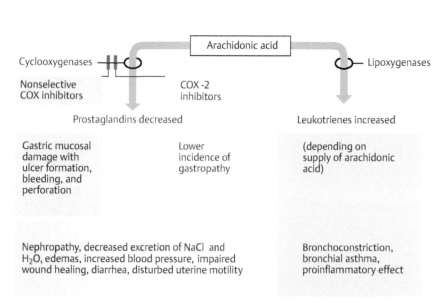

Fig. 33.2 Adverse effects of NSAIDs.
NSAID-induced inhibition of cyclooxygenase (COX) enzymes leads to decreased production of prostaglandins from arachidonic acid. This leads to gastric mucosal damage and its sequelae and nephropathy. COX-2 inhibitors show a lower incidence of gastropathy. Inhibition of this side of the arachidonic acid metabolic pathway may lead to increased leukotriene production, depending on arachidonic acid availability. This proinflammatory mediator can cause asthma and bronchoconstriction.

Fever and Antipyretic Drugs

Fever is produced by endogenous pyrogens (e.g., IL-1) released by infective bacteria. These pyrogens act on the anterior hypothalamus to increase prostaglandin synthesis, which in turn stimulates the thermoregulatory center to reset the new set point to a higher temperature. Because body temperature is cooler than the new set point, body temperature increases (heat production and conservation of heat) until it stabilizes at the new, elevated set point temperature. After the fever breaks and the new set point returns to 37 °C, the patient vasodilates and sweats to lose heat until body temperature returns to normal. Aspirin (and other NSAIDs) and acetaminophen are effective in suppressing fever because they inhibit COX and therefore prostaglandin synthesis. In doing so, they lower the set point temperature and will cause activation of the heat loss mechanisms. Steroids may also be used to reduce fever by blocking the release of arachidonic acid (the precursor of prostaglandins) from membrane phospholipids.

Contraindications

- Gastric ulcers (gastric irritation may aggravate ulcers).
- Asthma (NSAIDs can induce bronchospasm in asthmatics).
- Influenza-like illnesses in children or teenagers (up to 19 years of age). There is an increased risk of developing Reye syndrome in children with influenza or chickenpox.
- Pregnancy (third trimester). NSAIDs may cause premature closure of the ductus arteriosus.

The NSAIDs vary only slightly in their relative strength in producing anti-inflammatory, analgesic, and antipyretic actions. The major differences among the agents are in their pharmacokinetics and in the therapeutic responses and adverse reactions of individual patients to the various agents. The unique features of specific NSAIDs are discussed in the following section.

33.2.2 Salicylates

Aspirin (Acetylsalicylic Acid)

Pharmacokinetics

- Well absorbed following oral administration.
- Rapidly metabolized by plasma esterases to salicylic acid and acetic acid.
- Salicylate ion is highly bound (80–90%) to plasma proteins.
- Conjugation in the liver is the primary route of metabolism.
- Metabolites are excreted in the urine.

Effects

- Cardiovascular system: at low doses, aspirin inhibits platelet COX-1 and prevents thrombosis. Aspirin does not affect blood pressure.
- Blood: increased bleeding time due to inhibition of platelet aggregation.
- Kidney: no nephrotoxicity.

- Liver: there may be dose-dependent alterations in liver function with salicylate use. These changes usually are subclinical and reversible.

Contraindications/Precautions

- Influenza-like illnesses or chickenpox in children or teenagers (up to 19 years of age), as there is an increased risk of developing Reye syndrome.
- Asthma and nasal polyps, as there is an increased likelihood of hypersensitivity reaction.
- Bleeding disorders such as hemophilia, as aspirin may increase bleeding.
- Alcohol use (three or more drinks per day) or peptic ulcer, as there is an increased risk of GI bleeding.
- Decreased hepatic function.

Toxicity

- Acute toxicity may occur in children and teenagers (Reye syndrome) which is life threatening.
- Overdose progressively leads to tinnitus, hyperventilation, respiratory alkalosis, fever, metabolic acidosis, shock, coma, and death. Treatment is gastric lavage for acute cases, alkaline diuresis with sodium bicarbonate to increase excretion, and supportive measures.

33.2.3 Salicylic Acid Salts and Derivatives

Mesalamine, Olsalazine, and Sulfasalazine

Mechanisms of Action

These agents do not irreversibly inhibit COX enzymes and are much less effective than aspirin as COX inhibitors. They also do not inhibit platelet aggregation.

Clinical Correlation

Reye Syndrome

Reye syndrome is a rare disorder that affects all organs of the body, but liver and brain involvement is the most serious. It initially presents following a viral infection. Signs and symptoms progress from vomiting, lethargy, hyperventilation, and confusion to severe mental state changes, coma, respiratory failure, multiple organ failure, and death. Treatment is supportive and includes mechanical ventilation (if necessary), insulin (to increase glucose metabolism), corticosteroids (to reduce brain swelling), and diuretics (to increase fluid loss).

Pharmacokinetics

These agents are taken orally or rectally.

Uses

- Ulcerative colitis (local effect on the GI tract).
- Crohn's disease.
- RA (sulfasalazine).

VIII

Side Effects

Less frequent and minor compared with aspirin.

33.2.4 Other Salicylates

Choline Magnesium Salicylate, Salsalate, and Diflunisal

Salsalate is the salicylate ester of salicylic acid; in vivo, the drug is hydrolyzed to two molecules of salicylate.

Diflunisal is a salicylic acid derivative but is not metabolized to salicylate.

Pharmacokinetics

Given orally but also found in over-the-counter creams, gels, and patches for topical use.

Uses

Treatment of fever, pain, and arthritis in patients who cannot tolerate or are unresponsive to aspirin or other NSAIDs.

33.2.5 Acetic Acids

Indomethacin

Mechanism of Action

Similar to aspirin.

Uses

- Indomethacin has been the agent of choice for gout; however, there is no evidence that it is superior to other NSAIDs for acute gout.
- To accelerate closure of patent ductus arteriosus (see Chapter 32).

Side Effects

- A very high percentage (35–50%) of patients receiving usual therapeutic doses of indomethacin experience untoward symptoms, and ~ 20% must discontinue its use because of the side effects.
- The most frequent central nervous system (CNS) effect (indeed, the most common side effect) is severe frontal headache, occurring in 25 to 50% of patients who take the drug for long periods. Dizziness, vertigo, lightheadedness, and mental confusion may occur. Seizures have been reported, as have severe depression, psychosis, hallucinations, and suicide.
- GI complaints are common and can be serious. Diarrhea may occur and sometimes is associated with ulcerative lesions of the bowel. Acute pancreatitis has been reported, as have rare but potentially fatal cases of hepatitis.
- Neutropenia, thrombocytopenia, and, rarely, aplastic anemia.

Note: Most adverse effects are dose-related.

Contraindications

Underlying peptic ulcer disease.

Note: Caution is advised when administering indomethacin to elderly patients or to those with underlying epilepsy, psychiatric disorders, or Parkinson disease because they are at greater risk for the development of serious CNS adverse effects.

Clinical Correlation

Thrombocytopenia

Thrombocytopenia is a condition in which the platelet count is low. It can be caused by the decreased production of platelets, such as in bone marrow failure, and from the destruction or consumption of platelets, for example, in disseminated intravascular coagulation (DIC), hypersplenism, and viral infections, and from drugs (e.g., indomethacin). There may be no signs and symptoms of thrombocytopenia, and it may be diagnosed incidentally when the patient's blood count is measured, or there may be signs such as spontaneous bleeding from mucous membranes (e.g., gums and nose), easy and excessive bruising, and petichiae (superficial bleeding into the skin). The underlying cause should be treated if necessary.

▸ Table 33.1 summarizes other NSAIDs.

33.2.6 COX-2 Selective Inhibitor

Celecoxib

Mechanism of Action

Celecoxib is a selective COX-2 inhibitor and as such inhibits the production of vascular prostaglandins, which are inhibitors of platelet aggregation and vasodilators. Unlike the nonselective NSAIDs, which inhibit both COX-1 and COX-2, celecoxib does not reduce the endogenous production of thromboxane A_2, a potent activator of platelet aggregation and a vasoconstrictor. Thus, inhibition of prostacyclin without inhibition of thromboxane A_2 creates a prothrombotic state. However, the fact that it does not inhibit COX-1 leads to fewer GI side effects because it does not inhibit prostaglandins in the GI tract which maintain the normal lining of the stomach.

Side Effects

Adverse cardiovascular and cerebrovascular events are more likely due to the prothrombotic state.

Table 33.1 Summary of NSAIDs

Drugs	Comments
Diclofenac, etodolac, ketorolac, sulindac, tolmetin	These NSAIDs have greater potency against COX-2, have some COX-2 selectivity, and have less anti-inflammatory activity than other NSAIDs
	They are similar to indomethacin
Ibuprofen, fenoprofen, flurbiprofen, ketoprofen, naproxen, oxaprozin	Propionic acid derivatives that differ mainly in pharmacokinetics
Piroxicam, meloxicam	Major advantage is long duration of action
Nabumetone	Unique structure but similar activity to other NSAIDs

Note: Rofecoxib and valdecoxib have been withdrawn from the market because of the increased risk of cardiovascular events. Although celecoxib also carries such risks, it remains available, and its benefits (i.e., the reduced GI side effects) may outweigh the risks in properly selected and informed patients.

33.3 Other Analgesic-Antipyretic Drugs

Acetaminophen is excluded from the NSAID group of drugs because it does not have significant anti-inflammatory activity, although it is analgesic and antipyretic.

33.3.1 Acetaminophen

Mechanism of Action

Acetaminophen is a weak inhibitor of COXs. Its mechanism of action is not well understood.

Pharmacokinetics

- Well absorbed following oral administration.
- The primary route of metabolism is conjugation in the liver.
- Elimination is by filtration and active proximal tubular secretion into the urine.

Effects

- Antipyretic effects: comparable to aspirin.
- Analgesic effects: comparable to aspirin.
- Cardiovascular system: no effects at therapeutic doses.
- Respiratory system: no effects at therapeutic doses.
- Blood: no antiplatelet effects.
- Acetaminophen has no significant anti-inflammatory properties, which may be accounted for by the fact that it has greater activity against CNS COX than peripheral COX.

Uses

- Mild-to-moderate pain and pyrexia in patients for whom aspirin is contraindicated.
- Analgesic of choice in pregnancy.

Note: Acetaminophen does not cause Reye syndrome and may be used in children.

Toxicity

Acetaminophen has a high therapeutic index, requiring ≥ 6 g to be ingested for toxicity to occur. Hepatotoxicity is the most serious toxic effect, which is caused by the accumulation of *N*-acetyl-*p*-benzo-quinone imine (NAPQI), a toxic compound produced in small amounts during the metabolism of acetaminophen. Normally, it is immediately detoxified in the liver by conjugation with glutathione. In cases of acetaminophen overdose, glutathione may be depleted, and NAPQI may accumulate and damage the liver. Concurrent ethanol use may worsen the hepatic effect. Treat with acetylcysteine, which both replenish glutathione stores and may conjugate directly with NAPQI by serving as a glutathione substitute (only effective within 10 to 24 hours of overdose).

33.4 Drugs Used in the Treatment of Rheumatoid Arthritis

RA is a chronic inflammatory disorder that is mainly characterized by inflammation of the synovium of joints, especially the small joints of the hands and feet. This causes all of the signs of inflammation: pain, swelling, stiffness, redness, and loss of function. The synovium thickens as the disease progresses, and inflammatory mediators erode bone and cartilage, causing deformation of the joints. There is also a systemic component to RA that is thought to be mainly due to vasculitis (inflammation of blood vessels). Weight loss, fever, and malaise are often present, and there may be cardiovascular and respiratory disease, as well as problems with the skin and eyes.

33.4.1 Disease-Modifying Antirheumatic Drugs

NSAIDs and corticosteroids can provide symptomatic relief for patients with RA, but NSAIDs do not affect the progression of the disease and side effects limit the long-term use of systemic corticosteroids. DMARDs are drugs that do slow progression of the disease, reducing both symptoms and joint damage. They are commonly used with NSAIDs for the treatment of RA (▶ Fig. 33.3). Corticosteroids may be used in conjunction with these agents.

Methotrexate

This agent is discussed in detail in Chapter 27.

Mechanism of Action

Methotrexate is a folic acid analogue that competitively inhibits dihydrofolate reductase, the enzyme that normally converts folate to tetrahydrofolate. This is needed for purine and thymidine synthesis.
   Note: The mechanism of action in RA is unknown.

Pharmacokinetics

- Administered orally for the treatment of RA.
- Fifty percent is bound to plasma proteins (displaced by salicylates, sulfonamides, etc.).
- Excreted unchanged in urine (caution in patients with renal damage).

Uses

Methotrexate is generally the DMARD of choice for the treatment of RA. Not recommended in women of child-bearing age or in pregnancy due to teratogenic effects.

Side Effects

Side effects include oral and GI ulceration, bone marrow depression (dose-limiting toxicity), hepatic damage, and renal damage. May cause fetal damage.

Hydroxychloroquine

Mechanism of Action

Its mechanism for RA is unknown.

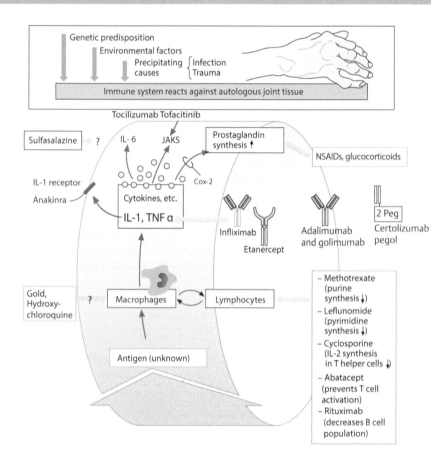

Fig. 33.3 Rheumatoid arthritis.
Refer to call-out box in section 33.3 for a description of the pathogenesis of rheumatoid arthritis (RA). NSAIDs (COX inhibitors) and glucocorticoids inhibit prostaglandin synthesis, which provides acute relief from the inflammatory symptoms. Disease-modifying agents slow disease progression. Methotrexate and leflunomide reduce purine and pyrimidine synthesis in lymphocytes, which prevents them from replicating (due to inhibition of DNA and RNA synthesis). Cyclosporine decreases interleukin-2 (IL-2) synthesis in T helper cells. Abatacept binds to CD80 and CD86 on antigen-presenting cells and prevents them from binding to CD28 on T cells, thereby preventing T-cell activation. Rituximab induces apoptosis of B cells. Decreasing the B-cell population decreases inflammation by decreasing the activation of T cells and the secretion of inflammatory cytokines. Adalimumab, certolizumab pegol, etanercept, golimumab and infliximab all intercept tumor necrosis factor-α (TNF-α) molecules (which is a major proinflammatory cytokine) and prevent them from interacting with membrane receptors on target cells (see ▶ Fig. 33.4). Tocilizumab binds to IL-6 receptors and blocks the actions of endogenous IL-6, thereby decreasing IL-6-mediated inflammatory responses. Tofacitinib inhibits JAKs and interrupts JAK-STAT signaling, thereby inhibiting the immune response. Anakinra is an analogue of endogenous IL-1 antagonists. The mechanisms of action of sulfasalazine, gold, and hydroxychloroquine are unknown.

Pharmacokinetics

- Administered alone (in mild cases) or in combination with other anti-inflammatory agents.
- Clinical improvement may require 3 to 6 months of therapy.

Clinical Correlation

Pathogenesis of Rheumatoid Arthritis

In RA, the immune system pathologically reacts to insults on the body by trigger factors, which may be genetic, environmental, infection, or trauma. The initial noxious stimulus causes inflammation of synovial membranes. The antigens released in this process are taken up by antigen-presenting cells, and this, in turn, activates lymphocytes and macrophages. The macrophages release further proinflammatory mediators, including cytokines and TNFα. Cytokines activate COX-2 and induce prostaglandin synthesis. This inflammatory response leads to a vicious circle of lymphocyte and macrophage activation. Synovial fibroblasts also proliferate during this time and release destructive enzymes. These enzymes are responsible for the characteristic, inflamed, pannus tissue of RA, which progressively invades joint cartilage and bone, cumulating in ankylosis and connective tissue scar formation. This causes loss of joint motion (▶ Fig. 33.3).

Clinical Correlation

Purines

Purines are a group of extremely biochemically significant organic compounds. The nucleic acids adenine and guanine, which comprise 50% of our DNA and RNA, are derived from purines, as well as several other important substances, for example, adenosine triphosphate (ATP), guanosine triphosphate (GTP), cyclic adenosine monophosphate (cAMP), the reduced form of nicotinamide adenine dinucleotide (NADH), and coenzyme A.

Side Effects

Serious ocular toxicity is associated with this agent but is rare at doses used for RA.

Sulfasalazine

Mechanism of Action

Sulfasalazine is a prodrug that is metabolized to 5-aminosalicylate (5-ASA). 5-ASA acts within the intestinal tract (mainly the terminal ileum and colon) to inhibit prostaglandin and leukotriene synthesis, thus reducing the inflammatory reaction (see Chapter 27).

The mechanism of action of sulfasalazine in RA is unknown.

Uses

Mild cases of RA.

Side Effects

- Nausea, vomiting, diarrhea, headache, and abdominal pain.
- Bone marrow suppression.

Gold Salts

Mechanism of Action

Gold salts have anti-inflammatory properties and inhibit prostaglandin synthesis. They have no analgesic or antipyretic effects.

Uses

- Used infrequently for the treatment of inflammatory conditions.
- May induce remission of RA, but the duration is highly variable. The mechanism by which they induce remission is unknown.

Side Effects

Mucocutaneous lesions, blood dyscrasias, and anaphylactoid reactions.

Leflunomide

Mechanism of Action

Leflunomide is an inhibitor of pyrimidine synthesis. Its mechanism to relieve symptoms of RA is unclear, but it may inhibit the proliferation of T cells to reduce inflammation.

Pharmacokinetics

Orally effective.

Uses

Initial monotherapy for RA instead of methotrexate, or added to methotrexate for patients who have not responded.

Effects

Reduces symptoms and improves function.

Side Effects

- Diarrhea occurs frequently.
- Reversible alopecia and skin rash are common.
- Hypertension.
- Hepatotoxicity.

Contraindications

Should not be administered in pregnancy.

33.4.2 Tumor Necrosis Factor-α Inhibitors

Adalimumab, Certolizumab pegol, Etanercept, Golimumab, and Infliximab

- Adalimumab and golimumab are human monoclonal antibodies to TNF-α.
- Certolizumab pegol is the pegylated Fab fragment of a human monoclonal antibody to TNF-α.
- Etanercept is a soluble recombinant TNF-α receptor:Fc fusion protein.
- Infliximab is a chimeric monoclonal antibody that binds to TNF-α. The use of infliximab as an immunosuppressant is discussed in Chapter 34.

Mechanism of Action

These agents bind to TNF-α, a proinflammatory cytokine, and prevent it from attaching to its receptor (▶ Fig. 33.4).

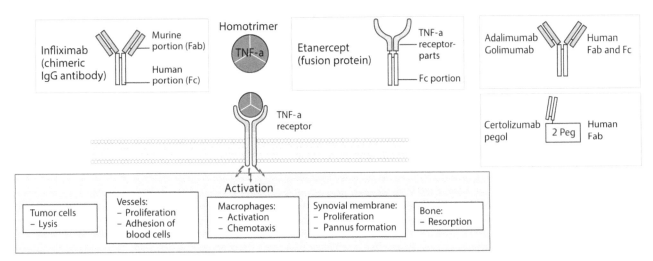

Fig. 33.4 TNF-α and inhibitors.
TNF-α receptor activation produces a number of effects that can worsen rheumatoid arthritis (RA). TNF levels are elevated in the synovial fluid of patients with RA. Infliximab is a chimeric monoclonal antibody to TNF-α. Etanercept is a soluble recombinant TNF receptor:Fc fusion protein. Adalimumab and golimumab are human monoclonal antibodies to TNF-α that work like infliximab. Certolizumab pegol is the pegylated Fab fragment of a human monoclonal antibody to TNF-α. All of these drugs bind to TNF-α and prevent it from interacting with its receptor.

Pharmacokinetics

- Adalimumab, certolizumab pegol, and etanercept are administered subcutaneously.
- Golimumab and infliximab require intravenous administration.

Uses

Use of a TNF-α inhibitor concurrently with methotrexate is more effective for treating RA than either one alone. These drugs provide symptomatic relief in 60% of patients, but they are not curative.

Clinical Correlation

Blood Dyscrasia

Blood dyscrasia is a general term for a pathologic disorder of the blood in which the cellular constituents of the blood are abnormal or are present in abnormal quantities. Examples of this include idiopathic thrombocytopenic purpura, hemophilia, sickle cell anemia, and leukemia.

Side Effects

- Minor irritation at injection sites is the most common side effect of etanercept and adalimumab.
- Increased susceptibility to bacterial and fungal infections. Serious and fatal infections have occurred.

33.4.3 Other Biologics for RA

IL-1 Antagonist

Anakinra

Anakinra is a recombinant form of the human IL-1 receptor antagonist (IL-1 Ra).

Mechanism of Action

Anakinra blocks the actions of endogenous IL-1, thereby decreasing IL-1-mediated inflammatory responses. It has shown moderate effectiveness.

Pharmacokinetics

Given by daily subcutaneous injection.

Side Effects

Side effects of anakinra are the same as TNF-α inhibitors: injection site reactions and increased susceptibility to infections.

IL-6 Antagonist

Tocilizumab

Tocilizumab is a monoclonal antibody to IL-6 receptors.

Mechanism of Action

IL-6 is a proinflammatory cytokine. Tocilizumab binds to IL-6 receptors and blocks the actions of endogenous IL-6, thereby decreasing IL-6-mediated inflammatory responses. It has shown moderate effectiveness.

Pharmacokinetics

Given intravenously every 4 weeks or subcutaneously every week.

Side Effects

Side effects are the same as TNF-α inhibitors: injection site reactions and increased susceptibility to infections.

Foundations

Clusters of Differentiation—Cell Surface Markers

The cell surface proteins expressed by lymphocytes vary depending on the type of lymphocyte, stage of differentiation, and/or activation state of the cell. These proteins can be used as cell surface markers to identify different types of cells and are called clusters of differentiation (CD).

33.4.4 T-cell Activation Inhibitor

Abatacept

Abatacept is a fusion protein consisting of a cytotoxic T lymphocyte antigen linked to a modified region of human IgG1.

Mechanism of Action

Abatacept binds to CD80 and CD86 on antigen-presenting cells and prevents them from binding to CD28 on T cells, thereby preventing T cell activation.

Pharmacokinetics

Initially given intravenously every 2 weeks and then monthly or SC weekly.

Side Effect

Side effects are the same as TNF-α inhibitors: injection site reactions and increased susceptibility to infections.

33.4.5 CD20 Antagonist

Rituximab

Rituximab is a recombinant chimeric monoclonal antibody to CD20, a B-cell-specific cell surface antigen.

Mechanism of Action

It is used in combination with methotrexate in patients who have not responded to TNF-α inhibitor therapy.

Pharmacokinetics

Given intravenously every 16 to 24 weeks. Premedication with acetaminophen, antihistamine, and methylprednisone is used to reduce infusion-related adverse effects.

Side Effects

Side effects are the same as TNF-α inhibitors: injection reactions and increased susceptibility to infections.

33.4.6 Janus Kinase Inhibitor

Tofacitinib

Tofacitinib is a small molecule inhibitor of the Janus kinases (JAKs).

Mechanism of Action

By inhibiting JAKs, tofacitinib interrupts JAK-STAT signaling. Normally, the JAK-STAT pathway influences transcription of several genes involved in the immune response. By inhibiting this signaling, tofacitinib inhibits the immune response.

Pharmacokinetics

Effective orally. May be used as monotherapy or in combination with a nonbiologic DMARD.

Side Effects

Increased susceptibility to infections. May increase cholesterol levels with long-term treatment.

33.5 Drugs Used in the Treatment of Gout

Gout is an arthropathy caused by hyperuricemia and the deposition of uric acid crystals in the joints. It may be precipitated by trauma, surgery, starvation, infection, or diuretic therapy. It often occurs in the metatarsophalangeal joint of the great toe (hallux). Symptoms include severe pain, redness, and swelling of the affected joints. The therapy of gout involves treatment of the acute attack with colchicine and NSAIDs, and chronic treatment of the hyperuricemia.

33.5.1 Treatment of Acute Gout

Colchicine

Mechanism of Action

Colchicine inhibits mitotic activity, neutrophil migration, and phagocytic activity in inflamed tissue (▶ Fig. 33.5).

Side Effects

GI irritation, bone marrow depression, myopathy, and alopecia with long-term use.

Indomethacin and Other NSAIDs

Indomethacin has been the traditional NSAID used for acute gout attacks, but there is no evidence that it is superior to other NSAIDs. Ibuprofen, naproxen, and celecoxib may be just as effective.

33.5.2 Treatment of Chronic Gout

Probenecid and Sulfinpyrazone

Mechanism of Action

These agents block the proximal tubular reabsorption of uric acid.

Pharmacokinetics

Rapidly absorbed orally.

Side Effects

GI irritation and allergic reactions.

Contraindications

Aspirin can impair the excretion of uric acid from the kidneys at the usual over-the-counter doses; however, low-dose aspirin taken for heart attack or stroke prevention should not significantly alter the uric acid level.

Allopurinol

Mechanism of Action

Allopurinol reduces the synthesis of uric acid by inhibiting xanthine oxidase, which is the enzyme that catalyzes the formation of uric acid from hypoxanthine via xanthine.

Side Effects

GI irritation, allergic reactions, and blood dyscrasias.

Febuxostat

Mechanism of Action

Febuxostat is a newer xanthine oxidase inhibitor.

Side Effects

Allergic reactions and altered liver function tests.

Pegloticase

Pegloticase is a recombinant uricase attached to polyethylene glycol.

Mechanism of Action

Pegloticase catalyzes the conversion of serum uric acid to allantoin, an inert metabolite that is readily eliminated by the kidneys.

Pharmacokinetics

The drug is given intravenously every 2 weeks.

Side Effects

Immune and allergic reactions.

VIII

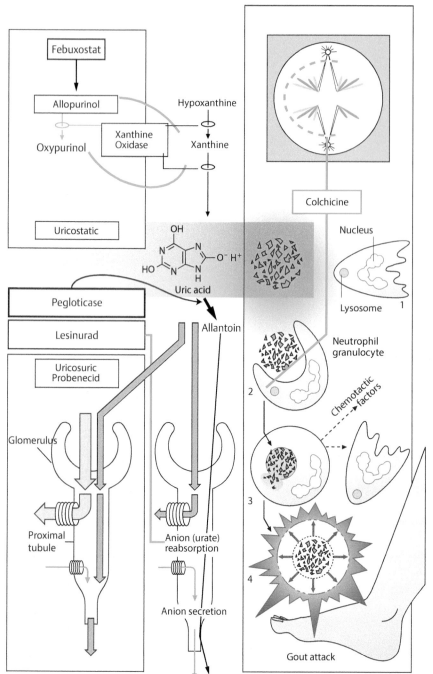

Fig. 33.5 Gout and its therapy.
Gout results from increased levels of uric acid (an end product of purine degradation). Uric acid tends to crystallize in the metatarsophalangeal joints and provides a strong stimulus for neutrophils and macrophages. Neutrophils are attracted (**1**) and phagocytose (**2**) the uric acid crystals. Neutrophils release proinflammatory cytokines (**3**). Macrophages also phagocytose the crystals and release lysosomal enzymes that promote inflammation. This results in an acute and very painful attack of gout (**4**). Colchicine and NSAIDs are used to treat acute attacks of gout. Colchicine binds to microtubular proteins and impairs their function, causing inter alia arrest of mitosis at metaphase ("spindle poison"). Its acute antigout activity is due to inhibition of neutrophil and macrophage reactions. Allopurinol along with its accumulating metabolite, oxypurinol, and the newer drug febuxostat are uricostatic agents that inhibit xanthine oxidase, the enzyme that catalyzes the formation of uric acid from hypoxanthine via xanthine. Uricosurics such as probenecid promote the renal excretion of uric acid by saturating the organic acid transport system in the renal proximal tubules, making it unavailable for uric acid resorption. Lesinurad promotes the renal excretion of uric acid by inhibiting the organic acid transport system. Pegloticase promotes the excretion of uric acid by catalyzing its conversion to allantoin.

Uses

This drug is reserved for patients unresponsive to other therapies.

Lesinurad

Lesinurad inhibits the uric acid transporters that are responsible for reabsorption of uric acid in the proximal tubule of the kidney.

Mechanism of Action

Inhibition of the reabsorption of uric acid results in increased uric acid excretion.

Pharmacokinetics

Once daily oral tablet.

Side Effects

Allergic reactions. Renal failure has been observed when the drug is used as monotherapy. It is approved for use in combination with a xanthine oxidase inhibitor.

Uses

This drug is reserved for patients unresponsive to other therapies.

Unit VIII Review Questions

1. A 42-year-old woman has been experiencing severe, unilateral throbbing headaches. The headaches are frequently preceded by flashing shapes of light in her vision. The headaches are accompanied by nausea, vomiting, and sensitivity to light. Which of the following might be suitable for treating this patient's headaches?
   A. Selective 5-HT$_3$ receptor antagonists.
   B. Selective D$_2$ receptor antagonists.
   C. Selective 5-HT$_{1B/1D}$ receptor agonists.
   D. Selective calcium channel antagonists.
   E. Selective H$_1$ receptor antagonists.

2. A 62-year-old woman has been experiencing an increased frequency of migraine headaches. She has also been experiencing dyspnea on exertion and mild peripheral edema. Which of the following would be contraindicated for migraine prophylaxis for this patient?
   A. Acetaminophen.
   B. Amitriptyline.
   C. Aspirin.
   D. Propranolol.
   E. Valproate.

3. Loratadine differs from most older H$_1$ antihistamines, in that it
   A. Inhibits gastric acid secretion.
   B. Has few CNS side effects, such as sedation.
   C. Has a much shorter duration of action.
   D. Does not have GI side effects.
   E. Has no tendency to induce impotence and gynecomastia in men.

4. Gynecomastia and impotence in men may occur with prolonged administration of which of the following?
   A. Diphenhydramine.
   B. Cimetidine.
   C. Ranitidine.
   D. Loratadine.
   E. Cromolyn sodium.

5. A 25-year-old Hispanic woman complains of itchy, watery eyes and an itchy, runny nose. The symptoms occur in the spring and summer and become worse if she mows the lawn. Which of the following might be useful for treatment of this patient's symptoms?
   A. Diphenhydramine.
   B. Ranitidine.
   C. Amantadine.
   D. Chlorpromazine.

6. A 36-year-old man has epigastric pain that he describes as burning. Which of the following drugs would be most useful to relieve the pain this patient is experiencing?
   A. Diphenhydramine.
   B. Ranitidine.
   C. Amantadine.
   D. Chlorpromazine.

7. A 58-year-old man with rheumatoid arthritis is taking anti-inflammatory doses of diclofenac. The drug is available in a combination with an analogue of prostaglandin E$_1$ (PCE$_1$).

What is the purpose of adding a PCE$_1$ analogue to diclofenac?
   A. To provide a synergistic anti-inflammatory effect.
   B. To prevent the breakdown of diclofenac in the gastrointestinal tract.
   C. To prolong the duration of action of diclofenac.
   D. To prevent diclofenac from causing nephritis.
   E. To protect the stomach lining from potential damage by diclofenac.

8. Which of the following promote platelet aggregation?
   A. Prostaglandins.
   B. Thromboxanes.
   C. Prostacyclins.
   D. Leukotrienes.
   E. Bradykinin.

9. Which of the following inhibits platelet aggregation by acetylating platelet cyclooxygenase?
   A. Aspirin.
   B. Acetaminophen.
   C. Celecoxib.
   D. Indomethacin.
   E. Ibuprofen.

10. A 5-month-old infant has been crying, has a decreased appetite, and has a fever of 39 °C (102 °F). Which of the following antipyretics should be used?
   A. Aspirin.
   B. Acetaminophen.
   C. Salicylate.
   D. Indomethacin.
   E. Ibuprofen.

11. A 48-year-old man attempts to commit suicide by taking an overdose of acetaminophen after consuming several shots of vodka. He is brought to the emergency room, and acetylcysteine is administered intravenously. What is the purpose of including acetylcysteine in the treatment regimen?
   A. To prevent cardiac failure.
   B. To increase urine flow.
   C. To block absorption of acetaminophen from the gastrointestinal tract.
   D. To enhance metabolism of ethanol.
   E. To prevent liver damage.

12. A patient has mild osteoarthritis (i.e., the disease is not progressing rapidly). Her pain is no longer effectively managed with aspirin, except by doses that cause unacceptable tinnitus. Which of the following would be the best course of action for treating this patient?
   A. Stop all medications for 4 weeks, then try aspirin again.
   B. Treat with acetaminophen.
   C. Treat with morphine.
   D. Treat with naproxen.
   E. Treat with an anti-inflammatory steroid.

13. Which of the following increases urinary excretion of uric acid?
   A. Probenecid.
   B. Colchicine.

C. Acetaminophen.

D. Allopurinol.

14. A 56-year-old man has pain, swelling, and redness in the first metatarsophalangeal joint of his right foot that began 2 days ago. He has a history of previous gout attacks. To treat the patient's symptoms, a drug may be given that does which of the following?

A. Decreases the production of uric acid.

B. Increases the excretion of uric acid.

C. Lowers the concentration of serum uric acid.

D. Inhibits the migration of leukocytes and interrupts the inflammatory response to uric acid by reducing phagocytosis.

15. Which of the following drugs is the best choice to treat severe chronic gout in the presence of impaired renal function?

A. Naproxen.

B. Sulfinpyrazone.

C. Allopurinol.

D. Probenecid.

E. Acetaminophen.

16. What is the mechanism of action of colchicine in gout?

A. It decreases the production of uric acid.

B. It increases the excretion of uric acid.

C. It lowers serum uric acid concentration.

D. It inhibits the migration of leukocytes and interrupts the inflammatory response to uric acid by reducing phagocytosis.

17. Which of the following increases urinary excretion of uric acid?

A. Probenecid.

B. Colchicine.

C. Acetaminophen.

D. Allopurinol.

18. The uricosuric action of probenecid may be decreased by

A. Colchicine.

B. Phenacetin.

C. Aspirin.

D. Acetaminophen.

E. Allopurinol.

19. Which of the following decreases the production of uric acid?

A. Probenecid.

B. Colchicine.

C. Acetaminophen.

D. Allopurinol.

E. Aspirin.

20. Sedation is a common side effect of which of the following?

A. Diphenhydramine.

B. Cimetidine.

C. Ranitidine.

D. Fexofenadine.

E. Cromolyn sodium.

21. Which of the following has no useful anti-inflammatory activity?

A. Aspirin.

B. Acetaminophen.

C. Salicylate.

D. Diflunisal.

E. Ibuprofen.

22. Which of the following is not a useful antipyretic?

A. Aspirin.

B. Acetaminophen.

C. Salicylate.

D. Gold salts.

E. Ibuprofen.

23. Aspirin irreversibly blocks the synthesis of this autacoid in platelets to decrease platelet aggregation.

A. Prostacyclin (PGI_2).

B. Thromboxane (TXA_2).

C. Misoprostol.

D. Prostaglandin F2a (PGF_{2a}).

E. Leukotriene C4 (LTC_4).

24. Which of the following may be used to produce closure of a patent ductus arteriosus?

A. Indomethacin.

B. Alcohol.

C. Tetracyclines.

D. Warfarin.

E. Propranolol.

25. The primary advantage of the oxicam class of nonsteroidal anti-inflammatory drugs (NSAIDs) is their

A. Increased oral bioavailability.

B. Long half-life.

C. Lower cost.

D. More effective analgesic properties.

26. A 54-year-old man has a history of previous gout attacks. He was treated for the most recent attack 2 weeks ago. To prevent further attacks, he is given a drug that acts by which of the following mechanisms?

A. Stimulates uric acid secretion by renal tubules.

B. Inhibits uric acid reabsorption.

C. Increases uric acid synthesis.

D. Inhibits the release of inflammatory mediators.

27. A 25-year-old Hispanic woman complains of itchy, watery eyes and an itchy, runny nose. The symptoms occur in the spring and summer and become worse if she mows the lawn. What advantage does a second-generation H_1 blocker have in this case?

A. It is less costly.

B. It has a longer half-life.

C. It is less sedating.

D. It produces less nausea.

E. It is less likely to produce headache.

28. A 68-year-old man has undergone coronary artery bypass graft surgery. For long-term antiplatelet therapy, he is given a drug that inhibits platelet aggregation by acetylating platelet cyclooxygenase. Which of the following drugs is this patient taking?

A. Diflunisal.

B. Acetaminophen.

C. Salicylate.

D. Aspirin.

E. Ibuprofen.

29. A 64-year-old man has osteoarthritis of the knee. At age 54, he had coronary artery bypass graft surgery. He is currently taking a thiazide diuretic and a β-blocker for hypertension. To treat his joint pain, he started 2 years ago on acetaminophen. Due to increased severity of pain, 6 months later his medication was changed to naproxen. Recently, the patient has once again been experiencing pain and is seeking further relief. Which of the following therapies could increase the patient's risk for myocardial infarction or stroke?

A. Intra-articular injections of a glucocorticoid.

B. Arthroscopic debridement and lavage.

C. Switch from naproxen to a selective cyclooxygenase-2 (COX-2) inhibitor.

D. Topical capsaicin cream.

E. Intra-articular injections of a hyaluronic acid.

30. A 40-year-old woman has just been diagnosed with rheumatoid arthritis. Her treatment plan includes methotrexate, which can be started immediately, and a second agent. Before starting the second agent, which of the following tests should be performed?

A. Prothrombin time and international normalized ratio test.

B. Serum alanine aminotransferase level.

C. Skin test for tuberculosis.

D. Serum uric acid level.

E. Von Willebrand factor antigen test.

Unit VIII Answers and Explanations

1. C. These are migraine symptoms that can be treated with triptans, which are selective 5-HT$_{1B/1D}$ receptor agonists.

A. Selective 5-HT$_3$ receptor antagonists are used to prevent nausea.

B. Selective D$_2$ receptor antagonists are antipsychotics.

D. Selective calcium channel antagonists are used to treat hypertension.

E. Selective H$_1$ receptor antagonists are used to treat allergies.

2. D. Although propranolol is used to treat migraines, it is a β-adrenergic receptor blocking agent that may have adverse effects in a patient with heart failure and/or difficulty breathing.

A, C. Acetaminophen and aspirin are for acute treatment of pain, not for prophylaxis.

B, E. Amitriptyline and valproate are used for migraine prophylaxis.

3. B. The main difference between loratadine and the first-generation antihistamines, such as diphenhydramine and chlorpheniramine, is that loratadine does not cross the blood–brain barrier. Thus, it has fewer CNS side effects.

A. Neither first- nor second-generation H$_1$ antihistamines inhibit gastric acid secretion; that is an H$_2$-mediated effect.

C. The duration of action of loratadine is longer than that of the H$_1$ agents.

D. Loratadine may have GI side effects.

E. None of the H$_1$ agents have a tendency to induce impotence and gynecomastia in men. These are rare side effects of cimetidine.

4. B. These side effects have been reported with cimetidine, an H$_2$ receptor blocker, but not with the other agents listed.

5. A. The patient is experiencing symptoms of allergic rhinitis. Diphenhydramine is a first-generation H$_1$ antihistamine useful for alleviating these symptoms.

B. Ranitidine is an H$_2$ antihistamine used in the treatment of peptic ulcers or gastroesophageal disease.

C. Amantadine is an antiviral agent.

D. Chlorpromazine is an antipsychotic agent.

6. B. The patient is having heartburn from gastroesophageal reflux, which can be treated with an H$_2$ antihistamine, such as ranitidine, which inhibits gastric acid secretions.

A. Diphenhydramine is an H$_1$ antihistamine that has no effect on gastric acid production.

C. Amantadine is an antiviral agent.

D. Chlorpromazine is an antipsychotic agent.

7. E. The PCE$_1$ analogue is an inhibitor of gastric acid secretion. It is used for prophylaxis of gastric ulcers induced by nonsteroidal anti-inflammatory agents, such as diclofenac.

8. B. Thromboxanes stimulate platelet aggregation.

A, C, E. Prostaglandins, prostacyclins, and bradykinin inhibit platelet aggregation.

D. Leukotrienes do not promote platelet aggregation.

9. A. Aspirin inhibits the cyclooxygenase enzymes by acetylating a single serine residue. This is an irreversible covalent modification that inactivates both cyclooxygenase-1 and -2 (COX-1 and COX-2). Inhibition of platelet COX-1 prevents thrombosis.

B. Celecoxib is a COX-2 selective inhibitor.

C. Acetaminophen is a weak inhibitor of COX.

D, E. Indomethacin and ibuprofen are competitive inhibitors of the cyclooxygenases.

10. B. Although most of the nonsteroidal anti-inflammatory drugs have some antipyretic action, aspirin is usually the antipyretic of choice. In patients younger than 19 years of age, however, aspirin and other salicylates are contraindicated in cases of fever associated with viral illness, due to an association of Reye syndrome with aspirin use in such cases. Acetaminophen is recommended to reduce fever in these cases.

11. E. Acetylcysteine protects against hepatic injury from the acetaminophen overdose.

A–D. The other choices are not applicable.

12. D. Although aspirin and acetaminophen can be used as initial treatment for osteoarthritis pain, an agent with greater analgesic activity, such as naproxen, is often required.

A, B. In general, aspirin and acetaminophen have equal analgesic activity.

C. Morphine is for severe pain and has numerous side effects.

E. Long-term use of anti-inflammatory steroids is not recommended due to side effects.

13. A. Probenecid blocks the proximal tubular reabsorption of uric acid, thus increasing its excretion.

B. Colchicine inhibits mitotic activity, neutrophil migration, and phagocytic activity in inflamed tissue. It does not affect production, excretion, or serum levels of uric acid.

C. Acetaminophen is an analgesic and antipyretic.

D. Allopurinol reduces the synthesis of uric acid by inhibiting xanthine oxidase.

14. D. The therapy of gout involves treatment of the acute attack with NSAIDs or colchicine. Colchicine inhibits mitotic activity, neutrophil migration, and phagocytic activity in inflamed tissue. NSAIDs inhibit cyclooxygenase to reduce inflammation.

A–C. Drugs that affect uric acid production, excretion, and/or serum concentration are not effective for acute attacks but are used to treat chronic gout.

15. C. Allopurinol is the correct choice because it reduces the synthesis of uric acid.

A. Naproxen is a nonsteroidal anti-inflammatory agent that may be used to treat symptoms of an acute attack of gout.

B, D. Sulfinpyrazone and probenecid block the proximal tubular reabsorption of uric acid and would be less effective in cases of impaired renal function.

E. Acetaminophen is an analgesic but not an anti-inflammatory agent, so it is generally not used in treating chronic gout.

16. D. Colchicine inhibits mitotic activity, neutrophil migration, and phagocytic activity in inflamed tissue.

A–C. It does not affect production, excretion, or serum levels of uric acid.

17. A. Probenecid blocks the proximal tubular reabsorption of uric acid, thus increasing its excretion.

B. Colchicine inhibits mitotic activity, neutrophil migration, and phagocytic activity in inflamed tissue. It does not affect production, excretion, or serum levels of uric acid.

C. Acetaminophen is an analgesic and antipyretic.

D. Allopurinol reduces the synthesis of uric acid by inhibiting xanthine oxidase.

18. C. Aspirin can impair the excretion of uric acid from the kidneys at the usual over-the-counter doses. Because probenecid works by blocking the proximal tubular reabsorption of uric acid, its effectiveness may be decreased by aspirin.

A, B, C, E. The other agents do not affect the uricosuric action of probenecid.

19. D. Allopurinol reduces the synthesis of uric acid by inhibiting xanthine oxidase.

A. Probenecid blocks the proximal tubular reabsorption of uric acid.

B. Colchicine inhibits mitotic activity, neutrophil migration, and phagocytic activity in inflamed tissue. It does not affect production, excretion, or serum levels of uric acid.

C. Acetaminophen is an analgesic and antipyretic agent.

E. Aspirin is a nonsteroidal anti-inflammatory agent used to treat mild to moderate pain, pyrexia, and certain inflammatory conditions, and as a thrombolytic agent.

20. A. Sedation is a common side effect of the first-generation H_1 receptor blockers, including diphenhydramine, as they are able to cross the blood-brain barrier into the CNS.

B, C. Cimetidine and ranitidine are H_2 receptor blockers. They do not produce sedation.

D. Fexofenadine, as a second-generation H_1 receptor blocker, is unable to cross the blood-brain barrier and therefore does not produce sedation.

E. Cromolyn sodium is a mast cell stabilizer. It does not produce sedation.

21. B. All of the drugs listed have antipyretic, analgesic, and anti-inflammatory properties, except for acetaminophen.

22. D. All of the drugs listed have antipyretic activity except for gold salts.

23. B. The antiplatelet activity of aspirin is due to irreversible block of cyclooxygenase-1 (COX-1), which blocks TXA_2 formation, which decreases platelet aggregation.

A, D. The prostacyclins and prostaglandins are the two other major groups of eicosanoids that are formed by COX activity, but decreasing their synthesis does not decrease platelet aggregation.

C. Misoprostol is a synthetic prostaglandin (PGE_1) methyl ester.

E. Leukotriene synthesis is catalyzed by lipoxygenase.

24. A. Prostaglandin E_2 is responsible for keeping the ductus arteriosus open during fetal development. The ductus arteriosus begins to close shortly after birth. If it fails to close, indomethacin, a nonsteroidal anti-inflammatory agent that inhibits prostaglandin synthesis, may be administered to produce closure.

B–E. None of the other drugs listed have this effect.

25. B. Piroxicam and meloxicam have a long duration of action that allows once-daily dosing.

A, C, D. They do not have an advantage with respect to bioavailability, cost or greater analgesic properties.

26. B. The goal of treatment of chronic gout is to decrease serum uric acid. This can be done by blocking the tubular reabsorption of uric acid or by decreasing uric acid synthesis.

27. C. The patient is experiencing symptoms of allergic rhinitis. Second-generation antihistamines will alleviate the symptoms without causing sedation as they do not cross the blood–brain barrier.

28. D. Of the drugs listed, aspirin is the one that inhibits platelet aggregation by acetylating platelet cyclooxygenase. It is also the only one used for antiplatelet therapy.

A. Diflunisal is a salicylate that is a reversible inhibitor of platelet aggregation.

B. Acetaminophen is a weak inhibitor of cyclooxygenases.

C. Salicylate is a class of drug which includes aspirin, choline magnesium salicylate, salsalate, and diflunisal.

E. Ibuprofen is a competitive inhibitor of cyclooxygenases.

29. C. COX-2 inhibitors produce an increased risk of adverse cardiovascular events, such as myocardial infarction and stroke. Some selective COX-2 inhibitors have been withdrawn from the market because of this. Although celecoxib, a highly selective

COX-2 inhibitor, also carries such risks, it remains available, and its benefits may outweigh the risks in properly selected and informed patients.

30. C. Methotrexate is more effective for treating rheumatoid arthritis when combined with a tumor necrosis factor-α (TNF-α) inhibitor. TNF-α inhibitors, however, may increase the susceptibility to bacterial infections. Thus, a skin test for latent tuberculosis is required prior to starting TNF-α inhibitor therapy.

A, E. Neither methotrexate or a TNF-α inhibitor will have an effect on blood clotting or clotting factors.

B. Methotrexate and TNF-α inhibitors are not contraindicated in liver disease so a serum alanine aminotransferase level is not necessary.

D. Methotrexate and TNF-α inhibitors do not affect serum uric acid levels.

Unit IX

Cancer Chemotherapy, Toxicology and Vitamins

By Dennis M. Peffley

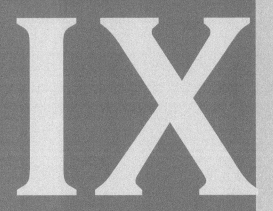

IX

34 Cancer Chemotherapy and Immunosuppressants

Summary

Chemotherapeutic drugs include alkylating agents, antimetabolites, antibiotics, topoisomerase inhibitors, and taxanes. Alkylating agents (mechlorethamine, cyclophosphamide and ifosfamide, melphalan, carmustine and lomustine, platin drugs [cisplatin, carboplatin, and oxaliplatin], chlorambucil, busulfan, procarbazine, dacarbazine, temozolomide, streptomycin, and mitomycin C) alkylate or otherwise modify tumor cell DNA. Antimetabolites (methotrexate, pemetrexed, pralatrexate, 6-mercaptopurine, thioguanine, fluorouracil, floxuridine, capecitabine, fludarabine, cladribine, cytarabine, gemcitabine, and azacytidine) inhibit DNA synthesis. Antibiotics (dactinomycin, daunorubicin, idarubicin, epirubicin, mitoxantrone, hydroxyurea, and bleomycin) inhibit DNA and RNA synthesis. Topoisomerase inhibitors (etoposide, teniposide, irinotecan, and topotecan) cause DNA strand breakage. Antimitotic agents (vincristine, vinblastine, paclitaxel, and docetaxel) arrest cell development in the M phase of the cell cycle. Monoclonal antibodies represent a rapidly evolving area for targeted therapy of various cancers. These include rituximab, tositumomab and iodine 131 tositumomab, indium 111 ibritumomab and yttrium 90 ibritumomab tiuxetan, trastuzumab, trastuzumab emtansine, pertuzumab, cetuximab, panitumumab, bevacizumab, atezolizumab, daratumumab, dinutuximab, elotuzumab, ipilimumab, nivolumab, obinutuzumab, ofatumumab, olaratumab, pembrolizumab, and ramucirumab. Tyrosine kinase inhibitors (imatinib, dasatinib, nilotinib, gefitinib, erlotinib, lapatinib, sorafenib, and sunitinib) inhibit receptor tyrosine kinases on membranes of cancer cells. Miscellaneous chemotherapeutic agents include bortezomib, thalidomide, asparaginase, and the differentiating agents, tretinoin and arsenic trioxide. Hormones (corticosteroids and prednisone) and hormone inhibitors (tamoxifen, anastrozole, letrozole, exemestane, triptorelin, bicalutamide, flutamide, and nilutamide) are effective for treating certain breast and prostate cancers (▸ Table 34.1).

Immunosuppressants are used to prevent rejection in patients receiving organ transplants and in patients with autoimmune diseases and include both small molecules (cyclosporine, tacrolimus, sirolimus, mycophenolate mofetil, azathioprine, everolimus, and temsirolimus) as well as monoclonal antibodies (basiliximab, infliximab, muromonab-cd3, belatacept, and daclizumab).

Keywords: antineoplastics, alkylating agents, antibiotics, antimetabolites, monoclonal antibodies, taxanes, topoisomerase inhibitors

34.1 Introduction

It is estimated that about 1,700,000 new cases of cancer are expected to be diagnosed in the United States in 2017. Over the past 30 decades, improvements in treatment as well as earlier diagnosis have increased the 5-year survival rates, due in part to the application of standard chemotherapeutic regimens as well as the more recent application of targeted therapies such as tyrosine kinase inhibitors and monoclonal antibodies. Cancer chemotherapy has undergone a revolution of sorts recently, with specifically targeted therapies directed to novel molecular targets and the use of pharmacogenomics testing to assess tumor susceptibility.

34.2 General Principles of Cancer Chemotherapy

34.2.1 Cell Cycle

An understanding of the cell cycle is essential for the effective use of anticancer agents (▸ Fig. 34.1). Most anticancer drugs kill dividing cells (they are proliferation dependent); thus, tumors with a high cell turnover are most susceptible (certain leukemias and lymphomas, small proliferating tumors, "recruited"

Table 34.1 Summary of monoclonal antibodies

Antigen	Agent	Uses
CD20	Rituximab	B cell lymphoma and chronic lymphocytic leukemia
CD20	Obinutuzumab	Chronic lymphocytic leukemia and follicular lymphoma
CD20	Ofatumumab	Chronic lymphocytic leukemia
CD20	Tositumomab and iodine 131 tositumomab	B cell lymphoma
CD20	Indium 111 ibritumomab and yttrium 90 ibritumomab tiuxetan	B cell lymphoma
HER2/neu (ErbB-2)	Trastuzumab	Breast cancer
HER2/neu (ErbB-2)	Pertuzumab	Breast cancer
EGFR (ErbB-1)	Cetuximab	Colorectal, head and neck cancers
EGFR (ErbB-1)	Panitumumab	Colorectal cancer
PDGFR-α	Olaratumab	Soft tissue sarcoma
VEGF	Bevacizumab	Colorectal, lung, breast, pancreatic cancers
VEGF	Ramucirumab	Gastric, gastroesophageal, colorectal, and non-small cell lung cancers
PD-L1	Atezolizumab	Bladder and non-small cell lung cancers
CD33	Gemtuzumab ozogamicin	Acute myeloid leukemia
CD38	Daratumumab	Multiple myeloma
GD-2	Dinutuximab	Neuroblastoma
SLAMF7	Elotuzumab	Multiple myeloma
CTLA-4	Ipilimumab	Melanoma
PD-1	Nivolumab	Hodgkin, melanoma, liver, colorectal, urothelial, renal, head and neck
PD-1	Pembrolizumab	Hodgkin, melanoma, colorectal, urothelial, stomach, head and neck

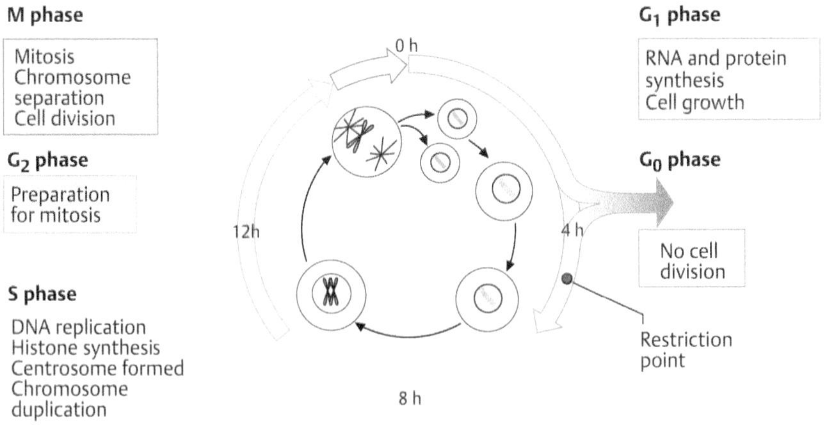

M phase

Mitosis
Chromosome separation
Cell division

G₂ phase

Preparation for mitosis

S phase

DNA replication
Histone synthesis
Centrosome formed
Chromosome duplication

0 h

12h

8 h

4 h

G₁ phase

RNA and protein synthesis
Cell growth

G₀ phase

No cell division

Restriction point

Fig. 34.1 Cell cycle.
The cell cycle describes the cellular events that take place, cumulating in cell division. It is divided into four phases: G_1, S, G_2, and M. Fully differentiated cells are in the G_0 stage when further cell division does not usually occur (hence, it is not part of the cell cycle). However, cells in the G_0 phase can reenter the G_1 phase if acted upon by certain mitotic signals (e.g., tumor viruses and cytokines). In the G_1 phase, the cell is growing and accumulating proteins and RNA. The restriction point in the G_1 phase is a control point that ensures that everything is ready for DNA synthesis, which occurs in the S phase. In the G_2 phase, the cell is preparing for mitosis, which occurs in the M phase, producing two daughter cells.

tumor cells, and micrometastases). The killing of tumor cells follows first-order kinetics. To produce a cure, therapy must continue until the final tumor cell has been eradicated. There is an inverse relationship between tumor cell number or tumor size and the ability of chemotherapy to fully eradicate the tumor. Agents that act preferentially on tumor cells in a given phase of the cell cycle are called *cell cycle specific*. Agents that act during several stages of the cell cycle are called *cell cycle nonspecific*.

34.2.2 Anticancer Drugs

Several neoplastic diseases can be cured with drugs alone or with a combination of drugs and other treatment modalities. Examples of these neoplastic diseases include choriocarcinoma, Hodgkin's disease, acute lymphocytic leukemia, Burkitt lymphoma, and testicular carcinoma. Adjuvant chemotherapy in combination with surgery and/or radiotherapy has increased survival rates for several solid tumors; however, the most prevalent forms of human cancer respond poorly or not at all to chemotherapy.

Drug treatment regimens for cancer usually involve combinations of agents given intermittently. Combining drugs with different mechanisms of action can produce larger therapeutic effects with fewer side effects. Intermittent therapy allows the patient to recover from drug toxicities, such as bone marrow suppression, between courses.

Foundations

Tumor Development

Tumors develop when the normal regulation of the balance between cell proliferation (mitosis) and programmed cell death (apoptosis) or autophagy is lost. Tumor initiation is the process by which normal cells are changed so that they are able to form tumors. This involves DNA damage of multiple genes (6–10). Substances that cause cancer can be tumor initiators or substances that can initiate DNA mutations in proto oncogenes or tumor suppressors. Tumor promotion is the process by which existing tumors are stimulated to grow. Tumor promoters are not able to cause tumors to form but increase the frequency of tumor formation in tissue previously exposed to the tumor initiator.

Clinical Correlation

Chemical Carcinogenesis

Many chemicals that are present as industrial or environmental pollutants, dietary components, combustion by-products, or therapeutic agents may increase the risk of cancer development. Genotoxic carcinogens are thought to initiate tumorigenesis by interacting with DNA. Chemicals may be inherently genotoxic, but many chemical carcinogens are metabolized to highly reactive metabolites, which in turn damage DNA. Alternatively, chemicals could act by altering DNA replication or repair. Epigenetic carcinogens do not appear to interact directly with DNA, but instead appear to augment neoplastic growth by poorly defined mechanisms. This class of carcinogens includes various hormones (e.g., estrogen and diethylstilbestrol), immunosuppressive drugs (e.g., azathioprine), solid-state carcinogens (e.g., asbestos), and promoting agents (agents that increase tumor development when given after a genotoxic chemical).

Foundations

Cancer Critical Genes

The two main types of genes that are now recognized as playing a role in cancer are oncogenes (e.g., HER-2, KRAS) and tumor suppressor (e.g., retinoblastoma, *p16*) genes. Most oncogenes are mutations of normal genes called *proto-oncogenes*. The mutant proteins coded by oncogenes (oncoproteins) are overactive and allow cells to proliferate when they should not. The protein products of tumor suppressor genes are normal genes that slow down cell division, repair DNA mistakes, and indicate when to undergo apoptosis (programmed cell death). These genes are deleted or inactivated in cancer cells, allowing unregulated proliferation.

Foundations

P53 Gene

P53 is a tumor suppressor gene that codes for a transcription factor that regulates the expression of other genes and arrests the cell cycle. It is the most frequently mutated gene in human cancers. *P53* is considered to be a central monitor of cellular stress and induction of DNA damage results in *p53* activation and cessation of cell cycle progression. Mutations in *p53* have been associated with carcinogenesis at multiple sites within the body.

34.3 Toxicity of Anticancer Drugs

Anticancer drugs generally have low therapeutic indices and potentially lethal toxicities. Many of the toxic effects of anticancer drugs are due to cytotoxic effects on normal tissues that have high proportions of dividing cells (▶ Fig. 34.2).
- Anticancer drugs frequently produce nausea and vomiting that can be ameliorated with phenothiazines or cannabinoids.
- The release of nucleic acid breakdown products following a very large cell kill from anticancer drugs can result in hyperuricemia and renal damage. Hyperuricemia is prevented with allopurinol (see Chapter 33).
- Many anticancer drugs are mutagenic and carcinogenic.

34.3.1 Combination Therapy

When selecting a combination of anticancer drugs, they should ideally have the following attributes:
- They should be effective when used alone.
- They should have different mechanisms of action.
- They should have minimally overlapping toxicities.
- There should be no cross-resistance.

Tumor Markers

Tumor markers are substances that can be detected in the peripheral blood and are derived from neoplastic populations, but lack functional hormonal or other physiologic activity. They include carcinoembryonic antigen (CEA), seen in colon, gastric, pancreatic, and breast carcinoma; prostate-specific antigen (PSA), seen in prostate carcinoma; cancer antigen 125 (CA-125), seen in ovarian carcinoma; alpha fetoprotein (AFP), seen in hepatocellular carcinoma and germ cell neoplasms, especially yolk sac carcinoma; and human chorionic gonadotropin (hCG), seen in choriocarcinoma testicular germ cell neoplasms. In general, serum tumor markers are characterized by low sensitivity and low specificity. Nonetheless, they are employed routinely for several purposes, including screening, monitoring therapy, and detection of recurrences.

Clinical Correlation

Radiotherapy and Its Systemic Effects

Radiotherapy involves the use of focused ionizing radiation to treat malignant cancer cells by damaging their DNA. It can be curative, used as an adjuvant therapy, or employed in palliative therapy to limit disease progression or to provide symptomatic relief. The systemic effects of radiation include several syndromes. Hematopoietic syndrome (200–500 rads) is

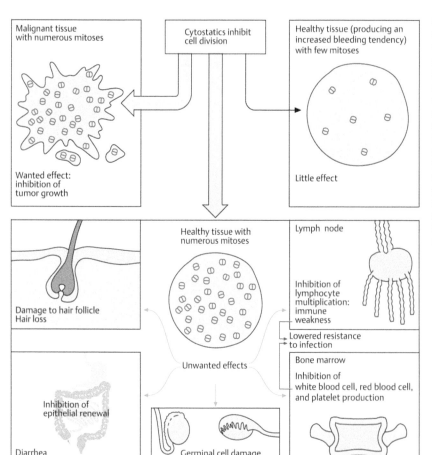

Fig. 34.2 Chemotherapy of tumors: principle and adverse effects.
Chemotherapeutic agents lack specificity and thus affect both malignant and endogenous cells. Because cytostatic agents act on proliferating or dividing (mitotic) cells, rapidly dividing malignant cells are preferentially injured (growth is retarded, and apoptosis is initiated). Endogenous tissues with a high mitotic rate (hair and epithelial cells) are also injured. In bone marrow, inhibition of mitosis causes neutropenia (producing a lowered resistance to infection), thrombocytopenia (producing an increased bleeding tendency), and anemia (producing fatigue, shortness of breath, dizziness, etc.). Infertility is also common due to suppression of spermatogenesis and follicle maturation. Healthy tissues and those with a low mitotic rate are largely unaffected by cytostatic agents.

development of a pancytopenia within a few weeks of exposure. Bleeding and infection are the major complications. Gastrointestinal (GI) syndrome (500–1000 rads) reflects injury to the GI epithelium, resulting in the development of nausea, vomiting, and severe diarrhea within several days of exposure. This may lead to severe metabolic disturbances, vascular collapse, sepsis, and death. Cerebral syndrome (> 2500 rads) is caused by vascular endothelial damage, resulting in cerebral edema, convulsions, coma, and death within hours of exposure.

Clinical Correlation

Local Effects of Radiotherapy

Depending on the tissues involved, acute radiation injury may manifest as an acute dermatitis, pneumonitis, and/or enteritis. Chronic changes reflect organ ischemia due to vasculopathy (endothelium is highly radiation sensitive). Neoplasms (primarily sarcomas) may develop even after an interval of 10 years or more. Acutely, blood vessels may dilate, thrombose, or rupture. Over time, however, reactive endothelial cell proliferation and mural scarring may lead to narrowing or even obliteration of the vessel lumens, causing tissue ischemia. The chronic effects of radiation injury, therefore, include interstitial fibrosis of various tissues and strictures of hollow organs.

This means that doses close to the regular doses for each drug as a single agent can be used to optimize the cytotoxic effects without additive toxicity. Drug resistance is the greatest obstacle to successful chemotherapy.

34.3.2 Drug Resistance

When tumor cells lack sensitivity to a drug, the drug resistance is termed *primary* or *endogenous*. Acquired drug resistance occurs when tumor cells undergo genotypic and phenotypic changes during therapy that render them insensitive to the drug (▶ Fig. 34.3).

The Goldie–Coldman hypothesis states that the probability of tumor containing a cell resistant to a specific drug is related to both tumor size and mutation frequency. Even the smallest detectable cancer would be expected to contain at least one drug-resistant cell. Drug exposure then provides the selection pressure for growth of a resistant cell population. Drug resistance may be to single or multiple drugs. Common mechanisms include decreased drug uptake, increased drug metabolism, and increased drug efflux from the cell. Increased drug efflux results from increased expression of P-glycoprotein and multidrug resistance protein and leads to multidrug resistance.

34.4 Cancer Chemotherapy Drugs

34.4.1 Alkylating Agents

Mechanism of Action

Alkylating agents bind covalently to the N7 position of guanine nucleotides of DNA and cross-link DNA strands. This prevents DNA replication and transcription, resulting in cytotoxicity and cell death (▶ Fig. 34.4). They are proliferation dependent but cell cycle nonspecific.

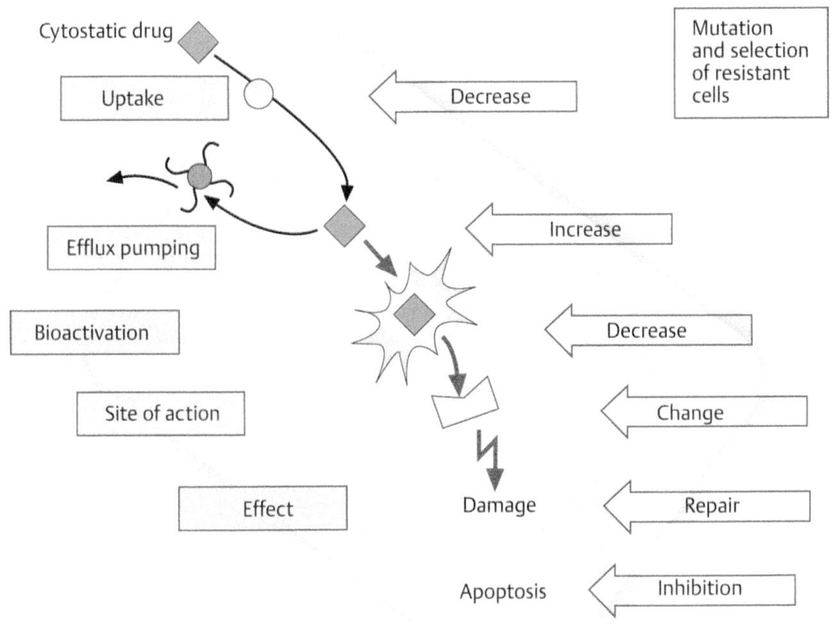

Fig. 34.3 Mechanisms of cytostatic resistance. The initial success of cytostatic agents can be followed by diminution of effect because of the emergence of resistant tumor cells. Genotypic and phenotypic changes may lead to reduced uptake of the drug into cancer cells, increased efflux of the drug from cells, diminished activation of prodrugs, and increased DNA repair.

IX

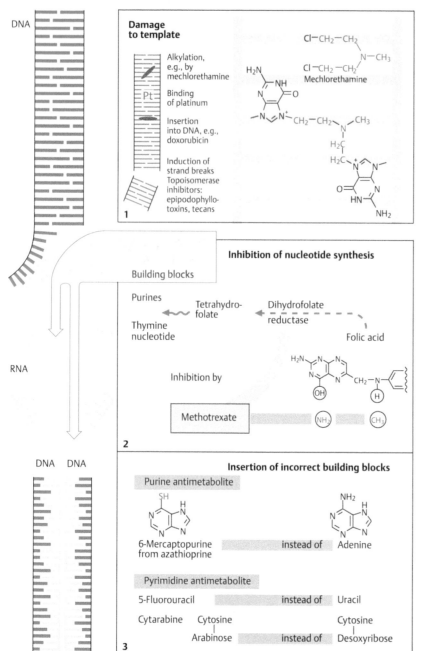

Fig. 34.4 Cytostatic: alkylating agents and cytostatic antibiotics (1), inhibitors of tetrahydrofolate synthesis (2), and antimetabolites (3). Mitosis is preceded by protein synthesis (RNA synthesis) and chromosomal replication (DNA synthesis). Existing DNA (*gray*) acts as a template for new DNA (*blue*). Alkylating agents (1) form covalent bonds with DNA, cross-linking it, and thus rendering it impossible to "unzip" and replicate. DNA strand breakage may also occur with some cytostatic antibiotics and topoisomerase inhibitors. Methotrexate is an antimetabolite (2) that inhibits dihydrofolate reductase, suppressing the production of purine and thymine nucleotides. Other antimetabolites (3) are purine and pyrimidine analogues that inhibit DNA/RNA synthesis or lead to the production of incorrect nucleic acids.

Clinical Correlation

Benign Versus Malignant Neoplasms

The distinction between benign and malignant tumors is based on their microscopic appearance, which predicts their clinical behavior. It reflects the degree of cellular differentiation, the extent to which neoplastic cells resemble their mature counterparts. Benign neoplasms are well differentiated (i.e., closely resemble mature cells of origin); hence, features such as gland formation are retained. Malignant cells, however, exhibit incomplete or lack of differentiation (anaplasia), and thus resemble stem cells. Anaplasia is characterized by cellular and nuclear pleomorphism (due to alterations in the cell cytoskeleton), increased nuclear/cytoplasmic ratio, increased nuclear chromatin density and bizarre mitoses (due to chromosomal aneuploidy), and loss of cellular orientation. Rate of growth tends to parallel the degree of differentiation of the neoplastic cells, as well as the cell turnover rate of the cell of origin. Thus, benign neoplasms have slow growth. Malignant neoplasms are characterized by a wide range of growth rates. Neoplasms derived from rapidly cycling populations (e.g., bone marrow and GI tract) grow much more rapidly than slowly proliferating tissues (e.g., prostate and salivary gland).

Resistance

High rates of DNA repair may be a cause of resistance.

Mechlorethamine

Mechlorethamine was the first anticancer drug to be used clinically, but it has largely been replaced by drugs that are better tolerated.

Pharmacokinetics

- Administered intravenously (IV).
- Highly reactive (the active drug has a very short half-life).
- A potent vesicant (i.e., it can cause chemical burns, resulting in large water blisters on contact with skin).

Uses

Mechlorethamine's main use is in the mechlorethamine, oncovin, procarbazine, and prednisone (MOPP) regimen for treatment of Hodgkin's disease.

Side Effects

- Bone marrow depression (leading to leucopenia and thrombocytopenia) is dose limiting.
- Severe nausea and vomiting may occur.

Cyclophosphamide and Ifosfamide

Cyclophosphamide is the most widely used alkylating agent. Ifosfamide is an analogue of cyclophosphamide.

Pharmacokinetics

- Effective orally or IV.
- Require cytochrome P-450-mediated metabolism to 4-hydroxycyclophosphamide and aldophosphamide for activation; nonenzymatic cleavage of aldophosphamide forms the toxic products phosphoramide and acrolein.
- Nonvesicant.

Uses

- Used for treatment of leukemia, lymphoma, ovarian cancer, breast cancer, and solid tumors in children (cyclophosphamide in combination with other drugs).
- Prevention of organ rejection after transplantation (cyclophosphamide).
- Immune disorders, such as Wegener granulomatosis, rheumatoid arthritis, and systemic lupus erythematosus (cyclophosphamide).
- Ifosfamide is approved as third-line therapy for testicular cancer, but it can also be used to treat the diseases for which cyclophosphamide is indicated.

Side Effects

- Bone marrow depression is dose limiting.
- Alopecia and immunosuppression are prominent.
- Renal excretion of metabolites causes hemorrhagic cystitis. This can be prevented with adequate prophylactic hydration and administration of 2-mercaptoethane sodium sulfonate (MESNA).

- Ifosfamide has greater myelosuppressive, renal, and neurologic side effects.

Melphalan

Melphalan is derived from nitrogen mustard and phenylalanine and functions as a bifunctional chloromethylating agent. Its mechanism of action is formation of DNA cross-links similar to that of other alkylating agents.

Pharmacokinetics

- Available in both oral and IV preparations.
- Oral bioavailability is variable with 20 to 50% being excreted in the stool.
- Poor oral absorption can account for lack of melphalan response in treatment of myeloma patients.
- Half-life is approximately 90 minutes.

Uses

- Its major use is in the treatment of multiple myeloma.
- The IV formulation is used for isolated limb perfusion in melanoma.

Side Effects

- Dose-limiting toxicity is myelosuppression.
- Nausea, vomiting, and alopecia are uncommon and mild.
- Amenorrhea and azoospermia, pulmonary fibrosis, and secondary malignancies have been noted with long-term use.

Carmustine and Lomustine

These drugs have a nitrosourea structure.

Pharmacokinetics

- These agents are highly lipophilic and cross the blood–brain barrier.
- Carmustine is given IV, and lomustine is given orally.

Uses

- Central nervous system (CNS) malignancies, i.e., malignant gliomas.
- Hodgkin's disease.

Side Effects

Bone marrow depression is delayed and may be prolonged.

Clinical Correlation

Hodgkin's Disease

Hodgkin's disease is a type of lymphoma (tumor of lymphocytes). On histological examination, there are characteristic cells (Reed–Sternberg cells) that have mirror image nuclei. Patients present with enlarged, painless lymph nodes in the neck or axillae, as well as fever, weight loss, night sweats, and general malaise (in 25% cases). Treatment depends on the stage of the disease but may involve radiotherapy and/or chemotherapy. This is one of the more treatable forms of cancer, with survival rates of up to 90% if detected early.

IX

Clinical Correlation

Chemotherapy Wafer Implants

Chemotherapy wafer implants are a new way of administering chemotherapy for certain brain tumors (gliomas and glioblastoma multiforme). Brain surgery is performed to remove all or most of the tumor, and the wafer is placed in the resulting space, where the drug (carmustine) slowly leaches out and treats the tumor locally. All of the usual chemotherapy side effects are still seen with this method of drug delivery.

Cisplatin, Carboplatin, and Oxaliplatin

Mechanism of Action

Each of these agents consists of a complex of inorganic platinum ions. They act by forming DNA cross-links, which prevents DNA replication and transcription.

Pharmacokinetics

- Administered IV.
- Bind to plasma proteins (90%).
- Concentrate in the liver, kidneys, intestines, and ovaries.
- Excreted in the urine.

Uses

Solid tumors, especially testicular, ovarian, and bladder cancer.

Side Effects

- Renal damage (dose-limiting). This can be decreased by prehydration and concomitant mannitol diuresis.
- Moderate bone marrow depression, ototoxicity (damage to the inner ear and acoustic nerve by a toxin), peripheral neuropathy, hypomagnesemia, and hypocalcemia.

Chlorambucil

Mechanism of Action

It is an alkylating agent that damages DNA and interferes with DNA replication.

Pharmacokinetics

- Administered orally.
- Hydrolyzed to inactive products.

Side Effects

- Bone marrow suppression.
- Neutropenia.

Busulfan

Pharmacokinetics

Given orally.

Uses

Chronic granulocytic leukemia.

Side Effects

- Bone marrow depression is selective for granulocytes (neutrophils, basophils, and eosinophils).
- Leukopenia (decreased number of white blood cells) and skin pigmentation may occur.

Procarbazine and Dacarbazine (Nonclassic Alkylating Agents)

Mechanisms of Action

Procarbazine acts by
- Inhibiting DNA, RNA, and protein synthesis.
- Prolonging interphase and general chromosome breaks.
- Oxidative metabolism of procarbazine by microsomal enzymes generates azoprocarbazine and hydrogen peroxide (oxidative damage of DNA).

Dacarbazine mechanism of action:
- Conversion to an alkylating agent requires metabolic activation in the liver by N-demethylation to a monomethyl triazeno metabolite.
- The monomethyl derivative generates a cytotoxic methyl carbonium ion and acts as a methylating agent.

Pharmacokinetics

- Procarbazine is administered orally; dacarbazine is administered IV.
- Both procarbazine and dacarbazine must undergo metabolic activation.
- These agents are not cross-resistant with other alkylating agents.

Uses

- Procarbazine is used in combination regimens for Hodgkin's and non-Hodgkin's lymphoma as well as brain tumors.
- Dacarbazine is used for treatment of malignant melanoma and Hodgkin's disease.

Side Effects

- Bone marrow depression is dose limiting (leukopenia and thrombocytopenia).
- CNS depression may occur (synergistic with phenothiazines and barbiturates).

Temozolomide

Mechanism of Action

- The parent drug is not active but undergoes rapid nonenzymatic conversion at physiological pH to the reactive compound monomethyl 5-triazino imidazole carboxamide (MITC).
- The tumor killing effects of temozolomide is alkylation of DNA, primarily at the O6 and N7 positions of guanine.

Pharmacokinetics

- Temozolomide is administered orally and is absorbed completely in the GI tract.
- Temozolomide is spontaneously hydrolyzed to MITC which is further hydrolyzed to 5-amino-imidazole-4-carboxamide (AIC), an active alkylating species.

Uses

- Temozolomide is used in the treatment of both acute myeloid leukemia and acute lymphocytic leukemia.

Side Effects

- Toxicity includes bone marrow depression that includes neutropenia, lymphopenia, anemia, and thrombocytopenia.
- Mild transaminase elevations and hyperbilirubinemia can occur in some patients.
- Mild-to-moderate headache is among the most commonly reported adverse effects.

Streptomycin

Mechanism of Action

- A nitrosourea derived from *Streptomyces achromogenes.*
- It is a glucosamine-1-methyl-nitrosurea that methylates DNA and mediates toxicity through induction of mismatch repair.

Pharmacokinetics

- Administered IV.
- It is rapidly metabolized with a half-life of 40 hours.

Uses

- Used in the initial treatment of Hodgkin's disease and sometimes for non-Hodgkin's lymphoma.

Side Effects

- Nausea and vomiting are severe and can be limiting toxic effects.
- Nephrotoxicity is considered the principal dose-limiting effect.
- Aggravation of duodenal ulcers.
- Mild myelosuppression.
- Some increase in hepatic enzymes.

Mitomycin C

Mechanism of Action

- An antibiotic isolated from *Streptococcus caespitosus.*
- Has been replaced by less toxic and more effective drugs but is known to be curative for anal cancer.
- Functions as a bifunctional and trifunctional alkylating agent after reduction of the quinone and loss of the methoxy group.
- Mitomycin C inhibits DNA synthesis and cross-links DNA at the N6 position of adenine and the O6 and N7 positions of guanine.

Pharmacokinetics

- Administered IV.
- The drug has a half-life of 25 to 90 minutes.
- The drug is widely distributed throughout the body but does not cross the blood–brain barrier.

Uses

- Used in combination with 5-fluorouracil and cisplatin for anal cancer.
- Used in the management of malignant and nonmalignant ophthalmic pathologies.

Side Effects

- Myelosuppression is the major toxic side effect and includes leukopenia and thrombocytopenia.
- Nausea, vomiting, diarrhea, stomatitis, and fever are also observed.
- Hemolytic uremic syndrome is considered the most dangerous toxic side effect.
- Doses > 50 mg/m^2 can result in hemolysis, neurological abnormalities, interstitial pneumonia, and glomerular damage leading to renal failure.

34.4.2 Antimetabolites

Mechanism of Action

These drugs include purine, pyrimidine, and folate analogues that act primarily by inhibiting DNA synthesis. They inhibit cells in the S phase (except fluorouracil, which has no clear-cut phase specificity) and may be incorporated into DNA and RNA. These drugs are converted by the cells to lethal metabolites (▶ Fig. 34.4).

Methotrexate

Methotrexate is also discussed in Chapters 27 and 33.

Mechanism of Action

Methotrexate is a folic acid analogue that competitively inhibits dihydrofolate reductase (DHFR), the enzyme that normally converts folate to tetrahydrofolate, which is needed for purine and thymidine synthesis. This results in reduced DNA, RNA, and protein synthesis (▶ Fig. 34.4).

Notes

Bone Marrow Function

There are two types of bone marrow: red and yellow. Red bone marrow contains myeloid tissue and produces red blood cells, most white blood cells, and platelets. Yellow bone marrow is largely made up of fat cells. At birth, all bone marrow is red, but in adults, it has been reduced by approximately half and is generally found in the fat bones, such as the hip, skull, vertebrae, and sternum, along with the cancellous ends of the long bones.

Pharmacokinetics

- Administered orally, IV, or intrathecally.
- It is poorly transported across the blood–brain barrier unless given in high concentrations or administered intrathecally.
- Fifty percent is bound to plasma proteins (displaced by salicylates, sulfonamides, etc.).
- Excreted unchanged in urine (so it should be used with caution in patients with renal damage).

Uses

- Drug of choice for gestational choriocarcinoma.
- Acute lymphocytic leukemia (in children).
- Burkitt lymphoma.
- Breast cancer.
- Psoriasis.
- Head and neck cancer.
- Rheumatoid arthritis.
- Inflammatory bowel disease.

Note: It is sometimes used in very high doses with leucovorin (5-formyltetrahydrofolate), an active form of folate, to prevent damage to normal cells (rescue therapy).

Side Effects

- Bone marrow depression (dose-limiting toxicity).
- Oral and GI ulceration.
- Hepatic damage.
- Renal damage (due to precipitation of crystallized metabolites in the kidney).

Pemetrexed

Mechanism of Action

- A pyrrolopyrimidine antifolate analogue that is a cell cycle-specific antitumor agent.
- Similar to methotrexate, it is transported into the cell through a reduced folate carrier.
- Activation requires folylpolyglutamyl synthase (FPGS) for polyglutamination.
- Targets DHFR but its main mechanism of action is thymidylate synthase inhibition.

Pharmacokinetics

- Administered IV as a single-agent in various doses infused over a 10-minute period.
- Pemetrexed is not metabolized appreciably and 70 to 80% of the dose is recovered unchanged in the urine after the first 24 hours following infusion.
- Plasma clearance decreases as renal function decreases.

Uses

- Approved for use in combination with cisplatin in mesothelioma treatment.
- Used as a second-line treatment for non-small cell lung cancer (NSCLC).

Side Effects

- The major side effects are myelosuppression skin rash, mucositis, diarrhea, fatigue, and hand-foot syndrome.
- Supplementation with folic acid and vitamin B_{12} is used to reduce toxicities associated with pemetrexed use.
- Dexamethasone treatment has been demonstrated to reduce hand-foot syndrome.

Pralatrexate

Mechanism of Action

- A 10-deaza-aminopterin antifolate analogue.
- Similar to methotrexate it requires reduced folate carrier and is activated by FPGS to form polyglutamated forms.
- Inhibits DHFR, an enzyme mediating de novo purine nucleotide synthesis, and thymidine synthase.

Pharmacokinetics

- Administered IV as a single agent.
- No significant metabolism by the phase I hepatic CYP450 enzymes or phase II hepatic glucuronidases.
- Excretion occurs through both the kidneys and liver.
- In patients with normal renal function, approximately 34% of pralatrexate is excreted unchanged into urine following a single dose; dose modification is required in renal dysfunction.

Uses

Approved for treatment of relapsed or refractory T-cell lymphoma.

Side Effects

- Main adverse effects include myelosuppression, skin rash, mucositis, diarrhea, and fatigue.
- Toxicities can be reduced with folic acid and vitamin B^{12} supplementation.

6-Mercaptopurine

Mechanism of Action

Mercaptopurine is a purine analogue that causes pseudofeedback inhibition of the first step in purine biosynthesis and inhibition of purine interconversions. This leads to the insertion of the incorrect bases into DNA (▶ Fig. 34.4).

Pharmacokinetics

- Administered orally.
- 6-Mercaptoprine is inactive in its parent form.
- It is converted to 6-thioinosinic acid by the action of hypoxanthine guanine phosphoribosyl transferase (HGPRT).

Mechanism of Action

- 6-Thioinosinic acid inhibits several enzymes of de novo purine nucleotide synthesis.

- The monophosphate form of 6-thioinosinic acid is metabolized to the triphosphate form, which is incorporated into RNA and DNA.
- High levels of thioguanylic acid and 6-methyl mercaptopurine ribotide also form 6-mercaptopurine and also contribute to its cytotoxic action.
- 6-Mercaptopurine is converted to the inactive metabolite 6-thiouric acid by xanthine oxidase.
- Allopurinol, a xanthine oxidase inhibitor, is used with acute leukemias to prevent hyperuricemia.
- Use of both 6-mercaptopurine and allopurinol requires that levels of 6-mercaptopurine be reduced to avoid drug toxicity.

Uses

Childhood acute lymphoid leukemia.

Side Effects

Bone marrow depression (major toxicity) and liver damage.

Thioguanine

Thioguanine has similar pharmacological properties to mercaptopurine except that allopurinol does not interfere with its inactivation.

Thiopurines are also metabolized by the enzyme thiopurine methyl transferase (TPMT).

Patients who have a genetic syndrome involving partial or complete deficiency of this enzyme develop severe toxicities in the form of myelosuppression and GI toxicity with mucositis and diarrhea.

Fluorouracil

Mechanism of Action

Fluorouracil is a pyrimidine analogue that is converted to 5-fluodeoxyuridine monophosphate, causing inhibition of thymidylate synthesis. DNA synthesis is therefore reduced due to a lack of thymidine. It also forms 5-fluodeoxyuridine triphosphate, which is incorporated into RNA and blocks translation. There is no cell cycle phase specificity.

- Leucovorin is also used in combination with fluorouracil. While it protects normal cells from damage by methotrexate, leucovorin potentiates the effectiveness of fluorouracil, presumably by providing active folate as a cofactor for the interaction of fluorouracil with thymidylate synthase.

Pharmacokinetics

- Administered IV.
- Able to enter the cerebrospinal fluid (CSF).
- Rapidly metabolized in the liver by dihydropyrimidine dehydrogenase (DPD); partial or complete deficiency of DPD results in severe 5-FU toxicity in the form of myelosuppression, diarrhea, nausea, and vomiting as well as neurotoxicity.

Uses

For treatment of breast, pancreatic, colorectal, and gastric cancer.

Side Effects

- Oral and GI ulcers.
- Bone marrow depression (dose-limiting toxicity).
- Neurologic defects (cerebellar).
- Hyperpigmentation.
- Alopecia.

Floxuridine

Mechanism of Action

- A pyrimidine analogue that acts as an inhibitor of S-phase cell division.
- Acts as a pyrimidine-like molecule that prevents normal pyrimidine from being incorporated into DNA during the S-phase of cell division.
- Floxuridine is catabolized to 5-fluorouracil following administration.
- The monophosphate of the drug (FUDR-MP) inhibits thymidylate synthetase and inhibits methylation of deoxyuridylic acid to thymidylic acid. This causes a thymineless death (see 5-fluorouracil discussion).

Pharmacokinetics

- Floxuridine is converted to 5-fluorouracil following IV administration.
- 5-fluorouracil requires conversion to the nucleotide for cytotoxic activity (see discussion on 5-fluorouracil).

Uses

- Used for palliative management of colorectal carcinoma metastatic to the liver that is recalcitrant to other treatments.
- Has been used for carcinoma of the breast, ovary, cervix, urinary bladder, kidney, and prostate that has not responded to other antimetabolites.

Side Effects

See discussion on 5-fluorouracil.

Capecitabine

Mechanism of Action

Capecitabine is a prodrug for fluorouracil and therefore acts similarly.

Uses

Advanced colon and breast cancer, either as a single agent or in combination with other agents.

Fludarabine and Cladribine

Mechanism of Action

These agents are purine analogue antagonists that cause a reduction in DNA synthesis.

Fludarabine (phosphate):
- Rapidly dephosphorylated to 2-fluoroarabinofuranosyladenosine and then phosphorylated by deoxycytidine kinase to the triphosphate.
- The triphosphate metabolite interferes with DNA synthesis and DNA repair through inhibition of DNA polymerase. The triphosphate can be incorporated directly into DNA—inhibits DNA synthesis and function.
- The diphosphate inhibits ribonucleotide reductase (RNR) and leads to inhibition of essential deoxyribonucleotide triphosphates.

Cladribine (2-chlorodeoxyadenosine):
- High specificity for lymphoid cells.
- Phosphorylated by deoxycytidine kinase to the monophosphate and eventually converted to the triphosphate form.
- The triphosphate form is incorporated into DNA.
- The triphosphate form also interferes with DNA synthesis and DNA repair by inhibiting DNA synthesis and DNA repair by inhibiting DNA polymerases.

Uses

- Chronic lymphocytic leukemia and some non-Hodgkin's lymphomas (fludarabine).
- Hairy cell leukemia (cladribine).

Nelarabine

Mechanism of Action

- Nelarabine is a prodrug of the deoxyguanosine analogue of arabinofuranosyl guanine (Ara-G).
- Accumulation of ara-GTP in leukemic blasts leads to accumulation of this analogue into DNA, which inhibits DNA synthesis and causes cell death.
- Adenosine deaminase converts nelarabine to ara-G, which is then monophosphorylated by deoxyguanosine kinase and deoxycytidine kinase. This metabolite is subsequently converted to the active 5′–triphosphate, or ara-GTP.

Pharmacokinetics

- Administered by IV.
- Elimination occurs through the kidneys.

Uses

- Nelarabine is used for treatment of T-cell acute lymphoblastic leukemia (ALL), T-cell lymphoma, and T-cell lymphoblastic lymphoma.

Side Effects

- Bone marrow suppression that includes anemia, leucopenia, thrombocytopenia, and neutropenia.
- Neurologic effects include asthenia, altered mental states, convulsions, and peripheral neuropathy.
- Demyelinating disease has been reported in cancer patients treated with nelarabine.

Clofarabine

Mechanism of Action

- A purine nucleoside antimetabolite.
- Inhibits DNA synthesis by inhibiting RNR and reducing cellular deoxynucleotide triphosphate pools.

Pharmacokinetics

- Clofarabine is phosphorylated to the cytotoxic form (clofarabine triphosphate) through deoxycytidine kinase.
- The majority of clofarabine triphosphate is excreted unchanged in the urine.
- Must be used with extreme caution in patients with renal dysfunction.

Uses

- Effective in the treatment of acute lymphocytic leukemia.
- Used sometimes in combination with cytarabine.

Cytarabine and Gemcitabine

Mechanism of Action

Cytarabine (S-phase specific for the cell cycle) and gemcitabine are metabolized to cytidine analogues that block DNA synthesis by inhibiting DNA polymerases α and β by becoming incorporated into DNA when phosphorylated to the triphosphates, preventing further elongation of the DNA.

Pharmacokinetics

- Administered IV.
- Rapidly deaminated in the liver, plasma, and other tissues.

Uses

- Acute lymphoid leukemia, acute myeloid leukemia, chronic myeloid leukemia, and meningeal leukemia (cytarabine).
- Advanced pancreatic, breast, and ovarian cancer, and NSCLC (gemcitabine).

Side Effects

- Bone marrow depression (major toxicity).
- Oral ulceration.
- Liver dysfunction.

Azacytidine

Mechanism of Action

- An analogue of the nucleoside cytidine that differs from the parent agent because of nitrogen at the 5′ position of the heterocyclic ring.
- Transportation across the cell membrane by facilitated nucleoside diffusion where it is converted to its monophosphate form, 5′-aza-CMP.
- 5′-aza-CMP is converted to its lethal derivative, 5′-aza-CTP, which is incorporated into RNA and, to a limited extent, DNA.
- Lethal action of 5′-azacytidine is mediated through reduced protein synthesis and disruption of RNA processing.

Pharmacokinetics

- Administered either IV or subcutaneously.
- The drug is extensively deaminated in the plasma and liver.
- The $t_{1/2}$ of the parent drug is 4 hours. It is rapidly converted to various other derivatives.
- Penetrance into the CNS is minimal.

Uses

- Primarily used to treat refractory acute myeloid leukemia.
- Produces clinical responses in some patients with myelodysplastic syndrome.

Side Effects

- The major toxicity is leukopenia.
- Nausea and vomiting.
- GI toxicity has been noted.
- In patients with preexisting hepatic disease, hepatotoxicity can occur.

34.4.3 Antibiotics

Antibiotic treatment of infections is discussed in Chapter 29. The agents discussed in this section are used to treat cancer. They act by binding to DNA (noncovalently by intercalation) and altering its function. They are cycle nonspecific (▶ Fig. 34.4).

Clinical Correlation

Tumor Grading

Grade refers to a microscopic pathologic determination of tumor aggressiveness based on the degree of differentiation of the neoplastic cells and the number of mitoses. Most tumors are graded from 1 (low grade, well differentiated) through 3 (high grade, undifferentiated). Some malignant neoplasms progress to a higher grade over time as less differentiated clones of cells become dominant. Criteria for grading include mitotic rate, nuclear pleomorphism, and architectural features (e.g., preservation of gland formation).

Clinical Correlation

Tumor Staging

Stage refers to a clinical and pathologic determination of tumor extent based on the size of the neoplasm, the presence or absence of regional lymph node metastases, and the presence or absence of distant metastases. This is the basis of the tumor size, node involvement, metastasis (TNM) staging system. Tumors are staged numerically from 0 through IV as follows:
- 0: in situ.
- I: small, organ confined.
- II: large or regional node metastases.
- III: invasion of adjacent organs.
- IV: distant metastases.

In general, stage has greater prognostic value than grade.

Dactinomycin (Actinomycin D)

Mechanism of Action

Dactinomycin intercalates between G-C pairs in double-stranded DNA and inhibits DNA-directed RNA synthesis. It is equally cytotoxic to proliferating and stationary cells.

Pharmacokinetics

- Administered IV (can cause local inflammation and phlebitis).

Side Effects

Side effects include bone marrow depression (toxicity is dose-limiting), oral and GI ulceration, and alopecia.

Uses

- Treatment of rhabdomyosarcoma and Wilms tumor in children.
- Used as a single agent or in combination with vincristine and cyclophosphamide.

Doxorubicin

Mechanism of action

- Inhibition of DNA and RNA synthesis due to intercalation.
- DNA fragmentation from reactive oxygen species.
- Inhibition of DNA topoisomerase II.
- Interaction with cell membranes, causing a broad spectrum of antitumor activity.

Pharmacokinetics

- Administered IV (extravasation leads to severe local reaction and necrosis).
- Extensively metabolized in the liver and excreted into the bile (decreased dose in the presence of hepatic dysfunction).
- Drug and metabolites color urine red.

Uses

Doxorubicin has a broad spectrum of activity and is used in the following cancers:
- Acute lymphoid leukemia, chronic lymphoid leukemia, and acute myeloid leukemia.
- Breast, stomach, bone, thyroid, kidney, liver, and pancreatic cancers.

Side Effects

- Bone marrow depression is their major toxicity (except for bleomycin). This is dose limiting.
- Cardiotoxicity (refractory congestive heart failure). This is due to avid uptake by and oxidative damage to heart muscle. The damage caused is potentially irreversible and can be delayed by many months. It is related to the total dose administered.
- Alopecia, stomatitis (inflammation of the mucosa of the mouth), fever, and chills.

IX

Daunorubicin

Daunorubicin is similar to doxorubicin but has a narrower spectrum of activity; used primarily for acute leukemias.

Idarubicin

Idarubicin is an analogue of daunorubicin used in combination with therapy for acute lymphoid leukemia.

Epirubicin

An anthracycline used for adjunctive therapy for breast cancer treatment. Cardiotoxicity can be increased significantly with this drug and the toxicity profile is the same as that of doxorubicin.

Mitoxantrone

Mechanism of Action

- Contains an azauridine group and a quinone group as well as a mitosane ring; each of these components participate in alkylation reaction with DNA.
- Binds to DNA to produce strand breakage and inhibits both DNA and RNA synthesis.

Pharmacokinetics

- Administered IV.
- Excretion occurs mainly through the kidney.

Uses

- Treatment of advanced, hormone-refractory prostate cancer and low-grade Hodgkin's lymphoma.
- Used in the treatment of breast cancer and in pediatric and adult acute myeloid leukemias.

Side Effects

- Myelosuppression with neutropenia is a dose-limiting toxicity.
- Cardiotoxicity is a dose-limiting effect and is similar to that observed with doxorubicin.

Hydroxyurea

Mechanism of Action

- Inhibits RNR, an enzyme that catalyzes the rate-limiting step in de novo biosynthesis of purine and pyrimidine deoxyribonucleotides.
- An antimetabolite that is an S phase-specific agent.
- Cells treated with hydroxyurea have depleted pools of deoxyribonucleotide triphosphate and DNS synthesis is inhibited.

Pharmacokinetics

- Administered orally.
- Readily absorbed from the GI tract.
- Penetrates CSF.
- Excretion occurs through the kidneys.

Uses

- Represents a mainstay therapy along with interferon-alpha for chronic or accelerated phase chronic myeloid leukemia.
- Used to treat myeloproliferative disorders that include myeloid metaplasia and myelofibrosis, polycythemia vera, and essential thrombocytosis.
- Hydroxyurea reduces the incidence of painful crises in individuals with sickle cell anemia.

Side Effects

- Common adverse effects include myelosuppression.
- GI symptoms include nausea and vomiting.
- Dermatologic toxicity includes rashes, skin ulcerations, and facial erythema.

Bleomycin

Mechanism of Action

Bleomycin is a mixture of complex glycopeptides that causes strand scission of DNA by producing reactive oxygen species. It is unusual in that it produces very little bone marrow depression.

Pharmacokinetics

- Administered IV.
- Enzymatically inactivated in several tissues (toxicity occurs in tissues with low inactivating activity, i.e., lungs and skin).
- Fifty percent is excreted unchanged in the urine.

Uses

- Hodgkin's and non-Hodgkin's lymphomas.
- Testicular cancer.
- Squamous cell carcinomas of the head, neck, nasopharynx, penis, vulva, and cervix.

Side Effects

- Pulmonary toxicity (pneumonitis and fibrosis) is dose limiting.
- The more common toxic effects involve the skin and mucous membranes.
- Alopecia and stomatitis.

34.4.4 Topoisomerase Inhibitors

Etoposide and Teniposide

Mechanism of Action

These agents inhibit topoisomerase II, which acts on single-stranded DNA to cause strand breakage (▶ Fig. 34.4). The drugs are most active in the late S and early G2 phases of the cell cycle.

Pharmacokinetics

- Available for both oral and IV administration.
- Elimination is through the kidneys and dose reduction is required with compromised renal function.

Uses

- Small cell lung cancer, testicular carcinoma, acute nonlymphocytic leukemia, and malignant lymphoma (etoposide).
- First-line therapy for neuroblastoma and retinoblastoma in combination with other agents.
- Refractory leukemias (teniposide).

Side Effects

- Nausea and vomiting (short term).
- Alopecia and myelosuppression (longer term).

Irinotecan and Topotecan

Mechanism of Action

Irinotecan and topotecan inhibit topoisomerase I, which acts on double-stranded DNA to induce strand breakage.

Pharmacokinetics

Irinotecan is a prodrug that is converted to the SN-38 metabolite. SN-38 is 1000-fold more potent as a topoisomerase I inhibitor than the parent compound.

Pharmacogenetic Note: SN-38 is eliminated through glucuronidation. Allelic variation of UGT1A1 alleles coding for glucuronyltransferase has been associated with reduced glucuronidation of SN-38 and severe drug toxicity.

Uses

- Metastatic colorectal cancer (irinotecan).
- Ovarian and small cell lung cancers (topotecan).

Side Effects

Same as for etoposide and teniposide.

34.4.5 Antimitotic Agents

Mechanism of Action

Antimitotic agents bind to tubulin, inhibiting mitotic spindles and arresting cell development in the M phase of the cell cycle.

The vinca alkaloids vincristine and vinblastine are structurally similar but have different activities and toxicities and show no cross-resistance.

Pharmacokinetics

- Administered IV (extravasation and subsequent local reactions may occur).
- Excreted into bile (use with caution in patients with obstructive jaundice).

Vincristine

Uses

- Acute leukemia.
- Hodgkin's disease.
- Nephroblastoma (Wilms tumor).
- Rhabdomyosarcoma.

Topoisomerase

DNA is arranged as in a double helix formation, which is then supercoiled or knotted in chromosomes. This is a very stable and efficient way to store our genetic information. To avoid having to uncoil and unwind entire lengths of DNA, topoisomerase enzymes bind to DNA and cut the phosphate backbone, thus allowing specific sections to uncoil and unwind for transcription and replication to occur. They reconnect the DNA strands when the process is finished.

Clinical Correlation

Nephroblastoma (Wilms Tumor)

Nephroblastoma (Wilms tumor) is a malignant renal tumor composed of mixed embryonal cell elements. Increased mature elements and decreased anaplastic cells are indicative of the best prognosis. Signs and symptoms include painless hematuria, abdominal pain, an enlarged abdomen, and a palpable abdominal mass. Computed tomography scans or magnetic resonance imaging of the abdomen is diagnostic for a mass. Hematuria is seen with urinalysis. Treatment includes surgery (nephrectomy), radiation therapy, and chemotherapy. The prognosis for 2-year survival (with favorable histology) is 95% for stage I, II, and III tumors and 50% for stage IV tumors.

IX

Side Effects

- Neurologic toxicities are dose-limiting. Suppression of the Achilles tendon reflex and paresthesias appear first, followed by other peripheral neuropathies, neuritic pain, constipation, and disorders of cranial nerve function.
- Alopecia.
- Mild bone marrow depression (vincristine is considered to be marrow-sparing compared with other agents).

Vinblastine

Uses

Some lymphomas and solid tumors.

Side Effects

- Bone marrow depression (dose limiting).
- Neuropathy is less frequent and less serious than with vincristine.
- Alopecia, stomatitis, and peripheral neuropathy.

Vinorelbine

Vinorelbine is a semisynthetic derivative of vinblastine.

Pharmacokinetics

Given orally.

Uses

For treatment of NSCLC.

Side Effects

They are similar to vinblastine.

34.4.6 Taxanes

Paclitaxel and Docetaxel

Mechanism of Action

These drugs promote the assembly of microtubules from tubulin dimers and stabilize microtubules by preventing depolymerization. This prevents reorganization of the microtubule network for mitosis.

Uses

- Breast cancer.
- Lung cancer.
- Ovarian cancer.

Side Effects

- Bone marrow suppression.
- Moderate nausea and vomiting.
- Alopecia.
- Sensory neuropathy.
- Hypersensitivity to the drug.

34.4.7 Monoclonal Antibodies

Mechanism of Action

Monoclonal antibodies bind specifically to proteins on cancer cells, resulting in inhibition of growth and antibody-dependent cellular cytotoxicity. Labeling the antibodies with radioactive isotopes allows the bound antibody to specifically deliver the radioactivity to target cells.

Pharmacokinetics

These agents must be given IV.

> **Notes**
>
> **Achilles Tendon Reflex**
>
> The Achilles tendon reflex is plantar (downward) flexion extension of the foot resulting from contraction of the calf muscles following a sharp blow to the Achilles tendon. This reflex is suppressed by vincristine.

Rituximab

Mechanism of Action

Rituximab binds to CD20, which is found on pre-B and mature B lymphocytes. It is also expressed on > 90% of B cell non-Hodgkin's lymphomas, but not expressed on hematopoietic stem cells, pro-B cells, normal plasma cells, or other normal tissues.

Pharmacokinetics

Given by slow IV infusion to prevent adverse reactions.

Uses

- B cell lymphoma.
- Chronic lymphoblastic leukemia.

Side Effects

- Changes in blood pressure.
- GI upset: nausea and vomiting.
- Neurologic effects including weakness, dizziness, headache, and sensory neuropathy.
- Fever and shivering.

Tositumomab and Iodine 131 Tositumomab

Mechanism of Action

Tositumomab and iodine 131 tositumomab bind to CD20.

Uses

B-cell lymphoma.

Side Effects

Diarrhea.

Indium 111 Ibritumomab and Yttrium 90 Ibritumomab Tiuxetan

Mechanism of Action

Composed of monoclonal antibody ibritumomab linked to tiuxetan:
- Tiuxetan is a linker for the radioisotopes Indium-111 or Yttrium-90.
- Ibritumomab binds to the CD20 antigen, which is found on the surface of malignant B lymphocytes in patients who have B cell non-Hodgkin's lymphoma.
- Beta emissions from the attached isotope induce cell death.
- The antibody alone can induce cell-mediated cytotoxicity, complement-dependent cytotoxicity, and apoptosis.

Uses

- Treatment of patients with relapsed or refractory grade, follicular or transformed B cell Hodgkin's lymphoma.
- Included treatment of patients with Rituximab-refractory follicular B cell Hodgkin's lymphoma.

Side Effects

- Severe allergic reactions have been observed.
- Severe hematological reactions, including anemia, leukopenia, thrombocytopenia, and bone marrow suppression.

- Nausea and vomiting.
- Weakness, dizziness, headache, and sensory neuropathy.
- Fever and shivering.

Trastuzumab

Mechanism of Action

Trastuzumab binds to subdomain IV of the HER2/neu (ErbB-2) protein, which is overexpressed in 25 to 30% of primary breast cancers.

Binding of trastuzumab disrupts ligand-mediated HER2/neu dimerization with other members of the HER family (▶ Fig. 34.5).

Uses

- Breast cancer.

Side Effects

- Edema.
- Rash.
- Diarrhea, nausea, and vomiting.
- Weakness, dizziness, headache, and backache or muscle pain.
- Fever and shivering.
- Cough, dyspnea, rhinitis, and pharyngitis.

Trastuzumab Emtansine (Ado-trastuzumab Emtansine)

Mechanism of Action

- A conjugate of trastuzumab linked to the cytotoxic emtansine (DM1).
- Trastuzumab binds to the HER2/neu receptor and prevents dimerization of the receptor with other members of the HER family. Emtansine is released into the tumor cells where it binds to the ends of microtubules and thereby inhibits cell division.

Uses

Treatment of HER2/neu-positive breast cancer in patients resistant to trastuzumab alone.

Side Effects

Similar to trastuzumab.

Pertuzumab

Mechanism of Action

A humanized monoclonal antibody that binds to the extracellular domain 2 of HER2/neu. It inhibits ligand-mediated HER2 and HER3 dimerizations. Activation of phosphatidylinositol 3-kinase/Akt is attenuated.

Uses

- Used in conjunction with trastuzumab to treat HER2-positive breast cancer.
- Trastuzumab and pertuzumab act in a complementary fashion and provide a more complete blockage of HER2-mediated signal transduction.

Side Effects

Similar to those for trastuzumab.

Cetuximab

Mechanism of Action

Cetuximab binds to epidermal growth factor receptor (EGFR), which has been detected in many human cancers, including those of the colon and rectum.

Uses

- Colorectal cancer.
- Head and neck cancers.

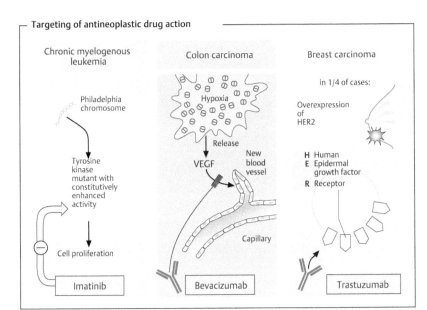

Fig. 34.5 Targeting of the chemotherapeutic drugs imatinib, bevacizumab, and trastuzumab. Targeted treatment of cancer can be utilized when cancer cells display metabolic properties that are different from those of healthy cells. **Imatinib:** Patients with chronic myelogenous leukemia almost always possess the Philadelphia chromosome. This recombinant gene encodes a tyrosine kinase mutant with unregulated, enhanced activity, causing cell proliferation. Imatinib specifically inhibits this mutant tyrosine kinase, thus inhibiting cell proliferation. **Bevacizumab:** Binds to vascular endothelial growth factor (VEGF). This prevents the proliferation of endothelial cells and formation of new blood vessels, thus starving tumors of their blood supply from lung. This drug may also be used in breast, lung, and pancreatic cancers. **Trastuzumab:** Trastuzumab binds to subdomain IV of the HER2 protein, which is overexpressed in 25% to 30% of primary breast cancers.

IX

Side Effects

- Rash.
- Hypomagnesemia.
- Constipation, diarrhea, nausea, and vomiting.
- Fatigue, pain, headache, and insomnia.
- Fever and shivering.
- Cough, dyspnea, and pharyngitis.

Panitumumab

Mechanism of Action

- A humanized antibody that binds to the extracellular domain of the EGFR.
- Mechanism of action is similar to that for cetuximab except that panitumumab does not mediate antibody-dependent cell-mediated cytotoxicity.

Uses

Improves progression-free survival in patients with metastatic colorectal carcinoma.

Side Effects

Similar to those for cetuximab.

Bevacizumab

Mechanism of Action

Bevacizumab binds to vascular endothelial growth factor (VEGF) and prevents the proliferation of endothelial cells and formation of new blood vessels, thus starving tumors of their blood supply.

Uses

- Colorectal cancer.
- Lung cancer.
- Breast cancer.
- Pancreatic cancer.

Side Effects

- Hypertension.
- Alopecia.
- Hypokalemia.
- Constipation, diarrhea, nausea, anorexia, and stomatitis.
- Fatigue, pain, headache, and sensory neuropathy.
- Epistaxis.
- Hemorrhage.

Atezolizumab

Mechanism of Action

- A fully humanized monoclonal antibody against the protein programmed cell death-ligand l (PD-L1), a negative regulator of the immune system.
- PD-L1 is overexpressed in many human cancer cell types and limits expansion and survival of CD8+ T cells.
- Atezolizumab inhibits activation of PD-1 and enhances T-cell-mediated immune response to neoplasms.

Uses

- Metastatic bladder cancer previously treated with platinum-based chemotherapy.
- Metastatic NSCLC previously treated with platinum-based chemotherapy.

Side Effects

- Fatigue, decreased appetite, nausea, and infections.

Daratumumab

Mechanism of Action

- A human IgG1 monoclonal antibody directed against the CD38 molecule.
- Binding of daratumumab to CD38 on multiple myeloma cells induces rapid tumor cell death through programmed cell death as well as other immune-mediated mechanisms such as complement-dependent cytotoxicity and antibody-dependent cellular toxicity.

Uses

- Approved in combination with lanalidomide and dexamethasone as well as bortezomib and dexamethasone for the treatment of multiple myeloma in patients who have received at least one prior therapy for treatment of multiple myeloma.

Side Effects

- Infusion reactions, fever, chills, back pain, and upper respiratory infection.

Dinutuximab

Mechanism of Action

- A monoclonal antibody targeting glycolipid GD-2, which is expressed on neuroblastoma cells and on normal cells of ectodermal origin.
- Dinutuximab binds to the ganglioside GD-2 and induces antibody-dependent cell-mediated cytotoxicity and complement-dependent cytotoxicity.

Uses

- Approved for high-risk neuroblastoma in pediatric patients who have responded to other first-line treatment.
- Used in combination with the granulocyte-macrophage colony stimulating factor, interleukin-2, and 13-cis-retinoic acid.

Side Effects

- Causes severe pain because of nerve cell irritation.
- Can cause nerve damage and severe infusion reactions.

Elotuzumab

Mechanism of Action

- A humanized IgG1 monoclonal immunostimulatory antibody that targets the Signaling Lymphocytic Activation Molecule Family member 7 (SLAMF7).

- SLAMF7 is expressed on myeloma and natural killer cells. It is not expressed on normal tissue and this enables selective killing of myeloma cells.
- Elotuzumab directly activates natural killer cells through the SLAMF7 pathway and Fc receptors.
- Antibody targeting of SLAMF7 on myeloma cells mediates the interaction with natural killer cell and facilitated myeloma cell death via antibody-dependent cellular cytotoxicity.

Uses

- Approved for use in combination with lenalidomide and dexamethasone for treatment of multiple myeloma in patients who have received one to three prior therapies.

Side Effects

- Fatigue, diarrhea, fever, constipation, peripheral neuropathy, and upper respiratory tract infection.

Ipilimumab

Mechanism of Action

- A monoclonal antibody that targets CTLA-4, a protein receptor that downregulates the immune system.
- Ipilimumab binds to CTLA-4 and suppresses an inhibitory mechanism that allows cytotoxic T lymphocytes to recognize and destroy cancer cells.

Uses

- Approved for treatment of patients with late-stage melanoma that has spread or cannot be resected through surgery.

Side Effects

- Associated with severe immunological effects resulting from T-cell activation and proliferation.
- Additional adverse effects are associated with GI tract disturbances that include stomach pain and either constipation or diarrhea.

Nivolumab

Mechanism of Action

- A fully human immunoglobulin IgG4 monoclonal antibody that interacts with the negative immunoregulatory human cell surface receptor programmed death-1 (PD-1) with immune checkpoint inhibitory and antineoplastic activities.
- Nivolumab binds to PD-1 and prevents its activation by its ligands PD-L1 and PD-L2.
- The antibody-mediated activation of T-cells and cell-mediated immune responses against tumor cells.

Uses

- Used as a first-line treatment for inoperable or metastatic melanoma in combination with ipilimumab if there is no BRAF mutation.
- Can be used as a second-line treatment for metastatic melanoma after ipilimumab treatment if there is a BRAF mutation.

- Hodgkin's disease after other therapies have failed.
- Liver cancer in patients previously treated with sorafenib.
- It is also used to treat metastatic squamous non-small cell lung, head and neck, colorectal, or urothelial cancer after platinum-based drugs.
- Renal cell carcinoma.

Side Effects

- Risk of severe immune-mediated inflammation of the lungs, colon, liver, and kidneys, and possibly immune-mediated hypo- and hyperthyroidism.

Obinutuzumab

Mechanism of Action

- A humanized anti-CD20 monoclonal antibody directed against CD20 on the surface of normal and cancerous B cells.
- Obinutuzumab binding to CD20 on B cells results in destruction of these cells by engaging the adaptive immune system and activating apoptosis pathways.

Uses

- Obinutuzumab is used as a first-line treatment for chronic lymphocytic leukemia in combination with chlorambucil.
- It is also used in combination with bendamustine for treatment of patients with follicular lymphoma.

Side Effects

- Infusion reactions, neutropenia, thrombocytopenia, and fever have been reported.
- Obinutuzumab has black box warnings that include hepatitis B reactivation and progressive multifocal leukoencephalopathy.

Ofatumumab

Mechanism of Action

- A fully human monoclonal antibody directed against the CD20 protein.
- Inhibits early-state B lymphocyte activation.
- It has an epitope distinct from that of rituximab and compared to rituximab, ofatumumab has greater affinity for CD20.
- Binding to CD20 results in cytotoxicity in CD20 expressing cells through complement-dependent cytotoxicity and antibody-dependent cellular cytotoxicity.

Uses

Used in treating chronic lymphocytic leukemia.

Side Effects

- Lower and upper respiratory tract infections, including pneumonia.
- Hepatitis B infection or reactivation and possible development of progressive multifocal leukoencephalopathy.

IX

Olaratumab

Mechanism of Action

- A human immunoglobulin G class 1 (IgG1) antibody that binds to platelet-derived growth factor receptor alpha (PDGFR-α) and blocks its activity.
- Olaratumab binds to PDGFR-α and prevents the binding of PDGF-AA and -BB ligands to the receptor and blocks tyrosine kinase-mediated signaling.

Uses

Used in combination with doxorubicin for treatment of advanced soft-tissue sarcoma that is incurable with surgery or radiation therapy.

Side Effects

- Neutropenia with the combination therapy of olaratumab and doxorubicin is one of the most serious side effects.
- Other effects include lymphopenia diarrhea, nausea and vomiting, and mucositis.

Pembrolizumab

Mechanism of Action

- A humanized monoclonal antibody that inhibits interactions between PD-1 and its ligands, PD-L1 and PD-L2.
- It acts as a programmed death receptor-1 (PD-1) blocking antibody and functions to enhance activity of the immune system.

Uses

Used to treat inoperable or metastatic melanoma, metastatic non-small cell lung cancer and head and neck squamous cell carcinoma, and refractory classical Hodgkin lymphoma.

Side Effects

- Infusion-related reactions.
- Lung inflammation and inflammation of endocrine organs that causes pituitary gland inflammation and pancreatitis.

Ramucirumab

Mechanism of Action

- A monoclonal antibody that inhibits the activity of VEGF.
- Ramucirumab blocks VEGF activity and prevents the growth of new blood vessels essential for providing tumor's source of nutrients.

Uses

- Used for advanced gastric cancer or gastroesophageal junction adenocarcinoma as a single agent after prior fluoropyrimidine or platinum-containing chemotherapy.
- Metastatic colorectal or NSCLC in combination therapies.

Side Effects

- Increased risk of hemorrhage and GI bleeding.
- Infusion reaction during or after IV administration.

- High blood pressure.
- Slower wound healing.

34.4.8 Tyrosine Kinase Inhibitors

Tyrosine kinase inhibitors target receptor tyrosine kinases on the membranes of cancer cells, inhibiting their activity and thus decreasing cancer cell growth.

Imatinib

Mechanism of Action

Imatinib is a selective inhibitor of the tyrosine kinase activity of the bcr-abl protein, which is the product of the Philadelphia chromosome or 9:22 translocation. It is present in virtually all patients with chronic myelogenous leukemia and some patients with acute lymphobastic leukemia (ALL).

Pharmacokinetics

Absorbed well after oral administration.

Uses

- Chronic myelogenous leukemia with the bcr-abl protein.
- ALL.

Side Effects

Edema, nausea, and vomiting.

Dasatinib

Mechanism of Action

Dasatinib is a tyrosine kinase inhibitor active against bcr-abl and Src family kinases. Dasatinib is more potent than imatinib, and it inhibits mutated forms of bcr-abl that are resistant to imatinib.

Uses

ALL and chronic myelogenous leukemia that is resistant to imatinib.

Side Effects

Same as imatinib.

Nilotinib

Mechanism of Action

- A selective tyrosine kinase inhibitor active against bcr-abl kinase.
- Similar to imatinib in that it binds to and stabilizes the inactive conformation of the kinase domain of the abl signal transduction protein.

Pharmacokinetics

- Administered orally in capsular forms.
- It is rapidly absorbed and reaches its peak concentration in 3 hours.

- Metabolism occurs through oxidation and hydroxylation and through CYP3A4-mediated metabolism.

Uses

Activity against chronic myeloid leukemia resistant to imatinib resulting from bcr-abl mutations.

Side Effects

Similar to that caused by imatinib.

Gefitinib and Erlotinib

Mechanism of Action

Gefitinib and erlotinib act as selective EGFR tyrosine kinase inhibitors through competitive blockade of ATP binding to the receptor. They block EGFR-mediated signal transduction pathways involved in tumor growth.

Uses

- NSCLC in patients with advanced forms for whom both platinum and docetaxel-based chemotherapies have failed.
- Pancreatic cancer (erlotinib).

Side Effects

- Rash.
- Diarrhea, nausea, and vomiting.

Lapatinib

Mechanism of Action

- A small molecule inhibitor of ErB2 (HER2/neu) kinase activity.
- Blocks both ErbF1 and ErbB2 by binding to the ATP-binding pocket.
- Lapatanib is capable of inhibiting truncated forms of the HER-2 receptor lacking a trastuzumab-binding domain.

Pharmacokinetics

- Administered orally.
- Metabolism occurs through CYP3A4 to a number of inactive products and an oxidized intermediate that has activity against ErbB1.

Uses

- Lapatinib is effective against HER2-amplified, trastuzumab-refractory breast cancer.
- It is used in combination with the fluoropyrimidine analogue, capecitabine.
- It crosses the blood–brain barrier and has been demonstrated to decrease the incidence of brain metastases.

Side Effects

- Toxicities include mild diarrhea and increased gastroesophageal reflux.
- In contrast to trastuzumab, lapatinib does not produce cardiotoxicity.

Sorafenib

Mechanism of Action

Sorafenib is a multiple kinase inhibitor that blocks the receptor tyrosine kinases VEGFR and PDGFR and the Raf serine/threonine kinases along the RAF/MEK/ERK pathway.

Uses

- Liver and renal cell carcinoma.

Side Effects

- Hypertension.
- Alopecia, rash, and chemotherapy-induced acral erythema (hand-foot syndrome).
- Abdominal pain, diarrhea, nausea, and anorexia.
- Headache and fatigue.
- Hemorrhage and arterial thromboembolic events.

Sunitinib

Mechanism of Action

Sunitinib is a multitargeting tyrosine kinase inhibitor that decreases tumor cell proliferation and angiogenesis. It competitively inhibits binding of ATP to the tyrosine kinase domain of the VEGF receptor-2. It also inhibits other protein tyrosine kinases.

Uses

- Advanced stomach and metastatic renal cell cancer.

Side Effects

- Hypertension and heart failure.
- Abdominal pain, constipation, diarrhea, nausea, anorexia, and stomatitis.
- Anemia, leukopenia, lymphocytopenia, and hemorrhage.
- Yellow discoloration of skin, hand-foot syndrome, and dry skin.

Bortezomib

Mechanism of Action

Bortezomib is an inhibitor of the 26S proteasome, a protease important for intracellular degradation of proteins involved in cell cycle control and cellular apoptosis. Disruption of the degradation of these proteins results in disruption of cell proliferation and increases cell death.

Uses

- Patients with multiple myeloma who have not responded to prior therapies.

Side Effects

- Serious dose-limiting effects on cardiovascular and hematological systems, along with the common skin, GI, neurologic, and respiratory effects of anticancer agents.

IX

Thalidomide

Mechanism of Action

Produces antiangiogenic and immunomodulatory effects through a number of possible mechanisms:
- Inhibition of the antiapoptotic effect of Bcl-2.
- Inhibition of interleukin-6, and tumor necrosis factor-α (TNF-α) synthesis, release, and signaling.
- Immunomodulation through enhancement of natural killer and T cell-mediated cytotoxicity.

Pharmacokinetics

Given orally; absorption from the GI tract is slow and variable.

Uses

Treatment of multiple myeloma.

Side Effects

Enhances sedative effects of barbiturates and alcohol.

Asparaginase

Mechanism of Action

- Hydrolyzes circulating asparagine to aspartic acid and ammonia. Tumor cells in acute lymphocytic leukemia lack asparagine synthase and require exogenous asparagine. Depletion of asparagine kills ALL tumor cells by inhibiting protein synthesis, a consequence of insufficient asparagine.

Pharmacokinetics

- Administered by IV.

Uses

- Treatment of childhood ALL.

Side Effect

- Hypersensitivity reaction characterized by fever, chills, nausea, and skin rash.

34.4.9 Differentiating Agents

Tretinoin

Tretinoin is an all-trans retinoic acid, which is a derivative of vitamin A.

Mechanism of Action

Tretinoin induces terminal maturation of leukemic promyelocytes into polymorphonuclear monocytes in acute promyelocytic leukemia.

Uses

Acute promyelocytic leukemia.

Side Effects

- Edema, arrhythmia, and blood pressure changes.
- Headache, pain, fatigue, and dizziness.

- Rash and dry skin.
- Hypercholesterolemia and hypertriglyceridemia.
- Abdominal pain, constipation, diarrhea, nausea, and vomiting.
- Leukocytosis.
- Upper respiratory tract disorders, dyspnea, and pneumonia.

Arsenic Trioxide

Mechanism of Action

Arsenic trioxide causes differentiation and apoptosis in acute promyelocytic leukemia refractory to tretinoin.

Uses

Acute promyelocytic leukemia refractory to tretinoin.

Side Effects

- Chest pain, edema, and hypotension.
- Headache, pain, fatigue, dizziness, and insomnia.
- Rash and dry skin.
- Hypo- or hyperkalemia, hyperglycemia, and hypomagnesemia.
- Abdominal pain, constipation, diarrhea, nausea, vomiting, and anorexia.
- Leukocytosis, anemia, and thrombocytopenia.
- Upper respiratory tract disorders, cough, dyspnea, and epistaxis.

34.4.10 Hormones

Hormonal therapy is effective for some cancers (e.g., breast cancer). They may inhibit tumor growth directly or oppose the effects of endogenous hormones. Toxicities are due to hormonal effects rather than cytotoxic effects.

Corticosteroids

Corticosteroids are also discussed in Chapters 16, 26, 27, and 32.

Prednisone

Mechanism of Action

Corticosteroids are useful in cancer chemotherapy due to their lymphocytic and antimitotic actions.

Uses

- Lymphomatous cancers (in conjunction with other agents).
- Used in conjunction with radiotherapy to reduce edema.

34.4.11 Hormone Inhibitors

Antiestrogens

Testing for the presence of estrogen receptors and progesterone receptors in tumor specimens from biopsy or surgery is recommended for all patients with primary invasive breast cancer. Up to 60% of patients with metastatic breast cancer will respond to hormonal therapy if their tumors contain estrogen receptors; however, less than 10% of patients with metastatic tumors that are estrogen receptor–negative respond to hormonal therapy. Up to 80% of patients with metastatic progesterone receptor–positive tumors respond to hormonal manipulation. The presence or absence of these receptors does not correlate with the response to other chemotherapies. Thus, adjuvant hormonal therapy, in combination with surgery, radiation, and/or chemotherapy, is recommended for all women whose breast cancer expresses hormone receptors.

Tamoxifen

Mechanism of Action

Tamoxifen is a partial agonist at the estrogen receptor. Its primary effect is to block the cell-proliferative effects of estrogen, but it also may inhibit replication by additional mechanisms (see ▶ Fig. 17.3). Many proteins and transcription factors interact with the estrogen receptor, so there are many downstream effects that occur because of tamoxifen's acting at the estrogen receptor, resulting in inhibition of growth-stimulatory factors, as well as activation of growth-inhibitory effects, including transforming growth factor beta (TGF-β).

Pharmacokinetics

Given orally.

Uses

- Adjuvant hormonal therapy in premenopausal women with invasive breast cancer, with or without ovarian suppression or ablation therapy.
- Adjuvant hormonal therapy in postmenopausal women with invasive breast cancer.

Side Effects

Nausea and vomiting, hot flashes, and hypercalcemia.

Aromatase Inhibitors

Anastrozole, Letrozole, and Exemestane

Mechanism of Action

Aromatase converts the adrenal androgen androstenedione in peripheral tissue to estrone and estradiol, the main source of estrogens in postmenopausal women.
- Anastrozole and letrozole are nonsteroidal competitive inhibitors.
- Exemestane is a derivative of androstenedione; thus, it is a steroidal compound that acts as a false substrate for the enzyme, binding to the active site and resulting in irreversible inactivation (▶ Fig. 34.6).

Uses

- For adjuvant treatment of postmenopausal women with hormone receptor–positive early breast cancer or for treatment of advanced breast cancer.

Note: When an aromatase inhibitor is used in premenopausal women, a gonadotropin-releasing hormone (GnRH) agonist (goserelin, leuprolide, or triptorelin) is given to block ovarian estrogen production, or the ovaries are removed surgically.

Side Effects

Nausea and vomiting, hot flashes, and musculoskeletal problems.

Gonadotropin-Releasing Hormone Agonist Agents

Leuprolide and Goserelin

Mechanism of Action

These agents are gonadotropin-releasing hormone (GnRH) agonists that desensitize pituitary GnRH receptors and inhibit the release of gonadotropins (follicle-stimulating hormone [FSH] and luteinizing hormone [LH]).

Uses

- Prostate cancer treatment (in combination with an antiandrogen) to prevent the initial flare-up of the disease.

Notes

Functions of the Prostate Gland

The prostate gland is responsible for producing a significant portion of the fluid that makes up semen. This fluid contains substances that aid sperm on their journey to the fallopian tubes during reproduction (e.g., fructose provides sperm with energy). Seminal fluid is alkaline, which neutralizes the acidity of the vagina and stops sperm death on contact. The prostate gland also plays a part in ejaculation and sealing off the urethra so that no urine is expelled at this time.

Triptorelin

Mechanism of Action

- A synthetic peptide that acts as a GnRH agonist that is a potent inhibitor of testosterone synthesis in men and estrogen in women.
- Mediates constant stimulation of the pituitary gland and through this action decreases secretin of gonadotropins, LH, and FSH.

Pharmacokinetics

- Administered IV.
- Pharmacokinetics follows a three-compartment model with half-lives of 6 minutes, 45 minutes, and 3 hours, respectively.
- Metabolism of triptorelin is not well understood.

Uses

- Used for the palliative treatment of advanced prostate cancer.

Side Effects

- Hot flashes.
- Loss of interest in sex or decreased libido.
- Inability to obtain or sustain an erection.

IX

A. Aromatase inhibitors

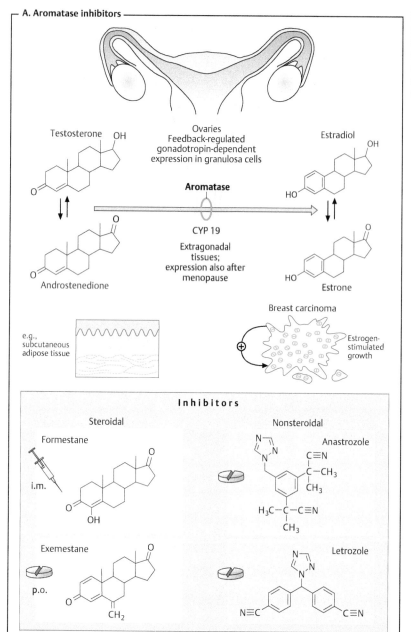

Fig. 34.6 Aromatase inhibitors.
Aromatase inhibitors block the conversion of androgens (testosterone and androstenedione) to estrone and estradiol in extragonadal tissue after menopause (when ovarian estrogen production ceases). In doing so, these agents inhibit the growth of estrogen-dependent breast cancers.

Antiandrogens

Bicalutamide, Flutamide, and Nilutamide

Mechanism of Action

These agents are competitive inhibitors of dihydrotestosterone (DHT) and testosterone at receptor binding sites.

Side Effects

- Hot flashes are common.
- Gynecomastia, nausea and vomiting, edema, and thrombophlebitis.

34.5 Immunosuppressants

Immunosuppressants are used to prevent rejection in patients receiving organ transplants and in autoimmune diseases. Although effective in such cases, they increase the risk of infections and cancers. ▶ Fig. 34.7 illustrates the normal immune reaction and the general steps that the immunosuppressant drugs may inhibit.

Immunosuppressants have been discussed in the sections on inflammatory bowel disease, cancer chemotherapy, and rheumatoid arthritis. Those agents that have not been discussed elsewhere are included below. ▶ Table 34.2 provides chapter and figure cross-references for all immunosuppressant drugs.

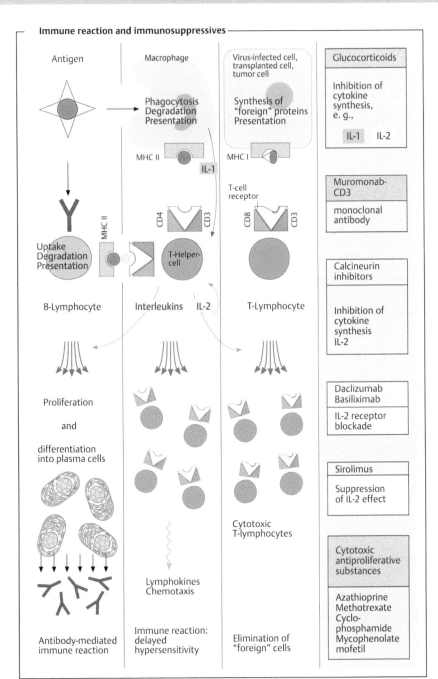

Fig. 34.7 Immune reaction and immunosuppressant drugs.
Humoral immunity (*left column*) and cell-mediated immunity (*middle two columns*) are described in the call-out box. The far-right column lists the actions of immunosuppressant drugs in inhibiting immune responses (MHC, major histocompatibility complex).

IX

Notes

Humoral and Cell-Mediated Immunity

Humoral immunity refers to the adaptive immune responses mediated by antigen-specific antibodies and cell-mediated immunity to those mediated by T cells. Both these responses begin with the binding of antigen by lymphocytes (B cells or T cells). B cells bind free antigen. Activated B cells differentiate into plasma cells and secrete antibodies that travel around the body and attack and destroy antigens identical to those that stimulated their production.

T cells require that antigens be on the surface of macrophages (for helper T cells) or other cells (for cytotoxic T cells) in conjunction with the major histocompatibility complex and CD proteins (MHC I and CD8 for cytotoxic T cells and MHC II and CD4 for helper T cells) to be recognized and bound. Following activation, cytotoxic T cells proliferate and travel to, bind, and destroy antigens identical to those that stimulated their production. Helper T cells do not attack antigens but instead assist in the activation and function of B cells and cytotoxic T cells. Once activated by binding antigen, helper T cells release cytokines which act on activated B and cytotoxic T cells. In most cases, this is essential for activated B cells and cytotoxic T cells to proliferate and function. In addition, some of the cytokines that helper T cells release mediate the inflammatory response.

Table 34.2 Summary of immunosuppressants

Drug class	Drugs	Chapter reference(s)	Figure reference(s)
Antimetabolites	Cyclophosphamide	Chapter 34	34.7
	Methotrexate	Chapter 27, Chapter 33, Chapter 34	27.13, 33.3, 34.4, 34.7
	Azathioprine	Chapter 27	27.13, 34.4, 34.7
Calcineurin inhibitors	Cyclosporine	Chapter 27	33.3, 34.8
	Tacrolimus	Chapter 34	34.8
Corticosteroids	Prednisone, budesonide, hydrocortisone (cortisol), methylpred- nisolone, triamcinolone, dexamethasone, betamethasone, beclomethasone, fluocinonide, ciclesonide, flunisolide, fluticasone	Chapter 16, Chapter 26, Chapter 27, Chapter 32, Chapter 34	16.8–16.11, 27.12
Monoclonal antibodies	Basiliximab	Chapter 34	34.7
	Infliximab	Chapter 27, Chapter 33, Chapter 34	33.4
	Muromonab-CD3	Chapter 34	34.7
	Daclizumab	Chapter 34	34.7
mTOR inhibitors	Sirolimus, everolimus, temsirolimus	Chapter 34	34.8
Other	Mycophenolate mofetil	Chapter 34	34.7
	Belatacept	Chapter 34	

34.5.1 Cyclosporine

Mechanism of Action

- Forms a complex with cyclophilin, a cytoplasmic receptor protein in cells (▶ Fig. 34.8).
- The cyclophilin–cyclosporine complex binds to calcineurin, thereby inhibiting Ca^{2+}-stimulated dephosphorylation of the transcription factor, NFAT.
- NFAT cannot be transported into the nucleus.
- Gene transcription is not activated and T lymphocytes fail to respond to specific antigenic stimulation.

Pharmacokinetics

Administered intravenously or orally.

Uses

Used for kidney, liver, heart, and other organ transplantations.

Side Effects

- Renal dysfunction.
- Hypertension.
- Hirsutism.
- Hyperlipidemia.

34.5.2 Tacrolimus

Tacrolimus is a macrolide antibiotic produced by *Streptomyces tsukubaensis*.

Mechanism of Action

- Binds to an FK binding protein (FKBP-12), an immunophilin (▶ Fig. 34.8).
- Inhibits calcineurin-catalyzed dephosphorylation.

- Prevents transport of NFAT into the nucleus.
- Inhibits T cell activation.

Pharmacokinetics

Given orally or IV.

Uses

Prophylaxis of organ transplant rejection.

Side Effects

- *Cardiovascular:* hypertension and edema.
- *Endocrine/metabolic:* hypomagnesemia, hyperglycemia, and diabetes.
- *GI:* nausea, vomiting, constipation, and diarrhea.
- *Hematologic:* anemia, leukopenia, and thrombocytopenia.
- *Neurologic:* headache, insomnia, pain, paresthesia, and tremor.

34.5.3 Sirolimus

Sirolimus, also known as rapamycin, is a macrocyclic lactone produced by *Streptomyces hygroscopicus*.

Mechanism of Action

- Binds FKBP-12 (▶ Fig. 34.8).
- The sirolimus–FKB-12 complex binds to the mammalian tar- get of rapamycin or mechanistic target of rapamycin (mTOR), a key enzyme in cell cycle progression.
- This inhibits activation and proliferation stimulation of T-lymphocytes by interleukin cytokines (IL-2, IL-4, and IL-15).

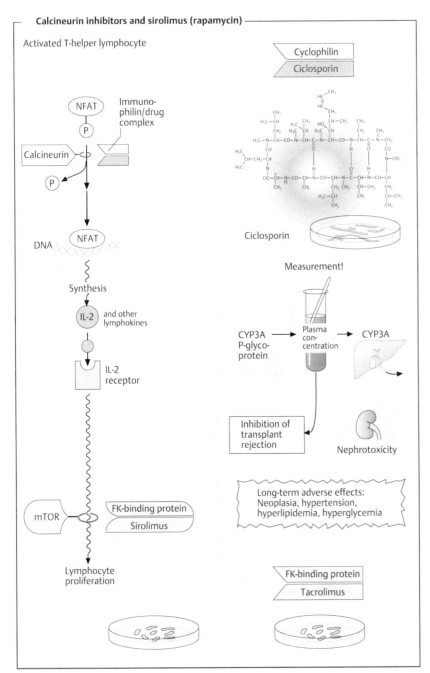

Calcineurin inhibitors and sirolimus (rapamycin)

Activated T-helper lymphocyte

NFAT
P
Immuno-philin/drug complex
Calcineurin
P
DNA
NFAT
Synthesis
IL-2 and other lymphokines
IL-2 receptor
mTOR
FK-binding protein
Sirolimus
Lymphocyte proliferation

Cyclophilin
Ciclosporin

Ciclosporin

Measurement!

CYP3A P-glyco-protein → Plasma concentration → CYP3A

Inhibition of transplant rejection

Nephrotoxicity

Long-term adverse effects: Neoplasia, hypertension, hyperlipidemia, hyperglycemia

FK-binding protein
Tacrolimus

Fig. 34.8 Calcineurin inhibitors and sirolimus (rapamycin).
In T-helper cells, nuclear factor of activated T cell (NFAT) promotes the expression of interleukin 2 (IL-2). NFAT is able to enter the nucleus following dephosphorylation of its phosphorylated precursor by the phosphatase calcineurin. Cyclosporine binds to the protein cyclophilin in the cell interior; this complex inhibits calcineurin, and thus the transcription and production of IL-2 are inhibited. Tacrolimus acts like cyclosporine, but it attaches to a so-called FK-binding protein instead of cyclophilin. Sirolimus forms a complex with the FK-binding protein, changing its conformation. This complex then inhibits mTOR (mammalian target of rapamycin), which operates the signaling path leading from the IL-2 receptor to the activation of mitosis in lymphocytes, thus inhibiting lymphocyte proliferation.

Pharmacokinetics

Given orally.

Uses

Prophylaxis of kidney transplant rejection.

Side Effects

- *Cardiovascular:* hypertension and edema.
- *Dermatologic:* acne and rash.
- *Endocrine/metabolic:* hyperlipidemias.
- *GI:* nausea, vomiting, constipation, and diarrhea.
- *Hematologic:* anemia and thrombocytopenia.
- *Neurologic:* headache, insomnia, and pain.

34.5.4 Everolimus and Temsirolimus

Mechanism of Action

- Congeners of sirolimus.
- Complex with FKBP-12, then bind to mTOR.
- Inhibit T lymphocyte activation and proliferation downstream of the IL-2 and other T-cell growth factor receptors.

Pharmacokinetics

- Administered orally.
- Everolimus has a shorter $t_{1/2}$ than sirolimus.
- Metabolism occurs through the same mechanism as sirolimus and rapamycin.

Uses

- Temsirolimus is approved for use in advanced renal cell carcinoma.
- Everolimus is used as a post-transplant immunosuppressant and for certain cancers.

Side Effects

Appear to be the same as those for sirolimus and rapamycin.

34.5.5 Mycophenolate Mofetil

Mycophenolate mofetil is a semisynthetic derivative of mycophenolic acid from the mold *Penicillium glaucum*.

Mechanism of Action

- Mycophenolate mofetil suppresses T and B lymphocyte responses.
- Inhibits inosine monophosphate (IMPDH), an enzyme in the de novo pathway of guanine nucleotide synthesis.
- B and T lymphocytes are highly dependent on this pathway for proliferation.

Pharmacokinetics

Given orally or IV.

Uses

Prophylaxis of organ transplant rejection.

Side Effects

- *Cardiovascular:* hypertension and edema.
- *Endocrine/metabolic:* hyperlipidemias.
- *GI:* nausea, vomiting, constipation, and diarrhea.
- *Hematologic:* anemia, severe neutropenia, and thrombocytopenia.
- *Neurologic:* asthenia, headache, insomnia, pain, and tremor.

34.5.6 Azathioprine

Mechanism of Action

- A purine antimetabolite that is an imidazolyl derivative of 6-mercaptopurine.
- Cleaved to 6-mercaptopurine, which is then converted to metabolites that inhibit de novo purine synthesis.
- The metabolite, 6-thio-IMP is converted to 6-thio-GTP that is incorporated into DNA.
- Inhibition of cell proliferation impairs lymphocyte function leading to immune suppression.

Pharmacokinetics

- Administered orally.
- Exposure to nucleophiles such as glutathione results in conversion to mercaptopurine.

- Both mercaptopurine and azathioprine are readily removed from the blood by oxidation or methylation in the liver or erythrocytes.
- Renal clearance has an insignificant impact on clearance.

Uses

- Used as an adjunct for prevention of organ transplant rejection.
- Used to treat rheumatoid arthritis

Side Effects

- Bone marrow suppression that includes leukopenia, thrombocytopenia, and anemia.
- Susceptibility to infections.
- Hepatotoxicity, alopecia, GI toxicity, and increased risk of neoplasia.

34.5.7 Basiliximab

Mechanism of Action

Basiliximab is a recombinant anti-IL-2 receptor antibody that binds to the CD25 antigen on the IL-2 receptor and prevents IL-2 binding, thus preventing IL-2-mediated activation of lymphocytes.

Pharmacokinetics

Given IV.

Uses

Prophylaxis of kidney transplant rejection.

Side Effects

- *Cardiovascular:* hypertension and edema.
- *GI:* pain and vomiting.
- *Hematologic:* anemia.
- *Neurologic:* headache and insomnia.

34.5.8 Infliximab

Mechanism of Action

Infliximab is an antibody to TNF-α that blocks TNF-α from binding to TNF receptors on inflammatory cell surfaces, resulting in suppression of downstream inflammatory cytokines such as IL-1 and IL-6 and adhesion molecules involved in leukocyte activation and migration.

34.5.9 Muromonab-CD3

Mechanism of Action

Muromonab-CD3 binds to the CD3 component of the T-cell receptor complex involved in antigen recognition, leading to rapid internalization of the T-cell receptor, thereby preventing subsequent antigen recognition.

Pharmacokinetics

Given IV.

Uses

Acute organ transplant rejection.

Side Effects

- *Cytokine release reactions:* fever, chills, nausea, vomiting, diarrhea, tachycardia, and changes in blood pressure. These reactions occur in many patients following the first few doses. Anaphylactic and anaphylactoid reactions may also occur, but fatalities are rare.
- *GI:* nausea, vomiting, and diarrhea.
- *Neurologic:* fever, headache, insomnia, and pain.

34.5.10 Belatacept

Mechanism of Action

- A fusion protein that consists of the Fc fragment of a human IgG1 immunoglobulin that is linked to the extracellular domain of CTLA-4.
- Belatacept is a T cell costimulation blocker that binds to CD80 and CD86 on antigen-presenting cells.
- Interaction with CD80 and CD86 blocks CD28-mediated costimulation of T lymphocytes.
- Belatacept treatment inhibits T lymphocyte proliferation and production of cytokines: interleukins, interferons, and TNF-α.

Pharmacokinetics

Administered IV.

Uses

Prolongs graft survival and decreased production of anti-donor antibodies.

Side Effects

Opportunistic infections have been reported in kidney transplant patients.

34.5.11 Daclizumab

A humanized monoclonal antibody that functions as an IL-2 receptor antagonist that bind to the Tac subunit of the high-affinity IL-2 receptor complex; it inhibits IL-2 binding.

Pharmacokinetics

- Administered through subcutaneous injection.
- It has a bioavailability of about 90% and has a biological half-life of 21 days.
- It is degraded by proteases to peptides.

Uses

Currently approved for treatment of adults with relapsing forms of multiple sclerosis.

Its use as an immunosuppressant in renal transplants has been discontinued.

Side Effects

- Opportunistic infections.
- There has been no increased risk of cancer with daclizumab.

IX

35 Toxicology and Poisoning

Summary

Nonspecific antidotes include gastric lavage (stomach pumping) with saline and activated charcoal for absorption of organic and inorganic compounds. Syrup of ipecac is used as an emetic agent but is now considered as a second-line agent for poisoning emergencies. Hemodialysis is used to filter waste products such as creatinine and urea or drugs from the blood in cases of kidney failure. Multiple specific antidotes are available and are used where the identity of the toxic substances is known or strongly suspected. Metal chelating agents are used to treat heavy metal poisoning by preventing or reversing the effects of a heavy metal or an enzyme. Dimercaprol protects essential sulfhydryl-containing enzymes and promotes excretion of metal in a stable complex form. Dimercaprol is an effective treatment for poisoning by mercury, arsenic, and other less common metals. Calcium disodium edetate is an efficient chelator of divalent and trivalent metals and is used to promote excretion of the lead chelate. Penicillamine is used for treatment of copper poisoning and can promote excretion of mercury and lead. Deferoxamine specifically chelates iron and promotes its excretions. Succimer represents a water-soluble analogue of dimercaprol and is indicated for lead poisoning in children.

Keywords: chelating agents, heavy metal toxicity, iron toxicity

35.1 Introduction

Although humans have endogenous mechanisms to protect themselves from the toxic effects of exogenous chemicals or xenobiotics, there are situations where either acute or chronic exposure can cause significant toxicity. In these cases, intervention with chemotherapeutic agents, which can limit or reverse these toxic effects and remove the xenobiotic, is necessary. This chapter reviews chemotherapeutic agents that are used to treat patients who have been exposed to various toxic agents. Most notable of these agents are those used to treat heavy metal poisoning. For example, environmental lead contamination is a common event because of its occurrence in lead-based paints as well as other industrial products such as batteries, ammunition, solder, plastics, and ceramics. Discussions are provided on chelating agents that selectively remove lead from the body. This chapter provides critical knowledge of how to treat heavy metal poisoning and other toxic exposures.

Toxic reactions to drugs and other agents can occur with acute exposure to a high dose of an agent, either accidentally or intentionally. Chronic toxicities can be observed with long-term exposure to an agent at lower doses. These reactions may be local, following skin contact or lung inhalation, or systemic, following absorption of the toxin. In some cases, the toxicity only develops following biotransformation of the absorbed substance to toxic metabolites. The resulting toxicities may be short- or long-term, they may appear immediately or may be delayed, and they may be reversible or irreversible.

Toxicities of specific agents have largely been dealt with along with the discussion of their pharmacological properties, but some of the more common toxic substances and poisonings are discussed in this chapter.

35.2 Nonspecific Antidotes

In cases of acute poisoning, the main goal is to minimize further exposure and enhance elimination of the toxin. Several procedures are used when specific antidotes are not available, and these are discussed below.

35.2.1 Gastric Lavage with Saline

Mechanism of Action

Gastric lavage (stomach pumping) involves fluid, usually saline, being sequentially administered and withdrawn via an orogastric or nasogastric tube.

Pharmacokinetics

Given orally as a suspension in doses of up to 100 g.

Note: During this procedure, the patient's airway is protected by an endotracheal tube to prevent aspiration of the ingested substances into the lung.

35.2.2 Activated Charcoal

Mechanism of Action

Activated charcoal adsorbs a large number of organic and inorganic compounds and prevents their absorption from the gastrointestinal (GI) tract.

Pharmacokinetics

Given orally or via gastric tube as a suspension in doses of up to 100 g.

35.2.3 Syrup of Ipecac

Mechanism of Action

This is an emetic agent. Emesis used to be primary therapy but is now becoming secondary to other therapies.

Pharmacokinetics

One ounce orally usually produces emesis within 30 minutes.

Contraindications

Emesis is contraindicated when there is a risk of perforation of the esophagus or stomach (corrosive agents), when ingested agents may be aspirated into the lung (e.g., if the patient is comatose), or if emesis is likely to induce seizures (strychnine or central nervous system [CNS] stimulants).

35.2.4 Hemodialysis

Mechanism of Action

Hemodialysis involves the use of a machine to filter waste products (e.g., creatinine and urea), salts, fluids, or drugs from the blood. The blood flows in the opposite direction to dialysis fluid, and these are separated by a semipermeable membrane. This allows substances to be cleared down their concentration gradient.

Emergency Treatment of the Poisoned Patient

The procedure for the emergency treatment of the poisoned patient is as follows: (1) check respiratory function, cardiovascular function, and CNS involvement; (2) stabilize the patient; (3) attempt to determine the identity and quantity of poison ingested and the time of exposure; and (4) treat with the appropriate antidote.

Hemoperfusion

Hemoperfusion is a technique in which large volumes of the patient's blood are passed over an adsorbent substance, such as resins or activated carbon, which attracts and removes toxic substances from the blood. It is used to treat overdoses of barbiturates, theophylline, digitalis, carbamazepine, methotrexate, acetaminophen, meprobamate, glutethimide, ethchlorvynol, and paraquat poisoning. Hemoperfusion may also be used to remove waste products in kidney disease and provide supportive treatment before and after liver transplantation.

Uses

Hemodialysis is not useful for poisons with large volumes of distribution or poisons that bind tightly to plasma proteins. It is generally reserved for extreme, life-threatening poisoning with alcohol, aspirin, or CNS-active drugs.

35.3 Specific Antidotes

When the identity of the toxic substances is known or strongly suspected, it may be desirable to treat with specific antidotes.

35.3.1 Metal Chelating Agents

These agents are used to treat heavy metal poisoning by preventing or reversing the effects of a heavy metal or an enzyme. These agents can also accelerate elimination of the metal from the body.

Dimercaprol (British Anti-Lewisite)

Mechanism of Action

Dimercaprol, or British anti-Lewisite (BAL), protects essential sulfhydryl-containing enzymes by forming a stable complex with circulating metallic poison. It promotes excretion of metal in a stable complex form (▶ Fig. 35.1).

Pharmacokinetics

Dispensed in a 10% solution of peanut oil and must be given intramuscularly.

Uses

Dimercaprol is an effective treatment following poisoning by mercury, arsenic, and some other less common metals, but it is not very effective for lead poisoning.

Side Effects

Increased blood pressure and heart rate, weakness, nausea, and pain at the injection site.

IX

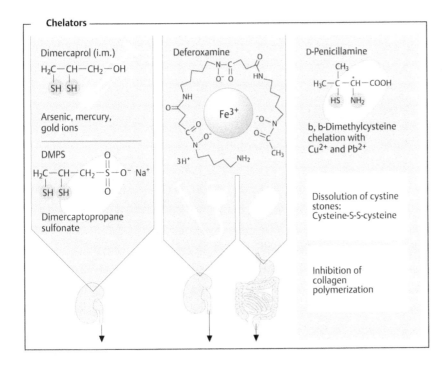

Fig. 35.1 Chelators.
Dimercaprol is given by intramuscular injection to chelate various metal ions. A related compound, dimercaptopropane sulfonate (DMPS), is suitable for oral administration. Deferoxamine is highly effective at chelating iron from hemoglobin or cytochromes.

Calcium Disodium Edetate

Mechanism of Action

Calcium disodium edetate is an efficient chelator of divalent and trivalent metals (or ethylenediaminetetraacetic acid [CaNa$_2$ EDTA]) and is used clinically to promote the excretion of the lead chelate.

Pharmacokinetics

Given by intravenous (IV) infusion, as it is not effective orally because of its highly polar ionic character limits and absorption. The calcium disodium salt form of EDTA is used to prevent potentially life-threatening calcium depletion.

Uses

Especially effective in lead poisoning, but may also be useful to chelate other less common metallic poisons such as zinc, manganese, and certain heavy radionuclides.

Side Effects

- Renal damage and hypersensitivity reactions.
- Contraindicated in anuric patients.

Penicillamine (d-Dimethyl Cysteine)

Penicillamine is a water-soluble derivative of penicillin.

Mechanism of Action

Penicillamine is used primarily for treatment of copper poisoning. It promotes excretion of mercury and lead but succimer has replaced penicillamine for this purpose.

Pharmacokinetics

Administered orally.

Uses

- Used to remove copper in hepatolenticular degeneration (Wilson's disease).
- Used in combination, usually following EDTA, for lead poisoning.
- Also useful in the treatment of rheumatoid arthritis (see Chapter 33).

Mercury Poisoning

The greatest danger with mercury poisoning is damage of the GI mucosa and kidneys. Fluid loss leads to shock and death. This tends to occur with acute intoxication. Symptoms of chronic intoxication include stomatitis, excessive salivation, blue gum line, renal toxicity, and CNS symptoms (e.g., depression, weakness, headache, insomnia, irritability, and hallucinations). This is treated by giving dimercaprol.

Arsenic Poisoning

Arsenic is considered to be a heavy metal and therefore has many toxic characteristics in common with lead and mercury. Signs and symptoms of arsenic poisoning include headache, confusion, drowsiness, abdominal pain, diarrhea, vomiting, convulsions, coma, and death. Treatment of acute arsenic poisoning is supportive, and chelation therapy with dimercaprol is used to bind the arsenic and hasten excretion in all symptomatic patients.

Lead Poisoning

Acute intoxication with lead is rare. Symptoms of chronic intoxication include spasm and hypermotility of the GI tract which causes intense cramping and lead encephalopathy (primarily a problem in children), the early symptoms of which are nonspecific and may include decreased appetite, irritability, fatigue, abdominal pain, and vomiting, followed by drowsiness, stupor, convulsions, and coma. This may lead to mental retardation and cerebral palsies, as well as myopathy, fatigue, weakness, wrist drop, foot drop, and involvement of extraocular muscles. Other results are anemia due to impaired heme biosynthesis, porphyrinuria, basophilic stippling of erythrocytes, and gingival lead line. Blood vessel constriction causes pallor and hypertension. Initial treatment is edetate administration. Penicillamine and dimercaprol (limited effectiveness) may also be used.

Side Effects

- Hypersensitivity reactions; use with extreme caution in patients with penicillin allergy.
- Rashes.
- Arthralgia.
- Nephrotic syndrome.

Trientine

Uses

Trientine is an alternative copper chelating agent for patients who are hypersensitive to penicillamine.

Deferoxamine

Mechanism of Action

Deferoxamine specifically chelates iron (ferric ions and ferrous ions) and promotes its excretion. It binds free and loosely bound iron, for example, from hemosiderin and ferritin, but does not chelate iron bound to hemoglobin or cytochromes.

Pharmacokinetics

This agent is orally effective in preventing iron absorption. It is given intramuscularly or IV for systemic toxicity. The iron-chelation complex is excreted in the urine and often imparts an orange red color to it.

Uses

Acute iron toxicity and iron storage diseases (e.g., hemochromatosis).

Side Effects

Hypertension, rashes, and GI upset.

Wilson's Disease

Wilson's disease is an autosomal recessive disease that results in the accumulation of copper (that is ingested) in the liver and brain, causing cirrhosis and basal ganglia destruction. It may present in a child or young adult with neurologic signs such as tremor, seizures, mental deterioration, and weakness; or there may be signs of cirrhosis, such as jaundice, hepatomegaly (swelling of the liver), edema, and fatigue. Treatment with penicillamine is effective if given early.

Iron Poisoning

Iron poisoning is the most common metallic poisoning, due to overdosage with oral supplements, multiple transfusions, or iron storage diseases. Acute symptoms of iron poisoning include vomiting (often bloody), gastric pain, and diarrhea. Chronic symptoms include metabolic acidosis, lethargy, which may progress to cardiovascular collapse, liver damage, and organ failure. Permanent scarring of the GI tract may occur with severe poisoning. Treatment is by desferoxamine.

35.3.2 Succimer (Dimercaptosuccinic Acid)

Pharmacokinetics

- Represents a water-soluble analogue of dimercaprol.
- Orally effective.

Uses

Succimer is indicated for lead poisoning in children. It may also be effective for mercury or arsenic.

▶ Table 35.1 summarizes other poisons and their antidotes.

Carbon Monoxide Poisoning

Carbon monoxide (CO) is a colorless, odorless, tasteless, nonirritant toxic gas that is produced from the incomplete burning of fossil fuels. It binds to hemoglobin, forming carboxyhemoglobin, and in doing so, it displaces oxygen. This results in a functional anemia. Symptoms of CO poisoning include headache, dizziness, weakness, confusion, lethargy, nausea, vomiting, seizures, and, at very high concentrations, coma and death. CO poisoning is the most common cause of death from poisoning. Treatment involves removing the source of CO, 100% oxygen therapy, and hyperbaric oxygen therapy (if severe).

Foundations

Electron Transport Chain

The electron transport chain consists of a group of complexes (CI–CV) that are located in the inner membrane of the mitochondria. It is the mechanism by which the energy needed to

IX

Table 35.1 Other poisons and their antidotes

Poison	Antidote	Mechanism of action of antidote
Belladonna (atropine)	Physostigmine (section 5.1.9)	Anticholinesterase action
Carbon monoxide	Hyperbaric O_2	Hyperbaric O_2 increases both O_2 delivery to tissue and CO elimination
Coumarin derivatives (e.g., warfarin)	Phytonadione (vitamin K_1)	Vitamin K promotes hepatic synthesis of factors II, VII, IX, and X, which are needed for coagulation of the blood
Cyanide	Sodium thiosulfate, amyl nitrite, and sodium nitrite	Sodium thiosulfate increases cyanide metabolism; amyl nitrite and sodium nitrite produce methemoglobin, which binds cyanide
Ethylene glycol and other glycols	Ethanol (section 15.6.1)	Ethanol is preferentially metabolized by alcohol dehydrogenase and prevents the occurrence of acidosis
Methanol	Ethanol (section 15.6.2)	Ethanol is preferentially metabolized by alcohol dehydrogenase and decreases the formation of both formaldehyde and formic acid from methanol
Iodine	Starch	Starch binds iodine
Opiates	Naloxone (section 13.5.1)	Naloxone is a narcotic antagonist
Nitrites	Methylene blue	Narcotic antagonist
Organophosphate	Pralidoxime	Pralidoxime is a cholinesterase reactivator
Insecticides	Atropine (section 5.2.4)	Atropine is an anticholinergic agent

drive the oxidative phosphorylation of adenosine triphosphate (ATP) is generated. NADH (the reduced form of nicotinamide adenine dinucleotide) and $FADH_2$ (or 1,5-dihydro-FAD [flavin adenine dinucleotide]), derived from carbohydrate and fatty acid catabolism, are electron donors. As electrons are passed along the chain of complexes, protons (H^+ ions) are pumped into the intermembrane space at certain points (CI, CIII, and CIV). These protons cause an electrochemical gradient to form. They flow back into the mitochondrial matrix through complex V (ATP synthase), which generates ATP from adenosine diphosphate (ADP) and P_i. The electron transport chain is disrupted by toxic substances such as cyanide and CO, thus decreasing the capacity for aerobic metabolism.

Organophosphate Poisoning

Organophosphates are commonly used insecticides and are one of the most common causes of poisoning worldwide. Organophosphates inhibit the action of acetylcholinesterase in nerve cells which results in excess acetylcholine. Signs and symptoms of organophosphate poisoning include salivation, lacrimation, sweating, vomiting, incontinence of urine and feces, convulsions, cyanosis, bradycardia, and hypotension. Treatment of organophosphate poisoning is with pralidoxime, a cholinesterase reactivator.

36   Water- and Fat-Soluble Vitamins

Summary

The vitamins include several chemically unrelated families of organic substances that are essential for the maintenance of metabolic homeostasis. Vitamins are divided into water-soluble type and fat-soluble type. Many of the water-soluble vitamins are coenzymes for enzymes and facilitate metabolic processes. Thiamine is a water-soluble vitamin also known as vitamin B_1. Riboflavin is vitamin B_2 and niacin is vitamin B_3. Pantothenic acid is vitamin B_5. Pyridoxine, vitamin B_6, refers to three biochemical entities—pyridoxine, pyridoxal, and pyridoxamine. Vitamin B_{12} includes the cobalamins—cyanocobalamin, hydroxycobalamin, methylcobalamin, and adenosylcobalamin. Ascorbic acid is vitamin C and biotin is vitamin H. The vitamin folate is converted to tetrahydrofolate by the action of dihydrofolate reductase.

Fat-soluble vitamins include vitamin A. There are two forms of vitamin A: provitamin A carotenoids, including β-carotene; and preformed vitamin A, including retinol, retinal, and retinoic acid. Vitamin D is calciferol. Vitamin E represents a mixture of lipid-soluble compounds that includes tocopherols and tocotrienols. Vitamin K consists of three compounds that are biologically active: K_1 (phylloquinone), the normal dietary source; K_2 (menaquinones), synthesized by bacteria in the intestine, and K_3 (menadiol diacetate), a synthetic compound that is metabolized into menaquinone.

Keywords: fat soluble, water soluble, beriberi, Wernicke-Korsakoff syndrome, megaloblastic anemia, peripheral neuropathy

36.1   Introduction

The vitamins include several chemically unrelated families of organic substances that are essential for the maintenance of metabolic homeostasis. The vitamins cannot be synthesized by the body and are obtained either through dietary sources or from supplements.

Vitamins are divided into those that are water-soluble and those that are fat-soluble. Absorption of these two classes is different. Water-soluble vitamins are readily absorbed in the intestine, but fat-soluble vitamins must associate with triglyceride-rich lipoprotein particles or bind to specific protein carriers to be absorbed (▶ Table 36.1).

Vitamin deficiencies are rare nowadays in developed, resource-rich countries, but diseases associated with insufficient vitamin levels can occur in cases of malnutrition or intestinal malabsorption. Notable examples of vitamin deficiency diseases include rickets (vitamin D), scurvy (vitamin C), beriberi (thiamine), and pellagra (niacin). The Food and Nutrition Board of the Institute of Medicine has developed Dietary Reference Intakes (DRIs) as a guide for vitamin intake. DRIs include the (1) recommended dietary allowance (RDA) that lists dietary vitamin intake need to meet daily nutrient requirements of 97% of individuals in a specific life stage; (2) adequate intake (AI) or vitamin intake needed to maintain good health; and (3) upper tolerable level or the maximum vitamin intake that will pose no risk of toxicity or adverse health effects.

36.2   Water-Soluble Vitamins

Many of the water-soluble vitamins are coenzymes for enzymes and facilitate metabolic processes.

36.2.1   Vitamin B_1 (Thiamine)

Metabolism and Mechanism of Action

Thiamine is a water-soluble vitamin also known as vitamin B_1. Thiamine is absorbed through two thiamine transport systems—THTR-1 and THTR-2—both of which are expressed and function in the small and large intestine. Thiamine is phosphorylated to its pyrophosphate form, thiamine pyrophosphate (TPP), once absorbed in the intestine and, in this form, it acts as a cofactor for multiple enzymes (e.g., transketolase, pyruvate dehydrogenase, α-ketoglutarate dehydrogenase, and branch-chain ketoacid dehydrogenase), thus modulating oxidative energy metabolism and ATP synthesis in mitochondria. TPP also has a role in modulating the function of membrane chloride functions by facilitating protein phosphorylation as well as initiation of nerve impulse propagation.

Sources

Important food sources include: yeast, legumes, brown rice, and whole grain cereals. Thiamine is low in polished rice and processed cereals because milling removes thiamine. Poor sources include milk products, fruits, and vegetables.

Requirements

The RDA for thiamine is 0.5 to 0.9 mg for children, 1.2 mg for adult men, and 1.1 mg for nonpregnant adult women.

Deficiency

Two clinical phenotypes are associated with thiamine deficiency, beriberi and Wernicke–Korsakoff syndrome.

Beriberi

- Two clinical phenotypes in adults—dry or wet.
- Dry beriberi is the development of a symmetrical peripheral neuropathy that includes sensory and motor impairments, and in certain cases it is associated with cardiac involvement.
- Wet beriberi involves the heart which leads to lower extremity edema.

Beriberi in Infants

- Acute or "fulminating" beriberi occurs primarily in infants between the ages of 2 and 3 months and occurs in women deficient in thiamine who are breastfeeding.
- Clinical symptoms include fulminant cardiac syndrome with heart failure, metabolic abnormalities, and some degree of neural involvement.

Table 36.1 Vitamin summary table

	Metabolism and mechanism of action	Sources	Requirements (RDA or AI)	Deficiency	Toxicity
Water-soluble vitamins					
Vitamin B$_1$ (thiamine)	Phosphorylated to form thiamine pyrophosphate Cofactor for enzymes modulating oxidative energy metabolism	Yeast, legumes, brown rice, and whole grain cereals Polished rice is low in thiamine because milling removes thiamine	0.5 to 0.9 mg for children, 1.2 mg for adult men, and 1.1 mg for nonpregnant adult women	Two clinical phenotypes: beriberi (dry or wet) and Wernicke–Korsakoff syndrome	None described
Vitamin B$_2$ (riboflavin)	Precursor of flavin adenine dinucleotide (FAD) and flavin mononucleotide (FMN) Functions in multiple metabolic pathways; Complexes with proteins to form flavoproteins	Liver, yeast, eggs, meat, enriched breads and cereals, milk	1.3 to 1.6 mg for adults	Degenerative changes in the nervous system, skin disorders, endocrine disorder, and anemia	None described
Vitamin B$_3$ (niacin)	Precursor for nicotinamide adenine dinucleotide (NAD) and nicotinamide adenine dinucleotide phosphate (NADP)	Meats, grains, legumes, and yeast; corn treated with alkali is a rich source	Children: 6 to 12 mg Adult males: 16 mg Nonpregnant adult females: 14 mg	Pellagra; deficiencies occur in chronic alcoholics and those with malabsorption disorders	Nicotinic acid and nicotinamide doses exceeding 500 mg/day can cause liver damage
Vitamin B$_6$ (pyridoxine)	Includes three biochemical entities: pyridoxine, pyridoxal, and pyridoxamine Phosphorylated forms are biologically active Act as cofactors for amino acid decarboxylation, synthesis of niacin from tryptophan, neurotransmitter synthesis, and carbohydrate metabolism	Meat, fish, starch vegetables, and non-citrus fruit	0.5 to 1 mg for children, 1.3 mg for young men and women, and 1.5 to 1.7 mg for men and women older than 50 years	Neurologic disorders or anemia	Doses over 250 mg/day associated with peripheral neuropathy, photosensitivity, and dizziness
Vitamin B$_5$ (pantothenic acid)	Functional group for coenzyme A, a coenzyme in the tricarboxylic acid cycle	Egg yolk, liver, broccoli, milk, and bacteria in the colon	AI ranges from 2 to 4 mg daily for children to 5 mg daily for adults	Deficiency is rare Symptoms of deficiency include paresthesias and dysesthesias collectively referred to as "burning feet syndrome"	No toxicity has been reported for high doses
Vitamin H (biotin)	Essential cofactor or carboxyl group carrier for carboxylase enzyme complexes	Egg yolk, liver, soy product, and yeast	8 to 12 µg for children and 30 µg for adults	Deficiencies are rare but consumption of large amount of raw egg whites can cause biotin deficiency	No toxicity is associated with consumption of large amounts of biotin
Vitamin C (ascorbic acid)	Reducing agent (antioxidant); acts as electron donor for enzymes in reactions that use iron and copper as cofactors	Citrus fruits, potatoes, tomatoes, cruciferous vegetables, and strawberries	15 to 45 mg for children and 75 to 90 mg for women and men Pregnant women and elderly require 120 mg	Clinical deficiency is known as scurvy, a syndrome characterized by impaired collagen synthesis	Consumption of large doses of vitamin C (gram quantities) can increase oxalate formation and the risk of calcium oxalate kidney stones
Vitamin B$_{12}$ (cobalamin)	Dietary B$_{12}$ becomes bound to R factors in gastric secretions Released from R factors in the intestine binds to intrinsic factor Required for transfer of methyl groups from tetrahydrofolate (FH4) to form methionine from homocysteine and as a coenzyme in conversion of methylmalonyl CoA to succinyl CoA	Meat and dairy products	5 to 7 µg	Megaloblastic anemia and neurological effects	No clear toxicity

Table 36.1 (*Continued*)

	Metabolism and mechanism of action	Sources	Requirements (RDA or AI)	Deficiency	Toxicity
Folic acid	Converted to FH4 by dihydrofolate reductase FH4 is the primary one-carbon carrier in the body One-carbon groups are used for de novo synthesis of purines, glycine to form serine and methyl groups for methylation of dUMP to TMP	Leafy green vegetables, nuts, fruits, and cereals; grains and flour in the United States and Australia are supplemented with folic acid	300 to 400 µg Increases to 600 in pregnant and 500 in lactating women	dUMP/dTMP ratios and an inhibition of DNA repair and fragmentation leading to macrocytic, megaloblastic anemia	None known
Fat-soluble vitamins					
Vitamin A	Provitamin A (beta-carotene) and pre-formed vitamin A (retinol, retinal, reti-noic acid, and retinyl esters) are metabolized to vitamin A In the eyes, vitamin A mediates photo-transduction and prevents xerophthalmia	Plants such as carrots, leafy green vegetables, and sweet potatoes	For adult males 3,000 IUs or 900 µg retinol; for females 2,300 IUs or 700 µg retinol	Night blindness, complete blindness, and xerophthalmia	Accumulation of free vitamin A results in membrane lysis and tissue damage Clinical symptoms include central nervous system effects such as ataxia and increased cerebrospinal fluid
Vitamin D	Ultraviolet light exposure converts 7-dehydrocholesterol to previtamin D, which is then converted into calcidiol, which is converted in the kidneys to the active form 1,25-dihydroxyvitamin D The vitamin D receptor regulates gene transcription Vitamin D mediates serum calcium concentrations	Major source is dermal synthesis of previtamin D from 7-dehydrocholes-terol Fatty fish livers are a rich source	Varies with age, pregnancy, sunlight exposure, and fat malabsorption issues For children 1 to 18 years, adults up to the age of 70 years, and pregnant or lactat-ing women is 15 µg Those with limited sunlight exposure require higher levels and for infants exclusively breastfed a daily supplement of 400 IUs is recommended	Rickets in children and osteo-malacia in adults	Toxicity has been associated with consumption of 60,000 IUs per day. Symptoms include hypercalcemia, polyuria, polydipsia, and anorexia and muscle weakness
Vitamin E	Mixture of lipid-soluble compounds collectively representing tocopherols; the bioactive form is alpha-tocopherol Reacts with free radicals forming a tocopherol-free radical complex that is reduced by vitamin C	Olive and sunflower oils, meat, eggs, and leafy vegetables	15 mg of dietary alpha-tocopherol for adolescents, men, and women	Deficiencies are not common but do occur in maladies that result in fat malabsorption Clinical symptoms of defi-ciency include neuromuscular disorders and neuropathy	The upper limit of alpha-tocopherol supplementation is 1,000 mg daily for adults and for children it is 200 mg daily Excessive intake of vitamin E is associated with mortality resulting from hemorrhagic strokes
Vitamin K	Consists of three biologically active compounds: phylloquinone, menaqui-nones, and menadiol diacetate Acts as a cofactor required for regulat-ing activity of proteins containing car-boxyglutamic acid residues Cofactor in the activation of clotting factors II, VII, IX, and X	Green leafy vegetables, broccoli, spi-nach, lettuce, herbs, and kale Gut microflora synthesis of menaqui-nones is an important source	AI is 90 µg for women and 120 µg for men	Deficiency of vitamin K is rare but acquired deficiency can occur because of fat malab-sorption issues and pancreatic secretion disorders Certain medications such as certain cephalosporins can interfere with vitamin K activity	Toxicity is rare and no upper level of intake has been identified for vitamin K supplementation

IX

421

Wernicke–Korsakoff Syndrome

- Wernicke's encephalopathy and Korsakoff's psychosis are often associated with chronic alcoholism. These can be manifested synchronously as Wernicke–Korsakoff syndrome in a patient with a thiamine deficiency. These are not separate pathologies, but are expressed as a spectrum of symptoms.
- Wernicke encephalopathy is an acute syndrome requiring immediate treatment with thiamine supplementation to prevent neurological issues.
- Korsakoff syndrome is a chronic neurological condition associated with Wernicke encephalopathy. It is associated with impairment of short-term memory and confabulation.

Toxicity

The kidneys rapidly clear excess thiamine and no real toxic syndrome of excess thiamine is known. The half-life of thiamine is approximately 10 to 20 days.

36.2.2 Riboflavin (Vitamin B$_2$)

Metabolism and Mechanism of Action

Riboflavin in the free base form exists as a dimethylisoalloxazine ring that is covalently bound to ribitol. Riboflavin is the precursor of flavin adenine dinucleotide (FAD) and flavin mononucleotide (FMN). Dietary riboflavin is bound to either albumin or riboflavin-specific carrier proteins, and release of riboflavin is accomplished by gastric acid or proteolysis. The free riboflavin is absorbed through RF transporters in the small and large intestine and is converted into FMN and FAD once it reaches the liver.

FMN and FAD form coenzyme complexes that have critical regulatory functions in multiple metabolic pathways that include energy-producing respiratory pathways. Riboflavin complexes with proteins to form flavoproteins that function in mitochondrial oxidative and reductive reactions as well as serving as electron transporters.

Sources

Dietary sources of riboflavin include liver, yeast, eggs, meat, enriched bread and cereals, and milk.

Requirements and Deficiency

The RDA of riboflavin for adults ranges from 1.3 to 1.6 mg.

Clinical symptoms of riboflavin deficiency are variable and include degenerative changes in the nervous system, skin disorders such as seborrheic dermatitis, endocrine disorders, and anemia. Riboflavin deficiency is often associated with inflammatory bowel disease and alcoholism.

Toxicity

Ingestion of high riboflavin doses has not been associated with any adverse effects. This may be a consequence of riboflavin's limited water solubility and the saturability of RF1 transporters in the small and large intestines.

36.2.3 Niacin (Vitamin B$_3$, Nicotinic acid, Nicotinamide)

Metabolism and Mechanism of Action

Niacin is a precursor for nicotinamide adenine dinucleotide (NAD) and nicotinamide adenine dinucleotide phosphate (NADP). Dietary NAD and NADP are converted to nicotinamide and nicotinic acid for intestinal absorption; both are converted back to NAD and NADP for cellular functions. Dietary tryptophan also serves as a source of the vitamin and is converted to nicotinamide in the liver.

NAD and NADP are critical for many biochemical reactions where the niacin moiety serves to either accept electrons or donate hydrogen ions. NAD-dependent reactions include oxidation of fatty acids and reactions generating compounds with high-energy bonds. NADP is involved in the hexose monophosphate shunt as well as fatty acid and steroid synthesis.

Sources

Niacin is widely distributed in plant and animal foods. Sources with high levels include meats, grains, legumes, and yeast. Corn treated with alkali is also a rich source.

Requirements and Deficiency

The RDA for children is 6 to 12 mg, for adult males it is 16 mg, and 14 mg for nonpregnant adult females.

Deficiency of niacin causes pellagra and is characterized as a photosensitive pigmented dermatitis on sun-exposed area, inflammation of mucous membranes, as well as diarrhea, dementia, and general weakness.

Niacin deficiencies can occur in chronic alcoholics, and those who have undergone bariatric surgery, Crohn's disease, and other malabsorptive disorders.

In resource-limited countries, niacin deficiency can occur with the consumption of corn not treated with alkali; niacin bioavailability in corn requires alkali treatment.

36.2.4 Pantothenic Acid (Vitamin B$_5$)

Metabolism and Mechanism of Action

Pantothenic acid represents the functional group for coenzyme A (CoA) and, therefore, has a fundamental role in energy-yielding metabolic processes. These include the tricarboxylic acid cycle, fatty acid synthesis and catabolism, as well as multiple mitochondrial and cytosolic reactions.

Pantothenic acid as CoA, the acetylation coenzyme, functions in the formation of a thioester bond between the sulfur of CoA and an acyl group (acetyl CoA, succinyl-CoA) in the TCA cycle.

Sources

Vitamin B$_5$ is found in many plant- and animal-based foods. It is found in high amounts in egg yolk, liver, broccoli, and milk.

Requirements and Deficiency

The recommended dietary intake of pantothenic acid ranges from 2 to 4 mg daily for children to 5 mg daily for adult men and women.

Deficiency is rare in humans, although it has been reported during famine where there is severe malnutrition. Symptoms of deficiency are characterized as paresthesias and dysesthesias that are collectively referred to as "burning feet syndrome."

Toxicity

No toxicity due to excess intake of pantothenic acid has been reported.

36.2.5 Pyridoxine (Vitamin B₆)

Metabolism and Mechanism of Action

Vitamin B_6 refers to three biochemical entities—pyridoxine, pyridoxal, and pyridoxamine—as well as their phosphorylated forms. Since the different forms can be readily interconverted, they are biologically equivalent.

The active form of vitamin B_6 is pyridoxal 5-phosphate (PLP). PLP functions as a coenzyme in transamination reactions. It is also a coenzyme in some decarboxylation reactions, synthesis of niacin from tryptophan, neurotransmitter synthesis, and carbohydrate metabolism.

Sources

Vitamin B_6 is widely distributed in food and rich sources include meat, fish, starchy vegetables, and noncitrus fruits.

Requirements and Deficiency

The RDA for vitamin B_6 ranges from 0.5 to 1 mg for children, 1.3 mg for young men and women, and 1.7 and 1.5 mg for men and women older than 50 years, respectively.

Significant deficiencies are rare but marginal deficiencies are more frequent. Deficiencies can lead to neurologic disorders or anemia. Disease-associated deficiencies can occur in chronic alcoholics, individuals with diabetes mellitus celiac disease, and those undergoing long-term isoniazid, penicillamine, hydralazine, or levodopa/carbidopa therapy.

Toxicity

Peripheral neuropathy, photosensitivity, and dizziness have been associated with pyridoxine doses over 250 mg/day.

36.2.6 Vitamin B₁₂ (Cobalamins)

The cobalamins are a series of related compounds with cobalt at the center of a ring structure. The forms depend on the ligand bound to the cobalt and include cyanocobalamin, hydroxycobalamin, methylcobalamin, and adenosylcobalamin (see ▶ Fig. 24.10).

Metabolism and Mechanism of Action

Dietary B_{12} is bound to proteins. It is released by the action of stomach acid and pepsin. Released B_{12} binds to intrinsic factor (IF) and the IF–B_{12} complex binds to transporter receptors in the ileum where it is absorbed into the blood stream. In the blood, B_{12} binds to transcobalamin II and is transported to tissues, mainly the liver.

Vitamin B_{12} is required for two essential enzymatic reactions: transfer of methyl groups from tetrahydrofolate (FH4) to form methionine from homocysteine and as a coenzyme in the conversion of methylmalonyl CoA to succinyl CoA, a reaction catalyzed by methylmalonyl CoA mutase.

Sources

Dietary B_{12} is obtained from meat and dairy products. B_{12} is synthesized only by bacteria and cannot be synthesized de novo by eukaryotic cells. B_{12} is absorbed by animals from bacteria in their food or their GI tracts, stored in their tissues or secreted into their milk, which is then absorbed once consumed by humans.

Requirements and Deficiency

The RDA for B_{12} is 2.4 µg for adults, 2.6 µg for pregnant women, and 2.8 µg for mothers who are breastfeeding.

There are two clinical manifestations of vitamin B_{12} deficiency. Hematopoietic effects result from effects on folate metabolism and are manifested as megaloblastic anemia.

Neurological effects result in progressive demyelination caused by an inability to convert methylmalonyl CoA to succinyl CoA in the brain. Methylmalonyl CoA accumulation interferes with myelin formation.

Toxicity

There is no toxicity associated with intake of B_{12}, probably because absorption is limited.

36.2.7 Vitamin C (Ascorbic Acid)

Metabolism and Mechanism of Action

Vitamin C acts as a reversible reducing agent and serves as a source of reducing equivalents in a number of reactions that utilize iron and copper. It reduces molecular oxygen by providing electrons. Reduced ascorbate can regenerate reduced forms of vitamin E by donating electrons in a redox cycle. Other functions of vitamin C in biological processes include

- Serving as a cofactor for reduction of folate to dihydro- and FH4.
- Facilitating enzymatic hydroxylation of proline and lysine in collagen. Ascorbic acid is a cofactor for propyl hydroxylase, and failure to hydroxylate these amino acids in collagen synthesis can impair wound healing, cause defective tooth formation, as well as compromise osteoblast and fibroblast function.
- Acting as a cofactor for the hydroxylation of dopamine by the enzyme dopamine-beta-monooxygenase.

Sources

Sources of vitamin C include citrus fruits, potatoes, tomatoes, cruciferous vegetables, and strawberries.

IX

Requirements and Deficiency

The RDA for vitamin C is 15 to 45 mg for children and 75 to 90 mg/day for women and men, respectively. Pregnant women and the elderly have a higher daily requirement of 120 mg.

Ascorbic acid is an essential vitamin in humans and clinical deficiency is known as scurvy. This syndrome is characterized by impaired collagen synthesis and disorganized connective tissues as well as bleeding and receding gums.

Toxicity

Consumption of large doses of vitamin C (gram quantities) can have a number of adverse effects. These can include an increase in oxalate formation and the risk of calcium oxalate kidney stones and a false-negative stool guaiac result.

36.2.8 Biotin (Vitamin H)

Metabolism and Mechanism of Action

Biotin represents an essential cofactor or carboxyl group carrier for carboxylase enzyme complexes in mammals. These include acetyl-CoA carboxylase, pyruvate carboxylase, proprionyl-CoA carboxylase, and beta-methylcrotonyl-CoA carboxylase.

Sources

Egg yolk, liver, soy products, and yeast have the highest biotin levels.

Requirements and Deficiency

The recommended dietary intake of biotin or AI is 8 to 12 µg daily for children, and 30 µg daily for adults.

Biotin deficiencies are rarely reported today. However, consumption of large amounts of raw egg whites can lead to biotin deficiency. Raw egg whites contain avidin, a compound that binds to biotin and limits it activity.

Toxicity

No toxicity has been associated with excess biotin intake.

36.2.9 Folic Acid

Metabolism and Mechanism of Action

Folic acid is derived from dietary sources in a polyglutaminated form and is absorbed in the small intestine as a monoglutamate. Folate enters intestinal cells through binding to a folate receptor and once inside of the cell it is polyglutaminated. The vitamin folate is converted to FH4 by the action of dihydrofolate reductase.

FH4 is the primary one-carbon carrier in the body. This vitamin obtains one-carbon units from serine, glycine, histidine, formaldehyde, and formate. The one-carbon groups are used for many biosynthetic reactions. Examples include carbons for the de novo synthesis of purine, glycine to form serine, and methyl groups for methylation of dUMP to TMP.

Sources

Folates are widely distributed in animal products, leafy green vegetables, nuts, fruits, and cereals. Grains and flour in both the United States and Australia are routinely supplemented with folic acid.

Requirements and Deficiencies

Minimum daily requirements range from 200 to 400 µg, but this increases to 500 and 800 µg per day in pregnant and lactating women. Because of routine folate supplementation of foodstuffs, folate deficiency is rare in the United States as well as other resource-rich countries. Dietary stores of folate range from 500 to 20,000 µg, and with dietary restriction of folate intake, stores of this vitamin do not fall for several weeks. Folate supplementation (0.8 to 1 mg/day) is recommended for women who are trying to conceive as well as pregnant women to prevent development of neural tube defects.

Deficiencies of folate are commonly associated with poor diet or alcoholism. Folates can also be inactivated during cooking. Chronic consumption of alcohol can significantly reduce serum folate within several days presumably through impairment of the enterohepatic cycle and inhibition of folate absorption.

Folate deficiency results in an increased dUMP/dTMP ratio and increased incorporation of uracil into DNA. This leads to an inhibition of DNA repair and DNA fragmentation.

The clinical manifestation of folate deficiency is macrocytic, megaloblastic anemia that results from the inability of hematopoietic and other cells to synthesize DNA and divide. This leads to formation of large cells with abundant cytoplasm as cells that persistently try but are unable to divide.

There are several important drug interactions that can interfere with folate metabolism. These include

- Sulfa Drugs and Trimethoprim: Both are inhibitors of dihydrofolate reductase and if given in high doses these can result in megaloblastic pancytopenia.
- Pyrimethamine: This is used in the treatment of malaria and toxoplasmosis and as an inhibitor of parasitic dihydrofolate reductase it has been associated with megaloblastic anemia due to FH4 deficiency.
- Methotrexate: This is a chemotherapeutic agent that is used to treat both leukemias and solid tumors. Its mechanism of action is inhibition of tumor cell dihydrofolate reductase. With methotrexate treatment oxidized or inactive dihydrofolate cannot be regenerated to the active FH4. Reversal of this untoward effect of methotrexate is accomplished through administration of the folate analogue leucovorin.

Toxicity

No toxic effects have been reported with elevated intake of folic acid that may occur by taking vitamin supplements.

36.3 Fat-Soluble Vitamins

36.3.1 Vitamin A

Metabolism and Mechanism of Action

Vitamin A represents a family (retinoic acids) of fat-soluble vitamins composed of four isoprenoid groups linked in a head-to-tail fashion. There are two forms of vitamin A—provitamin A carotenoids, including β-carotene, and preformed vitamin A, including retinol, retinal, and retinoic acid.

Vitamin A has important roles in vision, regulation of gene expression, and in cellular differentiation. In the photoreceptors of the retina, vitamin A is the source for retinal, the light-sensitive portion of rhodopsin. In cells, retinoid receptors regulate gene transcription and play a major role in regulating cell growth and differentiation.

Sources

Provitamin A carotenoids are found in plants such as carrots, leafy green vegetables, and sweet potatoes. β-Carotene is one of numerous carotenoids, but it is the only one metabolized to vitamin A by mammals.

Preformed vitamin A is found in animal sources such as eggs, liver, and butter.

Requirements and Deficiencies

The RDA for adult males is 3,000 IUs (900 µg) of retinol and for females, it is 2,300 IUs (700 µg) of retinol. There are special populations with fat malabsorption issues resulting from pancreatic insufficiency or other gastrointestinal maladies. Patients with pancreatic insufficiency such as those with cystic fibrosis are treated with supplements of vitamin A at doses several times higher than the RDA. Similarly, patients who have undergone bariatric surgery or suffer from short bowel syndrome generally have fat malabsorption issues and require vitamin A supplementation several-fold higher than the RDA.

Deficiencies of vitamin A are associated with night blindness, complete blindness, and xerophthalmia. Although vitamin A deficiencies are rare in the United States as well as other resource-rich countries, it is one of the leading causes of blindness in children in resource-poor countries.

Toxicities

The capacity to metabolize vitamin A is limited and excessive intake exceeds the binding capacity of intracellular binding proteins. Accumulation of free vitamin A results in membrane lysis and tissue damage. Symptoms of toxicity can include effects on the central nervous system that are manifested as headache, nausea, ataxia, and increased cerebrospinal fluid pressure. Other clinical symptoms include disruption of calcium homeostasis that results in hypercalcemia and calcification of soft tissues as well as thickening of the long bones.

36.3.2 Vitamin D

Metabolism

Vitamin D (calciferol) is derived from 7-dehydrocholesterol, an intermediate product of cholesterol synthesis that accumulates in the skin. On exposure to ultraviolet light, 7-dehydrocholesterol is converted nonenzymatically to previtamin D. Previtamin D is converted through thermal isomerization into cholecalciferol and this form is absorbed into the bloodstream. Cholecalciferol, either derived from the skin from dietary sources, is hydroxylated to form a 25-hydroxycholesterol derivative termed calcidiol. Calcidiol is released into the blood

stream where it is bound to vitamin D binding globulin, a main storage form of vitamin D. Metabolism of calcidiol also occurs in the kidney where it undergoes two reactions: 1-hydroxylation to form the active metabolite 1,25-dihydroxyvitamin D (calcitriol) or 24-hydroxylation to produce an inactive metabolite 24, 25-dihydroxyvitamin D (See ▶ Fig. 16.5).

Mechanism of Action

The active metabolite 1,25-dihydroxyvitamin D binds to an intracellular nuclear receptor, the vitamin D receptor (VDR). Vitamin D bound to the VDR mediates its effects and modulates gene transcription. The most important biological action of vitamin D is to regulate serum calcium concentrations. This effect is achieved in three ways: increased intestinal absorption of calcium, reduction of calcium excretion via the kidneys, and mobilization of bone calcium.

Sources

The major source of vitamin D is dermal synthesis of previtamin D from 7-dehydrocholesterol, an intermediate in the synthesis of cholesterol. There are a limited number of foods that naturally contain vitamin D with fatty fish livers representing a rich source.

Requirements and Deficiencies

The RDA for vitamin D varies with age, pregnancy, sunlight exposure, and fat malabsorption disorders. The RDA for children 1 to 18 years, adults up to the age of 70 years, and pregnant or lactating women is 15 µg. The RDA increases to 20 µg after age 71 years and for older individuals confined indoors with limited sunlight exposure who may have low-serum 25-hydroxyvitamin D, supplemental vitamin D should be increased to 600 to 800 IUs daily. For infants who are exclusively breastfed, a daily supplement of 400 IUs daily is recommended because breast milk is low in vitamin D.

Inadequate vitamin D levels are manifested as rickets in children and as osteomalacia in adults. These clinical manifestations result from reduced intestinal absorption of both calcium and phosphorus. When vitamin D deficiency is persistent, blood calcium levels decrease resulting in hyperparathyroidism. As a consequence, phosphaturia develops resulting in demineralization of bones.

Toxicities

An exact intake of vitamin D that produces toxicity is unknown. A tolerable upper limit for intake of vitamin D has been established as 100 µg daily for healthy adults and children up to 18 years. In patients with malabsorptive issues, up to 10,000 to 50,000 units per day may be administered.

Excessive intake of vitamin D has been reported in individuals consuming in excess of 60,000 IU/day. Symptoms of acute vitamin D intoxication result from hypercalcemia and are manifested as polyuria, polydipsia, anorexia, and vomiting and muscle weakness. Chronic consumption of toxic vitamin D levels can cause nephrocalcinosis, bone demineralization, and hyperalgesia.

36.3.3 Vitamin E

Metabolism and Mechanism of Action

Vitamin E represents a mixture of lipid-soluble compounds that includes tocopherols and tocotrienols. Vitamin E is a membrane-bound peroxyl radical scavenger. It prevents free radical degradation of membrane lipids and the formation of free radical-induced membrane damage. Vitamin E reacts with free radicals forming a tocopherol-free radical complex that is reduced by vitamin C. Through this process, vitamin E is restored to its antioxidant activity. It has also been reported that vitamin E may induce antioxidant enzymes such as superoxide dismutase and glutathione peroxidase.

Sources

Vitamin E is derived from plant chlorophyll and tyrosine. Sources include oils, meat, eggs, and leafy vegetables. Olive and sunflower oils are especially rich sources of alpha-tocopherol.

Requirements and Deficiencies

The RDA for vitamin E is 15 mg of dietary alpha-tocopherol.

Vitamin E deficiency is not common because of the abundance of tocopherols in a variety of foodstuffs. However, deficiencies do occur in certain pathologies. These are generally associated with maladies that result in fat malabsorption. Such causes can include pancreatic exocrine insufficiency with insufficient lipase to enable fat absorption, cholestatic liver disease where bile is insufficient to permit fat solubilization and absorption, and extensive resection or disease impacting the small intestine.

The clinical consequences of vitamin E deficiency are variable and in adults and children these are manifested as neuromuscular disorders and hemolysis. The neuromuscular disorders are neuropathic and myopathic, with neuropathy manifested as spinocerebellar syndrome. Vitamin E deficiency is known to cause hemolytic anemia in premature infants because of a shortened lifespan of red blood cells.

Toxicities

Excessive intake of vitamin E is associated with mortality resulting from hemorrhagic strokes. Vitamin E can interfere with vitamin K absorption and cause an increased risk of bleeding for those taking warfarin.

36.3.4 Vitamin K

Metabolism and Mechanism of Action

Vitamin K consists of three compounds that are biologically active: K_1 (phylloquinone), the normal dietary source; K_2 (menaquinones), synthesized by bacteria in the intestine; and K_3 (menadiol diacetate), a synthetic compound that is metabolized into menaquinone.

Vitamin K functions as a cofactor for regulating activity of proteins containing carboxyglutamic acid residues. Specifically, vitamin K mediates vitamin K-dependent (VKD) protein carboxylation through the VKD carboxylase. VKD carboxylase catalyzes the oxygenation of vitamin K hydroquinone to vitamin K epoxide and carboxylation of glutamate residues to gamma-carboxyglutamate on VKD proteins. This results in their activation, an essential step in synthesis of clotting factors II, VII, IX, and X. Osteocalcin, a protein related to bone calcification, is also carboxylated by VKD carboxylase.

Sources

Major dietary sources include green leafy vegetables, broccoli, spinach, lettuce, herbs, and kale. Another important source is gut microfloral synthesis of vitamin K_2, which has approximately 60% of the activity of vitamin K_1.

Requirements and Deficiencies

The dietary requirement for vitamin K acquired from leafy green vegetables is expressed as AI and is 90 µg daily in women and 120 µg daily in men.

Deficiency of vitamin K is relatively rare because of the extensive distribution of phylloquinone in plants and the synthesis of menaquinone by intestinal microflora. However, acquired deficiency can result from a number of causes. Vitamin K deficiency is manifested clinically as easy bruisability, mucosal bleeding, splinter hemorrhages, upper GI bleeding, tarry black stools, blood in the urine, and other impaired coagulation-related disorders.

Because Vitamin K is fat-soluble, fat malabsorption may result in vitamin K deficiency. As discussed previously with other fat-soluble vitamins, malabsorption can be a consequence of bile or pancreatic secretion disorders or disease or resection of the intestinal mucosa. Liver failure can also result in coagulation disorders because VKD coagulation factors are produced in the liver. Certain medications can also contribute to vitamin K deficiency, including antibiotics and high doses of vitamins A or E. Broad spectrum antibiotics reduce bacterial gut populations and suppress menaquinone production. Certain cephalosporin antibiotics have been associated with hypoprothrombinemia and have a weak coumarin-like effect in patients with low vitamin K.

Clinical Correlation

Of clinical significance is vitamin K-deficient bleeding in newborns and infants. This is a consequence of low vitamin K levels and the risk for vitamin K-deficient bleeding can result without hemorrhagic disease.

An important pharmacological note relates to coumarin-like anticoagulants. Coumarin and warfarin have a structure similar to vitamin K and these anticoagulants interfere with VKD carboxylation by blocking reduction of inactive vitamin K 2,3-epoxides to active vitamin K.

Toxicities

Vitamin K toxicity is rare and an upper limit for vitamin K intake has not been defined.

36.4 Vitamin Poisoning and Treatment

Vitamins are essential for many processes in the body, but some are highly toxic when ingested in excessive amounts. ▶ Table 36.2 lists the toxic effects of some vitamins and the treatment that may be given.

Table 36.2 Toxic effects of vitamins and treatment

Vitamin	Toxic effects	Treatment of toxic effects
Vitamin A (retinol)	Acute toxicity: dizziness, vomiting, erythema, and desquamation Chronic toxicity: skin and hair changes, liver damage (in infants and children); can cause pseudotumor cerebri (increased CSF fluid pressure)	Symptomatic and supportive (i.e., treatment is given to prevent, control, or relieve complications and side effects)
Vitamin D (ergocalciferol D_2, cholecalciferol D_2)	Hypercalcemia, and both mental and physical retardation	Terminate exposure to vitamin D Initiate a low-calcium diet Monitor urine volume, sodium, and potassium and replace lost fluids, sodium, and potassium by IV infusions
Vitamin E (tocopherol)	Nausea, muscular weakness, fatigue, headache, blurred vision, and GI upset	None
Vitamin K	Hemolytic anemia and hyperbilirubinemia may occur in newborns and persons with glucose-6-phosphate dehydrogenase deficiency	None
Niacin (vitamin B_3, nicotinic acid, nicotinamide)	Flushing, headache, pruritus, GI irritation	Symptomatic and supportive
Pyridoxine (B_6)	Sensory neuropathy and interference with levodopa therapy	There is no known treatment for the sensory neuropathy produced by high doses of pyridoxine. Spontaneous recovery usually occurs slowly over several months or years
Ascorbic acid (vitamin C)	Kidney stones and rebound scurvy (seen only with huge amounts ingested)	None

Note: The vitamins that are not included here have no known toxicity.
Abbreviations: CSF, cerebrospinal fluid; GI, gastrointestinal; IV, intravenous.

Unit IX Review Questions

1. Renal toxicity is associated with which of the following?
   A. Doxorubicin.
   B. Fluorouracil.
   C. Vincristine.
   D. Cisplatin.
   E. 6-Mercaptopurine.

2. The antineoplastic action of which drug is related to its high affinity for dihydrofolate reductase?
   A. Fluorouracil.
   B. Methotrexate.
   C. Mechlorethamine.
   D. Dactinomycin.
   E. Vincristine.

3. A 62-year-old African American man undergoes a hemicolectomy to remove an invasive adenocarcinoma from his ascending colon. Pathology shows pericolic lymph node involvement but no liver metastases. Based on the stage of the tumor, a course of treatment with leucovorin calcium, fluorouracil, and irinotecan hydrochloride is undertaken. What is the purpose of including leucovorin calcium?
   A. To provide normal cells with an active form of folic acid.
   B. To decrease nausea and vomiting produced by fluorouracil.
   C. To activate irinotecan.
   D. To increase the effectiveness of fluorouracil.
   E. To increase the uptake of drug into bone to prevent metastases.

4. Cardiac toxicity is associated with which of the following?
   A. Doxorubicin.
   B. Fluorouracil.
   C. Vincristine.
   D. Cisplatin.
   E. 6-Mercaptopurine.

5. Which one of the following drugs acts by inhibiting DNA topoisomerase?
   A. Cyclophosphamide.
   B. Methotrexate.
   C. Etoposide.
   D. Leuprolide.
   E. Fluorouracil.

6. A 58-year-old woman noticed a lump in her right breast ~ 1 month ago. She has no pain, nipple discharge, itching, or swelling of the breast. The patient is postmenopausal and had a mammogram 2 years ago. She takes several supplements, including calcium/vitamin D and vitamin C. She also takes iron tablets for occasional mild anemia. Breast examination reveals a hard 1 cm mass in the upper right quadrant of her breast. Right axillary lymph nodes are enlarged. The mass is confirmed by mammography and needle biopsy. A test to show the level of expression of which of the following antigens would assist in determining susceptibility of the tumor to trastuzumab?
   A. CD20.
   B. CD52.
   C. Epidermal growth factor receptor (EGFR).

D. HER2/neu.
E. Vascular endothelial growth factor (VEGF).

7. A 78-year-old male patient has hepatocellular carcinoma. The tumor is unresectable due to portal vein invasion. Sorafenib tosylate is a multiple tyrosine kinase inhibitor used in advanced kidney or bladder cancer that can increase survival by 6 to 9 months. What is the advantage of inhibiting multiple kinases as opposed to a single kinase?
   A. To account for genetic differences in kinases.
   B. To inhibit both angiogenesis and tumor cell growth.
   C. To inhibit multiple stages of blood vessel growth.
   D. To inhibit multiple sites on the Raf serine/threonine kinase.
   E. To ensure the drug is effective in both slow and rapid acetylators.

8. A 60-year-old man reports difficulty starting his urination and poor urinary stream for the last 4 months. A digital rectal exam of the prostate reveals masses in both lobes. Serum prostate-specific antigen (PSA) is elevated. The patient is referred to a urologist, who conducts a needle biopsy and histologic grading. The decision is made to use a combination of radiotherapy and hormonal therapy. Why is flutamide administered prior to leuprolide?
   A. It prevents the breakdown of leuprolide by liver cytochrome P-450 enzymes.
   B. A positive response to flutamide may obviate the need for giving leuprolide.
   C. It induces receptor desensitization.
   D. It increases absorption from the gastrointestinal tract.
   E. It blocks the effect of the initial surge of hormones produced by leuprolide.

9. A 29-year-old patient has a lymph node biopsy and is diagnosed as having Hodgkin's lymphoma, nodular sclerosis type. A course of therapy with doxorubicin, bleomycin, vinblastine, and dacarbazine is recommended. Before beginning chemotherapy, what steps might be taken to alleviate the most common acute toxicity of this regimen?
   A. Use behavioral modification therapy.
   B. Administer morphine as needed after the chemotherapy session.
   C. Administer ondansetron prophylactically.
   D. Soak the patient's arm in epsom salts.
   E. Administer milk of magnesia.

10. A 28-year-old female patient had ingested a toxic overdose of phencyclidine, a weak base. Because of the severity of her symptoms, you rightfully conclude that almost all of the phencyclidine had been absorbed by the time she was brought to the emergency room. Which of the following actions may be effective?
    A. Induce vomiting with apomorphine.
    B. Alkalinize the urine with sodium bicarbonate.
    C. Perform hemoperfusion.
    D. Acidify the urine with ammonium chloride.
    E. Perform gastric lavage with charcoal.

11. A patient who has received multiple blood transfusions may require chelation therapy with which of the following?
    A. Dimercaprol.
    B. Succimer.
    C. Ethylenediaminetetraacetic acid (EDTA).
    D. Trientine.
    E. Deferoxamine.

12. A person is brought to the hospital in a coma with severely depressed respiration, no response to pain, and small pupils. A friend says the patient took some kind of drug, or drugs, but he does not know what kind. An injection of naloxone makes the pupils larger and only slightly improves respiration. Injecting more naloxone causes no further change. Of the following, what is the most probable cause of this reaction to naloxone?
    A. This is probably a mixed overdose from an opioid plus another drug.
    B. The patient probably is also an amphetamine user, is tolerant to amphetamine, and would thus be cross-tolerant to the respiratory stimulation caused by naloxone.
    C. This is an addict who is in a postictal state, having just suffered an opioid withdrawal convulsion.

13. A college student is brought to the emergency room. She is unconscious, with no response to painful stimuli. Deep tendon reflexes are hyperactive. Respirations are 4/minute. Blood pressure is 80/50 mm Hg. The skin is cool and cyanotic. Pupils are slightly dilated with sluggish reaction to light. Her roommate reports that the patient took "about 10 or 20" capsules of chloral hydrate and "lots" of pills of codeine. An endotracheal tube is inserted. Gastric washing reveals many partially digested capsules. The resident on duty injects naloxone intravenously. After giving naloxone, respirations are still inadequate. Which one of the following measures is most appropriate to correct respiratory function?
    A. Inject strychnine.
    B. Inject pentylenetetrazol.
    C. Inject dopamine.
    D. Mechanically assist respirations.
    E. Force-feed caffeine.

14. A woman is found unconscious near a bottle hand-labeled "roach poison." She is having convulsive movements and is covered with urine and feces. In the emergency room, she is cyanotic, has a pulse of 50 beats/minute, blood pressure of 70/20 mm Hg, and cold, wet skin. Immediate action should include instituting artificial ventilation and which of the following?
    A. Administering atropine intravenously.
    B. Administering edrophonium intravenously.
    C. Administering neostigmine intravenously.
    D. Ordering an assay of serum cholinesterase activity.
    E. Ordering a blood toxicology panel.

15. Which of the following agents is useful in treating cyanide toxicity?
    A. Carbon monoxide.
    B. Trientine.
    C. Sodium nitrite/sodium thiosulfate.
    D. Pralidoxime.
    E. Dimercaprol.

16. A 3-year-old child has accidentally ingested tablets that she found in the medicine chest. The child develops symptoms that include severe gastrointestinal distress, vomiting with blood, and severe epigastric distress. The patient is brought to the emergency department where it is determined that she has metabolic acidosis and leukocytosis. Based on this clinical scenario what is the best treatment regimen for this child?
    A. Calcium disodium edetate.
    B. Deferoxamine.
    C. Dimercaprol.
    D. Penicillamine.
    E. Succimer.

17. A 35-year-old woman employed in a dental laboratory complains of conjunctivitis, skin irritation, and hair loss. Blood tests confirm that she has organic arsenic poisoning. Which one of the following agents represents the best treatment for this condition?
    A. Calcium disodium edetate.
    B. Deferoxamine.
    C. Dimercaprol.
    D. Penicillamine.
    E. Succimer.

18. Recent research has shown that neural tube defects such as anencephaly and spinal bifida are more frequent in certain populations and may have an environmental cause. Deficiency of which of the following vitamins is most likely associated with these defects?
    A. Ascorbic acid (vitamin C).
    B. Folic acid.
    C. Niacin (vitamin B_3).
    D. Riboflavin (vitamin B_2).
    E. Thiamine (vitamin B_1).

19. Cobalamin or vitamin B_{12} deficiency results in which of the following disorders?
    A. Beriberi.
    B. Pellagra.
    C. Pernicious anemia.
    D. Rickets.
    E. Scurvy.

20. Which of the following vitamins represents a major electron acceptor in the oxidation of various metabolites?
    A. Niacin.
    B. Riboflavin.
    C. Thiamine.
    D. Vitamin B_{12} (cobalamin).
    E. Vitamin B_6 (pyridoxine).

21. Which of the following binds with tubulin and inhibits formation of the mitotic spindle?
    A. Fluorouracil.
    B. Methotrexate.
    C. Mechlorethamine.
    D. Dactinomycin.
    E. Vincristine.

IX

22. Which of the following functions by being converted to a metabolite that inhibits the synthesis of thymidine monophosphate?
    A. Cyclophosphamide.
    B. Methotrexate.
    C. Fluorouracil.
    D. Vincristine and vinblastine.
    E. 6-mercaptopurine.

23. Which of the following is relatively selective for granulocytes?
    A. Mechlorethamine.
    B. Cyclophosphamide.
    C. Carmustine.
    D. Busulfan.
    E. Cisplatin.

24. Which of the following is effective only in treating estrogen receptor–positive breast cancer?
    A. Doxorubicin.
    B. Tamoxifen.
    C. Methotrexate.
    D. Dactinomycin.
    E. Fluorouracil.

25. The antineoplastic effect of which of the following is potentiated by allopurinol?
    A. Doxorubicin.
    B. Fluorouracil.
    C. Vincristine.
    D. Cisplatin.
    E. 6-mercaptopurine.

26. Which of the following is activated by the cytochrome P-450 mixed function oxidase system?
    A. Cyclophosphamide.
    B. Mechlorethamine.
    C. Carmustine.
    D. Lomustine.
    E. Cisplatin.

27. Mucocutaneous changes (hyperpigmentation, pruritic erythema, hyperkeratosis, desquamation, and mucositis) occur frequently with which of the following?
    A. Daunorubicin.
    B. Cyclophosphamide.
    C. Prednisone.
    D. Bleomycin.
    E. Vinblastine.

28. Which of the following may make tumor cells difficult to eradicate?
    A. They may develop resistance very slowly.
    B. Normal host cells will develop resistance to chemotherapeutic drugs.
    C. Tumor cells may become genetically resistant to a variety of cytotoxic drugs (a phenomenon known as pleiotropic, or multidrug, resistance).
    D. Many lymphoma cells are known to express the antigen CD20.
    E. Tumor cells complete the cell cycle in less time than is necessary for the normal host counterpart cells.

29. Irritability, hallucinations, and blue gumline are symptoms of chronic poisoning with which of the following?
    A. Lead.
    B. Arsenic.
    C. Mercury.
    D. Iron.
    E. Carbon monoxide.

30. Which chelating agents should be used to treat copper toxicity (e.g., in Wilson disease)?
    A. Calcium disodium ethylenediaminetetraacetic acid (EDTA).
    B. Deferoxamine.
    C. Dimercaprol.
    D. Penicillamine.
    E. Pralidoxime.

31. During a military crisis, several people injected themselves with syrettes containing a total of 4.2 mg of atropine, believing that they had been, or were about to be, exposed to a nerve gas. If no exposure to nerve gas occurred, 4 mg of atropine would be a toxic dose for adults. Which of the following drugs is most appropriate for treating atropine toxicity?
    A. Neostigmine.
    B. Physostigmine.
    C. Edrophonium.
    D. Propantheline.
    E. Acetylcholine.

32. Military troops are dispatched to a country that is known to have stocks of nerve gas. The soldiers are provided with syrettes containing 2.1 mg of atropine and 600 mg of pralidoxime. What is the purpose of pralidoxime?
    A. To act as an antagonist at the neuromuscular junction.
    B. To reactivate (restore to original activity) acetylcholinesterase.
    C. To reactivate (restore to original activity) choline acetyltransferase.
    D. To act as an antagonist at muscarinic sites.
    E. To act as an anticonvulsant.

Unit IX Answers and Explanations

1. D. Cisplatin concentrates in the kidneys and produces renal toxicity.

A–C, E. None of the other agents concentrate in the kidney and therefore do not produce renal toxicity.

2. B. Methotrexate is a folic acid analogue that competitively inhibits dihydrofolate reductase and thus suppresses the production of purine and thymine nucleotides.

A. Fluorouracil is a pyrimidine analogue that inhibits thymidylate synthesis.

C. Mechlorethamine is an alkylating agent that binds covalently to guanine nucleotides of DNA, cross-linking DNA strands, thus preventing DNA replication and transcription.

D. Dactinomycin intercalates between C–C pairs in double-stranded DNA and inhibits DNA-directed RNA synthesis. E Vincristine is an antimitotic agent that inhibits cell development.

3. A. Leucovorin is folinic acid, the active form of folic acid that does not require dihydrofolate reductase. Leucovorin enhances the efficacy of fluorouracil, possibly by inhibiting thymidylate synthase. When given with methotrexate, leucovorin is used to provide normal cells with the active form of folic acid.

4. A. Doxorubicin is taken up by cardiac muscle, leading to oxidative damage of heart muscle and refractory congestive heart failure.

B–E. These agents are not cardiotoxic.

5. C. Etoposide inhibits DNA topoisomerase II, which acts on single-stranded DNA to cause strand breakage.

A. Cyclophosphamide is a widely used alkylating agent that binds covalently to guanine nucleotides of DNA, cross-linking DNA strands, thus preventing DNA replication and transcription.

B. Methotrexate is a folic acid analogue that competitively inhibits dihydrofolate reductase and thus suppresses the production of purine and thymine nucleotides.

D. Leuprolide is a gonadotropin-releasing hormone (GnRH) agonist that desensitizes pituitary GnRH receptors and inhibits gonadotropin (follicle-stimulating hormone and luteinizing hormone) release.

E. Fluorouracil is a pyrimidine analogue that inhibits thymidylate synthesis.

6. D. Trastuzumab is a monoclonal antibody directed against HER2/neu. HER2/neu is a member of the epidermal growth factor family of cell membrane receptors. Trastuzumab is approved for treatment of metastatic breast cancer when HER2/neu is overexpressed.

A. Rituximab, tositumomab, ^{131}I-tositumomab, ^{111}In-ibritumomab, and ^{90}Y-ibritumomab tiuxetan bind to CD20, which is found on pre-B and mature B lymphocytes.

B. Alemtuzumab binds to CD52, which is present on the surface of essentially all B and T lymphocytes, a majority of monocytes, macrophages, and NK cells, as well as a subpopulation of granulocytes.

C. Cetuximab binds to EGFR, which has been detected in many human cancers, including those of the colon and rectum.

E. Bevacizumab binds to VEGF and prevents the proliferation of endothelial cells and formation of new blood vessels, thus starving tumors of their blood supply.

7. B. Sorafenib inhibits VEGF receptor and platelet-derived growth factor receptor to inhibit angiogenesis and the Raf serine/threonine kinases that mediate growth and differentiation of tumor cells.

8. E. The growth of prostate cells is stimulated by testosterone. Production of testosterone by Leydig cells of the testes is increased by luteinizing hormone (LH) released from the pituitary. The release of LH is regulated by gonadotropin-releasing hormone (GnRH) from the hypothalamus. Leuprolide is a GnRH-receptor agonist that initially stimulates and then desensitizes pituitary GnRH receptors. This leads to decreased gonadotropin release, decreased testosterone production, decreased prostate growth, and a beneficial effect in prostate cancer. The initial stimulation produced by leuprolide results in an initial surge in LH and testosterone release, which would have an adverse effect on prostate cancer. To block the effects of this initial surge of hormones, flutamide is given. Flutamide is a competitive antagonist of testosterone for binding to androgen receptors in the prostate gland. By doing so, it prevents them from stimulating the prostate cancer cells to grow.

9. C. Nausea and vomiting are the most common side effects of this chemotherapy. Of the listed choices, the only one that could be used to address nausea and vomiting is ondansetron, which is a 5-HT$_3$ receptor antagonist.

10. D. Weak bases are excreted faster ("ion-trapped") if the urine is acidified with ammonium chloride.

A, E. Inducing vomiting with apomorphine and performing gastric lavage with charcoal are unlikely to be effective, as the drug has already been absorbed.

B. Alkalinization of the urine with sodium bicarbonate will retard elimination because phencyclidine is a weak base.

C. Phencyclidine is not effectively extracted by hemoperfusion.

11. E. Multiple drug transfusions can lead to iron poisoning. Deferoxamine specifically chelates iron and promotes its excretion.

A. Dimercaprol is an effective treatment following poisoning by arsenic, gold, lead, and mercury.

B. Succimer is used for lead poisoning.

C. Calcium disodium EDTA is used for lead poisoning.

D. Trientine is a copper chelating agent.

12. A. Depressed respiration, nociception, and miosis are symptoms of opiate poisoning. As a competitive antagonist of opiates, naloxone should block all of the effects of opiates, with increasing effectiveness at higher doses. The lack of further effect of naloxone suggests multiple drug use.

B–D. The other possibilities are not indicated by the response to naloxone.

13. D. Although naloxone will block the effects of codeine, it will not block the effects of chloral hydrate, a central nervous system depressant drug. Because there are no specific antidotes for chloral hydrate, life support measures, such as mechanical assistance of respiration, must be taken.

A. Strychnine is a pesticide agent that acts by inhibiting glycine. This agent causes seizures and contractions of voluntary muscle that lead to respiratory paralysis.

B. Pentylenetetrazol is an experimental drug used to induce convulsions.

C, E. Neither dopamine nor caffeine would be expected to have a benefit here.

14. A. These are symptoms of organophosphate poisoning. Atropine is a muscarinic receptor antagonist given to relieve the overactivation of muscarinic receptors.

B, C. Edrophonium and neostigmine are acetylcholinesterase inhibitors and would worsen the symptoms.

D, E. Because this is an emergency situation, you would not have time to wait for laboratory results.

15. C. Sodium nitrite produces methemoglobin, which binds cyanide. Sodium thiosulfate increases cyanide metabolism.

A. Carbon monoxide is a poisonous gas.

B. Trientine is a copper chelating agent.

D. Pralidoxime is a cholinesterase reactivator used in organophosphate poisoning.

E. Dimercaprol is an effective treatment following poisoning by arsenic, gold, lead, and mercury.

16. B. The child has iron toxicity acquired by an overdose of her mother's iron supplement tablets. Deferoxamine is an iron chelator that can be used to enhance excretion of the excessive iron.

A. Calcium disodium edetate is an efficient chelator of divalent and trivalent metals and is used clinically to promote the excretion of lead chelate.

C. Dimercaprol is an effective treatment following poisoning by mercury, arsenic, and other heavy metal.

D. Penicillamine is used primarily for treatment of copper poisoning.

E. Succimer represents a water-soluble form of dimercaprol and is indicated for lead poisoning in children.

17. C. Dimercaprol is an injectable, fat-soluble chelator used for arsenic poisoning.

A. Calcium disodium edetate is an efficient chelator of divalent and trivalent metals and is used clinically to promote the excretion of lead chelate.

B. Deferoxamine is an iron chelator that can be used to enhance excretion of the excessive iron.

C. Penicillamine is used primarily for treatment of copper poisoning.

E. Succimer represents a water-soluble form of dimercaprol and is indicated for lead poisoning in children.

18. B. Folic acid is necessary for the development of the neural tube in the first few weeks of embryonic life, and children of women with nutritional deficiencies have higher rates of neural tube defects.

A. Ascorbic acid (vitamin C) deficiency leads to scurvy, which causes bleeding gums and bone disease.

C. Niacin (vitamin B_3) deficiency leads to pellagra, a disorder that produces skin rash, weight loss, and neurologic changes that include depression and dementia.

D. Riboflavin deficiency leads to mouth ulcer, scaly skin, and photophobia.

E. Thiamine (vitamin B_1) deficiency is related to beriberi as well as Wernicke–Korsakoff syndrome in alcoholics.

19. C. Pernicious anemia results from the inability to absorb cobalamin (vitamin B_{12}) from the gastrointestinal tract and its deficiency in vegetarian diets causes megaloblastic anemia and neurologic symptoms. The presence of neurologic symptoms led to the term "pernicious anemia" because the symptoms are progressive and eventually irreversible.

A. Beriberi results from deficiencies in thiamine.

B. Pellagra is a consequence of niacin or vitamin B_3 deficiency.

C. Rickets is softening and deformation of the bones and is due to vitamin D deficiency.

E. Scurvy is a result of vitamin C deficiency.

20. A. Nicotinamide adenine dinucleotide (NAD^+) is the functional coenzyme derivative of niacin. It is the major electron acceptor in the oxidation of molecules, generating NADH, which is the major electron donor for reduction reactions.

B. Riboflavin functions in the coenzyme forms of FMN or FAD.

C. Thiamine occurs functionally as TPP and is a coenzyme for enzymes such as pyruvate dehydrogenase.

D. Vitamin B_{12} or cobalamin is involved in the transfer of methyl groups from FH4.

E. Vitamin B_6 or pyridoxine has multiple functions that include amino acid decarboxylation, synthesis of niacin from tryptophan, and neurotransmitter synthesis.

21. E. Vincristine is an antimitotic agent that binds to tubulin, inhibiting mitotic spindles and arresting cell development in the M phase of the cell cycle.

A. Fluorouracil is a pyrimidine analogue that inhibits thymidylate synthesis.

B. Methotrexate is a folic acid analogue that competitively inhibits dihydrofolate reductase and thus suppresses the production of purine and thymine nucleotides.

C. Mechlorethamine is an alkylating agent that binds covalently to guanine nucleotides of DNA, cross-linking DNA strands, thus preventing DNA replication and transcription.

D. Dactinomycin intercalates between G-C pairs in double-stranded DNA and inhibits DNA-directed RNA synthesis.

22. C. Fluorouracil is a pyrimidine analogue that is converted to 5-fluodeoxyuridine monophosphate, causing inhibition of thymidylate synthesis. DNA synthesis is therefore reduced due to a lack of thymidine. Fluorouracil also forms 5-fluodeoxyuridine triphosphate, which is incorporated into RNA and blocks translation.

A. Cyclophosphamide is the most widely used alkylating agent that binds covalently to guanine nucleotides of DNA, cross-linking DNA strands, thus preventing DNA replication and transcription.

B. Methotrexate is a folic acid analogue that competitively inhibits dihydrofolate reductase and thus suppresses the production of purine and thymine nucleotides.

D. Vincristine and vinblastine are antimitotic agents that inhibit cell development.

E. 6-mercaptopurine is a purine analogue that causes pseudo-feedback inhibition of the first step in purine biosynthesis and inhibition of purine interconversions.

23. D. Busulfan, used for treatment of chronic granulocytic leukemia, is selective for granulocytes (neutrophils, basophils, and eosinophils).

A. Mechlorethamine, used in the mechlorethamine, oncovin, procarbazine, and prednisone (MOPP) regimen for treatment of Hodgkin disease, is not selective for granulocytes.

B. Cyclophosphamide, used to treat a variety of neoplastic conditions and as an immunosuppressant agent, is not selective for granulocytes.

C. Carmustine, used for central nervous system malignancies and Hodgkin disease, is not selective for granulocytes.

E. Cisplatin, used to treat solid tumors, is not selective for granulocytes.

24. B. Tamoxifen is a partial agonist at the estrogen receptor. Its primary effect is to block the cell-proliferative effects of endogenous estrogen. It is effective only in treating estrogen receptor–positive breast cancer.

A. Doxorubicin has a broad spectrum of activity in treating leukemia and many solid tumors.

C. Methotrexate has a broad spectrum of antineoplastic activity and is used as an immunosuppressant agent.

D. Dactinomycin has a broad spectrum of activity against many solid tumors.

E. Fluorouracil is used to treat breast, pancreatic, colorectal, and gastric cancer.

25. E. 6-mercaptopurine is a purine analogue that causes pseudofeedback inhibition of the first step in purine biosynthesis and inhibition of purine interconversions. Metabolism to inactive products is inhibited by allopurinol, a xanthine oxidase inhibitor used in the treatment of gout.

A–D. The metabolism of the other agents is unaffected by allopurinol.

26. A. Cyclophosphamide is activated by cytochrome P-450–mediated metabolism.

B–E. These agents do not require activation by cytochrome P-450–mediated metabolism.

27. D. The more common toxic effects of bleomycin involve skin and mucous membranes.

A, B, C, and E. Mucocutaneous changes are not seen with the other choices.

28. C. A major problem in cancer chemotherapy is acquired drug resistance, which occurs when tumor cells undergo genotypic and phenotypic changes during therapy that render them insensitive to the drug.

29. C. These are symptoms of chronic mercury poisoning.

A. Chronic lead poisoning causes abdominal cramping, decreased appetite, irritability, fatigue, abdominal pain, and vomiting, followed by drowsiness, stupor, convulsions, and coma.

B. Arsenic poisoning causes headaches, confusion, drowsiness, abdominal pain, diarrhea, vomiting, convulsions, coma, and death.

D. Acute symptoms of iron poisoning include vomiting (often bloody), gastric pain, and diarrhea. Chronic symptoms include metabolic acidosis, lethargy, which may progress to cardiovascular collapse, liver damage, and organ failure.

E. Carbon monoxide poisoning causes headache, dizziness, weakness, confusion, lethargy, nausea, vomiting, seizures, and, at very high concentrations, coma and death.

30. D. Penicillamine is used to remove copper in hepatolenticular degeneration (Wilson disease).

A. Calcium disodium EDTA is used for lead poisoning.

B. Deferoxamine chelates iron specifically.

C. Dimercaprol is an effective treatment following poisoning by arsenic, gold, lead, and mercury.

E. Pralidoxime is a cholinesterase reactivator used in organophosphate poisoning.

IX

31. B. Physostigmine is a central nervous system (CNS)–penetrant cholinesterase inhibitor that will increase acetylcholine levels to counteract the effects of atropine.

A. Neostigmine is also a cholinesterase inhibitor, but it does not penetrate the CNS and would not relieve the CNS symptoms of atropine poisoning.

C. Edrophonium is also a cholinesterase inhibitor, but it is very short acting and therefore not indicated in this situation.

D. Propantheline is a muscarinic receptor antagonist that has actions similar to atropine.

E. Acetylcholine is rapidly hydrolyzed and not useful as a drug.

32. B. Pralidoxime is a cholinesterase reactivator. It is thought to reverse the inhibition of acetylcholinesterase by organophosphates by reactivating the phosphorylated cholinesterase enzyme and protecting the enzyme from further inhibition.

Index

Note: Page numbers set **bold** or *italic* indicate headings or figures, respectively.